Todd Cowell

AF676516

Fetal Sonography

Terry J. DuBose, B.B.A., A.S., R.D.M.S., R.R.T.
Founding Director, Diagnostic Medical Sonography Program
Austin Community College
Austin, Texas
Former Senior Sonographer
Austin Radiological Association
Austin, Texas

Artist: *Victoria Vescovo Alderman*

W.B. SAUNDERS COMPANY
A Division of Harcourt Brace & Company
Philadelphia London Toronto Montreal Sydney Tokyo

W.B. SAUNDERS COMPANY
A Division of Harcourt Brace & Company

The Curtis Center
Independence Square West
Philadelphia, Pennsylvania 19106

Library of Congress Cataloging-in-Publication Data

Fetal sonography / [edited by] Terry J. DuBose. — 1st ed.
p. cm.
ISBN 0-7216-5432-0
1. Fetus—Ultrasonic imaging. I. DuBose, Terry J.
[DNLM: 1. Ultrasonography, Prenatal—methods. WQ 209 F41946 1966]

RG628.3.U58F48 1996
618.2'07543—dc20
DNLM/DLC 95-5452

Fetal Sonography ISBN 0-7216-5432-0

Printed in the United States of America

Last digit is the print number: 9 8 7 6 5 4 3 2 1

Dedicated to the memory of my father, Jack C. DuBose, a master mechanic who taught me to use a micrometer caliper at an early age, and to my mother, Bobbie O. DuBose, a wonderful seamstress who makes beautiful three-dimensional clothing out of flat pieces of cloth; to my wife, Lucy Ramsey DuBose and daughter, Renée DuBose, for being supportive and patient when it seemed this book would never be finished; to Robert N. Snider, M.D., and Larry W. Hill, M.D., for mentoring me in medical imaging; and to all registered diagnostic medical sonographers and the fetuses they study in the hope and expectation that the future will be better.

Again, thank you all.
Peace, Terry

PREFACE

Fetal Sonography is a comprehensive reference for the ultrasonographic study of the normal human embryo and fetus. We have presented the fundamental ideas of the early researchers as well as building on their work to present many new, original concepts and observations. Starting with Section I, *Fetal Sonography* is a discussion of the history, safety, statistics, ethics, and methodology of this new and exciting field. The difficult questions of ethics, politics, and legal issues involving the fetus and sonography are discussed. Section II continues with organ by organ fetal anatomy using sonographs, illustrations, and discussions. Cross-sectional sonographs of all dimensions of fetal anatomy are presented along with tables, graphs, and formulas for analysis of the measurements. Many sonographs are accompanied by schematic drawings by a talented sonographer (RDMS) who also holds a Master's degree in medical illustration. Particular attention is paid to the head and neural axis, with an in-depth discussion of the 3-dimensional measurements and statistical analysis of cranial biometry and brain anatomy. Fetal size, age, and weight estimates are discussed in detail. Established methods of age and weight estimation are compared with new algorithms for true 3-dimensional volumetric estimates. The embryonic-fetal heart rate and maternal-fetal perfusion throughout pregnancy are also covered. There are chapters on the fetal heart and fetal Doppler imaging with 31 color plates. Section III concludes with comprehensive week-by-week sonographs of embryofetal anatomy and development through the first trimester and representative weeks throughout the second and third trimesters. This section should be particularly useful to students of sonography as well as for patient education. The last chapter ends with the current state of and future of fetal sonography and the use of computers in the sonographic laboratory.

Fetal Sonography is a dream come true for me. After returning from military service in Vietnam, I had a strong desire to find a profession helping people. I enrolled in the Seton Hospital School of Radiological Technology in Austin. While working on a physics paper about the double helix and the diffraction of x-rays by crystals, I kept encountering literature about wave motion as it related to ultrasound in medicine. This led me to read more, and in 1976, when the first sonographic machine (an articulated arm Rohé machine) came to Seton Medical Center, I was on the loading dock. I fell in love with diagnostic sonography. Observing and measuring the fetus infatuated me and still does.

When personal computers were developed in the late 1970s and early 1980s, I found a second love. Using a small Sinclair Z80A with 2K of RAM in 1982, I began trying to automate fetal growth analysis. The programming language was

Basic and therefore the software BASIC BABY was born. This may have been the first program for personal computers to automate data accumulation and analysis of the growth of human fetal parameters. I have continued to work on that program for over 13 years. In 1986 I made BASIC BABY II available for fetal growth analysis. BASIC BABY II is the only computer program to analyze 3-dimensional cranial measurements, the embryonic heart rate for age, and to perform age range analysis (ARA). The ARA gives the user an instant visual (graphic) analysis of the total fetal proportionality; it is based on the statistical Z scores of parameter ages. It is a simple concept that requires a lot of number crunching, but using a menu-driven program makes the process simple. Personal computers are perfect for this kind of analysis.

The concurrent development of diagnostic sonography and the personal computer made *Fetal Sonography* possible. This is not to discount the many hours my fellow sonographers spent measuring in every way imaginable the 10,000+ fetuses on which much of this book is based. But it is highly unlikely I could have ever convinced all of them to take up to 50 measurements per fetus over a period of 11 years if the accumulation of the data, archives, and analysis of the resulting mass of data had not been automated and simple. This process is what much of this book is about.

If you, the reader, have comments, suggestions, corrections, criticisms, or new research that should be included in subsequent editions, please send your information to the editor, Terry J. DuBose, 811 West 31st Street, Austin, Texas 78705-2109. This is also the address for information about BASIC BABY II.

I feel very fortunate to have been where I was when these technologies were being developed. I hope you enjoy this book and learn as much from it as I have in developing and editing it.

TERRY J. DUBOSE
Austin, Texas

CONTRIBUTORS

Adrian Anthony, B.S., M.A.
Assistant Professor, State University of New York, Health Science Center at Brooklyn, Brooklyn, New York
Biological Effects and Safety

Mimi C. Berman, Ph.D., R.D.M.S.
Acting Dean, State University of New York, Health Science Center at Brooklyn, College of Health Related Professions, Brooklyn, New York
History of Fetal Sonography

Mark S. Cartier, B.S., R.D.M.S., R.R.T.
Research Associate, University of Tennessee, Memphis, Tennessee; Chief Sonographer, The MED, Memphis, Tennessee
Fetal Doppler

Dale R. Cyr, B.S., R.D.M.S., R.D.C.S.
Clinical Instructor, Seattle University, Seattle, Washington; Chief Sonographer, University of Washington Medical Center, Seattle, Washington
Fetal Echocardiography

Julia A. Drose, B.A., R.D.M.S., R.D.C.S.
Instructor, Department of Radiology, University of Colorado School of Medicine, Denver, Colorado; Chief Sonographer, Division of Diagnostic Ultrasound, Department of Radiology, University of Colorado Health Sciences Center, Denver, Colorado
Fetal Echocardiography

Terry J. DuBose, B.B.A., A.S., R.D.M.S., R.R.T
Founding Director, Diagnostic Medical Sonography Program, Austin Community College, Austin, Texas; Senior Sonographer, Austin Radiological Association, Austin, Texas
Scope; Physics and Methodology of Obstetrical Sonography; Ethics and Legal Issues: Introduction; Size/Age Analysis; Cranial Biometry; Fetal Head and Spine; Fetal Thorax and Neck; Heart Rate; Extremities; Extrafetal Structures of Pregnancy; Biophysical Profile; First Trimester; Second and Third Trimesters; Conclusions

Larry W. Hill, M.D.
President, Austin Radiological Association, Austin, Texas
Physics and Methodology of Obstetrical Sonography

Marcus L. Lines, M.D.
Visiting Professor, University of Texas Health Science Center at San Antonio, San Antonio, Texas; Radiologist, Austin Radiological Association, Austin, Texas
Abdomen

William Meacham, B.A., M.A., Ph.D.
Ethics and Legal Issues: Ethical Sonography

Robert M. Milman, M.D.
Radiologist, Austin Radiological Association, Austin, Texas
Abdomen

Gilbert Ramírez, Dr.P.H.
Assistant Professor, Department of Medicine, University of Texas Health Science Center, San Antonio, Texas
Statistics

J. Neal Rutledge, M.D.
Clinical Assistant Professor, University of Texas at Austin, Austin, Texas; Chief, Section of Neuroradiology, Austin Radiological Association, Austin, Texas
Fetal Head and Spine

CONTENTS

Fetal Sonography

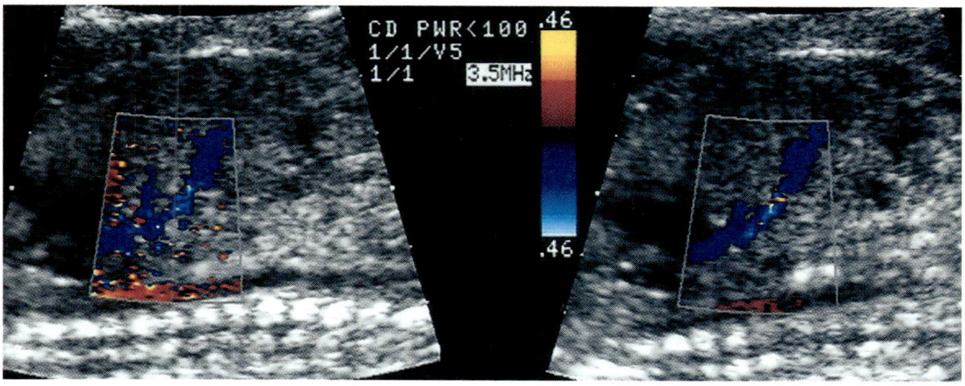

B C

COLOR FIGURE 13–1.
(see Color Figure 13–1*B*), *B*, Sagittal color Doppler image of umbilical vein and ductus venosus in a 20-week fetus. The inappropriately high gain setting exaggerates flow and vessel boundaries. *C*, Appropriate color gain setting in the same fetus provides more accurate flow data and depiction of vascular anatomy. With the proper gain setting, it is now possible to recognize the aliasing occurring in the ductus venosus as a result of normal high-velocity flow.

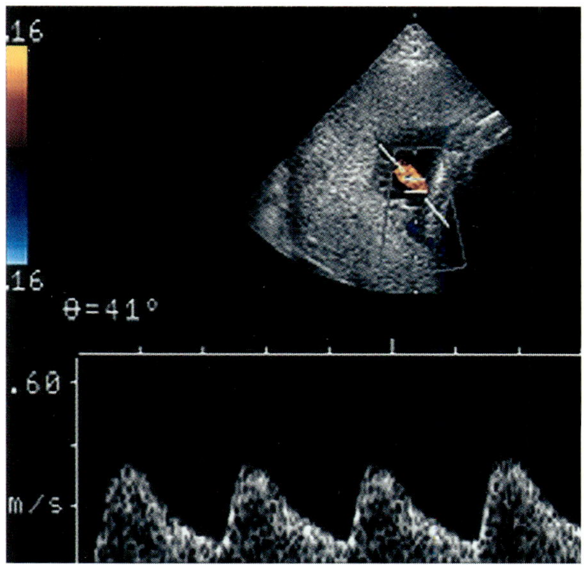

COLOR FIGURE 13–2.
View of the umbilical artery with optimal gate and angle placement for proper pulsed Doppler interrogation. Demonstration of flow on the color Doppler flow map allows for more precise Doppler angle setting.

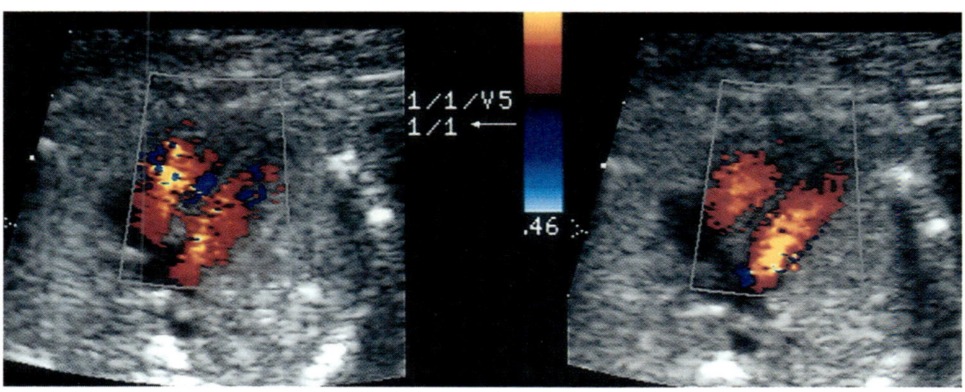

COLOR FIGURE 13–4.
Color Doppler images of a fetal heart (apical four-chamber view) demonstrating use of the high-pass filter. The image on the left was obtained with the filter set for a low-frequency cutoff, resulting in distortion of flow information. The image on the right is the same view but with the filter set for a higher-frequency cutoff. The color flow information is well defined and interpretable.

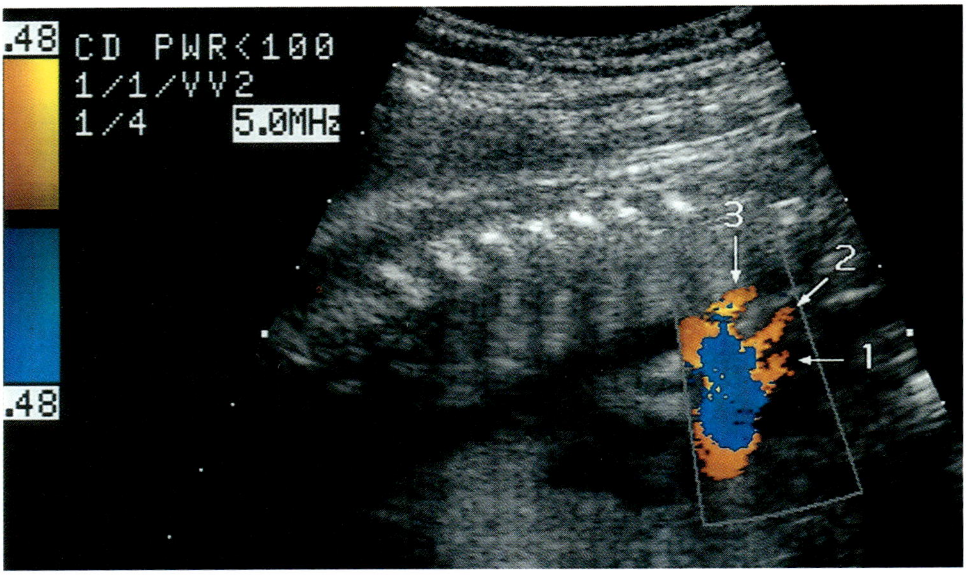

COLOR FIGURE 13–11.
Sagittal color flow image of the fetal aortic arch demonstrating aliasing in the color coding of flow. Much of the arch is color coded blue, which incorrectly indicates retrograde flow. Higher pulse repetition frequency was not possible with this transducer at this distance between the transducer and the interrogated vessel. Solutions include lowering the base line of the color scale or changing to a lower-frequency transducer. The three head and neck branches—(1) the innominate artery, (2) the left carotid artery, and (3) the left subclavian artery—are clearly seen branching off the top of the arch.

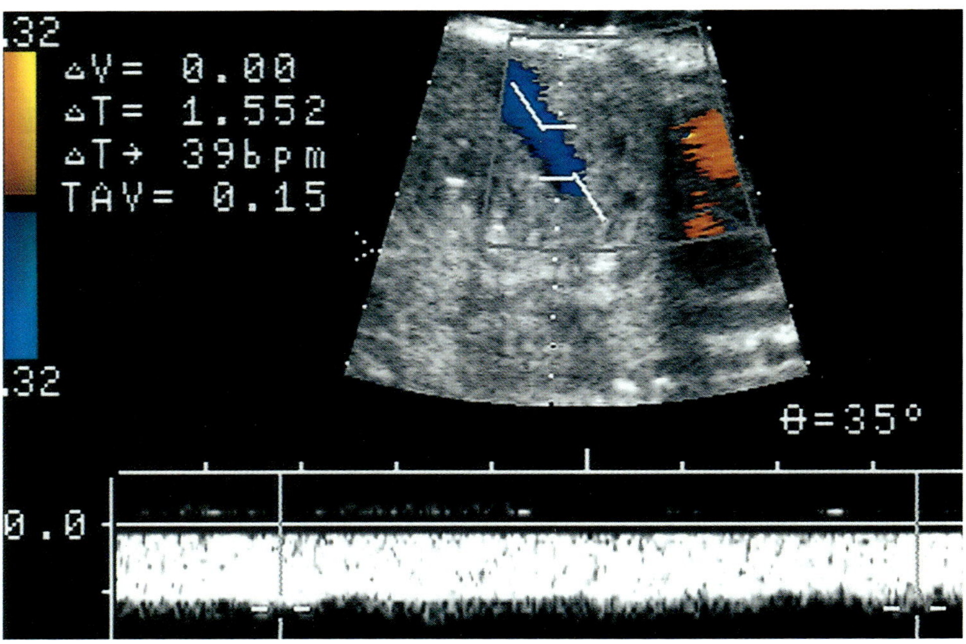

COLOR FIGURE 13–13.
Calculation of mean umbilical venous flow in a 25-week fetus. Doppler angle is set at 35 degrees to minimize error in this calculation. Color Doppler flow map assists rapid and accurate determination of the Doppler angle. The pulsed Doppler spectral tracing demonstrates a venous waveform with a time-averaged mean velocity of 15 cm/sec. Unlike the time-averaged maximum velocity, which averages the peak velocities throughout the cycle (see Fig. 13–10), the time-averaged mean velocity averages the mean velocities throughout the cardiac cycle.

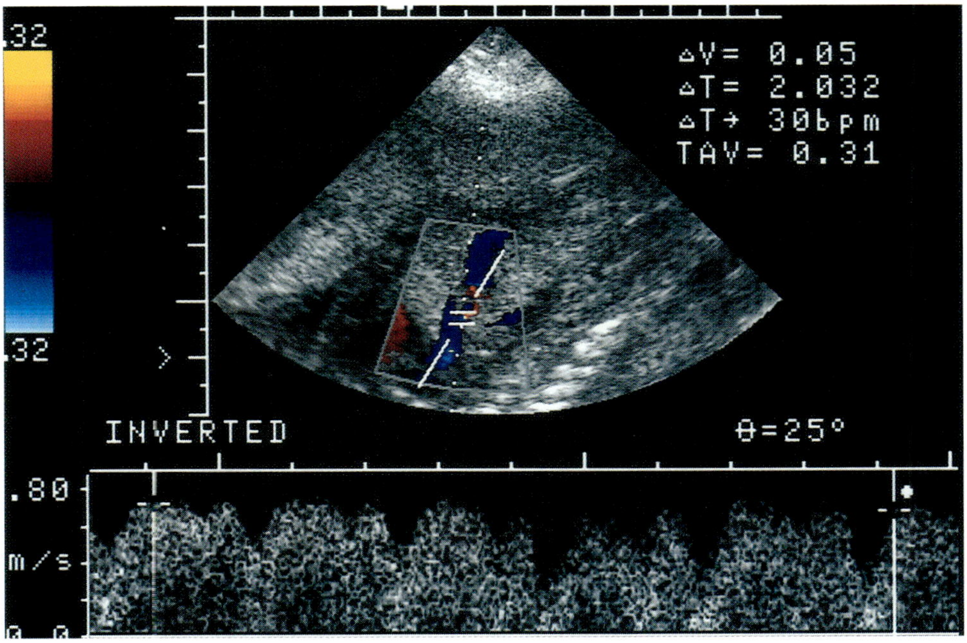

COLOR FIGURE 13–14.
Flow through the ductus venosus (DV) with color and pulsed Doppler in a 20-week fetus. The color map indicates higher velocities through the DV than through the umbilical vein (UV). As demonstrated on the pulsed Doppler tracing, DV flow is pulsatile. This derives from pressures reflected down from the right atrium. The maximal velocity is 75 cm/sec, and the time-averaged mean velocity is 31 cm/sec.

A 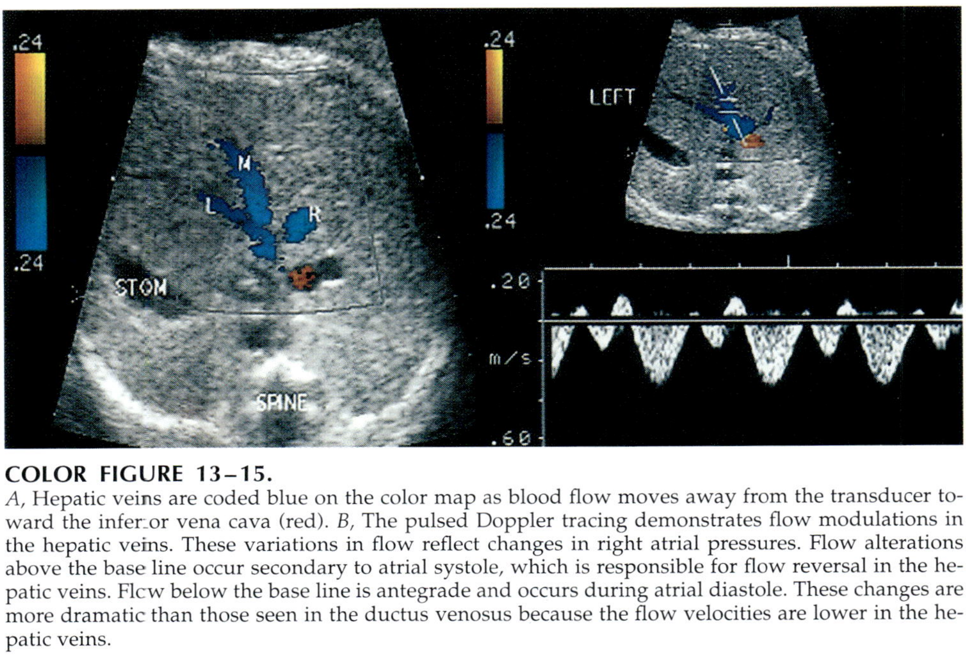 B

COLOR FIGURE 13–15.
A, Hepatic veins are coded blue on the color map as blood flow moves away from the transducer toward the inferior vena cava (red). *B*, The pulsed Doppler tracing demonstrates flow modulations in the hepatic veins. These variations in flow reflect changes in right atrial pressures. Flow alterations above the base line occur secondary to atrial systole, which is responsible for flow reversal in the hepatic veins. Flow below the base line is antegrade and occurs during atrial diastole. These changes are more dramatic than those seen in the ductus venosus because the flow velocities are lower in the hepatic veins.

A 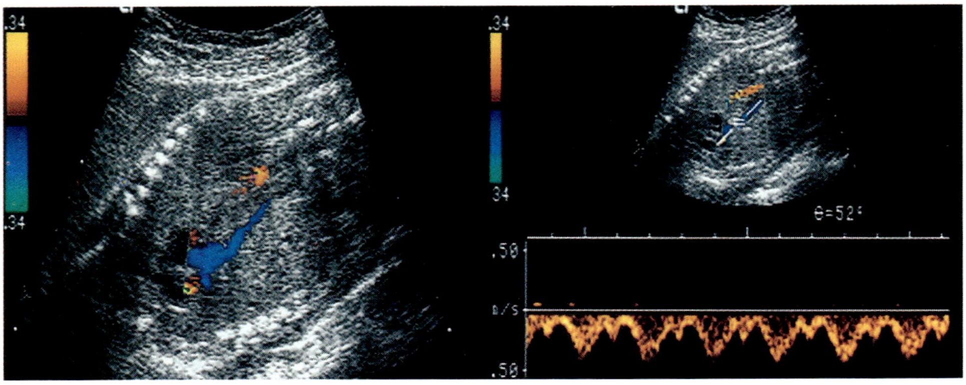 B

COLOR FIGURE 13–16.
A, Inferior vena cava (IVC) flow is seen traveling in a cranial direction through the liver and continuing into the right atrium. *B,* Modulations in venous waveform of the IVC due to changing atrial pressures during cardiac cycle. Additional changes in the waveform occur as a result of fetal breathing motion.

A 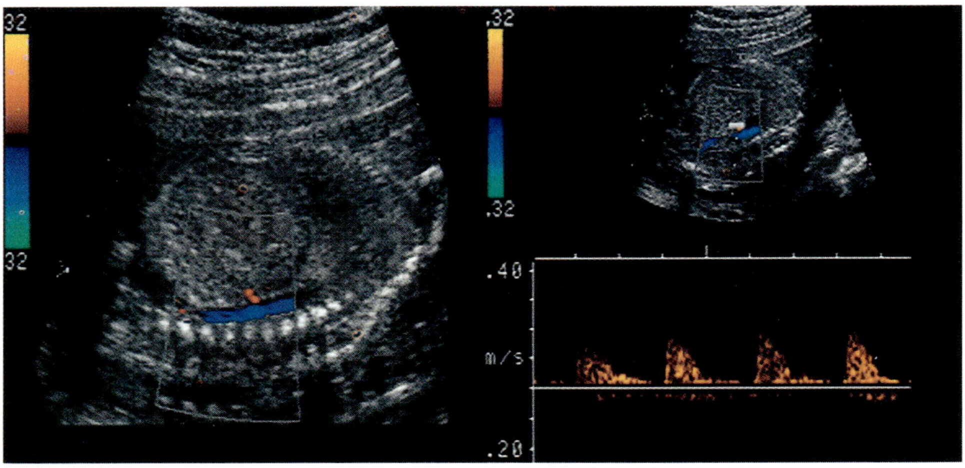 B

COLOR FIGURE 13–17.
Superior mesenteric arterial flow in a 16-week fetus. *A,* Color Doppler flow map with a fetus in the sagittal plane demonstrates flow in the abdominal aorta (coded blue) and the superior mesenteric artery (coded red). *B,* Pulsed Doppler interrogation reveals low-velocity flow with minimal diastolic component in the superior mesenteric artery.

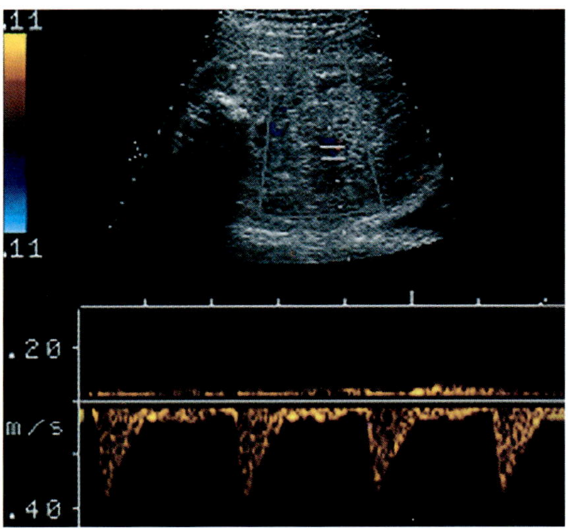

COLOR FIGURE 13–18.
Doppler flow in the mesentery of fetal bowel seen in a 36-week fetus. The color Doppler flow map permits detection of this flow, and pulsed Doppler interrogation reveals the waveforms. The arterial signal is seen below the base line, and the venous signal is above the base line.

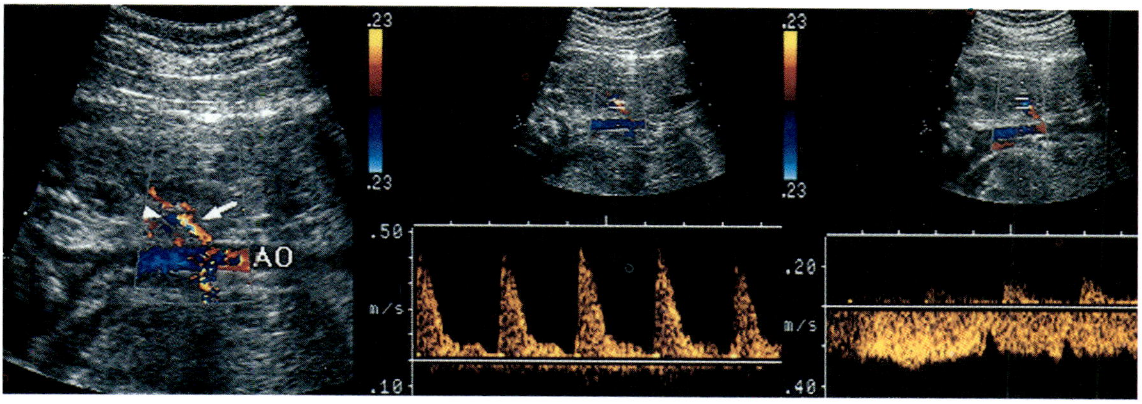

A B C

COLOR FIGURE 13–19.
Color and pulsed Doppler sonography of fetal renal arteries and veins. *A,* The renal arteries and veins are clearly seen on the color Doppler flow map. The renal artery (large arrow), seen exiting the aorta (AO) and traveling toward the kidney, is color coded red with its flow directed toward the transducer. The renal vein (coded blue, arrowhead) is seen next to the artery. *B,* The pulsed Doppler time–velocity tracing confirms the color Doppler information, revealing the renal artery waveform. *C,* Pulsed Doppler spectral tracing reveals venous waveform of the renal vein below the base line. Some renal arterial signal is seen above the base line, indicating oppositely directed flow.

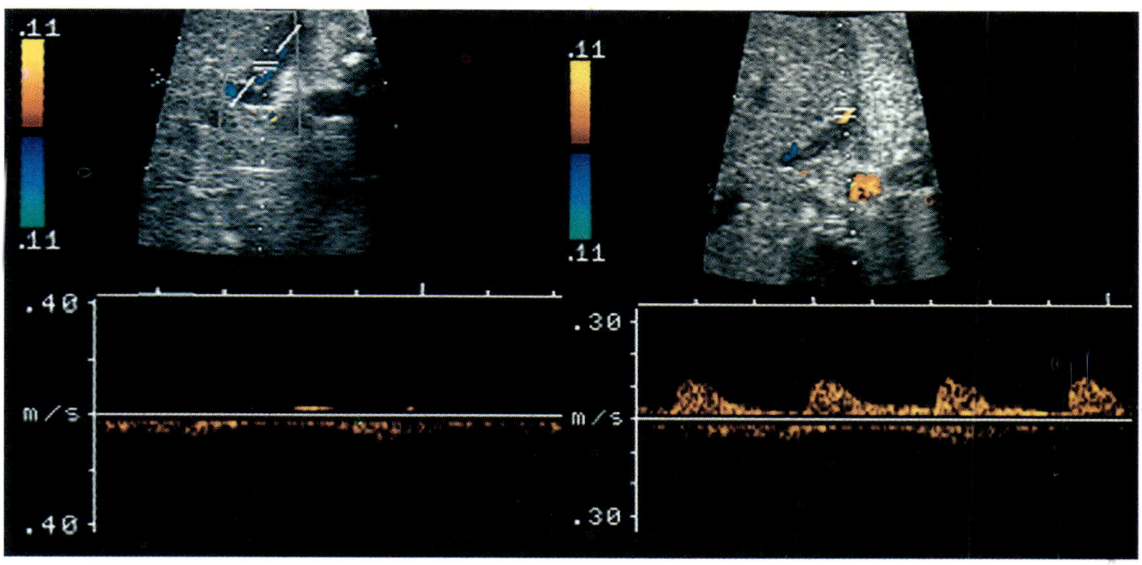

A B

COLOR FIGURE 13–20.
Color and pulsed Doppler of a fetal adrenal artery and vein. *A,* Very low-velocity flow is seen in the adrenal vein. *B,* Adrenal arterial flow has a relatively low velocity, typically between 10 and 20 cm/sec, similar to that of mesenteric arterial branches.

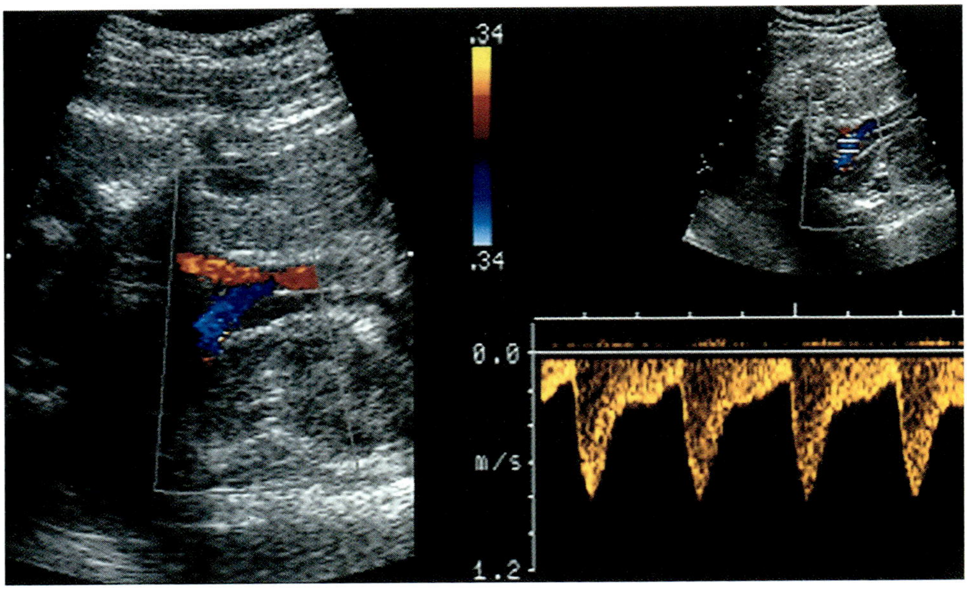

A B

COLOR FIGURE 13–21.
A, The common iliac arteries are best visualized in the coronal plane, bifurcating off the long axis of the aorta. They are easily identified with color mapping. One of the arteries is heading toward the transducer, and the other is heading away. This is reflected in the color coding of flow. *B,* The pulsed Doppler spectrum reveals a high-velocity arterial waveform with low end-diastolic velocity in one of the common iliac arteries.

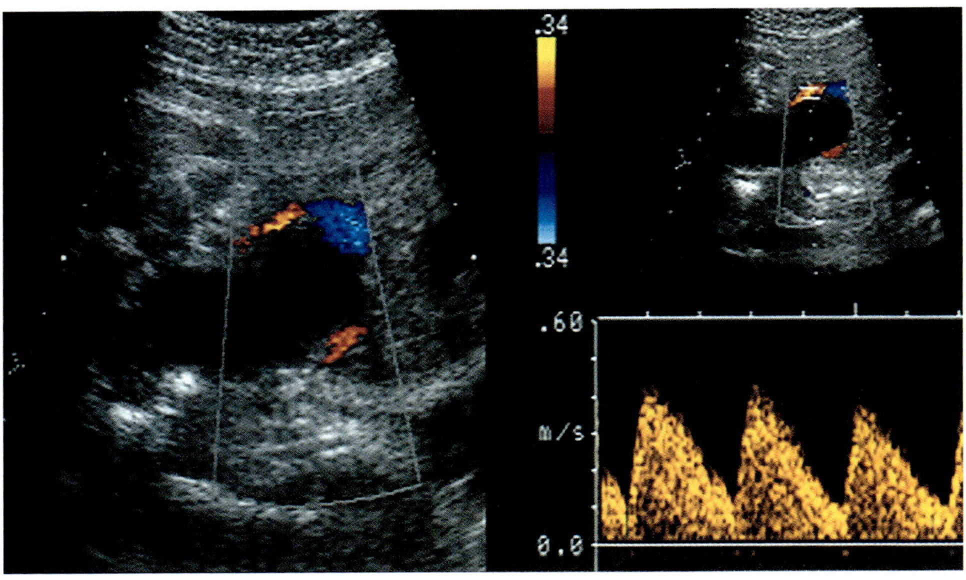

A B

COLOR FIGURE 13–22.
A, Color flow map reveals umbilical arteries coursing around the bladder. They are very useful anatomical landmarks for identifying bladder location when visualization is poor and the bladder is empty. *B,* Pulsed Doppler demonstrates a typical umbilical artery waveform. Pulsed Doppler of the umbilical arteries for determination of placental resistance is generally performed at the umbilical cord.

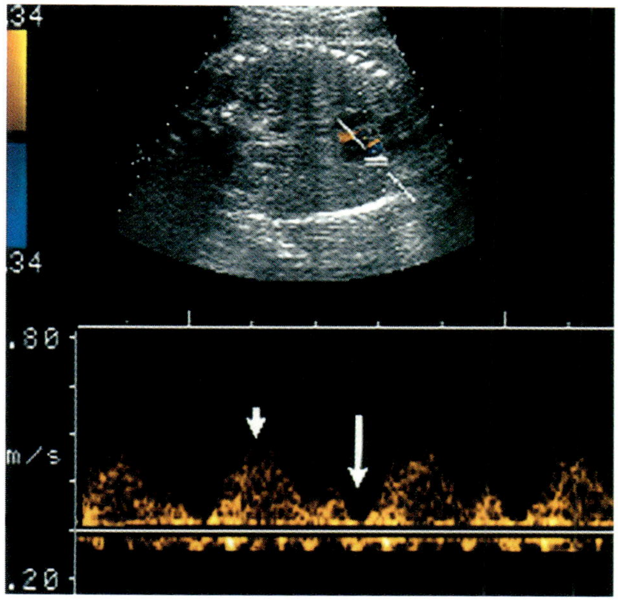

COLOR FIGURE 13–23.
Pulsed Doppler tracing of flow in the superior vena cava (SVC). Arrows indicate modulations in the SVC due to atrial systole and diastole.

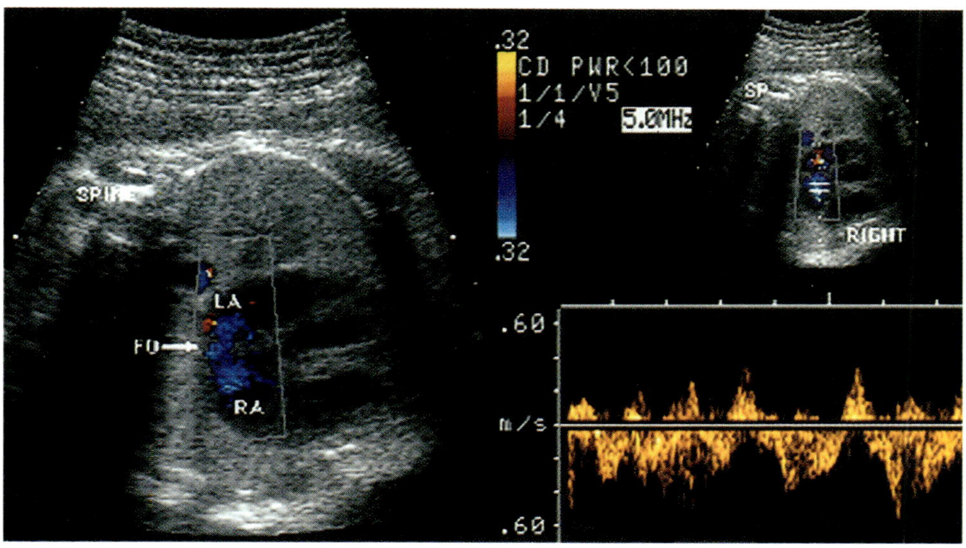

COLOR FIGURE 13–24.
Color and pulsed Doppler sonography of interatrial flow via the foramen ovale (FO). The color flow map on the left shows flow between the left and right atria (LA, RA) through the normally patent foramen ovale. Flow is coded blue, indicating movement away from the transducer. Although this suggests an abnormal left-to-right shunt at this level instead of the expected right-to-left shunt, it should be remembered that this image represents only one frame from a cine of the entire cardiac cycle. In reality, bidirectional flow often occurs at the FO, as can be seen on the pulsed Doppler spectral tracing on the right.

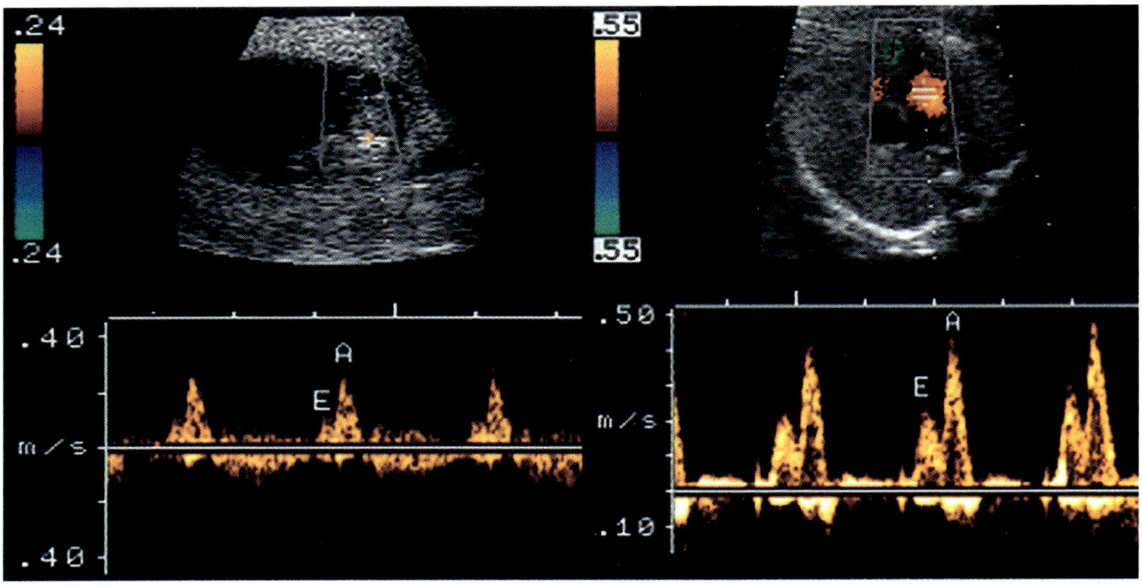

A

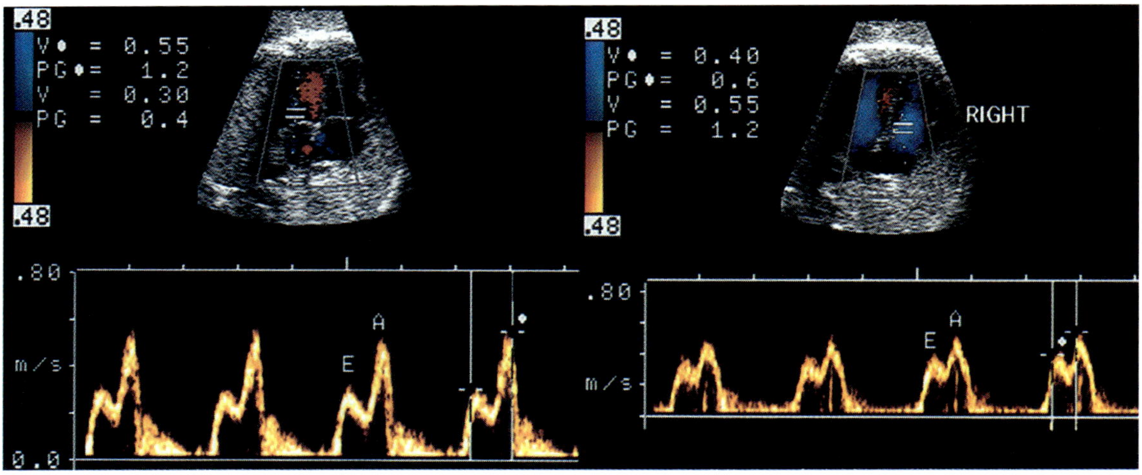

B

COLOR FIGURE 13–25.
A, Pulsed Doppler waveforms across the atrioventricular valves. The typical M-shaped waveform is seen in both the 9.5-week fetus (left) and the 25-week fetus (right). A/E ratio represents peak velocity at atrial systole (A) divided by the peak velocity at early diastole (E). *B*, Although M-shaped waveform is seen across both atrioventricular valves, there are differences in flow velocity and therefore in the A/E ratios. In this case, the peak velocity during atrial systole, 5 cm/sec, is the same for the mitral valve (left) and the tricuspid valve (right). The peak velocity at early diastole (E) is lower at the mitral valve (30 cm/sec) than at the tricuspid valve (40 cm/sec).

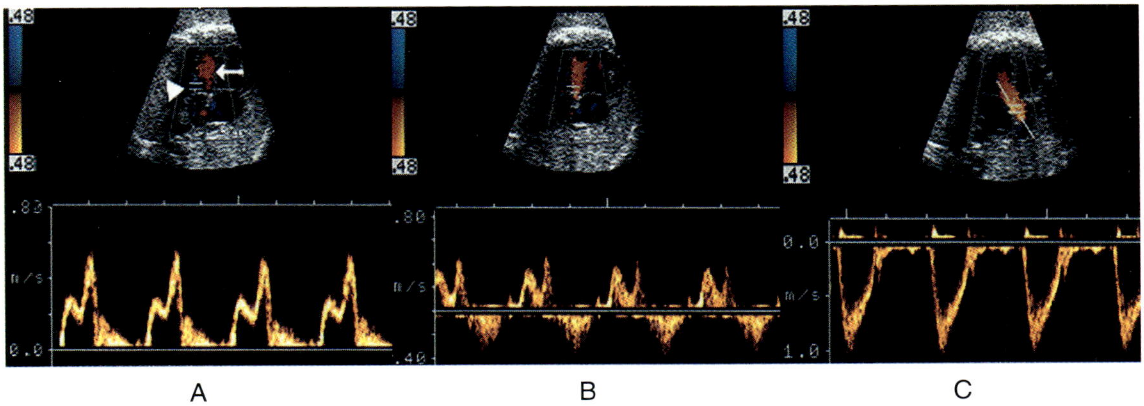

COLOR FIGURE 13–26.
Pulsed Doppler sampling of mitral and aortic flow. *A*, The Doppler range gate (arrowhead) is appropriately placed for an accurate representation of mitral flow. *B*, Doppler range gate straddles both the inflow and outflow tracts of the left ventricle, yielding imperfect Doppler waveforms of both mitral and aortic flow on opposite sides of the base line. *C*, Further positioning of the range gate into the ascending aorta produces a clean and accurate aortic outflow waveform.

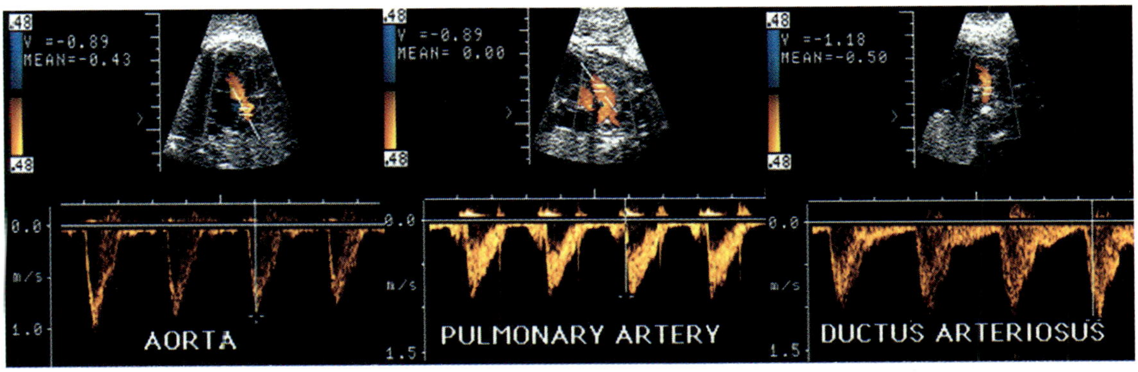

COLOR FIGURE 13–27.
Pulsed Doppler waveforms of the aorta, pulmonary artery, and ductus arteriosus. The aorta and pulmonary artery have little diastolic flow compared with that of the ductus arteriosus. Peak velocities are lower in the aorta (89 cm/sec) and pulmonary artery (89 cm/sec) than in the ductus arteriosus (118 cm/sec). Color Doppler expedites accurate placement of the pulsed Doppler range gate and determination of the Doppler angle adjustment.

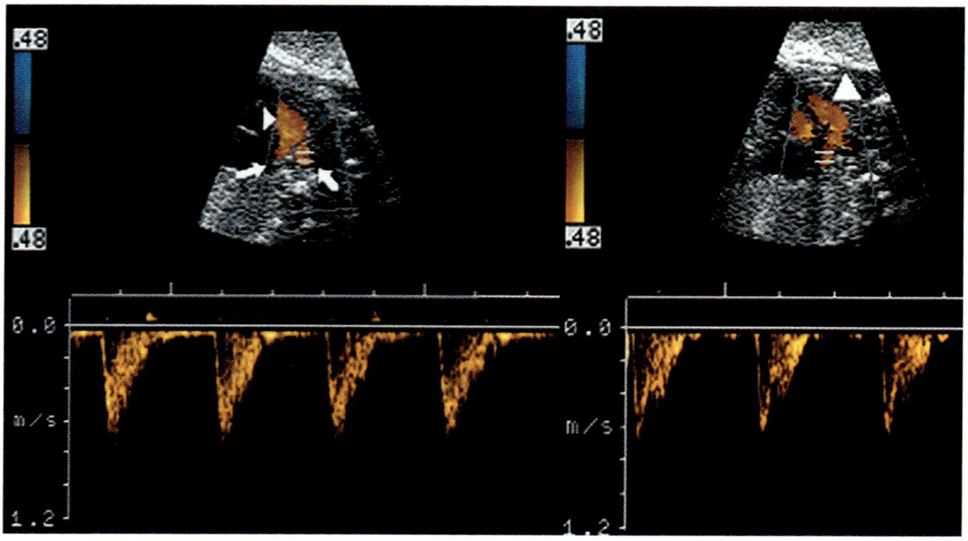

A B

COLOR FIGURE 13–28.
Although flow within right and left pulmonary artery branches (arrows) of the main pulmonary artery (arrowhead) is seen clearly on the color map, pulsed Doppler sampling can be performed even without color Doppler. *A*, Left pulmonary artery. *B*, Right pulmonary artery.

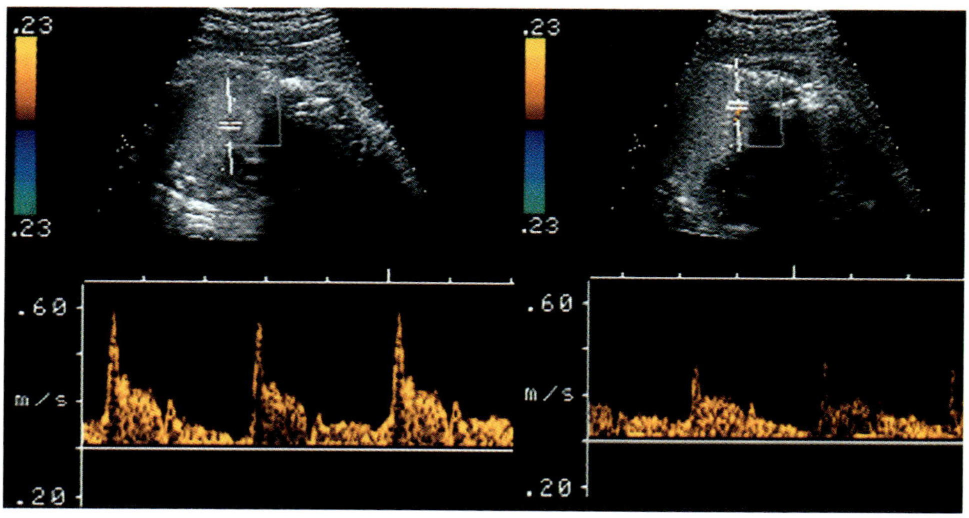

COLOR FIGURE 13–29.
Waveforms of the distal pulmonary arterial branches of the lungs demonstrate an initial needlelike systolic peak and a rapid diastolic decay. This appearance suggests the effects of high vascular resistance in the pulmonary bed. The shape of the waveform remains unchanged as pulsed Doppler sampling moves farther into the periphery of the lungs, although peak systolic velocities decrease.

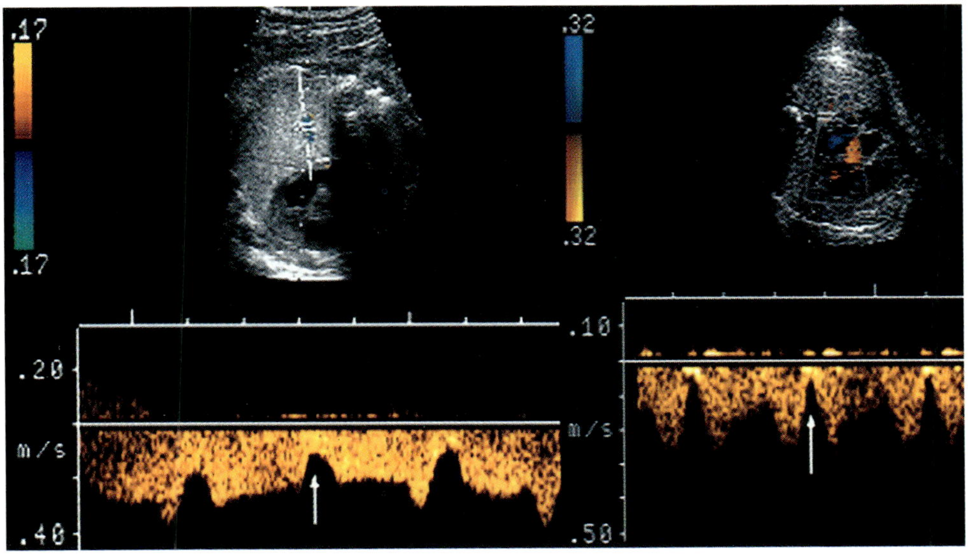

A B

COLOR FIGURE 13–30.
The pulmonary veins may be followed with color flow Doppler from the periphery of the lungs (*A*) to the left atrium (*B*). Similar modulations in the venous waveform due to changes in atrial pressures are seen in the pulmonary veins as in the inferior vena cava, hepatic veins, and ductus venosus. Arrows indicate slowing of forward flow due to atrial contraction.

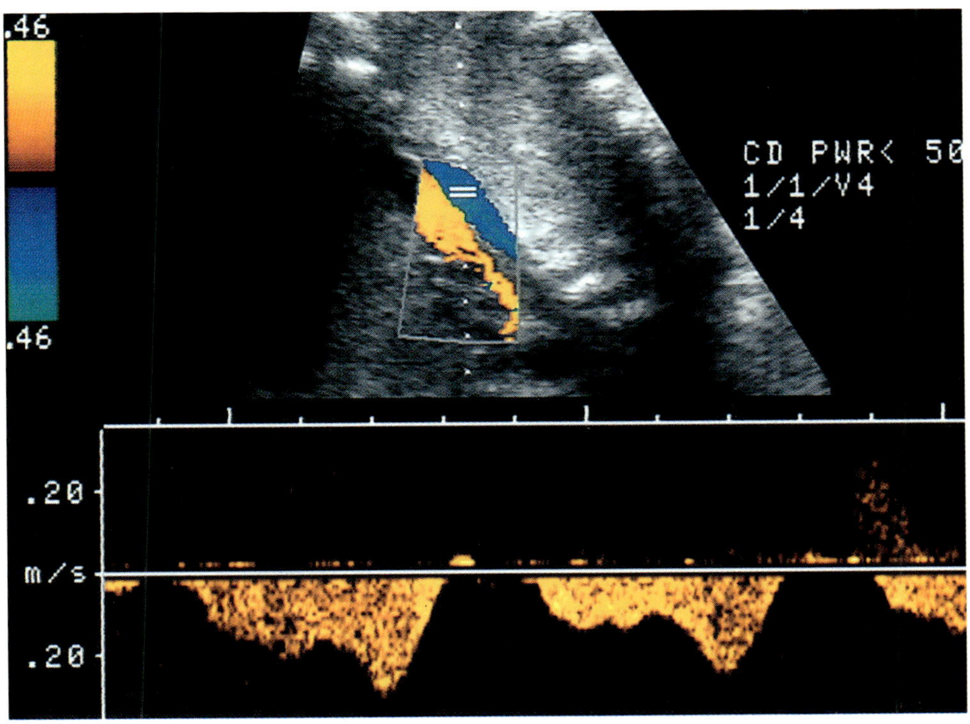

COLOR FIGURE 13–31.
Color Doppler map demonstrates azygos vein coded blue, indicating opposite flow from that of the aorta, which is coded red-yellow because of aliasing. Pulsed Doppler interrogation reveals the venous waveform with low-frequency modulations produced by fetal breathing.

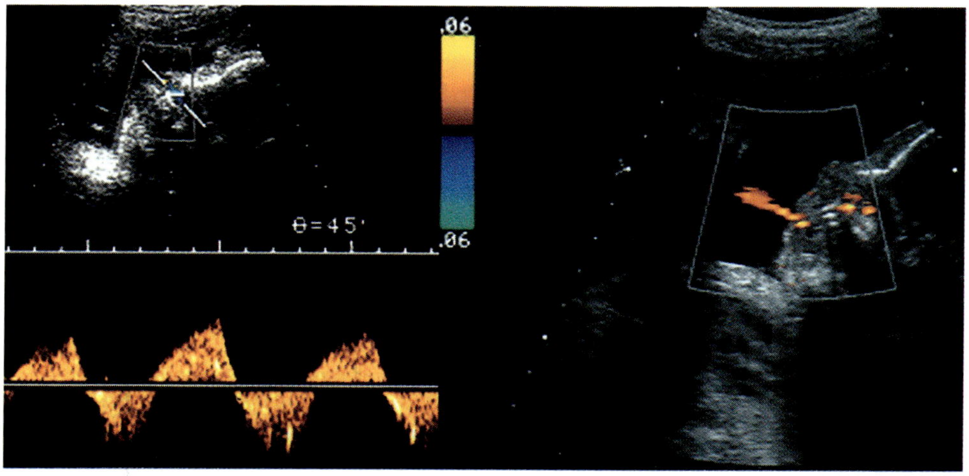

A B

COLOR FIGURE 13–33.
Fetal breathing motion on Doppler in a 32-week fetus. *A,* Pulsed Doppler demonstrates a waveform of the amniotic fluid movement in the nasopharynx. Inspiration is plotted below the base line, and expiration is plotted above the base line. *B,* Sagittal view of a fetal face with a color Doppler map demonstrating movement of amniotic fluid during breathing motion.

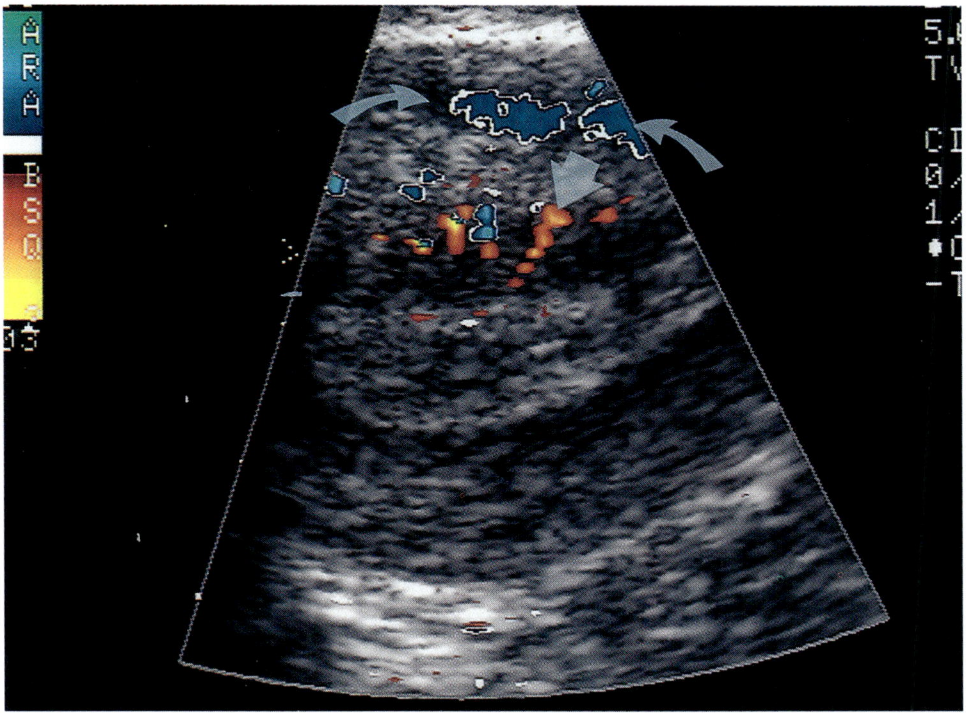

COLOR FIGURE 16–2.
Transvaginal sonogram of uterine cross section. Arcuate myometrial vessels are blue (curved arrows) around the periphery of uterus. The spiral artery, shown spiraling toward the endometrium (large arrow), is unusually well demonstrated. Compare the anatomy with Figure 16–1*A*. In this case, a left ectopic pregnancy was diagnosed in the fifth LMP week; therefore, it is hypothesized that the hormones of pregnancy were dilating the vessels, making them easier to visualize. (LNMP 5.1 weeks, TD)

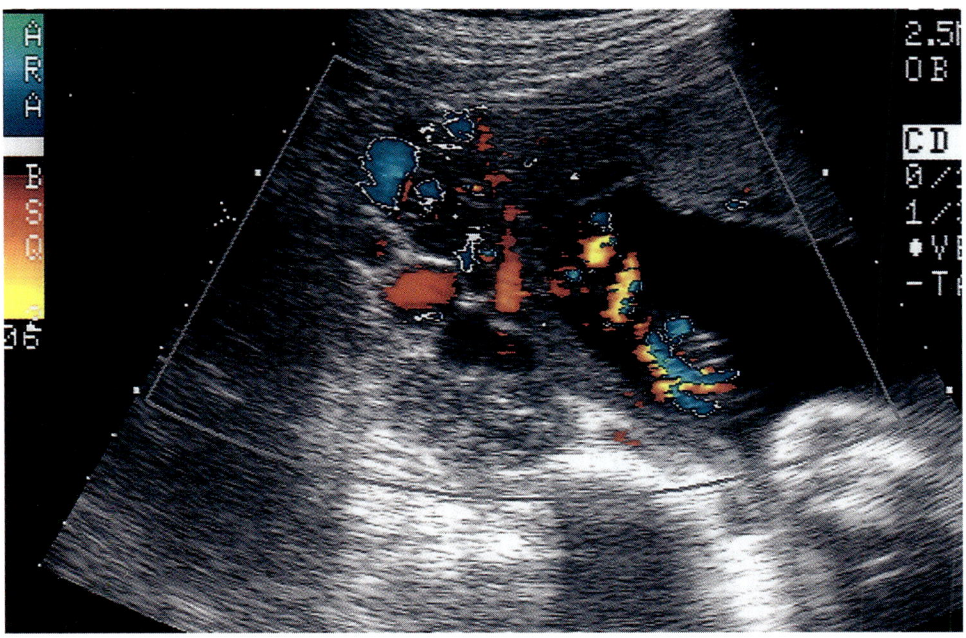

COLOR FIGURE 16–5.
Transverse right lateral section of the uterus showing a mass of vessels. Color Doppler proves these to be vessels and not cysts. In this case, a slow-flow velocity tag was used to outline blood flowing toward the transducer so that direction can be distinguished in black-and-white images. The free-floating umbilical cord is seen within the amniotic fluid. (AA = 25.1 LMP weeks, range = 3.1 weeks, n = 9, TD)

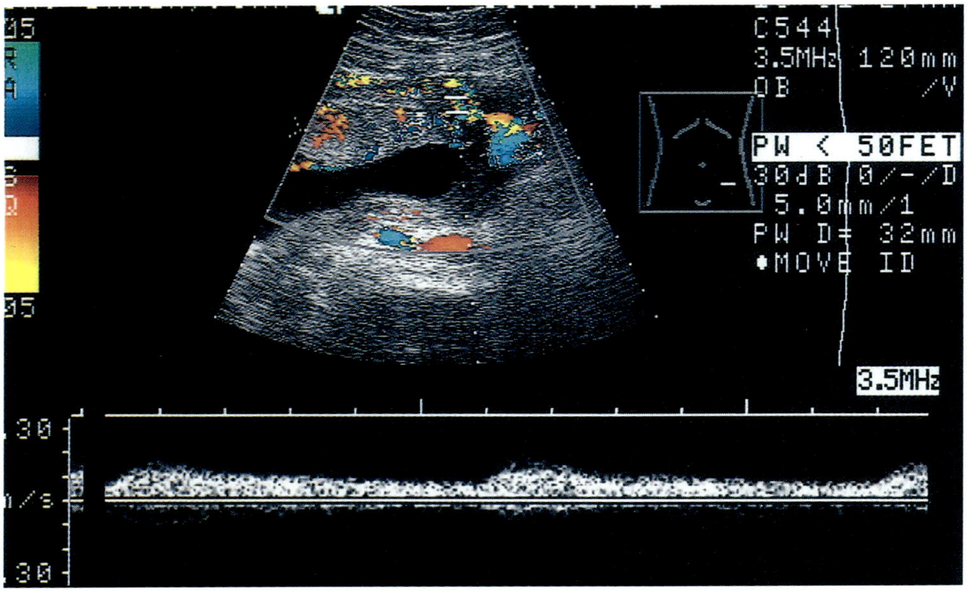

A

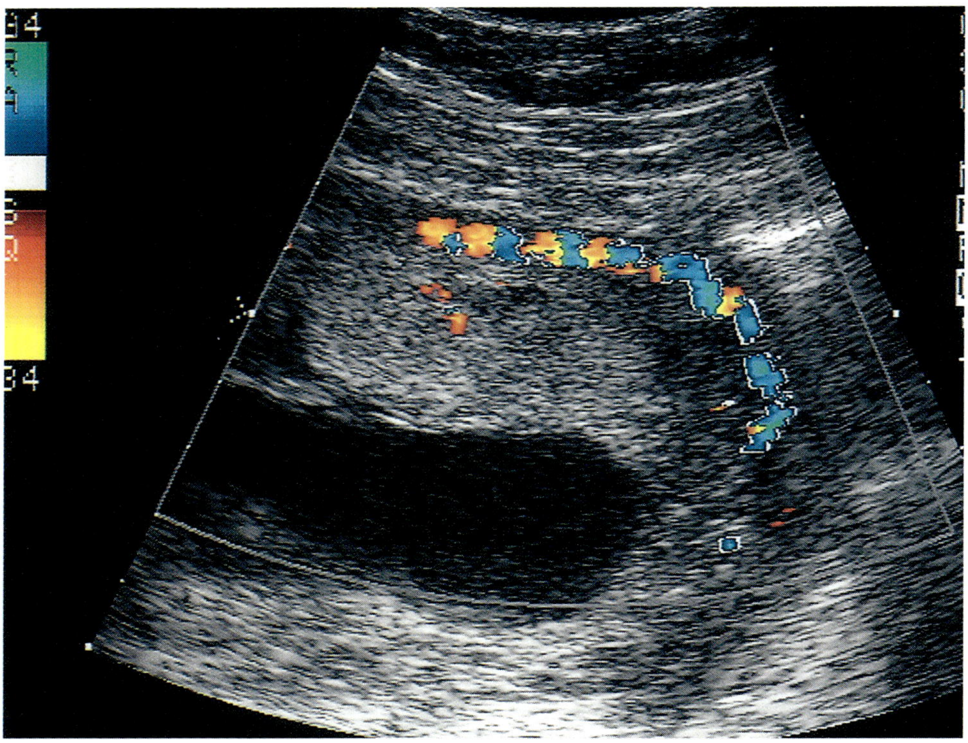

B

COLOR FIGURE 16–9.
Subplacental complex of vessels. *A*, Color and spectral Doppler show this to be a low-resistance arterial flow. This type of flow has been documented as originating from spiral arteries.[26] *B*, Color Doppler from the same region of the uterus as in *A*. Note the spiraling effect of color flow. It is believed that these are spiral myometrial arteries, which are stretched from their normal penetrating angle before pregnancy to more horizontal positions with uterine growth. (AA = 17.7 LMP weeks, range = 1.3 weeks, n = 9, TD)

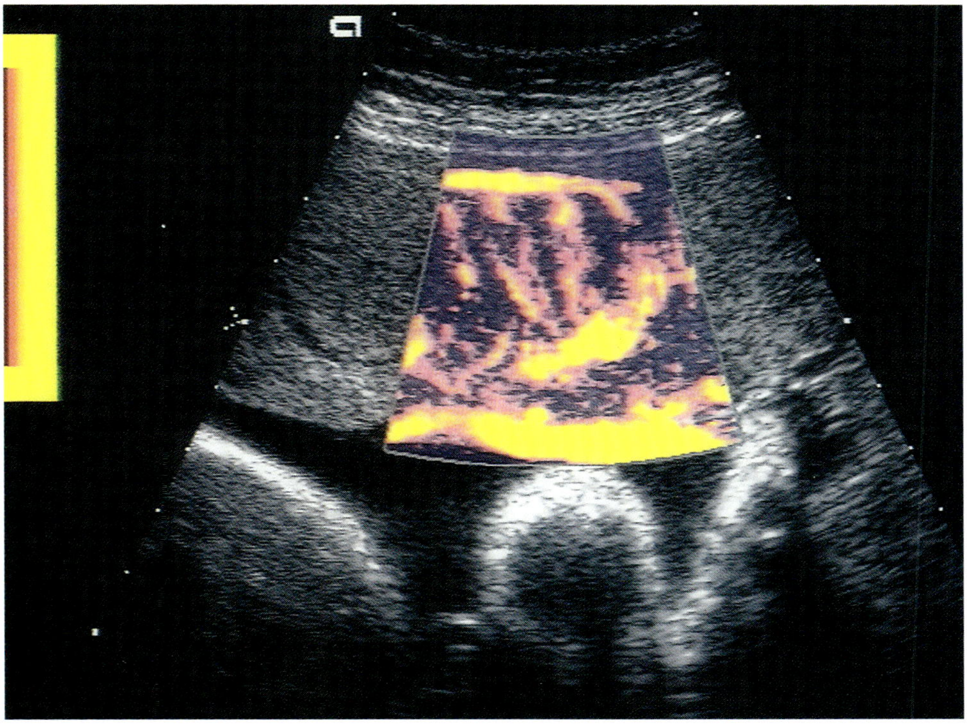

COLOR FIGURE 16–10.
This image demonstrates the use of Doppler energy or amplitude imaging. This new modality does not show direction or velocity of blood flow, only the amplitude of the Doppler echoes. With more research, this type of Doppler should provide more information about placental perfusion. (Image courtesy of ACUSON Corp.)

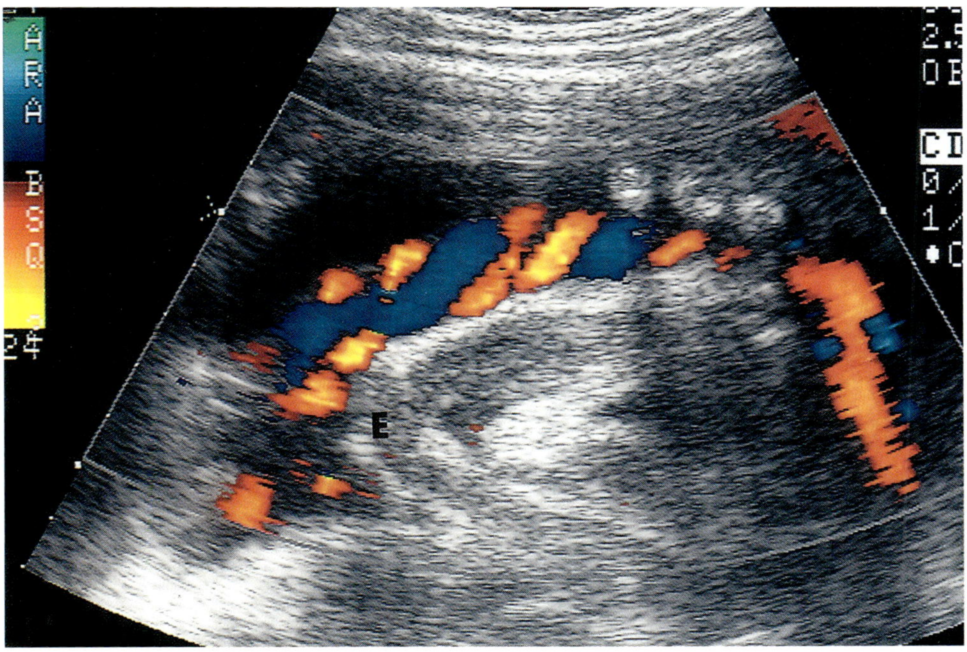

COLOR FIGURE 16–22.
The two arteries and vein. Where flow is toward the transducer, the shorter Doppler shift is shown as blue, and flow away as red. Three fetal fingers can be seen to grasp and press the cord against the other wrist, with the cord passing along the forearm to the elbow (E). (LNMP = 31.9, AA = 31.6 LMP weeks, range = 2.5 weeks, n = 9, TD)

CHAPTER 1

SCOPE

Terry J. DuBose

This book is a basic reference for the sonographic study of the normal human embryo and fetus. In order to qualify as a basic reference work, it must be comprehensive and must contain material that will help a novice enter the field of diagnostic medical sonography as well as information that will continue to serve as a convenient reference as a reader moves from the student phase into the practitioner phase of the profession.

As the founding Program Director and Instructor of Diagnostic Medical Sonography at Austin Community College, I perceived a need for a textbook that would discuss the physical use of sonographic equipment as well as the normal embryofetal sonographic anatomy as it develops throughout pregnancy. Although some texts detail abnormal fetal anatomy[1,2] and congenital anomalies, it is a fact that until one has a thorough grasp of normal anatomy, abnormal anatomy will be difficult to recognize. At this time there are several good obstetrical sonographic books[3–9] but few books specific to the fetus, especially early embryonic development, which has become accessible in just the past 5 years with the advent of transvaginal transducers. Some individual books cover the use of transvaginal sonography in obstetrics, but these are not comprehensive in that they do not deal with the fetus after it is too large to be imaged transvaginally.[10,11]

The field of medical sonography is in the early years of development, and to date there has been no textbook, to my knowledge, that defines the physical movement of the transducer. Through my experience in teaching and thinking about this book, the Austin Community College Diagnostic Medical Sonography (ACC-DMS) 1991–1992 class and I developed a working vocabulary that describes the motions used for acquiring the various image planes necessary for the study and measurement of a fetus. This unique approach to transducer manipulation helps students and teachers to communicate more effectively about the practice of obstetrical sonography. This same way of thinking and communicating about sonography is also applicable to abdominal and other types of sonography.

Fetal measurement and size/age analysis is currently stuck in "flatland." Almost all of the standard measurements of the fetus are either linear or two-dimensional diameters and circumferences of the head, abdomen, or long bones. In reality, the fetal organs are three-dimensional (3-D) structures, and 3-D measurements provide more accurate evaluation of fetal size. In December 1983, I devised a method of estimating the vertical diameter of the fetal cranium (VCD). By using this measurement with the standard two-dimensional measurements, it was possible to estimate the calvarial volume or brain mass of a fetus. This method was published in 1985, and in 1986, the Society of Diagnostic Medical Sonographers (SDMS) presented me with the Kenneth Gottesfeld Award for the research. However, because the statistical proof was lacking, it was said, "Despite the theoretical probability that a volume measurement is better for evaluating brain mass and overall head size, this method has not yet been proved. It should, therefore, at present not be considered in the routine examination of the fetal head."[12, 13] The proof of the accuracy of the 3-D head measurements is now presented here in Chapter 8.

The use of the embryonic heart rate to estimate age is another new topic. During the writing of this book, my group analyzed our 1993 data. By performing regression analysis for the mean age and 95% confidence intervals, we noted that six embryos were below the lower interval line. Follow-up found that at least four and possibly five of the six ended in first-trimester spontaneous abortions. During our research, we also found a surprising visual similarity in the heart rate curve and the shape of the human chorionic gonadotropin curve, both having a peak at approximately 9.0 last menstrual period (LMP) weeks. Our observations on the heart rate are included in Chapter 12. Although they are compelling, much more research is required to understand these relationships. As Cliff Stoll says in his intriguing book about InterNet espionage, "You look at things that occur close together in time, and try to find the probability that they're somehow connected."[14]

An additional unique topic for this book is age range analysis (ARA). This new way of looking at multiple fetal measurements provides a comprehensive analysis of the total fetal proportions without the use of numerous confusing ratios and tables. Although the range of ages was first presented at the 1988 annual conference of the American Institute of Ultrasound in Medicine and SDMS in Washington, D.C., and again at the 1992 conference in San Diego, and at least two preeminent sonographic fetal biometricists have used the method, to date no other documentation of this useful method has been published.

Content and Organization

It was my intent to produce a useful resource book as well as one that can reduce rather complex, esoteric technical discussion into readable and enjoyable prose. Although this book includes detailed statistical and technical concepts, I hope that the relaxed style of writing makes reading it an enjoyable experience. Readers will be called on to use their mind's eye or imagination to visualize many parts of the discussion; this is not unlike the mental visualization required to interpret the two-dimensional "slices" of sonography as representations of the 3-D structures we are studying. It is hoped that this use of the mind's eye while reading this book will provide good practice for the imagination required in successful application of sonography.

This book is divided into three major sections. This first section is a discussion of fetal sonographic history, acoustic physics as is applicable, statistics, ethics, sonographic biological effects and safety, and the general aspects of the conduct of an obstetrical sonographic examination. This last part uses text and artwork to show the actual manipulation of the transducer and to provide a working vocabulary for describing the various motions involved.

The second section is a system-by-system description of the normal fetal anatomy, sonography, and measurements used to study fetal growth throughout pregnancy. The normal uterus, the ovaries, and the fertilization processes are addressed. The discussion then moves to the first trimester. In the late embryonic and the fetal periods, the discussion continues with the head and spine and then the trunk, including the thorax, heart and vascular system, and abdominal contents. Next is a discussion of the extremities, followed by a description of the extrafetal structures of pregnancy such as the placenta, umbilical cord, and amniotic fluid. Also included is some discussion of the maternal changes in the morphology of the uterus that may affect fetal growth, such as the changes in the uterine vessels and perfusion.

A large part of the second section is a discussion of the various approaches to sonographic fetal size/age analysis that have been used by others. This section uses graphs and tables to correlate fetal size and age. Many of the methods of fetal size/age measurements have been published by others and are reproduced here with permission. This is the first formal presentation of some of the parameters; these include 3-D head measurements and calculations and the use of the embryonic heart rate as an indicator of age and possibly cardiac development. This section documents two different ways of analyzing fetal growth and proportionality: the more traditional use of ratios is to study proportionality and age range analysis in looking at the proportional totality of a fetus.

The last section presents many images that show normal human pregnancy from start to term. The images are week by week for the first trimester, when the growth and changes in an embryo/fetus are most rapid. The second- and third-trimester images show only representative weeks to term. These highlight specific normal variations such as changes in the 3-D head shape due to molding toward term, which has received little attention in the sonographic literature. Changes in the amniotic fluid and uterine vascularity have not, in my opinion, been adequately addressed in the literature. This text uses images from representative normal pregnancies for various weeks and includes discussion of the fetal measurements and fetal size/age analysis for those weeks.

While reading and studying images in other sonography textbooks, I have found myself wondering, "At what fetal age does this organ appear like this?" For this reason, in many chapters a protocol has been followed at the end of the figure legends to give the mother's reported last normal menstrual period (LNMP), the average age of multiple fetal parameters (MFP AA or AA), the number of parameters used to calculate the MFP AA (n), the range of the parameter ages in weeks (range), and the initials of the sonographer who produced the image. In this way, it is hoped that the reader will get a better feel for the sonographic appearances at the various ages, as well as develop a better idea of how the fetal ages can be used to evaluate fetal proportionality by using age range analysis.

Conventions and Other Details

To avoid confusion, the following conventions have been followed for defining the dates of pregnancy. The rationale for these conventions is discussed in the first part of Chapter 7. For those who read books from the beginning, the following is provided up front: The date of the woman's reported last normal menstrual period is referred to as the LNMP age. The LMP is the date established by other methods such as fetal measurements and is also reported in menstrual weeks. The average age of multiple fetal parameters (MFP AA) is reported in equivalent menstrual weeks. The date of conception is called the *conceptual age* (Cage) and is the same as the LMP minus 2 weeks or 14 days.

The term *sonologist* refers to a licensed medical doctor who uses diagnostic medical sonography. A DMS is a diagnostic medical sonographer who is not a medical doctor. Unless otherwise noted, a DMS is a person who has successfully passed examinations by the American Registry of Diagnostic Medical Sonographers (ARDMS). The term *sonographer* is used interchangeably with both sonologist and DMS.

Many of the black-and-white images were produced entirely in the sonographic laboratory. The images in Chapters 7 to 10, 12, and 15 to 17, and all in Section III were produced in a way that may particularly interest readers who publish. The sonographic films were produced and recorded using standard medical methods, but the photographs for the publisher were also produced in the laboratory. The negatives were exposed using Kodak 35-mm Cinefluorographic (#2476) or Linagraph Shellburst (CFHC 746) film. This film was provided by Matt Anderson, RT, Director of the Catheterization Laboratory (Angiography) from "tails" left over from the heart catheterization laboratory at South Austin Medical Center. Because it is considered poor practice to run out of film while a catheter is in a patient's heart, it is common practice to throw out tails of a film 100 feet or shorter. These tails were hand loaded into empty 35-mm photographic canisters in complete darkness. Do not use even a darkroom light when handling this film.

The negatives were then shot using a Nikon AF N8008 autofocus camera through a Nikkor AF 35–70 mm macrozoom lens with combinations of Tiffen +1, +2, and +3 close-up adapter lenses. The exposures were made with a ISO/ASA film speed rating of 200. This speed rating varies depending on the film processing and many require shooting a test roll of film at different ISO settings. After exposure, the film was developed through a standard 90-second Kodak Xomat radiographic processor. This was done by taping the leading edge of the 35-mm roll to a 5×7 film leader with hot water–proof tape. If the film is developed as soon as the Xomat is turned on, while it is still cool, the negatives have a longer scale of contrast. As the processor heat rises, the contrast increases.

The developed negatives were printed through a standard photographic enlarger on Ilford Multigrade III glossy resin-coated (RC) photographic paper, medium weight. The exposed enlargements were processed through the same radiographic Xomat processor as used for the film after it had reached standard operating temperature. Be sure to use RC paper, which is a sort of plastic-impregnated paper. Regular fiber photographic paper has a tendency to turn into something like papier-mâché in the hot chemicals and wash of the Xomat.

Experimentation is necessary to adjust exposure times in the camera and enlarger, depending on the time, temperatures, and chemicals used in the processor. The major problem is keeping the contrast in the negative low because of the high concentration of chemicals and temperatures used for rapid radiographic film processing. However, the convenience, speed, and economy of developing the end product are worth the effort.

Acknowledgments

I want to thank Lisa Biello, Vice President and Editor-in-Chief, W.B. Saunders Company, and her staff for the opportunity to edit this book. It is an honor. We are in an exciting time of new ways to peer into our body and marvel at its complexity, beauty, and magic.

The chapter authors are to be acknowledged and thanked for sharing their experience and understanding about this very interesting field of diagnostic medical sonography. Mimi Berman, PhD, RDMS, is one of the foremost of sonographers. Dr. Berman has been Editor of the *Journal of Diagnostic Medical Sonography* and is Director of Health-Related Professions at the State University of New York (SUNY), Brooklyn. Mark Cartier, University of Tennessee, Memphis, Julia Drose, Chief Sonographer, University of Colorado Health Sciences Center, Denver, and Dale Cyr, University of Washington, Seattle, have contributed greatly to the field of sonography through their research and observations of the developing human cardiovascular system. Julia, Dale, and Mark are respected educators and researchers in the field of obstetrical sonography and have always been eager to teach and share their knowledge. Adrian Anthony, RDMS, RDCS, also of SUNY, Brooklyn, has made the topic of bioeffects and safety pleasant and enjoyable. Dr. Gilbert Ramirez is an Assistant Professor, Department of Medicine, University of Texas Health Science Center, San Antonio. Dr. Ramirez has contributed a clear, comprehensive chapter on statistics; he also has helped by suggesting statistical methods for other chapters. Bill Meacham, PhD, studied philosophy in the turbulent 60s and 70s at the University of Texas at Austin and brings a particular interest in women's issues to the chapter on ethics. The contributions of Drs. L. W. Hill, M. L. Lines, R. M. Milman, and J. N. Rutledge, with whom I worked for many years, are also acknowledged.

The discussions of statistical issues and the guidance of Charles Johnson, PhD, and Richard DeMouy, PhD, of the Health Research Program, Health Administration, Southwest Texas State University, San Marcos, Texas, are appreciated. Their suggestions have kept us from committing some tragic statistical blunders. Their cautions led me to use the term "voodoo statistics" for that section of Chapter 7. Neither they nor anyone else can be blamed for the possible statistical naiveté of this book—that is my sole responsibility.

This book, in large part, is a result of more than 10,000 sets of embryofetal measurements conscientiously collected and entered in a personal computer database between 1984 and 1994 in Austin, Texas. Fifty variables were collected, including names, ages, other identifying information, and specific observations such as heart chambers, umbilical vessels, amniotic fluid quantities, and placental grades, as well as embryofetal measurements such as the humerus, femur, abdominal, 3-D cranial, M-mode heart rates, and more. Other comments describing fetal motion and placental position and Doppler resistive indexes for umbilical and fetal aortic and middle cerebral arteries were occasionally made in selected cases. Much of this information has never been reported before, and this text is, in part, a presentation of these data.

Thanks is due to almost everyone in the Austin Radiological Association for their dedication to good health care and their organizational strengths, which allowed the delivery in a complex modern society and facilitated accumulation of the data we are discussing. A very special thanks to the Austin Radiological Association radiologists/sonologists who had the vision and curiosity about ultrasound to provide an environment for its practice and early study during the 20 years of the 1970s and 1980s. Particularly, Robert N. Snider, Larry Hill, Edward Poole, William DeGinder, James Cunyus, Robert Ellzey, and Walter Hennigan were among the first in Austin to embrace sonography and the use of personal computers to accumulate the mass of data these two technologies have made available. Their willingness to be open to the innovations of their staff and to provide finances, equipment, and the time to pursue this interesting research, for no other reasons than curiosity, good health care, and the knowledge that the medical community respects good work, made much of this text possible.

The Austin Radiological Association DMS crew, many of whom have worked in and around the Austin diagnostic imaging community for more than 20 years, includes both sonologists and sonographers. These people and their titles are listed later. It is this group who performed the examinations and discussed and interpreted many of the sonographic examinations used here.

We must not forget the support staff, who are too numerous to name individually, including the secretaries, file room clerks, couriers, and everyone who worked or helped in the darkroom to keep the whole routine going. None of this would have been possible without their good work.

We also acknowledge the referring physicians and their patients for the confidence, support, trust, and occasional feedback.

In addition to these groups, we would like to acknowledge the assistance of sonographers and sonologists throughout the Central Texas area who served as Clinical Instructors for the ACC-DMS program from its start in 1989 through 1994, particularly Sid Lister, RDMS, Senior Sonographer at Austin Regional Clinic, who proofread some of the chapters and was always willing to discuss concepts and make suggestions. Many of these instructors have freely shared their knowledge and images for the production of this text. These helpful people are also listed later. I must also thank Ms. Biello and W.B. Saunders for their patience; what was promised to them in 1 year has taken more than 2 and a half years.

And last but certainly not least is my gratitude to Victoria Vescovo Alderman, MA, RDMS, for her contribution to this book. It is rare that a teacher of diagnostic sonography has a student with the background, enthusiasm for the field, and creative talent that Ms. Alderman possesses. Ms. Alderman has a Master's degree in Medical Illustration from the University of Texas Southwestern Medical School in Dallas. After working as a freelance medical illustrator, she came to Austin Community College for sonography. This is probably the only sonographic textbook to be illustrated by a RDMS with such great artistic talent.

I have tried to include all those who contributed to this book in Table 1–1.

I had toyed with the idea of a comprehensive fetal sonography textbook for several years, but it was not until one evening in class that the possibility started to seem real. The lecture was about why two-dimensional measurements of the fetal head are more accurate than single biparietal diameter measurements and why 3-D would be even more accurate, as well as the difficulty of ex-

TABLE 1–1. **THANKS TO THE FOLLOWING FOR THEIR SUPPORT IN VARIOUS WAYS**

NAME		TITLE	IMAGES	CONTRIBUTIONS
Carmon	Alley	ACC-DMS student 91–92		Transducer motion discussion
Nora	Bird	Dr. VM, ACC-DMS student 93–94		Discussions
Valerie	Black	ACC-DMS student 93–94		Discussions
Mark	Bowens	ACC-DMS student 92–93		Discussions
Tracey	Buckner	ACC-DMS student 93–94		Discussions
Howard A.	Buell	Sonologist/radiologist		Discussions of sonography issues
Lou Ann	Buell	ARA-staff DMS	LAB	Former ARA Staff Sonographer
Chris M.	Butschek	Sonologist/radiologist		Uterine vessel research
Anna	Chan	Dr. VM, ACC-DMS student 93–94		Discussions
Pam	Clayton	ARA-staff DMS (current)	PC	Clinical Instructor, DMS-ACC
J.A.	Cunyus	Sonologist/radiologist		EHR regression (retired)
Dot	Davis	ARA-staff DMS (current)	DOT	Doppler sonography
Tamara	Deans-Barrett	ACC-DMS student 93–94	TDB	Images
William	DeGinder	Sonologist/radiologist		ARA #1 computer guru (retired)
Denise	Dickey	ARA-MAS, Chief DMS	DKD	Obstetrical sonography
William	Dietlein	ACC-DMS student 91–92		Transducer motion discussion
Terry	DuBose	ARA-senior DMS 1980–1994	TD	All research areas, founding director ACC-DMS program
Robert F.	Ellzey	Sonologist/radiologist		Senior radiologist, educator
T.	Fletcher	Sonologist/radiologist		Discussions of issues
Louie	Garza	ARA-staff DMS (current)	LG	Clinical instructor, DMS-ACC
Robin	Garza	ARA-staff DMS (current)	RRG	Color Doppler of urine jets
Douglas	Graham	ACC-DMS student 93–94	DG	Images
Mark B.	Gray	Sonologist/radiologist		Medical director, DMS program ACC
Robert	Green	ACC-DMS student 91–92		Transducer motion discussion
Carol	Greenwood	ARA-MPT, chief DMS	CG	Uterine vessel research and illustration
Sara	Guidry	ARA-staff DMS (current)	SG	Clinical instructor, DMS-ACC
Tamela	Hemphill	ACC-DMS student 91–92		Transducer motion discussion
H.W.	Hennigan	Sonologist/radiologist		Uterine vessel research
Larry W.	Hill	Sonologist/radiologist		ARA president, researcher, and grammarian
Susan	Hodges	ACC-DMS student 91–92		Transducer motion discussion
Holly	Hueth	ACC-DMS student 92–93		Discussions
J. J.	Jefferson	ACC-DMS student 91–92		Transducer motion discussion
Savadary	Lieou	ACC-DMS student 92–93		Discussions
M.L.	Lines	Sonologist/radiologist		Obstetrical sonography, educator
Sid	Lister	Sr. DMS Austin Regional Clinic	SL	Images, proofreading, discussion
Sue	Mankin	DMS Austin Diagnostic Clinic		Clinical instructor, DMS-ACC
Ellison	Marshall	ACC-DMS physics instructor		Clinical instructor, DMS-ACC
Michael B.	Martin	Sonologist/radiologist		Uterine vessel research
Mark	McLelland	Sonologist/radiologist		Discussions of issues
Gunar G.	Mezaraups	Sonologist/radiologist		Contributed to age range analysis research
Pam	Moore	ACC-DMS student 92–93		Discussions
David H.	Nichols	Sonologist/radiologist		Neonatal sonography
Penny	Parks	ARA-staff DMS (current)	PP	Clinical instructor, DMS-ACC
Virgil	Pascual	ACC-DMS student 93–94		Discussions
Tuyet	Pham	ACC-DMS student 93–94		Discussions
Lynnell	Pilgrim	ACC-DMS student 92–93		Discussions
Edward	Poole	Sonologist/radiologist		Austin, Texas' first sonologist (retired)

TABLE 1–1. THANKS TO THE FOLLOWING FOR THEIR SUPPORT IN VARIOUS WAYS—*Continued*

NAME		TITLE	IMAGES	CONTRIBUTIONS
Linda	Porter	ARA-BSQ, chief DMS	LP	All research areas, ideas, and moral support
JoJean	Ray	ARA-staff DMS (current)	JR	Clinical instructor, DMS-ACC
Chris	Richards	DMS Austin Regional Clinic		ACC-DMS student 90–91
Angela	Rogers	ACC-DMS student 93–94		Discussions
J. Neal	Rutledge	Neuroradiologist		Neurosonography
Rodney D.	Schmidt	Neuroradiologist		Uterine vessel research
Nipurna	Shah	ACC-DMS student 92–93		Discussions
Sharon	Shull	Dr. VM, ACC-DMS student 91–92		Transducer motion discussion (major portions)
R.N.	Snider	Sonologist/radiologist		ARA founder and educator (retired), age range analysis
Cheryl	Stewart	DMS Brackenridge Hospital		Clinical instructor, DMS-ACC
Mechala	Stewart	ARA-staff DMS		Former ARA staff sonographer
Victoria	Vescovo Alderman	ACC-DMS student 91–92		Transducer motion discussion, medical illustrator
Mary	Winsett	Sonologist/radiologist		Discussions of issues
Estala	Zavala	ARA-Stratum, chief DMS	EZ	Clinical instructor, DMS-ACC

plaining the 3-D concepts of sonography. Ms. Alderman enthusiastically blurted out, "Let's do a book!" Coincidentally, soon after Ms. Alderman's suggestion, Lisa Biello contacted me about the possibility of producing the book that I had conceptualized. Now it is a reality. I hope you, the reader, enjoy this book as much as we have enjoyed producing it.

REFERENCES

1. Romero R, Pilu G, Jeanty P, et al: Prenatal Diagnosis of Congenital Anomalies. Appleton & Lange, Norwalk, CT, 1988.
2. Divon MY: Abnormal Fetal Growth. Elsevier, New York, 1991.
3. Berman MC: Obstetrics and Gynecology, vol 1: Diagnostic Medical Sonography: A Guide to Clinical Practice. JB Lippincott, Philadelphia, 1991.
4. Fleischer AC, Romero R, Manning RA, et al (eds): The Principles and Practice of Ultrasonography in Obstetrics and Gynecology. 4th ed. Appelton & Lange, Norwalk, CT, 1991.
5. Goldberg BB, Kurtz AB: Atlas of Ultrasound Measurements. Year Book Medical Publishers, Chicago, 1990.
6. Kurtz AB, Goldberg BB: Obstetrical Measurements in Ultrasound: A Reference Manual. Year Book Medical Publishers, Chicago, 1988.
7. Hansmann M, Hackeloer JB, Staudach A: Ultrasound Diagnosis in Obstetrics and Gynecology. Springer-Verlag, New York, 1985.
8. Callen PW: Ultrasonography in Obstetrics and Gynecology. WB Saunders, Philadelphia, 1983.
9. Sabbagha RE: Diagnostic Ultrasound: Applied to Obstetrics and Gynecology, 2nd ed. JB Lippincott, Philadelphia, 1987.
10. Timor-Tritsch IE: Transvaginal Sonography, 2nd ed. Elsevier, New York, 1991.
11. Bernaschek G, Deutinger J, Kratochwil A: Endosonography in Obstetrics and Gynecology. Springer-Verlag, New York, 1990.
12. Kurtz AB, Goldberg BB: Obstetrical Measurements in Ultrasound: A Reference Manual. Year Book Medical Publishers, Chicago, 1988.
13. Goldberg BB, Kurtz AB: Atlas of Ultrasound Measurements. Year Book Medical Publishers, Chicago, 1990, p 278.
14. Stoll C: The Cuckoo's Egg. Doubleday, New York, 1989, p 132.

SECTION I

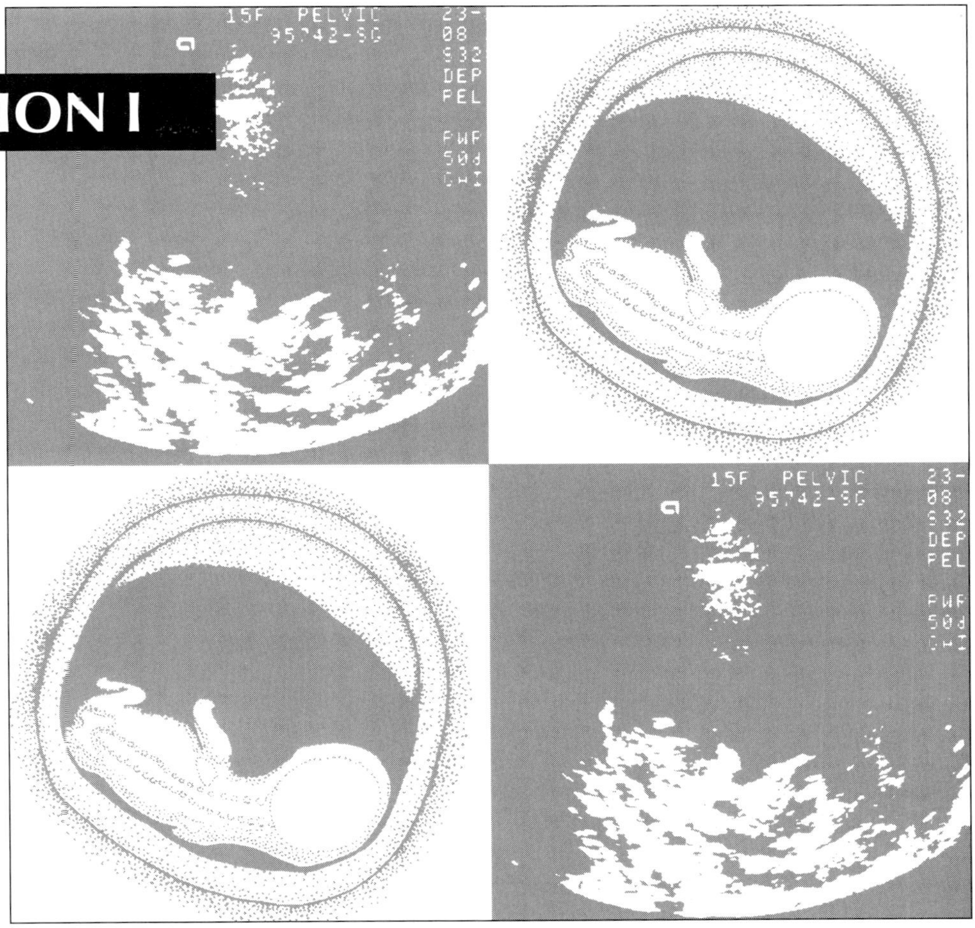

Sonographic History, Technique, Physics, Safety, and Statistics

CHAPTER 2

HISTORY OF FETAL SONOGRAPHY

Mimi Berman, PhD, RDMS

Diagnostic ultrasonography is largely responsible for our regarding the fetus as a human being. Today ultrasonography is used to investigate the anatomy and function of every fetal structure, from the fingernails to the optic nerve.[1] According to the founder of fetal ultrasonography, Ian Donald, before the use of ultrasonography, the mystery of the fetal state was created by a "veritable iron curtain which obscured all but a limited assessment of the state of fetal health."[2] Donald had already penetrated this iron curtain by 1959, when he reported having been able to confidently identify the fetal head and body.[3] His success in examining the fetus, even with equipment modified from metal flaw detectors, convinced him that fetal ultrasonography would create a specialty in fetal medicine.[2]

Physicians unanimously agree with Stuart Campbell, another pioneer of fetal ultrasonography, that diagnostic ultrasonography is "the single most important investigation in pregnancy."[4] It is estimated that a minimum of 80% of pregnant American women have at least one sonogram during each pregnancy,[5] and pregnant women in Britain, Germany, Austria, Norway, and Iceland are routinely scanned.[5,6] Most examinations are performed to obtain a base line study including determination of the age of the fetus and an assessment of fetal anatomy and well-being. Examinations now performed using real-time equipment and computer programs record and analyze parameters obtained during the study. Doppler and color Doppler are used when questions arise about normal implantation, embryonic viability, placental function, and fetal anomalies. The applications of three-dimensional imaging of the fetus are being evaluated.[7] A fetus is almost more accessible to probing than a child or adult, to the point that George Leopold believed that it was necessary to remind the medical community that "fetuses aren't small children."[8]

Intrauterine invasive procedures include amniocentesis, cordocentesis, fetal intravascular transfusion, and shunt placement for decompression of fluid in hydrocephalus and obstructive uropathy.[9] Corrections of diaphragmatic hernias have been performed, but fetal outcome is still being evaluated. Research is being conducted into the treatment of hematological genetic disorders by in utero transplantation of hematopoietic stem cells, and results seem promising.[10]

The primary role of sonography in prenatal health care has been to determine fetal age and to assess fetal health status. Knowledge of fetal age provides the framework for monitoring fetal growth. An awareness of fetal abnormalities allows parents to decide whether to abort a fetus, seek prenatal treatment sometimes including surgery, or be prepared to have the neonate treated immediately after delivery.

History of General Ultrasonography

The history of the first applications of high-frequency sound to the study of the body is well documented.[11–15] Significant breakthroughs did not occur until after World War II. During World War I, sound waves were used to detect submarines, and after the war they were used to locate schools of fish and to map the ocean floor.[11,16] After World War II, ultrasound was used to detect flaws in various materials including metal. The discovery that ultrasound could show structural changes piqued the imagination of physicians in several specialties including surgery, radiology, cardiology, obstetrics-gynecology, and ophthalmology. Physicians and engineers in the United States, Scotland, France, Sweden, Japan, and Australia were exploring clinical applications of ultrasound at about the same time.

As early as 1942, the Austrian physician Karl Dussik described using ultrasound to map the adult human brain.[17] He claimed to have identified abnormalities based on changes in attenuation. During the middle 1940s to early 1950s, teams of engineers and physicians, among whom were Drs. George Ludwig, Douglas Howry, and John Wild, were conducting experiments using ultrasound to investigate breast lesions, gallstones, the morphology of the eye, and the female pelvic viscera. Physiatrists in the United States were the first to use ultrasound in regular clinical practice, although they used it as a treatment modality for muscle disorders rather than a diagnostic tool.[17] In 1953, Cecil Bircher, a manufacturer of ultrasound equipment, supplied the physiatrist members of the original American Institute of Ultrasound in Medicine (AIUM) with ultrasound equipment for therapeutic use.[17] By 1964, members of the AIUM included engineers and physicians who were interested in the diagnostic application of this new energy source.

Early History of Fetal Diagnostic Ultrasonography

Ian Donald, working in Glasgow, a city where ultrasound was being used in the engineering industry to test metal for flaws, considered the possibility of using this imaging system to penetrate through soft tissue. X-rays were available for skeletal imaging, but he, as well as others, was seeking ways of detecting nonosseous lesions. By 1958, Donald and his colleagues had already progressed from A-scope presentations of interfaces to B-scope images on cathode-ray tubes. Donald found a way to eliminate the need for water tanks, in which a patient had to sit, or water containers, which were applied against the area being examined. After applying olive oil to a patient's abdomen, he rotated a probe (2.5 MHz) that moved along a measuring jig and produced cross sections of the abdomen (Fig. 2–1).

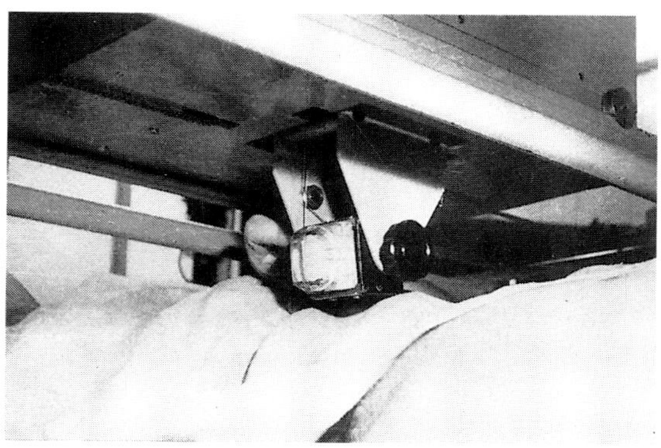

FIGURE 2–1.
The electronics and motor mechanisms of the first contact compound scanner designed by Dr. Ian Donald and engineer Tom G. Brown and constructed at Smith's Industrial Division, Glasgow, in 1957. The transducer was rotated by the clinician along the horizontal bar. (Reproduced with permission from the American Institute of Ultrasound in Medicine, From Medical Diagnostic Ultrasound: A Retrospective on Its 40th Anniversary. Archives, Eastman Kodak Company, 1988.)

Donald is credited with being the first to successfully use diagnostic ultrasonography to investigate the gravid uterus. It was obvious to him that ultrasound had tremendous potential in obstetrics. He wrote, "The pregnant uterus offers considerable scope for this kind of work because it is a cystic cavity containing a solid foetus."[18] The excitement he felt on seeing recognizable anatomy with ultrasound is expressed in the articles he wrote describing his discoveries. His approach was that of a true researcher. The first equipment in his laboratory was developed in the research department of the Hillington Factory in Glasgow.[3] Donald reported in Lancet in 1958 that he had scanned 100 clinic patients at the Royal Maternity Hospital and had identified twins, hydramnios, and the fetal skull, as well as gynecological pathology.[3] He further advanced ultrasonography in gynecology and obstetrics by discovering that a urine-filled bladder provided a means of displacing the gas-filled intestines, thus enabling the sound beam to reach the pelvic viscera.[2] His enthusiasm influenced Dr. Joseph Holmes in Denver and Dr. Louis Hellman in Brooklyn to explore ways to apply ultrasound to obstetrics and gynecology. One of his colleagues, Dr. Stuart Campbell, moved to London and in 1968 opened the first large obstetrical ultrasonography center in England.

Having learned the basics of scanning technique, such as the importance of keeping the ultrasound beam perpendicular to the surface and the effect of scanning with different megahertz transducers, and having developed usable instruments, Donald began focusing on the interpretation and use of the images. Respect for the potential and limitations of diagnostic ultrasonography was always evident in his reports. He also was careful to ascertain that ultrasound was safe, at least in the short term.

Before the advent of ultrasonography, the only part of a fetus that could be measured without the use of x-rays was the fetal head, which could be palpated. Recognizing that the biparietal diameter (BPD) measurement might be a means of measuring the growth of a fetus, Donald, along with Brown and Willocks, developed a technique using "A-scope" to obtain that measurement.[18] They used a modified commercial ultrasonographic flaw detector with a 2.5-MHz transducer that produced spikes at skull-brain interfaces. Donald determined that neonatal ultrasonographic measurements of the BPD were accurate to within 1 mm of caliper measurements. However, fetal BPDs resulted in a standard error of 25 days, which was too great to be able to rely on ultrasonographic measurements alone to estimate fetal age. But he was encouraged by the close correlation (0.77) between birth weight and ultrasonographic BPD measurements taken 7 days or less before delivery and believed that ultrasonography was useful at this stage of development for assessing presentation and fetal size, as well as monitoring growth after the 28th week of pregnancy.

Campbell incorporated B-mode scanning into cephalometry because he showed that A-scans were sometimes measuring two skull surfaces but not necessarily the greatest distance between parietal bones. By identifying the head first by B-scan, the location of the parietal bones could be established. A-mode could be angled perpendicular to them, ensuring that the spike representing the falx was at the appropriate level of the fetal head. Combining B-scans and A-scans improved the accuracy of BPD measurements when compared with postnatal caliper measurements to a difference of less than 2 mm. The combined B-scan and A-scan method also made it possible to measure the BPD even when the head could not be palpated, such as in the middle trimester and in cases of polyhydramnios[9,20] (Fig. 2–2).

The first BPD nomogram was published by Donald and was based on Campbell's measurements of 400 fetuses that were delivered within 3 days of the expected dates of confinement.[2] Obstetricians and gynecologists immediately proceeded to duplicate, test, and expand on this growth curve.

Donald actively encouraged others to use ultrasonography. In 1964, he brought an A-scope unit with him to Hellman's laboratory at Kings County Hospital in Brooklyn, New York. He demonstrated his techniques to Hellman and Lewis Fillisti, an engineer who had built Dr. Gilbert Baum's first ultrasound eye scanner. This particular unit did not function properly, so Fillisti went to Glasgow to learn Donald's techniques. When he returned,

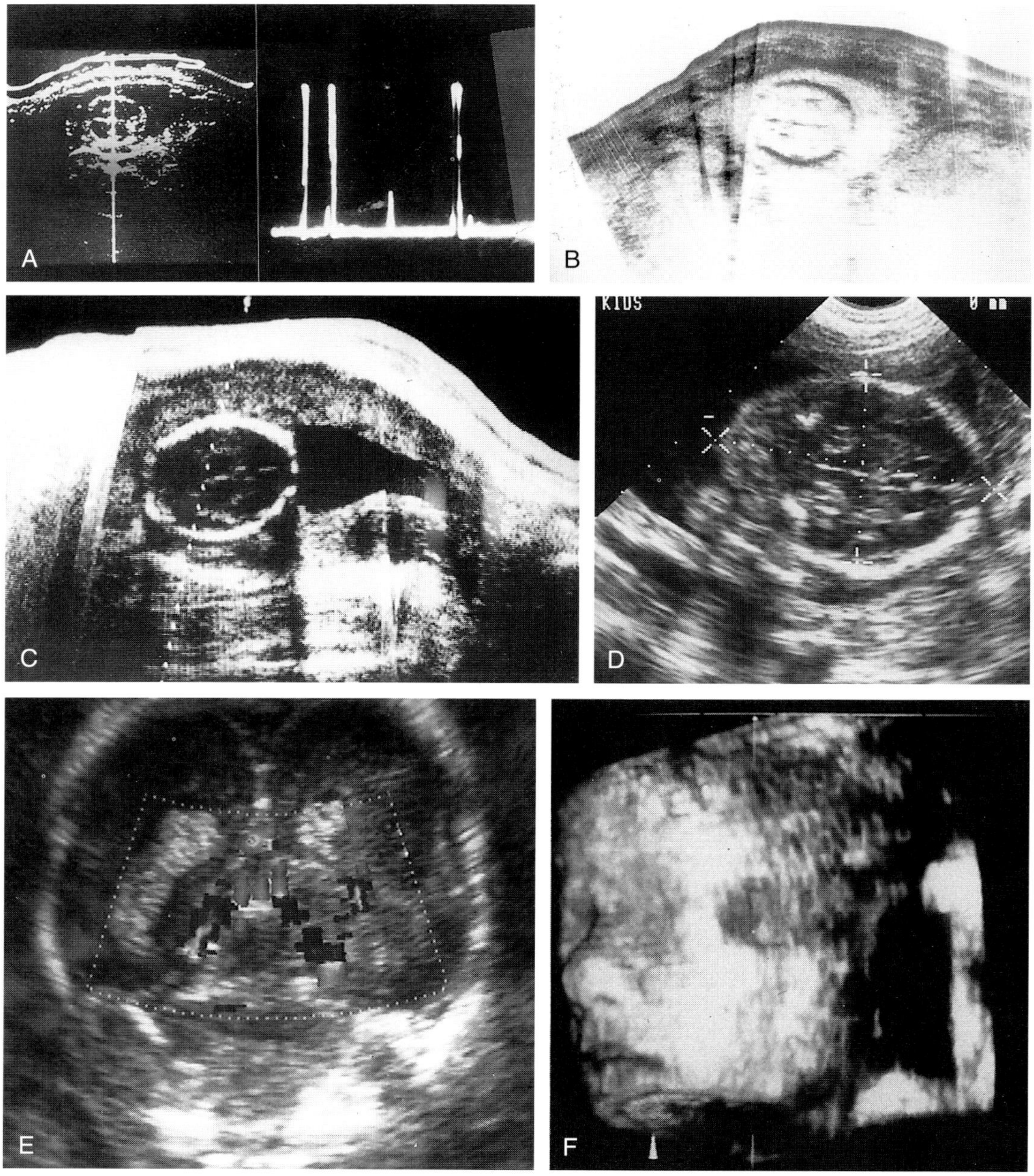

FIGURE 2–2.
A, A 1964 scan of a fetal head, showing the midline echo in the A-mode presentation at right and cross section of the fetal head in the bistable B-mode presentation at left. This scan was probably produced by Ian Donald's Diasonograph. (Reproduced with permission from the American Institute of Ultrasound in Medicine, From Medical Diagnostic Ultrasound: A Retrospective on its 40th Anniversary. Archives, Eastman Kodak Company, 1988.) *B*, Gray-scale scan at the level of the biparietal diameter created by an articulated arm scanner, displaying image with gray echoes against a white background. Scan taken in 1977. *C*, Gray-scale scan at the level of the biparietal diameter created by an articulated arm scanner but with echoes appearing in white against a black background. Scan taken in 1978. *D*, Real-time scan at the level of the biparietal diameter taken in 1993. *E*, Transvaginal coronal scan of a fetal head at 29 weeks of gestation. Color Doppler, seen here as gray and black blocks, outlines the circle of Willis and internal carotids. (Sonogram courtesy of Dr. Shraga Rottem, University Hospital of Brooklyn, State University of New York, Health Science Center at Brooklyn, NY.) *F*, Three-dimensional scan of a fetal head showing the face. (Sonogram courtesy of Dr. Horst Steiner, Salzburg General Hospital.)

the laboratory began scanning patients using a unit made by Physionics Engineering in Longmont, Colorado.* Fillisti described how Hellman, Dr. Kobayashi, and Ellen Cromb Campos, the sonographer, had to coerce physicians to obtain patients for scanning, but as residents and attendings became familiar with ultrasonography, requests began escalating for clinical purposes.

Hellman agreed with Donald that a single measurement, such as the BPD, did not yield the precision that physicians wanted.[11] Consequently, he decided to measure the uterus, the gestational sac, and the placental volume to analyze whether they correlated with fetal growth. The growth charts based on these measurements were quite accurate, and the gestational sac nomogram was adopted by many laboratories. Uterine size and the placental volume provided no usable results, however. While studying the growth of the gestational sac, Hellman also described its pattern of growth, concluding that the sac seemed to dissolve between the 11th and the 13th weeks of gestation, just as the head was becoming visible.[21]

Another mode of research on fetal ultrasonography was undertaken in Denver, Colorado. Involvement with medical applications of ultrasound to imaging the body began with the investigation by Howry into mapping soft tissue in the late 1940s. In 1951, Holmes contributed his administrative acumen to Howry's efforts to produce a practical ultrasound system not requiring a patient to be immersed in a tank of water. In the early 1960s, once the group had developed a compound contact scanner, Drs. Horace Thompson and Kenneth Gottesfeld joined Holmes's laboratory and began using ultrasound for obstetrics and gynecology[15] (Fig. 2–3).

Bistable imaging, although limited to seeing strong interfaces, could demonstrate most fetal anatomy including the fetal spine, aorta, umbilical vein, liver, kidneys, heart, and stomach.[22] Campbell and Wilkin believed that estimates of fetal weight could be improved by basing them not only on BPDs but also on the abdominal circumference (AC). They chose this section because it represented the

*Fillisti L: Written communication, November 1979.

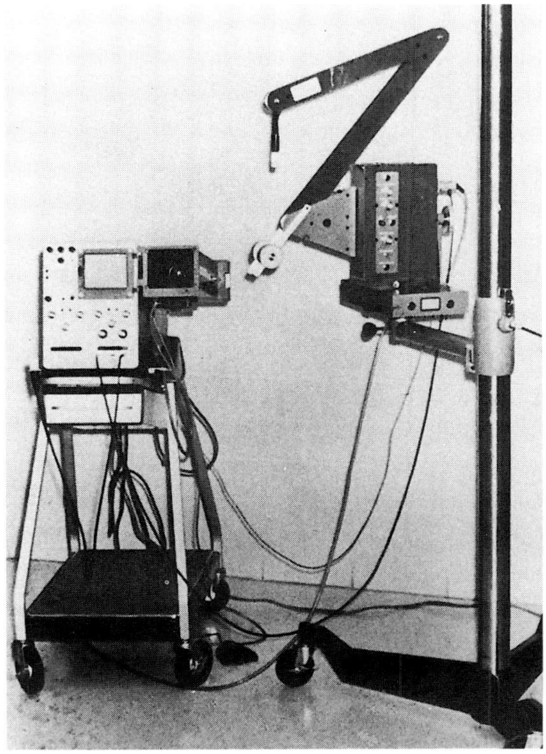

FIGURE 2–3.
Articulated arm hand-held scanner produced in 1964 in Denver by Physionics, the company founded by William Wright and Ed Meyer. (Reproduced with permission from the American Institute of Ultrasound in Medicine, From Medical Diagnostic Ultrasound: A Retrospective on Its 40th Anniversary. Archives, Eastman Kodak Company, 1988.)

total fetal body mass.[23] Furthermore, the sectional image was easy to obtain and could be used to screen for fetal pathology.

Bistable imaging limited diagnostic ultrasonography to the measurements described earlier and to visualizing gross fetal anomalies such as hydrocephalus, ascites, and fetal death (no heart motion seen). Multiple gestations could of course be studied.

Impact of Gray-Scale Imaging

The display of gray-scale images was dependent on the screen from which the permanent image was photographed. Wild's and Donald's machines were capable of producing images with multiple shades of gray, but the cathode-ray tubes displayed only the strongest echoes, producing bistable images.

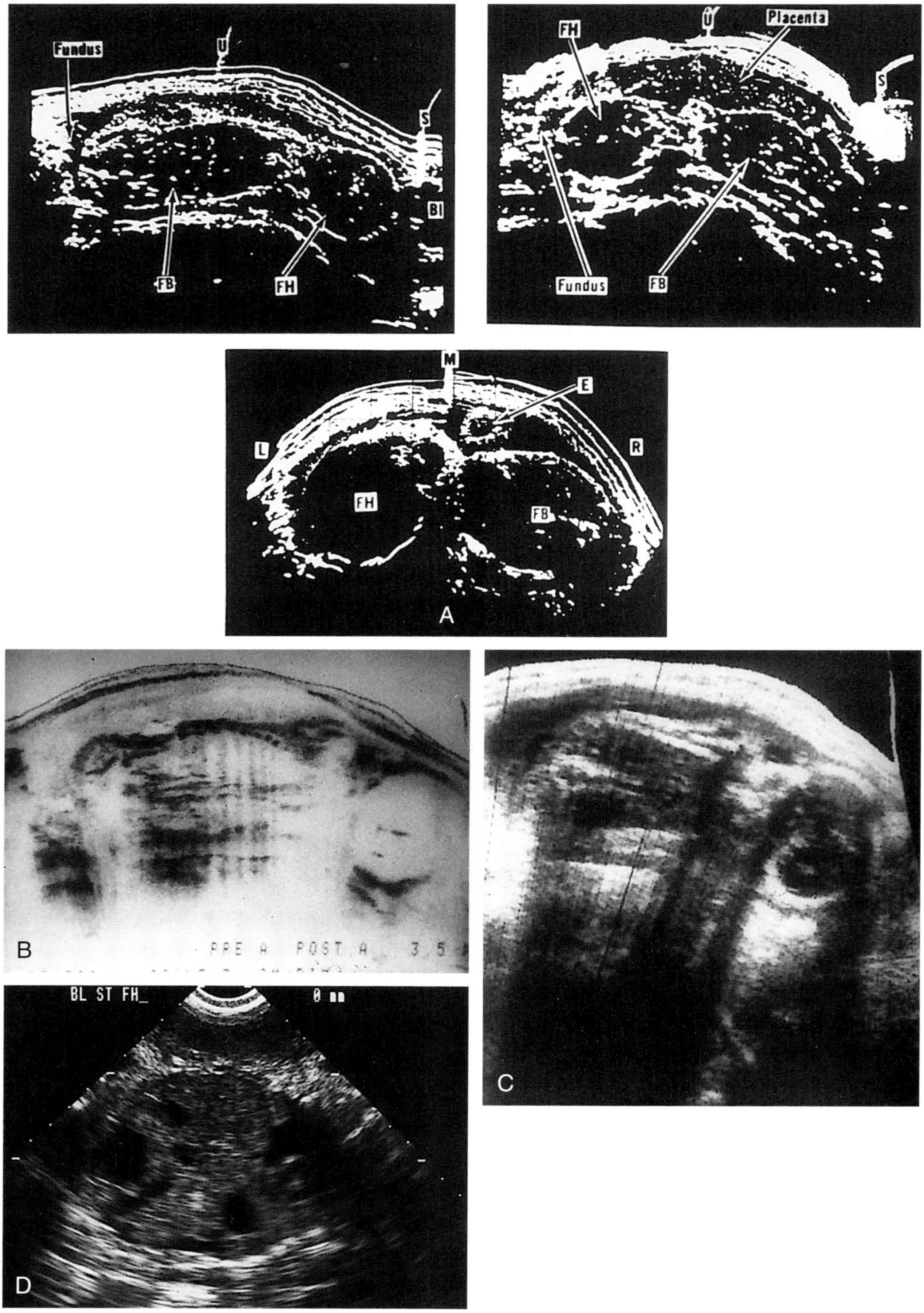

FIGURE 2–4. *See legend on opposite page*

By using a television monitor, many shades of gray corresponding to the amplitude of the echoes could be recorded.[24,25]

Kossoff and Garrett, in Australia, advanced the use and appreciation of gray-scale imaging of the fetus. In the mid-1960s, they were working on imaging techniques that they perfected by the early 1970s.[22,26] As early as 1970, use of the gray scale produced clear cross sections of a fetus showing ribs and vertebrae measuring only 2 mm apart.[27]

Until about 1978, images were produced on a white background. At about this time, multiformat cameras using x-ray film were introduced and probably led to reversing the polarity to that used for x-rays.

Once organ parenchyma could be visualized and detailed, every fetal organ was thoroughly investigated. The second edition of Sanders' textbook is a testament to the leap in fetal ultrasonography that occurred with the adoption of gray scale. In the first edition (1977), two chapters addressed the normal and abnormal fetus in the second and third trimesters; in the second edition (1980), five chapters were needed to describe the added sonographic information (Fig. 2–4).

Gray scale particularly enhanced the depiction of the fetal brain, thus refining the methods used to measure it. The thalamus, cavum septi pellucidi, falx cerebri, and thalamic nuclei were now easy to delineate and use as landmarks for measuring the BPD. Hadlock and Shepard developed nomograms based on measurements taken at sections through these landmarks. As confidence about the level of measurement increased, attention was also given to how the shape, dolicocephalic or brachycephalic, affected the measurement. Hadlock was thus led to introduce the head circumference measurement to estimate fetal age.[28]

After normal values for most organs were established, normal ratios began to be used to determine whether a fetus was growth retarded. Sabbagha developed an approach requiring two examinations of a fetus to establish whether it was small, average, or large for gestational age.[29] Fetal dating improved as the central age tendency of the various fetal parameters was analyzed. Averaging of fetal parameters in the first trimester was first suggested by Bovicelli and colleagues in 1981,[30] but the use of multiple parameters did not become widely applied until Hadlock and associates published their findings in 1983.[31] The availability of computers for analysis of data undoubtedly encouraged this approach.

Once fetal organs could be identified accurately, research was directed at which organs to use to estimate fetal weight. In 1977, Shepard and colleagues from Yale developed a table using the BPD and AC to determine fetal weight. It was revised in 1980[32] and is still in use today. Hadlock and colleagues in 1984[33] found that the femur length and AC measurements were more accurate than head and body dimensions as correlates of weight. After evaluating multiple studies predicting fetal weight from ultrasound measurements, Hadlock concluded in 1984 that accuracy is enhanced by using more than one body component, the choice of these depending on the characteristics of one's population and equipment.[33] Today, both Shepard's and Hadlock's weight tables are regarded as providing acceptable weight estimates.[34]

Gray scale also led to more accurate evaluation of the fetal urinary and gastrointestinal tracts. Sonographic evidence of renal disorders included oligohydramnios, missing kidneys, abnormal kidneys, or a nonfunctioning urinary bladder. Pathology of the esophagus,

FIGURE 2–4.
A, Bistable sonograms demonstrating cephalic, breech, and transverse fetal lie. Top sonograms are sagittal views; bottom is a transverse section of the uterus with the fetus in a transverse lie. FB, fetal body; FH, fetal head; E, extremity; M, midline; R, right; L, left; U = umbilicus; S = symphysis pubis. *B,* Early gray-scale sagittal sonogram produced by an articulated arm scanner. The image was recorded with gray echoes on a white background. Anatomical details such as the aorta, inferior vena cava, and fetal rib shadowing were demonstrable with this technology. *C,* A sonogram of a 33–34 week gestation taken with a Picker articulated arm scanner in 1979. The echoes appear as variations of white against a black background. Note the fetal aorta. *D,* A real-time sector scan of the abdomen of a 34-week fetus. Many fetal structures are identifiable (heart, stomach, diaphragm, urinary bladder, liver), but the entire fetus cannot be seen on one scan as was possible with the articulated arm scanners. (Sonogram courtesy of Judy Schwartz, BS, RDMS, Kings County Hospital Center, Brooklyn, NY.)

stomach, or upper gastrointestinal tract could be suggested by polyhydramnios, absence of stomach echoes, or various other signs, including the double-bubble sign, suggesting duodenal atresia.

Gray scale showed the placenta to be a dynamic, evolving structure not yet fully appreciated, although certainly imaged, with bistable ultrasonography. Grannum in 1979 classified maturation of the placenta into four stages. This classification is still used today to evaluate normal placental development, especially when intrauterine growth retardation is suspected, but its use as an indicator of pulmonic maturity has diminished.[35,36]

All organs and structures visible today, with the exception of vasculature demonstrated with color Doppler, were visible once gray scale was introduced.[37]

Impact of Real-Time Scanning

Automated scanners need to be differentiated from real-time transducers. One of Donald's earliest units had a transducer that traversed the body, scanning at preset intervals. Most of the early units, especially the ones requiring patients to sit in water baths or to be scanned through water-filled bags, had automated transducers. When articulated scanning arms were developed and it was recognized that patients did not have to be surrounded by fluid, manual scanning was adopted. Manual manipulation of the transducer produced better cross sections, even if they were less consistent. Attempts to eliminate the dependency on the skill of the operator and to automate scanning reappeared in the late 1960s. Kossoff and Garrett had completed the automated scanner, the UI Octoson, by 1970. Patients lay on a table, which had a plastic membrane covering the window to the water and transducer frame. The eight transducers arranged in an arc below the water could be manipulated to fire off sequentially, singly, or in other groupings and to move automatically to produce transverse or sagittal images[38] (Fig. 2–5). Doppler was incorporated into the scanning. This unit and a smaller version designed for breast scanning were used in the majority of ultrasound laboratories in Australia, but only a few physicians in the United States adopted them. The size, expense, and expertise required to manipulate them discouraged most potential users. When it was first introduced, automated scanning seemed to solve the problem of variability of images due to the operator's technical skill, but once real-time ultrasonog-

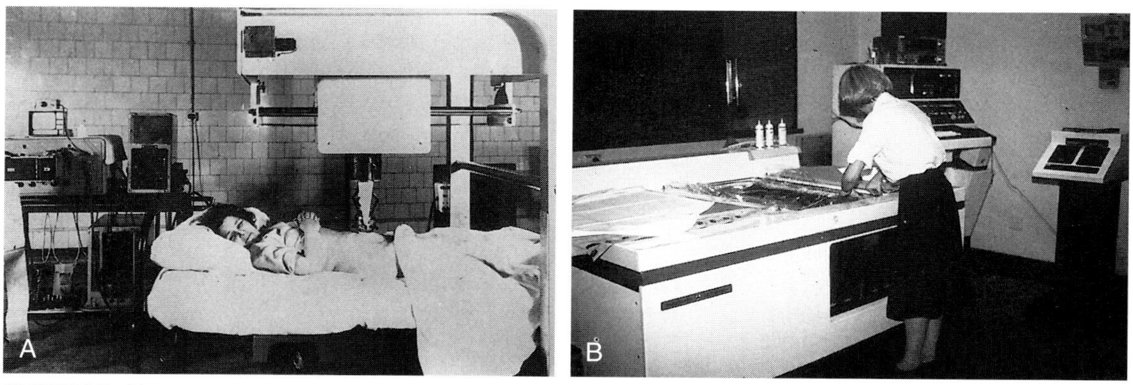

FIGURE 2–5.
A, The automatic mechanical sector scanner designed by Ian Donald and Tom Brown in 1960. The transducer sectored automatically as the transducer carriage moved across the pregnant woman's abdomen. It was hoped that by mechanically maintaining a constant scanning pattern, the variability of results obtained with the manual contact scanner could be overcome. After using it for 4 years, they concluded it was not superior to manually operated scanning. (Reproduced with permission from the American Institute of Ultrasound in Medicine, From Medical Diagnostic Ultrasound: A Retrospective on Its 40th Anniversary. Archives, Eastman Kodak Company, 1988.) *B*, Sonographer changing the membrane on the Octoson. The patient lay with the body part being scanned covered with gel and placed against the membrane. The transducers are housed underneath and controlled electronically from the panel in back of the sonographer. Photograph taken in 1986.

raphy became available, much of the artistic aspect of scanning was no longer relevant.

The advent of real-time made scanning easier and faster while not diminishing its accuracy and resolution. Fred Winsberg was one of the first to use real-time in North America.[39] Real-time equipment initially was cumbersome and produced crude images. When engineers reduced the size of the transducer and improved its resolution, real-time became attractive to obstetricians and gynecologists in private practices as well as to physicians who had previously been intimidated by the technology of the articulated arm scanners. Moving fetal anatomical structures, which had been difficult to record, could now be studied and measured. Fetal long bones could be scrutinized and measured. Queenan and colleagues were the first to measure them and to develop a nomogram based on the femur length. Investigators duplicated each other's findings using increasingly larger samples with increasingly sophisticated statistical analysis until Hadlock's study of 338 women allowed him to conclude that after 23 weeks of gestation, the variability in estimating age from femur length measurements was equivalent to that using the BPD, and thus, either could be used to date a pregnancy.[28,40]

With the introduction of real-time imaging, detailed fetal cardiac anatomy and physiology could be studied. Although M-mode could record wall and septal movement, gray scale could not capture images of a quickly beating fetal heart. By 1985, when Sanders' and James's third edition of their text *The Principles and Practice of Ultrasonography in Obstetrics and Gynecology* was published, they included a separate chapter on fetal cardiac ultrasonography and advised that long-axis and four-chamber views should demonstrate the majority of major cardiac anomalies.[41]

Impact of Transvaginal Scanning

Transvaginal ultrasonography, first introduced in 1966 but not broadly adopted clinically until the mid-1980s,[42] has had its greatest impact on ultrasonography during the first trimester and has prompted the new term, *sonoembryology*. The first trimester is now divided into three stages—4 to 6 weeks, 7 to 8 weeks, and 9 to 11 weeks[43] (Fig. 2–6). The gestational sac can be seen as early as 4 weeks after the last menstrual period; the embryo, adjacent yolk sac, and fetal heartbeats can be seen at 7 weeks. At the eighth week and thereafter, embryonic organs can be studied for normal growth and appearance and such physiologic changes as midgut herniation.[44] The contribution of transvaginal ultrasonography to dating a pregnancy resides in the ability to visualize the milestones in the first trimester. It has facilitated invasive procedures such as chorionic villus sampling, ovum retrieval for in vitro fertilization, follicular and other cyst aspirations, and gamete intrafallopian transfer.

Doppler and Color Doppler in Obstetrics

Doppler was used in the early days of ultrasound to detect fetal heart sounds.[45] Until the late 1970s, the audible Doppler signals and spectral waveform tracings of the signal from the fetal heart, placenta, and maternal vessels represented the extent of the use of Doppler in obstetrics.[46] The addition in the late 1980s of duplex Doppler to transvaginal probes and more recently color Doppler have facilitated the location and evaluation of fetal vessels.[42] Color Doppler is used to study umbilical artery and vein flow and to locate these vessels for blood sampling. It is used to locate and study flow patterns in the carotid and cerebral arteries that might denote brain sparing in cases of intrauterine growth retardation, to investigate anastomosis in twins, and to observe increased blood flow from trophoblastic tissue and angiogenesis related to the corpus luteum cyst in normal and ectopic pregnancies. We are just beginning to appreciate its capabilities.

Relationship Between Advancement in Technology and Clinical Applications of Diagnostic Ultrasonography—A Summary

Inexorable progress since 1959 has produced advances in technology that have

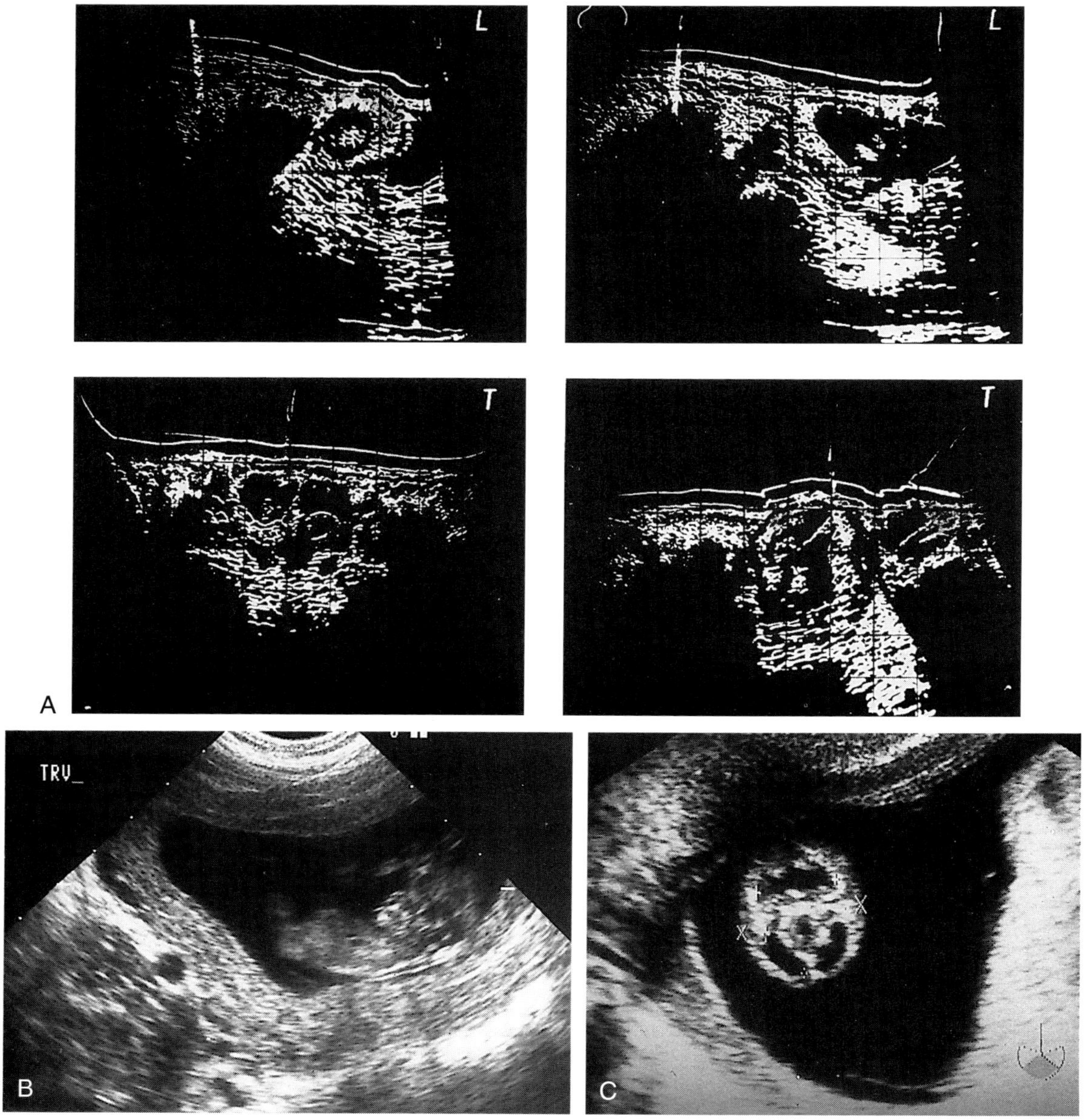

FIGURE 2–6.
A, Four bistable views of a 10-week gestation. The fetus is visible, a clump of echoes with no recognizable structures. *B*, Real-time sector sonogram of a 10-week gestation, allowing identification of the fetal heart, legs, facial bones, brain, and umbilical cord. *C*, Transvaginal scan of a 10-week fetal head. The lateral ventricles, thalami, and hindbrain can be identified. (Sonogram courtesy of Dr. Shraga Rottem, University Hospital of Brooklyn, State University of New York, Health Science Center at Brooklyn, NY.)

exposed more detailed anatomy as well as fetal physiology. Technology has obviously propelled these discoveries in fetal ultrasonography. Much progress has been made in looking at a fetus. Gray-scale imaging introduced in 1972 revealed the tissue makeup of organs. Real-time permitted easy measurement of the crown-rump length and femur length and identification of all fetal anatomy. Transvaginal ultrasonography has made it possible to observe more embryological milestones than seen before, without using invasive procedures. Doppler has added information on the physiology of fetal organs and facilitated evaluation of fetal well-being through analysis of blood flow in the umbilical vessels, carotid arteries, and other vasculature. Age-related charts describing the changes in flow patterns during pregnancy abound.

We have probably exhausted methods of reliably establishing fetal age based on size of organs or structures.[47] Although BPD nomograms based on bistable images were more reliable than estimates based on last menstrual period and physical examinations, those developed after the introduction of gray scale were more consistent. It was obvious from the early use of ultrasound that the measurements from one organ would not provide as accurate dating as that based on several measurements. Estimates of fetal weight were originally based only on BPDs, but the abdominal circumference was soon added to the formula to improve its accuracy.[47,48]

In contrast to the minimal improvements in the accuracy of fetal dating produced by innovations in ultrasound technology, enhanced visualization of fetal organs has resulted in improved assessment of fetal anomalies. Gray scale aided our analysis of tissue characteristics of the parenchyma of organs. Bistable imaging could display large morphological changes in size and even internal structure such as in multicystic kidneys, but gray scale gave us the ability to identify polycystic kidneys in utero. Its introduction particularly enhanced imaging of the fetal brain.

The use of real-time improved organ analysis by making it faster and easier to chase a floating embryo and later a fetus. It became possible to observe and study patterns of movement. The fetal heart could be charted. Real-time made it safer to perform invasive procedures such as chorionic villus sampling, intrauterine transfusions, and fetal surgery. Intrauterine surgery such as repair of diaphragmatic hernias, decompression of renal obstruction, and the placement of shunts for hydrocephalus has been facilitated by ultrasonography's continuous imaging capabilities.

Three-Dimensional and Contrast Ultrasonography

Three-dimensional reconstruction of obstetrical images is in the forefront of new developments in diagnostic ultrasonography. Its application is still being investigated, but early research suggests that it will help surgeons pinpoint their area of concern by allowing viewing of the whole fetus.[49]

Contrast agents such as Echovist have been used to image the uterus and fallopian tubes.[50] Applications to obstetrical scanning have not yet been reported, although contrast has been found to increase the sensitivity of color Doppler, which could, if proven safe, be applied to tracing vasculature in a fetus.[49,51]

Safety Considerations

As mentioned earlier, the safety of diagnostic ultrasonography has never been taken for granted. Before proceeding with the application of ultrasound on pregnant women, Donald, Hellman, and Kossoff researched ultrasonography's effect on tissue and chromosomes. Hellman conducted an extensive epidemiological study of 1114 women who had been examined with ultrasound during their pregnancy.[12,52] Results have always shown diagnostic ultrasound to be safe at the power levels used in normal obstetrical examinations, including Doppler and color Doppler. Epidemiological studies have demonstrated no long-term deleterious effects of in utero exposure to diagnostic ultrasound.[53]

Ultrasonography's reputation as a safe and easy-to-use modality has resulted in routine scanning of most pregnant women and even its abuse, as in the practice of photographic studios offering videotapes and sonograms of fetuses without concomitant diagnostic study. The Consensus Development Conference was convened in 1984 to bring together experts who could summarize the safety, indications, and ethical issues relevant to its use. One of the conclusions of the conference proceedings was, "With our current understanding of ultrasonically induced biological effects, it is scientifically impossible to support statements such as 'diagnostic ultrasound is not harmful to the conceptus,'"[54] but it is generally accepted that its call for caution has been disregarded. Diagnostic ultrasonography is considered by most women to be an integral part of obstetrical care, and many expect to receive copies of sonograms or videotapes for their future baby's album. However, government pressure to reduce health care expenditures, along with the rise in managed care plans, could change this practice, especially if clinical practice guidelines respond to the findings in such large-scale studies as that by Ewigman & colleagues. This study of 15,151 low-risk pregnant women, which reported that "screening ultrasound did not improve perinatal outcome,"[55] has been criticized by the AIUM as providing information on a select group of women who are not the ones to be the most affected by changes in health care policy.[55a]

Sonographers' Involvement in Development of Diagnostic Ultrasonography

In most instances, one can safely say that behind or next to every physician/researcher was a dedicated sonographer. Many of these sonographers' names are not known or acknowledged in articles reporting new findings, but their contributions should be noticed. Physicians have always voiced their appreciation for the importance of technical skill in using diagnostic ultrasonography, especially before real-time; however, seldom did they mention the names of their sonographers. Kobayashi stated in his 1974 textbook, "The role of the ultrasound technologist cannot be overemphasized in the practice of diagnostic ultrasound."[56] He was one of the first physicians to credit his sonographer, in this case, Ellen Cromb Campos, with expertise in producing and recognizing the images. In those early years, sonographers scanning alongside physicians were trying to identify the origins of the spikes and dots on the screen. Marveen Craig described a typical Friday at the University of Colorado with Drs. Holmes, Gottesfeld, Thompson, and E. Stewart Taylor: "We'd spread dozens of Polaroids out on the floor and the 'docs' would sprawl beside us trying to make sense of what we had found and thought we were seeing."* Also in the mid-1960s, Joan Baker was invited to come from England to the Stanford Medical Center to share her knowledge of ultrasound, but obstetrical scanning proved limited because the B-mode ultrasound unit required placing a water-filled tank on the pregnant patient's abdomen, resulting in vena cava compression syndrome.† Another pioneer was Shirley Staiano, who worked with Dr. L.I. von Micsky in New York City to explore the potential of the newly developed contact scanner and to develop new equipment. In the 1970s, Jean Lea scanned alongside Dr. Charles Hohler at Strong Memorial Hospital in Rochester, New York, to investigate patterns of fetal breathing[57] (Table 2–1).

By the early 1980s, sonographers were being named as coauthors and principal investigators in significant fetal research reports. Terry DuBose has been publishing regularly to report his research findings on the use of cranial volume to improve pregnancy dating and the incorporation of computers to report and analyze data derived from fetal sonographic studies.[58,59] Working with Drs. John Hobbins, Richard Berkowitz, Frank Chervenak, and Peter Grannum, Kara Mayden and Marge Tortora used sonography to investigate the umbilical vein diameter in Rh isoim-

*Craig M: Written communication, August 12, 1993.
†Baker J: Personal communication, September 1993.

TABLE 2–1. **PIONEERS IN FETAL ULTRASONOGRAPHY, 1950s–1960s**

PHYSICIANS	SONOGRAPHERS	MAJOR CONTRIBUTIONS
I. Donald (Glasgow)		Regarded as the father of fetal ultrasonography. Identified BPD using A-mode and developed first BPD nomogram. Discovered full-bladder technique.
K. Gottesfeld H. Thompson J. Holmes (Denver)	Marveen Craig	Sonographic characterization of normal and abnormal placenta (hydatidiform mole) and multiple gestations. Developed second- and third-trimester growth charts.
G. Kossoff D. E. Robinson W. J. Garrett (Australia)	Kaye Griffith	Introduced gray-scale imaging of fetus. Invented UI Octoson.
L. I. von Micsky (New York)	Shirley Staiano	Developed scanner with vacuum chamber to minimize weight of water on pregnant abdomen. Developed transvesical and transvaginal transducers.
S. Campbell (England)		Combined B-mode with A-mode to improve accuracy of BPD. Developed weight prediction formula based on BPD and AC.
L. Hellman M. Kobayashi (Brooklyn, New York)	Ellen Cromb Campos Lewis Fillisti	Developed gestation sac nomogram and growth chart nomogram and growth chart for pregnant uterus. Wrote first atlas of obstetrical ultrasonography.

BPD, biparietal diameter; AC, abdominal circumference.

munization, the usefulness of measuring the fetal orbital distances to date the pregnancy and evaluate whether a fetus suffered from hypotelorism or hypertelorism, the role of ultrasonography in evaluating pregnancies with elevated alpha-fetoprotein concentrations, and other obstetrical concerns.[60-62] One of Wayne Persutte's earliest contributions was the first sonographic identification of a fetal patent urachus.[63] Julia Drose participated in the development of a fetal lateral ventricular ratio nomogram in the second trimester and a study of ultrasonographic diagnosis of fetal infection.[64,65] Dale Cyr began conducting research as a student, when he was the first to report on the appearance of the intrahepatic vasculature and fetal pancreas. Since then, his contributions have included reports on fetal echocardiography and the demonstration of normal embryological processes such as midgut herniation.[66-69] More recently, Mark Cartier has been participating and reporting on research of Doppler applications in obstetrics. Many other sonographers have either collaborated with others or influenced others to become involved in developing the field of fetal ultrasonography. Among these individuals, we need to acknowledge several dedicated educators including Kathy McDiarmid, Marie DeLange, Sandra Hagen-Ansert, Andrea Skelly, and Diane Kawamura.

As sonographers obtain advanced degrees that equip them to conduct research, they will inevitably contribute more independent research findings to the field of sonography.

Unfortunately, the public has yet to recognize the important role of sonographers in clinical practice and in the growth of the profession. In a review I conducted of news reports and articles in magazines, I found little attention given to the sonographer. The physician was usually credited with both scanning and interpreting the sonograms. The growth of the field of sonography, along with the increasing involvement of sonographers in scholastic activities, should eventually change this situation.

Ethical Issues Associated with the Advancement of Diagnostic Ultrasonography

As sonography has become more incisive in its investigation of a fetus while at the same time becoming easier to use, ethical concerns have arisen. Sonography in obstetrical practice involves ethical issues when its unwarranted use wastes health care resources, but more complex dilemmas occur when sonography reveals anomalies that compel prospective parents to make decisions about treatment or abortion. The use of sonography to abet abortions has been controversial, and the reverse practice of using the image of a fetus to discourage abortion has also been questioned. As in many ethical dilemmas, there are no absolute answers, but sonographers and sonologists are becoming more sensitive to the ethical ramifications of their detailed observation of the human fetus.

REFERENCES

1. Jeanty P: Sonographic depiction of normal fetal anatomy. In: Fleischer A, Romero R, Manning F, et al, eds: The Principles and Practice of Ultrasonography in Obtetrics and Gynecology, 4th ed. Appleton & Lange, Norwalk, CT, 1991, pp 77–92.
2. Donald I: Sonar as a method of studying prenatal development. J Pediatr 1969;75:326–333.
3. Donald I, MacVicar J, Brown TG: Investigation of abdominal masses by pulsed ultrasound. Lancet 1958; 1:1188–1195.
4. Campbell S: The obstetric ultrasound examination. In: Chervenak FA, Isaacson GC, Campbell S, eds: Ultrasound in Obstetrics and Gynecology. Little, Brown & Co, Boston, 1993, p 1.
5. Weber DO: Practice Patterns in Diagnostic Ultrasound Market Trends and Clinical Practice in the U.S. Diagnostic Imaging Technology Report. Vol 2. San Francisco, Miller Freeman, Inc. 1993, p 2(1).
6. Eik-Nes SH. An overview of routine versus selective use of ultrasound. In: Chervenak FA, Isaacson GC, Campbell S, eds: Ultrasound in Obstetrics and Gynecology. Little, Brown & Co, Boston, 1993, p 1.
7. Kuo HC, Chang FM, Wu CH, et al: The primary application of three-dimensional ultrasonography in obstetrics. Am J Obstet Gynecol 1992;166(3): 880–886.
8. Leopold GR: Fetuses aren't small children. Clin Imaging 1990;14:271–279.
9. Harman CR: Ultrasound in the management of the alloimmunized pregnancy. In: Fleischer AC, Romero R, Manning FA, et al, eds: The Principles and Practice of Ultrasonography in Obstetrics and Gynecology, 4th ed. Appleton & Lange, Norwalk, CT, 1991, p 408.
10. Touraine JL: In utero transplantation of fetal liver stem cells in humans. Blood Cells 1991;17:379–387.
11. Hellman LM: Ultrasound in historical perspective. In: Sanders RC, James AE Jr, eds: Ultrasonography in Obstetrics and Gynecology. Appleton-Century-Crofts, New York, 1977.
12. Wells PNT: Physical Principle of Ultrasonic Diagnosis. Academic Press, London, 1969.
13. Kossof G, Garrett WJ, Robinson DE: An ultrasonic echoscope for visualizing the pregnant uterus. In: Kelly E, ed: Ultrasonic Energy. University of Illinois Press, Urbana, IL, 1965.
14. Hill CR: History—now and then. In: Cosgrove D, Hylton M, Dewberry K, eds: Abdominal and General Ultrasound. Churchill Livingstone, New York, 1993.
15. Medical Diagnostic Ultrasound: A Retrospective on its 40th Anniversary. Archives, Eastman Kodak Company, 1988.
16. Oakley A: The history of ultrasonography in obstetrics. Birth 1986;13:8–13.
17. Holmes JH: Diagnostic ultrasound during the early years of A.I.U.M. J Clin Ultrasound 1980;8:299–308.
18. Willocks J, Donald I, Duggan TC, et al: Foetal cephalometry by ultrasound. Obstet Gynaecol 1964; 71:11–20.
19. Campbell S: An improved method of fetal cephalometry by ultrasound. J Obstet Gynaecol Br Commonw 1968;75:568–576.
20. Campbell S: The accuracy of ultrasonic measurement of the fetal biparietal diameter during the Second Trimester. In: Rand E, ed: Recent Advances in Diagnostic Ultrasound. Charles C Thomas, Springfield, IL, 1971.
21. Hellman IM, Kobayashi M, Fillisti L, et al: Growth and development of the human fetus prior to the twentieth week of gestation. Am J Obstet Gynecol 1969;103:789–798.
22. Garrett WJ: Study of the fetus and placenta by grey scale echography. In: Donald I, Levi S, eds: Present and Future of Diagnostic Ultrasound. John Wiley & Sons, New York, 1976.
23. Campbell S, Wilkin D: Ultrasonic measurement of fetal abdomen circumference in the estimation of fetal weight. Br J Obstet Gynaecol 1975;82:689–697.
24. Kossoff G: Technical procedures and imaging. In: Donald I, Levi S, eds: Present and Future of Diag nostic Ultrasound. John Wiley & Sons, New York, 1976.
25. Ziskin MC: Basic physics of ultrasound. In: Sanders

RC, James AE Jr, eds: Ultrasonography in Obstetrics and Gynecology. Appleton-Century-Crofts, New York, 1980.
26. Garrett W, Kossoff G: Gray scale examination of the fetus. In: Sanders R, James AE, eds: Ultrasonography in Obstetrics and Gynecology. Appleton-Century-Crofts, New York, 1977, pp 173–179.
27. Kossoff G, Garrett WJ, Radovanovich G: Grey scale echography in obstetrics and gynaecology. Australas Radiol 1974; XVIII (1):62–111.
28. Hadlock FP: Evaluation of fetal dating studies. In: Deter RL, Harrist RB, Birnholz JC, et al, eds: Quantitative Obstetrical Ultrasonography. John Wiley & Sons, New York, 1986.
29. Sabbagha RE, Barton BA, Barton FB, et al: Sonar biparietal diameter, II. Predictive of three fetal growth patterns leading to a closer assessment of gestational age and neonatal weight. Am J Obstet Gynecol 1976;126:485.
30. Bovicelli L, Orsins LF, Rizzo N, et al: Estimation of gestational age during the first trimester by real-time measurement of the fetal crown-rump length and biparietal diameter. J Clin Ultrasound 1981; 9:71–75.
31. Hadlock FP, Deter RL, Harrist RB, et al: Computer-assisted analysis of fetal age in the third trimester using multiple growth parameters. J Clin Ultrasound 1983;11:313–316.
32. Shepard MJ, Richards V, Berkowitz R, et al: An evaluation of two equations for predicting fetal weight by ultrasound. Am J Obstet Gynecol 1982;142:47–54.
33. Hadlock FP: Evaluation of fetal weight estimation procedures. In: Deter RL, Harrist RB, Birnholz JC, Hadlock FP, eds. Quantitative Obstetrical Ultrasonography. John Wiley & Sons, New York, 1986.
34. Kurtz AB, Goldberg BB: Obstetrical Measurements in Ultrasound—A Reference Manual. Year Book Medical Publishers, Chicago, 1988, p 151.
35. Manning FA, Harrison MR, Rodeck C: Fetal surgery: Report of the international fetal surgery registry 1985. In: Berkowitz RL, ed: Contemporary Issues in Obstetrics and Gynecology. Churchill Livingstone, New York, 1988.
36. Grannum PA: Development of the placenta. In: Chervenak F, Isaacson G, Campbell S, eds: Ultrasound in Obstetrics and Gynecology, vol 1. Little, Brown & Co, Boston, 1993, pp 321–325.
37. Beach KW: A quarter century of ultrasound technology. Ultrasound Med Biol 1992;18(4):377–388.
38. Garrett WJ: Fetal organ imaging. In: Sabbagha RE, ed: Diagnostic Ultrasound Applied to Obstetrics and Gynecology. Harper & Row, Hagerstown, MD, 1980.
39. Goldberg B, Gramiak R, Freimanis A: Early history of diagnostic ultrasound: The role of American radiologists. AJR 1993;160:189–194.
40. Hadlock RP, Deter RL, Harrist RB, et al: Fetal biparietal diameter: A critical re-evaluation of the relation to menstrual age by means of real-time ultrasound. J Ultrasound Med 1982;1:97–104.
41. Allen LD: Fetal cardiac ultrasound. In: Sanders RC, James AE, eds: The Principles and Practice of Ultrasonography in Obstetrics and Gynecology, 3rd ed. Appleton-Century Crofts, Norwalk, CT, 1985, pp 211–217.
42. Rottem S: Transvaginal ultrasonography. In: Chervanek F, Isaacson G, Campbell S, eds: Ultrasound in Obstetrics and Gynecology, vol 1. Little, Brown & Co, Boston, 1993, pp 133–140.
43. Fleischer AC, Pennell RG, Sacks GA, et al: Pregnancy emphasizing transvaginal scanning. In: Fleischer AC, Romero R, Manning F, et al, eds: The Principle and Practice of Ultrasonography in Obstetrics and Gynecology, 4th ed. Appleton & Lange, Norwalk, CT, 1991, pp 39–55.
44. Timor-Tritsch IE, Blumenfeld Z, Rottem S: Sonoembryology. In: Timor-Tritsch IE, Rottem S, eds. Transvaginal Sonography. Elsevier, New York, 1991.
45. Donald I: Ultrasonic investigations in obstetrics and gynaecology. In: Wells PNT, ed: Ultrasonics in Clinical Diagnosis. Longman Group, London, 1972, pp 74–93.
46. Niebyl JR: Doppler monitoring techniques in pregnancy. In: Sanders RC, James AE, eds. The Principles and Practice of Ultrasonography in Obstetrics and Gynecology, 3rd ed. Appleton-Century-Crofts, Norwalk, CT, 1985.
47. Hadlock FP. Gestational age determination: Third trimester. In: Chervenak FA, Isaacson GC, Campbell S, eds: Ultrasound in Obstetrics and Gynecology, vol I. Little, Brown & Co, Boston, 1993.
48. Ott WJ: Accurate gestational dating. Obstet Gynecol 1985;66:311.
49. Goldberg B, Liu JB: Future trends. In: Goldberg B, ed. Textbook of Abdominal Ultrasound. Williams & Wilkins, Baltimore, 1993, p 504.
50. Schlief R, Ulrich D: Hysterosalpingo-contrast sonography of the uterus and fallopian tubes: Results of a clinical trial of a new contrast medium in 120 patients. Radiology 1991;178:213–215.
51. Goldberg BB, Ji-Bin L, Burns PN, et al: Galactose-based intravenous sonographic contrast agent: Experimental studies. J Ultrasound Med 1993;12: 463–470.
52. Hill CR: Biological effects of ultrasound. In: Wells PNT, ed. Ultrasonics in Clinical Diagnosis. Churchill Livingstone, New York, 1972.
53. Lyons EA, Dyke C, Toms M, et al: In utero exposure to diagnostic ultrasound: A 6-year follow-up. Radiology 1988;166:687–690.
54. Diagnostic Ultrasound in Pregnancy. National Institutes of Health, Washington, DC, 1984, p 667.
55. Ewigman BG, Crane JP, Frigoletto FD, et al: Effect of prenatal ultrasound screening on perinatal outcome. N Engl J Med 1993;329:821–827.
55a. AIUM Bioeffects Committee: Bioeffects Committee Reviews RADIUS Study. AIUM Reporter 1994;10:2. Issued by American Institute of Ultrasound in Medicine, Laurel, MD.
56. Kobayashi M: Illustrated Manual of Ultrasonography in Obstetrics and Gynecology. Igaku Shoin, Tokyo, 1974.
57. Hohler CW, Fox HE, Inglis J, et al: 24-Hour continuous observation of human fetal breathing using real time B-scan. In: White DN, ed. Ultrasound in Medicine, vol 5. Plenum, New York, 1979.
58. DuBose RJ: Basic baby—a computer algorithm for analysis of multiple fetal parameters. J Ultrasound Med 1988; 7S:206.
59. DuBose RJ: Coronal BPD revisited. J Ultrasound Med 1992;11:84.
60. Mayden KL: The umbilical vein diameter in Rh isoimmunization. Med Ultrasound 1980;4:119–125.
61. Mayden KL, Tortora M, Berkowitz RL, et al: Orbital diameters: A new parameter for prenatal diagnosis and dating. Am J Obstet Gynecol 1982;144:228.
62. Hobbins JC, Venus I, Tortora M, et al: Stage II ultrasound examination for the diagnosis of fetal abnormalities with an elevated amniotic fluid alpha-fetoprotein concentration. Am J Obstet Gynecol 1982; 142:1026.

63. Persutte WH, Lenke RR, Kropp K, et al: Antenatal diagnosis of fetal patent urachus. J Ultrasound Med 1988;7(7):399–403.
64. Pretorius DH, Drose JA, Manco-Johnson ML: Fetal lateral ventricular ratio determination during the second trimester. J Ultrasound Med 1986;5:121–124.
65. Drose JA, Dennis MA, Thickman D: Ultrasound diagnosis of in utero infection: A review of 19 cases. Radiology 1991;178:369–374.
66. Cyr DR: Ultrasonic visualization of the fetal pancreas and hepatic venous circulation. Med Ultrasound 1983;7:27–31.
67. Cyr DR, Guntheroth WG, Mack LA, et al: A systematic approach to 2D/real-time fetal echocardiography. J Ultrasound Med 1986;5:343–350.
68. Cyr DR, Mack LA, Schoenecker SA, et al: Bowel migration in the normal fetus: Ultrasound detection. Radiology 1986;l6l:119–121.
69. Guntheroth WG, Cyr DR, Winter T, et al: Fetal Doppler of pulmonary atresia. J Ultrasound Med 1993;5:281–284.

CHAPTER 3

BIOLOGICAL EFFECTS AND SAFETY

Adrian Anthony

Since 1966, diagnostic ultrasound as a clinical tool has had a profound effect on the practice of obstetrics. It has also expanded our knowledge of human embryonic and fetal development. Because the fetus is generally inaccessible to most clinical investigations, ultrasonography has been a most useful modality.[1]

Although the general belief today is that ultrasound produces no identifiable hazard, many investigators believe that the studies that have been carried out are not yet conclusive. Many of these researchers recall medicine's past experience with ionizing radiation. After radioactive sources were first discovered in the 1880s, they were soon used widely and freely both medically and commercially. It was not until much later that the nature and degree of the hazard—namely, genetic and carcinogenic effects—were discovered.[2,3] In 1934, limits regulating radiation exposure were finally created.[4] The example set by radiation hazard is not the only reason for judicious use of ultrasound. Opponents of the routine use of ultrasound also cite the cases of fetuses exposed to diethylstilbestrol, a steroidal compound that causes birth defects.[1]

In the 1970s, fear and ignorance propagated a rumor that insonating the fertilized eggs of certain chickens could cause them to grow to a height of 4 ft.[5] Although no confirmed identifiable hazards have been found in the routine use of diagnostic ultrasound, it is a fact that every type of energy has the potential of producing some biological effects.[5] Added to this is the fear that some effects may not be detectable because they are too subtle, too delayed, of an incidence that is too low, or almost the same as the natural occurrence rate.[6] If this were in fact true, we could be endangering the millions of women who undergo ultrasound examinations and the half million who have more than one such examination, not to mention their fetuses.[7]

Any approach to investigating the possible bioeffects of ultrasound must consider not only structural effects but also the possibility that the function and behavior of cells and whole organisms such as a human fetus can be modified. Another factor to consider is whether the damage imposed might be of a teratogenic or mutagenic nature.[5] Thus, most of the concern about adverse effects of ultrasound in humans has centered on the possibility that in utero exposure to ultrasound may harm a fetus.

In approaching the question of possible hazards in the use of diagnostic medical ultrasound, the basic questions that we must ask are as follows:

1. What physical effects can be properly observed and measured?
2. What doses of energy should be used and under what experimental conditions can they be produced?
3. What harm can be inflicted and by what mechanism?
4. Can the function of a cell or whole organism be modified?
5. Is there any genetic damage, and if so, is it manifested in teratogenic or mutagenic forms?

Those of us in clinical practice (e.g., physicians, nurses, sonographers, midwives) carry the responsibility of satisfying both ourselves and our patients that the use of diagnostic medical ultrasound is safe. Current research has not yet been able to conduct well-designed, controlled, and long-term prospective epidemiological studies; therefore, it has been necessary to resort to the application of in vitro and in vivo studies (using animals) in the laboratory.[8]

Basic Properties of Ultrasound

The fear of ultrasound exposure has grown from the fear of the unknown to the fear of effects of any radiation such as x-rays. Although sound and x-rays (electromagnetic radiation) are very different energy sources, they are viewed by laypersons as being similar because they appear to be used for similar reasons. However, they are in fact very different.

X-rays are a type of ionizing radiation. Ionizing radiation occurs when extremely energetic particles or electromagnetic waves travel at great velocities and interact in cells by depositing very small amounts of energy through energy exchanges with orbital electrons. Ultrasound, however, is a type of nonionizing radiation and consists of mechanical vibrations that do not deposit energy at the atomic level but at levels of greater complexity such as the cellular or macromolecular.

One of the first 20th century contributors to the study of ultrasound was the French physicist Paul Langevin, who, during World War I, was commissioned to explore the possibility of using high-frequency sound in underwater detection of German submarines. From the first uses of ultrasound by Langevin in Toulon, France, the lethal effects of ultrasound were documented. His experiments proved that sonar was capable of killing small aquatic species.[9]

Since Langevin's time, other in vivo experiments have been performed on animals, producing lethal effects. This information may or may not be relevant to humans, however, owing to the fact that the studies performed on animals generally deal with an intensity level much greater than that used in diagnostic ultrasound. Also, such data may not extrapolate to humans because of the differing physiologies. Furthermore, it is unethical to perform any clinical trials on human beings when any harm is expected.

To understand the possible hazards of diagnostic ultrasound, one must have an appreciation of some of the basic principles of ultrasound.

THE NATURE OF ULTRASOUND

The term *acoustic variables* is used to denote the category of reversible effects that ultrasound has on human tissue. As ultrasound waves travel through the soft tissue medium, changes in density, temperature, particle displacement, and pressure occur. Propagation of the ultrasonic mechanical force is caused by particle displacement, which transmits the force in a straight line and parallel to the axis of energy production. This straight-line phenomenon was explained by Huygens and is thus called Huygens' principle.[10] Thus, the ultrasound beam used in diagnostic medicine is propagated longitudinally.

When ultrasound moves through a medium, the particles of the medium are moved back and forth about a point of equilibrium or about the original resting point of that particle. It should be noted that the motion of the particle is not reflective of the speed of propagation of the mechanical force. The particle displacement is on the order of a few nanometers and is defined as the particle velocity, whereas the actual mechanical force velocity is defined as the phase velocity (Fig. 3–1).[11]

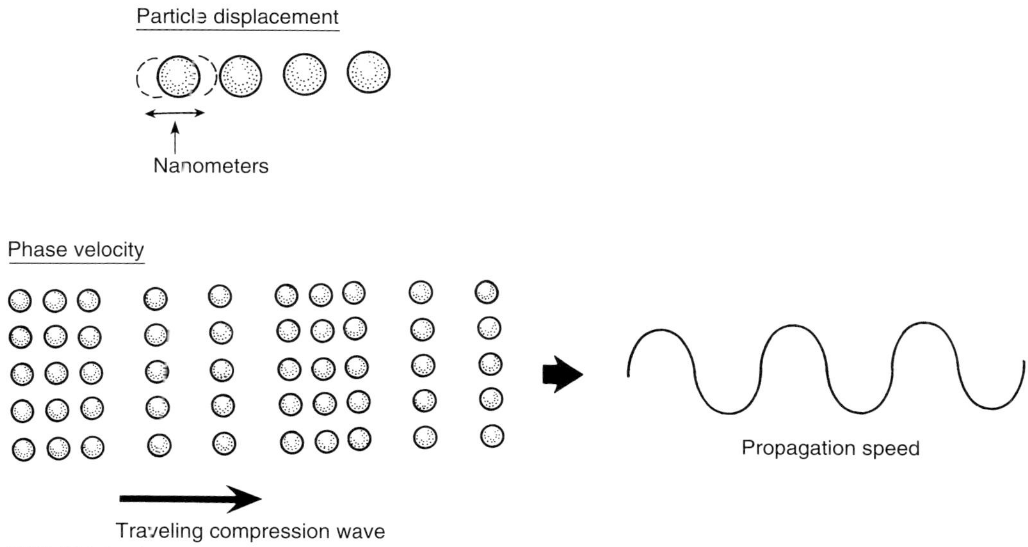

FIGURE 3–1.
Wave propagation. A graphic representation of compression wave propagation through a medium. The particles or molecules oscillate about the rest position. The wave travels as each particle bumps the adjacent particle, and the energy is transferred as a wave front. The sine wave represents the periodicity of the propagation.

The study of ultrasound bioeffects, although seated in the study of the normally reversible effects of temperature, pressure, density, and particle motion, is really focused on irreversible effects that might emerge. Reversible effects produce irreversible effects at high intensity levels. In particular, the most studied biological effects are those caused by changes in temperature and pressure.

Ultrasonic Beam Properties

The physical nature of the ultrasound pulse and beam must be appreciated in order to have some sense of the production of biological effects. The ultrasound beam is a longitudinal propagating mechanical phenomenon. Having this longitudinal characteristic means that it moves generally in a straight line unless it is reflected off an interface or spreads out via a scattering medium or a nonspecular reflector. The ultrasound beam is a force that fluctuates in sine wave cycles that are controlled by the frequency of the beam. Thus, a 1-MHz ultrasound beam causes the particles in the medium through which it travels to fluctuate about their points of equilibrium at one million times per second.

UNFOCUSED BEAM

Many of the schematics that demonstrate the behavior of ultrasound concentrate on the unfocused ultrasound beam because its behavior is more predictable and less variable than the focused beam. The focused beam can vary greatly depending on its method of focus. The unfocused beam is usually presented as a cylindrical beam generated from a circular piezoelectrical crystal. This cylindrical beam contains an area close to the crystal face, called the *near field* or the *Fresnel zone.* This beam diverges at some point distal from the crystal face. This area is called the *far field* or the *Fraunhofer zone*. The two zones are separated by a point called the *last intensity maximum*. Equations can predict the length of the near field. The relationships between the near field, the crystal diameter, the frequency, and the wavelength are as follows:

$$\text{Near-zone length (mm)} = \frac{[\text{transducer diameter (mm)}]^2}{4 \times \text{wavelength (mm)}}$$

$$\text{Near-zone length (mm)} = \frac{[\text{transducer diameter (mm)}]^2 \times \text{frequency (MHz)}}{6}$$

Note that the second equation solves for soft tissue.[12]

FOCUSED BEAM

All transducers used in diagnostic medical ultrasound use focused ultrasound beams. This focusing is desirable because it improves axial and lateral resolution. In general, a strongly focused beam has a shorter focal length and a narrower beam width at the focal point.[11] Ultrasound beams can be focused by a focusing mirror or by internal or external focus or can be focused dynamically as in crystal arrays (phased array).

Generation of Ultrasound

Ultrasound is generated by electrical stimulation of a crystal or ceramic that has piezoelectrical properties. This material, when shocked by an electrical potential, can deform and recover at a rate that is consistent with the high frequencies of ultrasound. Note that the thickness of the ceramic material used has an inherent frequency of resonation, and the alternating current that is used to stimulate the crystal is usually set to match that inherent frequency. The materials in use today are manufactured and are usually lead zirconate titanate or some derivative of this substance. Quartz and Rochelle salts are naturally occurring materials that also have piezoelectrical qualities, but they are not as effective for this purpose as the manufactured materials.

Measurement of Ultrasound

Ultrasound is a mechanical force that can be measured using various techniques. In general, the measurements are of physical radiation force or temperature increase (also called the thermal mechanism). The thermal mechanism measures the effect of heating, which is due to absorption of ultrasound by the medium that is being transversed. Both of these parameters are dependent on beam intensity and power, which are widely variable because of the complexity of the ultrasound beam itself.

Power, which also relates to the strength of the sound wave, is the rate at which work is performed or energy transferred. Power is determined by the sound source and not the medium. Power (watts) is proportional to the amplitude of the wave squared.

Intensity can be considered as a measure of the flow rate of energy through 1 cm^2 of material positioned at right angles to the beam. In an ultrasound beam, the more intense the beam, the greater the length of vibration of particles in the medium and the greater the pressure variation found at each point in the medium as the wave passes through it.

The intensity of the ultrasound beam can be measured in relationship to its peak intensity in space or the average intensity in space. Thus, the spatial peak intensity is a measurement of ultrasound in one point in space, and the spatial average intensity is the measurement of the ultrasound across a prescribed area. The beam duration must also be taken into consideration. Thus, the temporal peak intensity is the measurement of the ultrasound beam in one moment in time, and the temporal average intensity is the measurement of the ultrasound beam across a prescribed time period or the whole length of time that the medium is being insonated.

By combining spatial and temporal intensities, various intensities can be quantified to denote diverse exposure conditions. Thus, many intensity measurements have been developed for ultrasound. These measurements or intensities [I] have been labeled as follows: SPTP[I], spatial peak, temporal peak intensity; SPTA[I], spatial peak temporal average; SATP[I], spatial average, temporal peak intensity; and SATA[I], spatial average, temporal average intensity. The intensities most studied in diagnostic ultrasound are SPTA and SATA. SPTA[I] is the quantity most referred to when discussing data on biological effects, and SATA intensity (the lowest numerically) is the quantity most frequently quoted by manufacturers.

In pulsed systems, the parameter pulsed average has to be taken into account, thus creating two new quantities—SAPA[I], spatial average-pulse average; and SPPA[I], spatial peak-pulse average. SPPA[I] tends to be higher in imaging than in Doppler instruments, whereas SPTA[I] is generally higher in Doppler modes. The order of intensities in general from highest to lowest is as follows: (1) SPTP, (2) SPPA, (3) SPTA, (4) SATP, (5) SAPA, and (6) SATA. The Food and Drug Administration (FDA) has referred to both SPPA and SPTA quantities in regulating ultrasound devices.

DOSIMETRIC QUANTITIES

Dosimetry in ultrasound is the study of the effect of ultrasound at particular intensities. As described earlier, these intensities must be designated at either an SATA, SATP, SPPA, SAPA, SPTA, or SPTP intensity.

Improvements in ultrasound technology have encountered a common and consistent obstacle, and that is the limitation in power output that is allowable for imaging systems. It is known by manufacturers that increasing the power output increases the imaging capabilities. The old standards are still in place, however, and research, by being vague and inconclusive, has prevented the establishment of new and clear guidelines. In 1987, the American Institute for Ultrasound in Medicine (AIUM) and the Center for Devices and Radiological Health (CDRH) collaborated with the National Electrical Manufacturers Association (NEMA) and the FDA to develop a voluntary standard for the display of acoustic output information. The goal was to provide information that would improve the regulation of ultrasound instruments and would provide a method by which users of clinical devices would be able to apply the ALARA (as low as reasonably achievable) principle.[13]

Ultrasonic Detection and Measurement

Considerable variation in power output is noted between the many types of diagnostic ultrasound units and the diverse methods used to quantify differing power levels. Among these are hydrophones, radiation force balances, optical measuring techniques, and thermal techniques.

HYDROPHONE MEASUREMENTS

Hydrophones are used to take sound pressure measurements. A hydrophone is an ultrasound transducer much like a transmitting transducer; however, it is much smaller and can be moved about the ultrasound field produced by the transmitting ultrasound probe to measure the pressures at each point. In this way, a profile of the beam pressure and intensity can be derived (Fig. 3–2).[14]

RADIATION FORCE AND FORCE BALANCES

Radiation force balances are used to determine total radiating power. The radiating power is unidirectional and is caused by the alternating field. The transducer insonates a liquid into which a target object of specific acoustic properties is introduced. The aim is

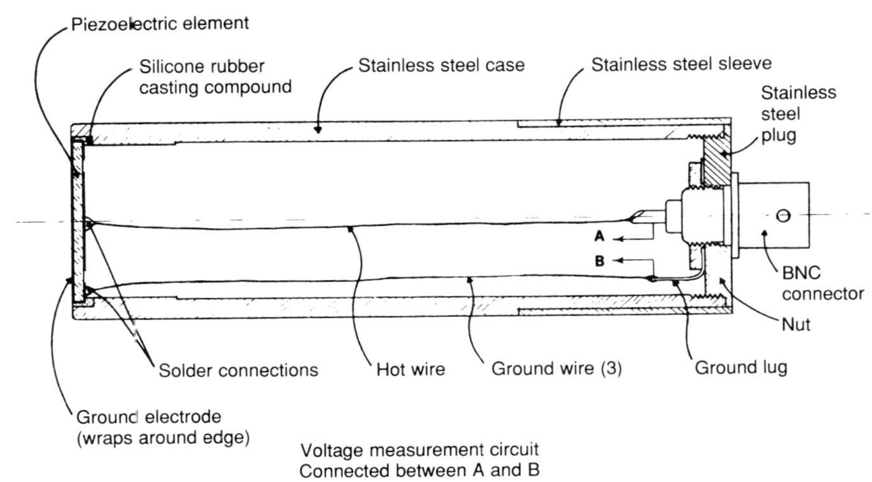

FIGURE 3–2.
Sectional view of transducer. (From Ziskin MC: Ultrasonic Exposimetry. CRC Press, Boca Raton, FL, 1993, p 176.)

to determine the time-average ultrasonic power. The two basic types are those devices based on gravimetric balance principles and those based on the float principles (Fig. 3–3).[11]

OPTICAL MEASURING TECHNIQUES

Optical measuring techniques allow scientists to measure a sound field without disturbing it. They also result in resolution of the ultrasound field, spatially and temporally. Thus, field or beam shape can be resolved. These techniques are not unlike Schlieren's methods used in medical ultrasound during its infancy. These techniques are based on the principle of optical refraction: When ultrasound passes through water, the pressure fluctuations alter its optical refractive index at specific points. These points can be visualized by shining light into the system and using a system of lenses and apertures.[15] The devices of today use a laser, and the sound field is created in degassed or deionized water (Fig. 3–4).[11]

THERMAL TECHNIQUES

Thermal techniques measure acoustic energy in a certain volume. A calorimeter is a device that uses a solution or fluid to transform the ultrasound power to heat and then mea-

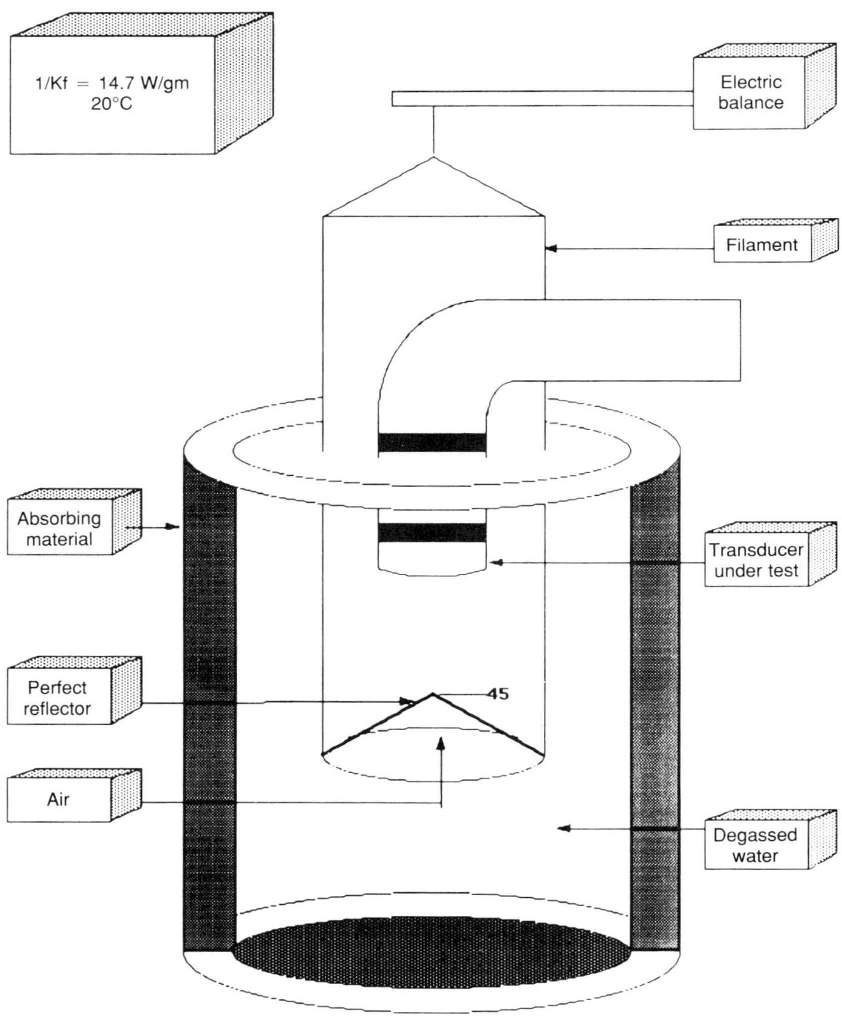

FIGURE 3–3.
The radiation force measurement principle. (From Ziskin MC: Ultrasonic Exposimetry. CRC Press, Boca Raton, FL, 1993, pp 144–160.)

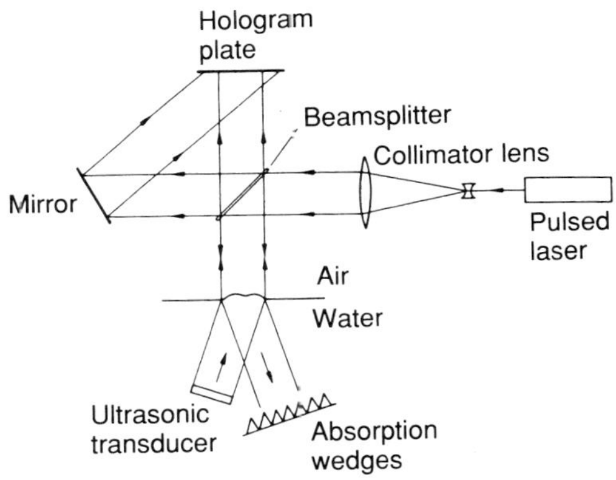

FIGURE 3–4.
Optical arrangement of the holographic system. (From Ziskin MC: Ultrasonic Exposimetry. CRC Press, Boca Raton, FL, 1993, p 145.)

sure the heat in the solution. The temperature increase in a calorimeter is reflective of the time-average ultrasonic power. If a calorimeter is not used a thermocouple or combination of calorimeter and thermocouple is used. The thermocouple is a thermoelectric probe designed to detect temperature changes.[11]

Physical Interactions with Tissue

When ultrasound enters the body, a bidirectional interplay occurs. The tissue affects the ultrasound beam, and the ultrasonic energies affect the tissue. The action of ultrasound on tissue is termed the *biological effect*. The effect of the medium on the sound beam is what is necessary to produce an image. Acoustic variables are the effect of the sound on the medium and are also called *reversible interactions of ultrasound*.

REVERSIBLE INTERACTIONS

The acoustic variables, which are particle displacement, tissue change in density, temperature increase, and pressure amplification, fluctuate sinusoidally with the passage of the ultrasound cycles. These changes immediately reverse themselves as the sonic effect passes. If the ultrasound intensity is high enough within its category of either SATA, SATP, SPTA, or SPTP intensities, some irreversible effect or interaction occurs.

Note, however, that heat is one acoustic variable that is created by absorption of the ultrasound by the tissue. Therefore, technically, some reversibility is not achieved.[7]

IRREVERSIBLE INTERACTIONS

In liquid and soft tissue media, a wide array of irreversible effects have been documented.[14] Many different terms are used to designate particular kinds of irreversible interactions. The categories discussed in this chapter include (1) force effects, (2) heating or thermal effects, and (3) cavitation.

Force Effect

At higher intensities, force effects, sometimes called *radiation forces* or *unidirectional forces*, are produced. This force is directly proportional to the intensity drop across the boundary (medium) and is related to the intensity of the wave and the reflection coefficient at the boundary (Fig. 3–5). Remember that the reflection coefficient is derived from the differing acoustic impedances from the two media. The acoustic impedances of each medium are determined by the medium's elasticity and the speed of sound in that medium. These radiation forces, categorized with names such as the *alternating force, radiation torque, acoustic streaming, Stokes's force, Oseen's force,* and *Bernoulli's force,* can occur in liquidlike media.

The alternating force is a force that exists along a half wavelength in the direction of the true wave, between pressure peak and pressure trough. Fatigue tearing of the tissues is possible as a result of this force. The radiation force can produce stasis of red blood cells when a standing wave is created along the direction of flow of the blood.[16] Oseen's force is the unidirectional average net force resembling a radiation force due to the nonlinearity of the medium. Bernoulli's force is the force experienced by two particles near each other along the beam axis. The pressure gradient produced by the insonation tends to draw them toward each other.

Heating

Heating of the medium via ultrasound is a result of absorption of the ultrasound due to friction within the medium. When consider-

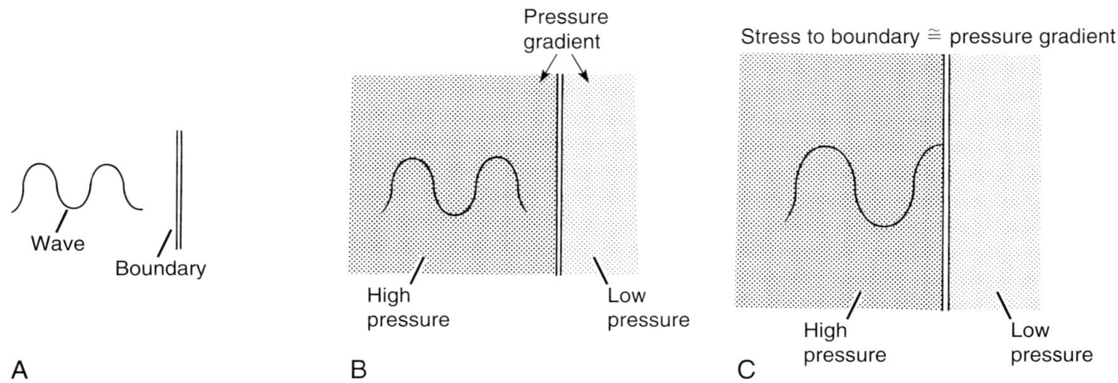

FIGURE 3–5.
Acoustic force effect. The force of the propagation of a wave across a boundary is proportional to intensity drop across the boundary.

ing the effect of the source of ultrasound, the amount of the tissue that is heated depends on the intensity, the frequency, beam focusing, tissue perfusion, and duration of insonation.[10] In terms of source-producing parameters, intensity is the most important in the production of heat. When considering the effect of the medium, the rate and extent of the absorption are dependent on the tissue's (1) heat storage capacity, or its ability to retain heat; (2) the absorption coefficient, or the tissue's ability to absorb ultrasound; and (3) the thickness of the tissue.[10] All three of these parameters affect the overall, final temperature increase.

Inanimate absorption models have been used to calculate the temperature rise in mammalian tissues. Heat, whether it is produced by ultrasound or any other source, is teratogenic and is dangerous to a fetus, particularly during organogenesis.[17] Most research indicates that temperature rises greater than 1°C are considered significant.[10]

The World Federation of Ultrasound in Medicine and Biology's 1992 Symposium on Safety and Standardization in Medical Ultrasound indicated that a rise up to 1.5°C could be used in clinical examination. However, any temperature rise to or above 41°C (105.8°F) should be considered hazardous in embryonic or fetal exposures.[18]

Most data on heating, however, have shown that heating is negligible under most diagnostically relevant conditions.[19] This is because for in vivo systems such as mammalian tissue, the heat generated by insonation is transported to cooler areas by conduction and via convective processes related to blood flow.[17] Also, the on-cycle of the ultrasound pulse is only 1% of the total time that sound traverses the system, thus allowing ample time for cooling of heated areas.

Cavitation, Stable and Transient

Cavitation is a category of ultrasound bioeffects that deals with the formation and behaviors of microscopic bubbles in fluidlike media. Cavitation consists of two types of bubble formation—namely, stable or noncollapse and transient or collapse.

Stable or noncollapse cavitation involves the growth of bubbles during the negative pressure phase of the acoustic cycle and the rapid contraction during the positive pressure phase. The resonating of bubbles causes transmission of energy to the surrounding medium, creating destructive effects such as acoustic streaming.

Transient or collapse cavitation involves the same bubble growth during the negative phase of the pressure wave, but during the positive phase contraction of the bubble is so rapid that implosion results (Figs. 3–5 and 3–6). This implosion gives rise to high pressure and temperature stresses that violently affect the surrounding medium. Note that noncollapse cavitation is associated with lower intensities and collapse cavitation with higher intensities.

A requirement for cavitation to occur is preexistence of small, stabilized gaseous nuclei. Within mammalian tissues, it is probable that such sites for the initiation of acoustic cavitation exist, but little conclusive information has

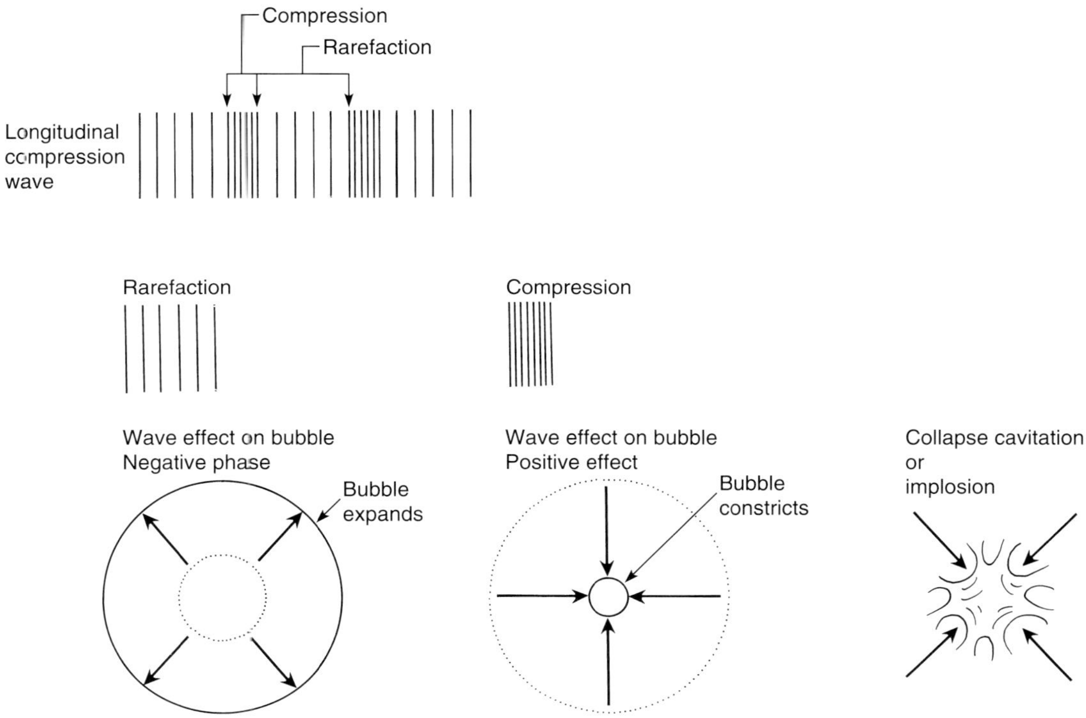

FIGURE 3–6.
Wave motion and cavitation. Graphic representation of compression and rarefaction of wave motion, which can cause formation of microbubbles (cavitation) and collapse.

been gained about their physical properties such as optimal size, chemical composition, and elasticity of the medium.[19] Some data indicate that cavitation potential is increased relative to the higher amplitude short pulses used in imaging than those used in Doppler modes.[19]

Genetics

Most of the measurements of genetic effects have been inconclusive Of these experiments, however, most attention has been drawn to sister chromatid exchange, which can be used as an indicator of chromosomal damage.

When a cell divides, the nuclear material (chromatin) loses its appearance and condenses to form a number of rod-shaped organelles called *chromosomes*. Each cell species has a characteristic chromosome constitution called a *karyotype*. The karyotype can be defined as the way in which the chromosome is organized. The chromosomes themselves are divided into subsets called *genes*, which have specific locations on a gene map. The term *genome* refers to the full DNA content of the chromosome set (remember that chromosomes are arranged in sets of two). Whereas the genotype is the genetic constitution with reference to a single locus, the phenotype is the expression of the genotype as a morphological and physiological characteristic.[20]

The two kinds of cell division are mitosis and meiosis. Mitosis is ordinary cell division by which the body grows and replaces dead or injured cells. It results in two daughter cells that are precisely identical to the parent cell in chromosome complement and genetic information. Meiosis occurs only once in a life cycle and results in the production of reproductive cells, gametes, each of which has a complement of 23 chromosomes. Gametes are haploid, n chromosomes number, whereas somatic cells are said to have the diploid or 2n chromosome.

In mitotic division, the cytoplasm of the cell simply cleaves into two approximately equal halves, whereas the nucleus undergoes a complicated sequence of activities. Four stages are required for chromosome replication and its associated cell division to be completed. These four stages are called *prophase, metaphase, anaphase,* and *telophase*. The stage before or between division is called *interphase*. It is during this stage that actual chromosome (DNA/chromatin) replication occurs, from a two-chromatid structure to a four-chromatid structure.[21]

It is during prophase that the chromosomes are discernible. Because replication has already occurred, 46 chromosomes are present. Each chromosome can be seen to consist of a pair of long, thin parallel strands or chromatids (sister chromatid), which are held together at one spot, the centromere. It is during metaphase that chromosomes are most easily studied.[20] During metaphase, the 46 pairs of chromatids and their centromeres begin to group in the cell center. In anaphase, the centromere divides, each daughter centromere attached to one of the two chromatids. The chromatids are no longer paired, and they are now called *chromosomes*. In telophase, the cytoplasm pinches and the dividing cell becomes two new cells (Fig. 3–7).

Sister Chromatid Exchange

Sister chromatid exchange is the crossing over between the sister chromatids of a single chromosome. This phenomenon was discovered by using a special staining technique and noting the frequency of the genetic disorder named *Bloom's syndrome*. The phenotype of Bloom's syndrome consists of low birth weight; dwarfism; hypersensitivity to light, causing a skin rash; a characteristic facial appearance; a high frequency of chromosome breakage and rearrangement in cell culture; and predisposition to leukemia.[20]

It is the association between frequency of sister chromatid exchanges and genetic disorders that generates this phenomenon as a possible marker for chromosomal damage. The study of ionizing radiation has shown the association between radiation exposure and radiation-induced chromosomal aberrations or cytogenetic damage. These types of damage are sometimes termed *main-chain scission, cross-linking,* and *point lesions*.[21] It is therefore logical that sister chromatid exchange would be one method of assessment for the study of ultrasound bioeffects.

Studies in sister chromatid exchange can be summarized as follows:

> Over a 10-year period, about two dozen reports have been published on this subject. Most studies have yielded negative results. Of importance is the fact that there is no independent confirmation of a published positive effect. Attempts to do so have led to the conclusion that the cause of small but statistically significant effects is unknown; however, it seems clear that the ultrasound exposure either does not produce increased

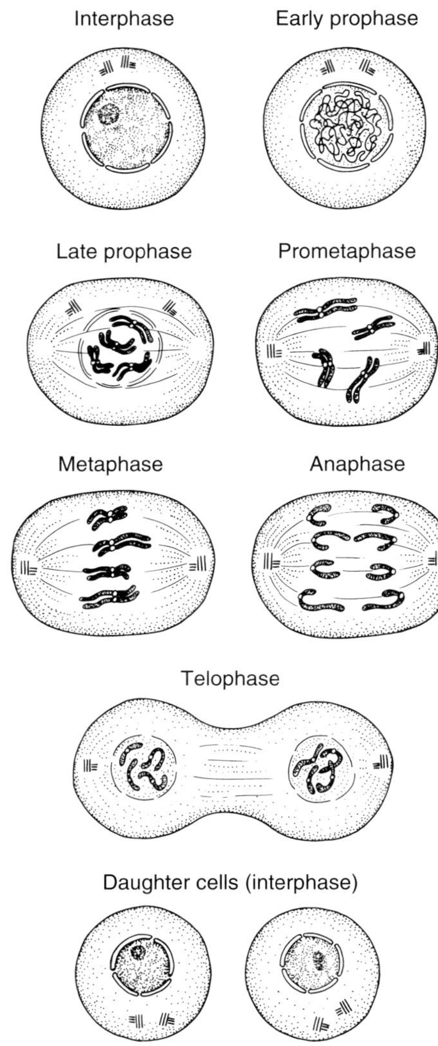

FIGURE 3–7.
Mitosis. The process of mitosis is in four phases: prophase, metaphase, anaphase, and telophase. The interphase is the period of cell existence between divisions.

exchanges or the effect is not reproducible and is too small to be consistently produced.[22]

Biological Effects of Ultrasound

The biological effects of ultrasound have been the subject of considerable interest. This is because of many factors such as (1) the continued concern over the well-being of the fetus; (2) the need for exposure criteria as assessed by organizations such as the National Council for Radiation Protection (NCRP), the AIUM, the World Federation for Ultrasound in Medicine and Biology, the FDA, the National Institutes of Health (NIH), and NEMA; (3) the need for assessment of the risk component of the risk-benefit relationship; and (4) the necessity for assessment of the dose-response relationship.

At present, the AIUM, FDA, and NEMA are the safety watchdogs in the study of the manufacture of diagnostic ultrasound equipment and the biological effects of diagnostic ultrasound. When looking at the manufacture of ultrasound systems, these organizations look at the power output as well as other parameters. This can be described as evaluating the *dose* of the dose-response relationship. When looking at the biological effects, these organizations study the mechanisms or the biological changes or damage. This can be described as evaluating the *response* in the dose-response relationship.

In looking at the history of equipment manufacture, the evaluation of power output can be summarized by three criteria: (1) the exposure values of instrument outputs before 1980, (2) the exposure values of instrument outputs after 1980, and (3) summaries of data published in 1979, 1985, and 1990.

The first quantification of exposure values for medical devices before 1980 was carried out by Hill and published in Vienna in 1971. The measuring devices used were a radiation force balance and ceramic hydrophone. A study of 15 pulse-echo transducers and 3 continuous wave Doppler transducers was performed. Before 1980, published reports of pulse-echo transducers described the range as 0.5 to 14.4 mW, whereas continuous wave Doppler powers reached the 37 mW range.[11]

EXPOSURE VALUES AFTER 1980

Since 1980, the FDA has made it mandatory that manufacturers of commercial equipment file exposure information. This has allowed us to witness the increasing intensities of these systems. Before the mid-1980s, values reached 180 mW SPTA. By the mid-1980s, the AIUM published reports[23] that not only evidenced the increasing trend toward higher outputs but drew attention to the considerably higher intensities used in pulsed Doppler beams, in which intensities reached 1.95 W cm^{-2}.

SUMMARY OF REPORTED DATA

The summaries of reported data published by the end of 1979, by 1985, and by 1990 are shown in Table 3–1.[11]

The study of the power intensity needed in diagnostic ultrasound can also be divided into three categories:

1. Medical diagnostic pulse-echo equipment
2. Medical diagnostic pulsed Doppler equipment
3. Medical diagnostic color flow Doppler equipment

Table 3–2 illustrates the maximum exposure in water from modern medical diagnostic pulse-echo equipment.[11]

It has been established that energy emitted by pulsed Doppler devices far exceeds that of pulse-echo equipment.[24] Note that the pulsed Doppler technique is similar to the imaging technique except for (1) ensemble length—the time and number of pulses needed to extract Doppler information; (2) pulse length—the number of cycles in one package of ultrasound; and (3) sonic intensity—the strength of the ultrasound beam. Note also that the intensity of pulsed wave is higher than continuous wave when all other things are equal (i.e., same power output, frequency, and so forth). Here the term SATA can be replaced by SAPA and SPTA can be replaced by SPPA.

Table 3–3 illustrates the maximum exposure in water from modern medical diagnostic pulsed Doppler equipment.[11]

As mentioned earlier, the power emitted from the continuous wave systems is much lower than that of pulsed Doppler ultra-

TABLE 3–1. **CHRONOLOGICAL DEVELOPMENT OF MAXIMUM EXPOSURE VALUES**

	TO 1978	1985	1990
Pulse-echo			
Power (mW)	0.3–21	1.0–80	0.5–350
SATA [I] source (mW cm^{-2})	0.05–7.1	1–37	<5–100
SPTA [I] scanning (mW cm^{-2})	<1–11	<1–37	0.3–177
SPTA [I] M-mode (mW cm^{-2})	0.01–169	<1–680	2.4–440
SPPA [I] (W cm^{-2})	0.5–200	<1–1100	21–930
p+ (MPa)	0.1–5.0	0.1–7.4	0.8–8.8
p− (MPa)		0.1–3.9	0.1–3.9
Pulsed Doppler			
Power (mW)	10.6*	2.8–70	8.7–210
SATA [I] source (mW cm^{-2})	150*		440 (max)
SPTA [I] (mW cm^{-2})		0.08–1.95*	0.11–4.52
SPPA [I] (W cm^{-2})		3.6–1270	1.1–770
p+ (MPa)			0.2–6.4
p− (MPa)			0.2–3.8
CW Doppler			
Power (mW)	1–105	1–250	2.3–90
SATA [I] source (mW cm^{-2})	0.24–840		320 (max)
SPTA [I] (mW cm^{-2})		39–1000	37–850
Pressure (kPa)			10–160

*Single value.
Adapted from Ziskin MC: Ultrasonic Exposimetry. CRC Press, Boca Raton, FL, 1993, p 320.

sound. Table 3–4 illustrates the maximum exposure in water from modern medical diagnostic continuous wave Doppler equipment.[11]

For ultrasound systems to be able to detect the small phase shifts in the assessment of velocity changes, a much higher intensity transmitted beam must be used. These transmitted intensities can be as much as five times the levels required in continuous wave and in B-mode imaging.[25] In general, the Doppler technique requires greater ensemble length and pulse length than that used in imaging. Pulses with relatively high SPPA intensities are delivered with low duty cycle, such that the intensity average over time is low.

The trend toward increased power output intensities, particularly for the best and newest devices with pulsed Doppler capability, has heightened interest in safety issues. Manufacturers are required to submit pre-

TABLE 3–2. **MAXIMUM EXPOSURE IN WATER FROM PULSE-ECHO EQUIPMENT**

	RANGE	MEAN	MEDIAN	n
Peak compression p+ (MPa)	0.75–8.8	4.13	4.1	108
Peak rarefaction p− (MPa)	0.58–4.3	2.09	2.1	108
SPPA [I] (W cm^{-2})	14–933	270	230	105
SPTA [I] stationary (mW cm^{-2})	2.4–440	98.7	86	81
SPTA [I] scanning (mW cm^{-2})	0.3–177	16.7	6.0	101
Acoustic power (mW)	0.5–350	19.1	7.1	51
Nonlinear propagation parameter σ_m	0.24≥3.2	2.26	2.20	99

Adapted from Ziskin MC: Ultrasonic Exposimetry. CRC Press, Boca Raton, FL, 1993, p 323.

TABLE 3–3. MAXIMUM EXPOSURE IN WATER FROM PULSED DOPPLER EQUIPMENT

	RANGE	MEAN	MEDIAN	n
Peak compression p+ (MPa)	0.2–6.4	3.53	3.1	36
Peak rarefaction p− (MPa)	0.2–3.8	1.61	1.5	36
SPPA [I] (W cm^{-2})	1.1–771	208	138	34
SPTA [I] (W cm^{-2})	0.11–4.52	1.43	1.07	35
Acoustic power (mW)	8.7–210	62	45	16
Nonlinear propagation parameter σ_m	0.26≥3.2	2.11	2.11	32

Adapted from Ziskin MC: Ultrasonic Exposimetry. CRC Press, Boca Raton, FL, 1993, p 323.

market notification to the FDA. The FDA then reviews this notification to determine if the device is substantially equivalent with regard to safety and effectiveness. Information about whether the higher intensities of commercially available Doppler insonation increase the risk of chromosomal aberrations or any other effects is conflicting.

Because color flow Doppler involves interweaving of pulse-echo information with Doppler information, quantification of power output is difficult. However, in general, color flow power can be considered slightly higher than pulse-echo but not nearly that of pulsed Doppler. Table 3–5 illustrates the maximum exposure in water from modern medical diagnostic color Doppler equipment.[11]

The AIUM has investigated the two major mechanisms of ultrasound biological effects—namely, thermal effects and cavitation—and has issued two sets of statements about these possible areas of danger. The first set, which consists of five statements, addresses the thermal mechanisms of ultrasound bioeffect as follows:

1. A thermal criterion is one reasonable approach to specifying potentially hazardous exposures to diagnostic ultrasound.
2. Based solely on the thermal criterion, a diagnostic exposure that produces a maximum temperature rise of 1°C above normal physiologic levels may be used without reservation in clinical examination.
3. An in situ temperature rise to or above 41°C is considered hazardous in fetal exposures; the longer this temperature elevation is maintained, the greater is the likelihood for damage to occur.
4. Analytical models of ultrasonically induced heating have been applied successfully to in vivo mammalian situa-

TABLE 3–4. MAXIMUM EXPOSURE IN WATER FROM CONTINUOUS WAVE DOPPLER DEVICES

	RANGE	MEAN	MEDIAN	n
PV and cardiac				
Acoustic power (mW)	2.3–90	25.7	16	19
SPTA [I] (mW cm^{-2})	8.5–850	159	99	21
Peak pressure (kPa)	18–160	60.1	54	21
Fetal heart				
Acoustic power (mW)	17–25			4
SPTA [I] (mW cm^{-2})	6–33			4
Peak pressure (kPa)	13–31			4

Adapted from Ziskin MC: Ultrasonic Exposimetry. CRC Press, Boca Raton, FL, 1993, p 334.

TABLE 3–5. MAXIMUM EXPOSURE IN WATER FROM COLOR DOPPLER SYSTEMS

	RANGE	MEAN	MEDIAN	n
Peak compression p+ (MPa)	2.4–6.4	3.94	3.7	11
Peak compression p− (MPa)	0.9–2.7	1.91	1.9	11
SPPA [I] (W cm^{-2})	60–670	258	193	11
SPTA [I] (mW cm^{-2})	25–256	95.6	55	11

Adapted from Ziskin MC: Ultrasonic Exposimetry. CRC Press, Boca Raton, FL, 1993, p 337.

tions. In those clinical situations where local tissue temperatures are not measured, estimates of temperature elevations can be made by employing such analytical models.

5. Calculations of ultrasonically induced temperature elevation, based on a simplified tissue model and a simplified model of stationary beams, suggest the following. For examinations of fetal soft tissue with typical perfusion rates, employing center frequencies between 2 and 10 MHz and beam widths (−6 dB beam width, according to AIUM/NEMA definition) less than 11 wavelengths, the computed temperature rise will not be significantly above 1°C if the in situ SATA intensity does not exceed 200 mW/cm^2 (SATA intensity refers to the spatial average value over the focal area); or if the beam width does not exceed 200 mW/cm^2; or if the beam width does not exceed eight wavelengths, the corresponding intensity is 300 mW/cm^2. However, if the same beam impinges on fetal bone, the local temperature rise may be much higher.[26]

The AIUM has also issued three statements regarding cavitation:

1. Acoustic cavitation may occur with short pulses and has the potential for producing deleterious biological effects.
2. Currently available information indicates that pulses with peak pressures greater than 10 MPa (3300 W/cm^2) can induce cavitation in mammals. (Evidence is from observations with lithotripters.)
3. With the limited data available, it is not possible to specify threshold pressure amplitudes at which acoustic cavitation will occur, in mammals, with diagnostically relevant pulse lengths and repetition rates.[26]

The statements listed are the synthesis of countless studies in the area of ultrasound biological effects. The sources can be categorized as follows:

1. In vitro: the study of macromolecules in solutions and suspension of cells
2. In vivo: the study of plants and experimental animals
3. The study of epidemiology in humans

Macromolecules in Solutions (In Vitro)

The study of macromolecules in solution involves assessment of the effect of insonation on the ultrastructure of cells. This includes the effect on cell permeability, the alteration of DNA, mitochondria, lysosomal membrane, and so forth. Studies have indicated the following:

1. In aqueous solutions, the degradation of DNA has been reported at intensity levels (SATA) of 4 kW m^{-2}.
2. Some studies have noted some change in membrane permeability and an associated swelling of mitochondria.
3. Some studies have shown that insonation of the liver of rodents causes some lysosomal damage.[25]

Although ultrastructure studies have shown that permeability of various membranes of the cells had been affected by insonation, the parameters of insonation in these experiments have been considerably greater than those involved in typical diagnostic studies.[27] As indicated earlier, the most reported in vitro endpoint is sister chromatid exchange.

Suspension of Cells (In Vitro)

The study of cells has demonstrated the following destructive effects of ultrasound:

1. Cell disruption
2. Thrombocyte disruption (clot initiation)
3. Dislodgement of ribosomes
4. Release of enzymes from lysosomes
5. Rupture of nucleolus
6. Disruption of mitochondrial cristae
7. Chromosomal abnormalities
8. Mitotic delay
9. Increase of cell membrane permeability
10. Intracellular streaming
11. Abnormal cell division
12. Cell surface changes[25]

At the intensities of 1 to 35 kW m^{-2} and exposure durations from 60 to 900 seconds, the suspension of cells, cell lysis, membrane permeability increases, electrophoretic mobility changes, altered growth properties, and chromosomal changes have been reported.[25]

Plants and Mammalian Tissues (In Vivo)

Plants are studied because they contain gas-filled channels. Thus, they serve as models to study cavitation. The irreversible effect demonstrated is cell death due to membrane damage. The reversible effects demonstrated are chromosomal abnormalities, reductions in miotic index, and growth rate reduction. The overwhelming majority of studies conducted with animals have used mice. Mice have demonstrated the most consistent deleterious effects. These include fetal weight reduction, postpartum fetal mortality, fetal abnormalities, tissue lesions, hindlimb paralysis, and blood flow stasis. Note that fetal weight reduction studies have been more or less consistent, however, with only one particular strain of mice.[6]

Other studies have shown that insonation of mice embryos during the period of active organogenesis demonstrated increased incidence of congenital abnormalities.[27] However, insonation after organogenesis did not produce any apparent damage. It can be extrapolated that after organogenesis is complete, evidence shows that the fetus becomes more resistant to ultrasonic damage.

The 1987 AIUM revised statement on In Vivo Mammalian Bioeffects is as follows:

> "In the low megahertz frequency range there have been (as of this date) no independently confirmed significant biological effects in mammalian tissues exposed in vivo to unfocused ultrasound with intensities below 100 mW/cm^2, or to focused ultrasound with intensities below 1 W/cm^2. Furthermore, for exposure times greater than 1 second and less than 500 seconds from unfocused ultrasound or 50 seconds for focused ultrasound, such effects have not been demonstrated even at higher intensities, when the product of intensity and exposure time is less than 50 joules/cm^2."[26]

EXTRAPOLATION FROM SMALL MAMMAL DATA

James, in *The Physical Basis of Medical Imaging*, describes the method of extrapolating animal data to humans:

> "The use of repetitive pulses for a longer duration (10 msec), however, showed that hemorrhage into the spinal cord and paraplegia could be produced by peak intensities in the region of only 25 W/cm^2. It was also found that insonation time for production of hemorrhage increased with increasing frequency to 5 MHz, at which frequency hemorrhage and paraplegia no longer occurred. This damage factor seemed to be inversely related to thermal changes."[27]

This series of experiments on the production of paraplegia and hemorrhage into the spinal cord of rats also produced evidence of dose accumulation. When the intervals between adjacent pulses were increased, the onset of damage was dependent only on the integrated dose-time. By extrapolating these data to the diagnostic parameters of dosage, one finds that many hours of continued insonation would be required to produce damage, even allowing for hypoxia in the fetus.[27]

Using measurements obtained in vitro and applying certain assumptions about attenuation of the ultrasound beam, these intensities may be estimated from typical clinical conditions.

APPLICATION TO HUMAN PATIENTS

To date, studies of the biological effects of ultrasound on the fetus have been limited to five major areas: (1) birth weight, (2) structural fetal anomalies, (3) neurological development, (4) cancer induction, and (5) hearing. The studies that concentrated on birth weight were those that attempted to extrapolate from mammalian studies of mice that indicated that some species of mice have shown a decrease in birth weight after insonation. These results have never been observed in the human population.

The studies that were concerned with fetal anomalies were focusing on the fact that it is during organogenesis that a fetus is most vulnerable to any deleterious effects. The period of major organogenesis is completed by the 10th week of pregnancy. The majority of ultrasound examinations are in fact performed after this period. A few studies, however, have supported the hypothesis that no deleterious effects result from diagnostic levels of ultrasound, and no studies prove that such effects occur.

The studies of deficits in neurological development are trials extrapolated from mice studies that demonstrated destruction to rat nerve fibers by ultrasound. This effect demonstrated paralysis of limbs. Some studies tried to associate dyslexia and tonic/grasp reflex deficits from ultrasound, but this has never been proved.

The cancer induction studies have demonstrated no evidence of an association between insonation and cancer.

Ultrasound is a mechanical form of energy different from sound that can be heard with the human ear only in that its frequency is higher. Some alarmists have tried to find an association between ultrasound and hearing loss. To date, this has not been proved.

Miller and Ziskin have studied the heating effect of ultrasound mainly because it has been shown to occur at lower intensities than does cavitation. They have used the model that the human body can safely withstand temperature elevations of 1° to 2°C. Therefore, temperature rises only above 2°C should be considered harmful.[28]

Sister Chromatid Exchange

Although a number of positive results have been noted, the overwhelming statistical results are inconclusive. At present, sister chromatid exchanges have not proved to have a genetic effect and therefore do not constitute risk.[6]

Epidemiology

Epidemiology can be used as a method of assessing the safety of ultrasound techniques. This science can be performed both prospectively and retrospectively. Retrospective studies are very limited but on the whole have found no appreciable hazard to a fetus. Widespread clinical use and the various randomized clinical studies have not established any adverse effect arising from exposure to diagnostic ultrasound. Criteria have been established for evaluating an allegation of danger from a particular agent: (1) repeatable epidemiological findings, (2) secular trends, (3) animal models, (4) dose-response relationships, and (5) biologically plausible explanations. Epidemiological findings have already been discussed. Secular trends are noted when evaluating for malformations and when correlating for introduction of an intervention. Studies have found no increase in malformations that correlated with the increased use of ultrasound.[29]

Animal models are used to note any correlation between animal studies and human studies. Obviously, with animal studies, empirical investigation can be continued to endpoint. To date no animal study has been able to be applied to humans because of the protective nature of the maternal environment, as well as the fact that the correlation of the exposure times and dosages needs more study.[29]

Dose-response relationship of ultrasound dosage is difficult to identify when the variability in pulse ultrasound equipment hampers this quantification. Finally, biological plausibility mandates transcending hypothesis and theory and looking at the truth of these proposals. At this point, most of the concentration in the study of the mechanism of bioeffects rests in analyzing cavitation and heating. According to Carstensen, the risk of cavitation is small and nonexistent at intensities less than 10 W/cm^2.[30]

Therefore, hyperthermia remains the final consideration. An exhaustive study by Miller and Ziskin identified no hazards as long as the temperature elevation does not exceed 2°C.[31]

The AIUM has issued a statement on epidemiology:

1. Widespread clinical use over 25 years has not established any adverse effect arising from exposure to diagnostic ultrasound.
2. Randomized clinical studies are the most rigorous method for assessing potential adverse effects of diagnostic ultrasound. Studies using this methodology show no evidence of an effect on birth weight in humans.
3. Other epidemiologic studies have shown no causal association of diagnostic ultrasound with any of the adverse fetal outcomes studied.[26]

Current State of the Safety Question

Ultrasound is a constantly evolving technology. Trends toward improved resolution and expanding application (particularly the endocavitary approaches) have led to transmission of higher energies into patients. Because of these changes, the safety question must be constantly reassessed.

The central question is whether in any situation or routine application of diagnostic ultrasound, the health and diagnostic benefits no longer outweigh the actual benefits.

The AIUM and NEMA have worked on establishing guidelines for the manufacture of ultrasound devices. These guidelines, along with the desire of manufacturers to use higher power outputs, have led to the display of power output of the ultrasound systems, specific labeling, and measuring criteria. Ultrasound units may display SPTA data (in water or derated—accounting for attenuation) that are related to thermal bioeffect mechanisms and a mechanical index that is related to cavitational bioeffect mechanisms.

PRUDENT USE AND STEPS TO MINIMIZE PATIENT EXPOSURE

Taylor and Kremkau outline some guidelines to follow in order to minimize exposure:

"1. Physicians and Sonographers should be aware of the potential for high intensity and for harm and avoid using Doppler 'just to see what the neonatal head and vessels look like.'
2. The operator should be aware of the intensity parameters, especially the SPTA, for the transducer at the frequency being used.
3. The operator must know how to reduce the SPTA to a prudent level. Some machines have a power output which is adjustable, so that a fraction of the maximum power can be used. For example, the properly calibrated power setting of 10% indicates only 100 mW/cm^2 if the maximum intensity is 1 W/cm^2. Maternal tissue attenuation will reduce this to about 40 mW/cm^2 at the embryo which is within the FDA guidelines [see FDA update[32]]. Check the power when the machine is turned on. Some machines power up to maximum intensity and should be reduced to minimum before scanning the patient.
4. For obstetric applications, the minimum power output should be used initially. If penetration is poor, the TGC should be increased first. Then the receiver gain should be fully increased, and only if penetration or the Doppler signal is still inadequate should the power output be increased.
5. There is a wide variation between equipment. Some equipment requires maximum output to achieve the signals that can be acquired at much lower intensities with a more sensitive and better designed device. We should not purchase equipment unless we are satisfied that the machine is of sufficient sensitivity and can be used at low intensities, within the FDA guidelines, for obstetric purposes.
6. Most obstetric Doppler procedures are experimental. Thus, the consent of a hu-

man experimental committee is appropriate, and this will involve patient consent [see Taylor[33]]. If the fetal exposure is estimated to be less than 94 mW/cm^2, the risk is considered to be nonsignificant. If it is above the FDA level, approval should be sought from the FDA. This will involve applying for an investigational device exemption (IDE).

7. Exposure time should be minimized, consistent with obtaining the necessary clinical data. A sensitive machine in the hands of a competent, well-trained sonographer will enable the data to be obtained expeditiously."[34]

REFERENCES

1. McGahan JP: Controversies in ultrasound. Clin Diagn Ultrasound 1987;20:114–118.
2. Bushong SC: Radiologic Science for Technologists: Physics, Biology, and Protection. JB Lippincott, New York, 1984.
3. Upron A: The biological effects of low-level ionizing radiation. Sci Am 1982;246(2):41–49.
4. Dotle E: Addressing the fear of radiation. RT Image 1991; May 6, 1991.
5. Donald I, Levi S: Present and Future of Diagnostic Ultrasound. John Wiley & Sons, New York, 1976.
6. Kremkau FW: Safety of ultrasound. In: Chervenack FA, Issacson GC, Campbell S, eds: Ultrasound in Obstetrics and Gynecology. Little, Brown & Co, Boston, 1993.
7. Hussey M: Basic Physics and Technology of Medical Diagnostic Ultrasound. Elsevier, New York, 1985.
8. Statement issued by the European Federation of Societies for Ultrasound in Medicine and Biology (EFSUMB) in 1989. Ultrasound Med Biol 1989; 15 (Suppl), Oct 22–23, 1988, Airlie, Virginia.
9. Craig M: The History of Ultrasound. Sonography Today, July–Sept, 1991, p 6.
10. Kremkau FW: Diagnostic Ultrasound: Principles and Instruments, 4th ed. WB Saunders, Philadelphia, 1993.
11. Ziskin M, Lewin P: Ultrasonic Exposimetry, CRC Press, Boca Raton, FL, 1993.
12. Kremkau FW: Diagnostic Ultrasound: Principles and Instruments, 4th ed. WB Saunders, Philadelphia, 1993.
13. American Institute of Ultrasound in Medicine and the National Electrical Manufacturers Association: Standard for real-time display of thermal and mechanical Acoustic Output Indices on Diagnostic Ultrasound Equipment, AIUM, Rockville, MD, 1992.
14. Hussey M: A Review of the Biological Effects and the Safety of Diagnostic Ultrasound. Department of Physics, Dublin Institute of Technology, Dublin, Ireland, 1991.
15. McDicken WN: Diagnostic Ultrasonics, Principles and Use of Instruments. Churchill Livingstone, New York, 1991.
16. American Institute of Ultrasound in Medicine: Bioeffects considerations for the safety of diagnostic ultrasound. J Ultrasound Med 1988;7:s1–s38.
17. Skelly AC: Beyond 100 mW/cm^2. A bioeffects primer: Part I—fundamentals. J Diagn Med Sonogr 1985;1: 190–199.
18. World Federation of Ultrasound in Medicine and Biology: Symposium on safety and standardization in medical ultrasound: Issues and recommendations regarding thermal mechanisms for biological effects. World Federation of Ultrasound in Medicine and Biology, June 12–16, 1992, Zagreb, Yugoslavia.
19. Carstensen EL: Acoustic cavitation and the safety of diagnostic ultrasound. Ultrasound Med Biol 1987;10:597–606.
20. Thompson JS, Thompson MW: Genetics in Medicine. WB Saunders, Philadelphia, 1980.
21. Bushong SC: Radiologic Science for Technologists: Physics, Biology, and Protection. CV Mosby, St Louis, 1984.
22. Kremkau FW: Biologic Effects and Safety. In: Rumack CM, Wilson SR, Charboneau JW, eds: Diagnostic Ultrasound. Mosby-Year Book, St Louis, 1991, pp 19–29.
23. American Institute of Ultrasound in Medicine: Acoustical Data for Diagnostic Ultrasound Equipment, AIUM, JUM, Rockville, MD, 1985.
24. Safety Considerations for Diagnostic Ultrasound, revised 1990. Prepared by the Bioeffects Committee of the American Institute of Ultrasound in Medicine, 1991.
25. Hussey M: A Review of the Biological Effects and the Safety of Diagnostic Ultrasound. Department of Physics, Dublin Institute of Technology, Dublin, Ireland, 1991.
26. American Institute of Ultrasound in Medicine: Bioeffects considerations for the safety of diagnostic ultrasound. J Ultrasound Med 1988;7(Suppl):S1.
27. James EA: Ultrasound: Certain considerations of equipment usage. The Physical Basis of Medical Imaging.
28. Merritt CRB: Bioeffect and safety of diagnostic ultrasound. Appl Radiol 1993; Jan:50–54.
29. Brent RL, Jensh RP, Bellman DA: Medical sonography: Reproductive effects and risks. In: Chervenick FA, Isaacson GC, Campbell S: Ultrasound in Obstetrics and Gynecology, vol 1. Little, Brown & Co, Boston, 1993, pp 11–132.
30. Carstensen EL: Acoustic cavitation and safety of diagnostic ultrasound. Ultrasound Med Biol 1987; 13:597.
31. Miller MW, Ziskin MC: Biological consequence of hyperthermia. Ultrasound Med Biol 1989;15:707.
32. Diagnostic Ultrasound Guidance Update. Food and Drug Administration, Rockville, MD, 1987.
33. Taylor KJW: A prudent approach to Doppler ultrasound. Radiology 1987;165:283–284.
34. Taylor KJW, Kremkau FW: Diminishing exposure to Doppler ultrasound: The sonographer's role. J Diagn Med Sonogr 1988;4:5–8.

CHAPTER 4

STATISTICS

Gilbert Ramírez, DrPH

When first asked to write this chapter, I contemplated many different approaches to the topic of statistics. I first envisioned a detailed description of general statistical techniques most often used by those who would be interested in this text. I also considered a technical discussion of specific statistical techniques of interest to the editor of this text and to me, which include methods for prediction such as linear and nonlinear regression analyses. I finally opted instead for a presentation of the statistical process. By process, I am referring to a series of steps that should be followed when analyzing data. I have found when teaching students that those who become familiar with the process (as compared with those who memorize details) tend to achieve higher grades simply because they are able to apply these steps to a multitude of analysis scenarios. The process is what is truly important to most researchers, particularly given the current state of computer and software technology.

A Review of Statistics

The statistical analysis of data proceeds best when carried out according to a detailed plan of action. Statistics is much more than a set of equations (or menu selections from a statistical software package)—it is a process. The process, often ignored or given little emphasis in introductory statistics classes, provides the basic structure for planning and implementing the statistical analysis and, if carried out properly, increases the likelihood of high-quality results when the analysis has been completed.

THE PROCESS

The process is very simple. First, you need to clearly understand the research question you are attempting to answer. Although at first this may seem somewhat ludicrous (surely researchers must understand what it is they are about to study), statistical results often do not answer the original research question because of various methodological factors. The methodological factor that most often affects the quality of a statistical analysis is the selection of an appropriate statistical test.

I personally believe the single most important reason why mistakes are made when a researcher selects a statistical test is the manner in which introductory statistics courses are taught, which often reflects the way introductory statistics textbooks are written. Most introductory texts begin with an overview of the importance of statistics (and how they are useful), follow with a discussion of descriptive statistics and an introduction to hypothesis formulation and testing, and culminate with the presentation of inferential statistics for various analysis situations. This is a piecemeal approach in which most students learn just enough to get by from one examination to the next. Many researchers receive only a single statistics course or, at most, two or three and are greatly influenced (perhaps handicapped) by this piecemeal approach to statistical analyses.

Rather than teaching statistics by a piecemeal approach, I prefer establishing a firm foundation in a systematic process from which students learn how to plan and carry out a statistical analysis. As each new analysis situation is revealed, the structure of the process is reintroduced, thereby ensuring what is learned is the process itself, which can then be applied to any analysis situation confronted by the student (and ultimately by the future researcher). Even if these students never conduct their own research, they become wiser consumers of statistical analyses when they evaluate research findings of their colleagues or when the need arises to hire the services of a statistical consultant.

The process begins with formulating the hypothesis. This is required whether you are attempting to collect and analyze new data (primary data analyses) or analyzing existing data (secondary data analyses). Once a hypothesis has been formulated, the analyst should then examine the types of data that are available and make a preliminary determination of which statistical tests are appropriate. I emphasize *preliminary* because once the data have been collected and perused, certain limitations may preclude the use of a preferred statistical test and require the use of an alternative.

For those collecting their own data, several concerns need to be addressed by the analyst, because they may affect data quality and subsequently influence the choice of the statistical test. For example, does the person who is filling out the data collection form (interviewer, respondent) fully understand what is being asked? If items are closed ended, have sufficient responses been provided or do the majority of respondents answer "not applicable" or some similar response? These types of concerns require pilot testing of data collection instruments—a step that often is left out because of either time or funds. When pilot testing has been omitted, errors often are not identified until they are too late to rectify, leaving the researcher too few options for the statistical analysis phase.

Once data collection has ended, the analyst can begin the descriptive statistical analysis phase. The importance of this step should not be overlooked, nor should the descriptive analysis be hurried along (in an effort to get to the inferential analysis). Descriptive analyses reveal much about the data, particularly in terms of outliers. The analyst should always be aware of outliers, because important decisions must be made about how to deal with these observations *before* proceeding with the inferential analysis. For example, should the outliers simply be omitted from the analysis, or should they be examined as a separate group? Descriptive analyses also aid the researcher in determining if important assumptions of specific statistical tests have been violated. For example, are the data normally distributed, and if not, should the data be transformed to a normal distribution? These questions are important in selecting an inferential statistical test and can be answered only by carefully carrying out the descriptive analyses.

If the analysis strategy has been properly designed and carried out, the researcher will often have a good idea of what to expect well before the inferential analyses are carried out. In this sense, the inferential statistical analysis only serves to confirm what has been gleaned from the descriptive analyses, and what remains is the interpretation of findings. When the research hypothesis is not confirmed, the analyst must avoid the temptation to apply other statistical procedures, thinking perhaps that there is a better way to analyze the data.

What has been presented thus far is an overview of the stages of the statistical analysis process. I next present a slightly more in-depth discussion of each stage, recognizing the inherent limitations when this subject is restricted to a single chapter. This presentation is intended only as a review of concepts that readers of this text should have already been exposed to. For more detailed discussion of these issues, readers are encouraged to refer to standard statistical texts such as those in the reference list or those that they are currently familiar with.

THE RESEARCH QUESTION

The research question needs to be clearly stated and should be as succinct as the particular situation allows. The research question is typically expressed in broad terms, such as, What is the relationship between gestational age and fetal head size? Even though this question appears clear and is definitely succinct, the reader should quickly observe three definitional problems: What exactly is meant by, first, gestational age; second, fetal head size; and third, relationship? The first two definitional problems are what researchers refer to as *constructs*. What is most important is how these constructs are operationalized, because that will greatly influence the choice of a statistical procedure. For example, gestational age could be operationalized as number of days, weeks, and so on, based on the last menstrual period. It could also be operationalized as simply preterm, term, or postterm. These two operationalizations result in two different scales of measurement, the former being ratio and the latter being ordinal. Scale of measurement is an important factor in selecting an appropriate statistical test. Fetal head size is also problematic, because one could measure it in various ways, of which the most commonly used is based on a two-dimensional measurement. A three-dimensional measurement also has been proposed, and it would present a different operationalization of the construct. Finally, the concept *relationship* also needs further clarification, which typically is more statistical in nature than the research constructs. Is the researcher interested in a cause-effect relationship or simply one of association? The two are quite different ways of looking at relationships and require different statistical techniques as well as different research designs.

A more specific research question, and one of interest to me and to the editor of this text, is, Does a three-dimensional measurement of fetal head size provide a more precise prediction of gestational age than a two-dimensional measurement? Although this question is more specific in terms of what is meant by *relationship*, notice that a definitional problem remains with the construct *gestational age* and additional problems now exist with *precise* and *prediction*.

FORMULATION OF HYPOTHESES

Once the research question has been clearly and succinctly stated to the satisfaction of the researcher, the stage has been set to formulate hypotheses. There are essentially two types of hypotheses—research and statistical. A research hypothesis simply states the outcome expected by the researcher in a narrative format. This projection is typically based on observations, for example, in a clinical setting or on reviews of the literature. [As a side note, literature reviews are typically qualitative in nature, but quantitative techniques for reviewing or synthesizing the literature are now available. These techniques, commonly referred to as *meta-analysis*, are described later in this chapter.] As with the research question, considerable effort should be given to formulating the research hypothesis because it determines the formulation of the statistical hypotheses. One should note that it is particularly important to describe the operationalization of constructs in the statement of the research hypothesis—for example, What is the relationship between gestational age *as measured by weeks of gestation based on the last menstrual period and weeks of gestation measured by LMP*?

There are basically two statistical hypotheses, both of which are simply mathematical statements: the null and the alternative hypotheses. In my statistics classes, I begin by explaining the alternative hypothesis (H_A) simply because it reflects (or should) exactly what has been stated by the research hypothesis, but in mathematical terms. As with any mathematical statement (equation) there are three possible relationships: equal, less than, or greater than; the latter two may also be summarized as not equal. When formulating statistical hypotheses, I constantly remind my students that all three mathematical relationships must be accounted for in the statement of statistical hypotheses. For example, if the research hypothesis reflects an expectation of change in a specified direction—for example, an increase or decrease in some value such as a reduction of average cholesterol level after administering a specified drug regimen—then the alternative hypothesis should reflect the same expectation:

$$H_A\colon \mu_{\text{after treatment}} < \mu_{\text{before treatment}}$$

The formulation of the null hypothesis then simply accounts for the mathematical relationships not reflected by the alternative hypothesis:

$$H_0\colon \mu_{\text{after treatment}} \geq \mu_{\text{before treatment}}$$

Similarly, if the alternative hypothesis suggests an increase, or $>$, then the null hypothesis would reflect the opposite, or $\leq$. Both of these situations are referred to as *directional hypotheses*, in which change is anticipated in a specified direction and the analyst wants to use a one-tail statistical test. When the research hypothesis is nondirectional—that is, when change is anticipated but the researcher is unsure about the direction in which it will occur—then a two-tail statistical test *must* be used. The mathematical relationships would be expressed as follows:

$$H_0\colon \mu_{\text{after treatment}} = \mu_{\text{before treatment}} \quad \text{and}$$

$$H_A\colon \mu_{\text{after treatment}} \neq \mu_{\text{before treatment}}.$$

Students often fail to see the importance of being able to take advantage of a one-tail statistical test. Quite simply, when the hypothesis is directional, the analyst is able to allow for error at one end of the probability distribution, resulting in a criterion for rejection of the null hypothesis that has a lower value than when using a two-tail statistical test, which could be the difference between confirming and failing to confirm a research hypothesis. The analyst is cautioned, however, that the use of a directional hypothesis must be theoretically justifiable. When in doubt or when the theoretical evidence underlying the directionality of the research hypothesis is weak, use a two-tail statistical test.

The notion of rejecting the null hypothesis having been introduced, there is no better time to elaborate on this all-important concept. The purpose of conducting statistical analyses is to determine if the evidence sufficiently supports the research hypothesis. *Sufficiently supports* is a far cry from absolute proof, and the goal of the researcher is to minimize the probability of making an incorrect decision with regard to the research hypothesis. Because it is generally easier to disprove than to prove a hypothesis, statistical decisions are made with regard to the null hypothesis. If sufficient evidence suggests that the null hypothesis is false, then the researcher can reject this statement and accept the alternative—which just happens to be consistent with the research hypothesis. If the evidence is insufficient to believe that the null hypothesis is a false statement (reject the null hypothesis), then that is the end of it—*there is insufficient evidence to reject the null hypothesis*.

What this boils down to is that the researcher is faced with two decisions: Reject the null hypothesis (and therefore accept the alternative) or fail to reject the null hypothesis. The decision that is made, given the evidence at hand, will be either a correct or incorrect decision. Incorrect decisions are errors, of which there are two types. A type I error occurs when a researcher rejects the null hypothesis based on the evidence when in fact the null hypothesis is true. A type II error occurs when a researcher fails to reject the null hypothesis (again based on the evidence) when the null hypothesis is actually false. Each of these errors can be described in terms of its probability of occurrence, *and* it is the researcher's responsibility to prescribe (before carrying out the statistical analysis) what degree or likelihood of errors is acceptable.

The probability of a type I error (rejecting the null hypothesis when it is actually true) is represented by α (alpha), and the probability of a type II error (failing to reject the null hypothesis when it is actually false) is represented by β (beta). The power of a study to detect a specified magnitude of effect (or difference) is also quantifiable as a probability and is equal to the quantity $(1-\beta)$. Although most students and other users of statistics become quite comfortable with α, they typically are less comfortable with β and the concept of power. Students tend to understand that if they wish to carry out a statistical analysis with a 95% degree of confidence, they must use an α of .05. Unfortunately, most also leave their first statistics course believing that all statistical tests are performed at the 95% confidence level, and this is simply not true. As stated earlier, it is the researcher's responsibility to determine α (and β); the level of probability chosen depends on several factors.

A type I error is generally the more serious of the two errors that a researcher can make; thus, it is generally advisable to use a small α. The reasoning behind this assertion is that when a type I error is committed (the null hypothesis is rejected when it is actually a true statement), clinicians are likely to believe there is evidence that the research hypothesis has been confirmed (because the null hypothesis has been rejected and the alternative, which is consistent with the research hypothesis, has been accepted), and that the clinical procedure is effective. On the other hand, when a type II error is committed (the null hypothesis is not rejected when it is actually a false statement), the researcher simply does not have any evidence that the procedure is effective (or ineffective).

Once students recognize the importance of minimizing type I errors, they often ask, "Why not use an α of .01 or .001?" The answer to this question is, There is a tradeoff: As α decreases, sample size increases, resulting in greater study costs. One should also understand that it is sometimes acceptable to increase α, for example, from .05 to .10 (and hence decrease the required sample size) when the impact of a type I error is not severe. For example, it is reasonable to imagine a study in which one is attempting to determine the degree to which different wall colors in a clinic waiting room affect patients' stress levels. Such a decision, although important, is certainly less critical than other decisions that medical researchers face and could be studied with a greater probability of a type I error.

LIMITATIONS PRESENTED BY THE DATA

The type of data also has an important role in selecting an appropriate statistical test. Data can be classified along two dimensions, the first of which simply categorizes the data as continuous or discrete. Continuous data are simply those in which between any two values another value can be found. For example, age is continuous because between any two values, such as 2 years and 3 years, an infinite number of values exist, such as 2.5 years, 2.25 years, and so on. An example of discrete data is number of live births—for example, 2.5 live births does not exist.

Data also can be classified by their scale of measurement, of which there are four categories. *Nominal data* do not reflect any numerical value but are simply used as labels. The best example of nominal data is gender, for even when the values 0 and 1 are used to reflect the two gender classifications, a 1 does not reflect a higher value than 0. The next scale of measurement is *ordinal*. Data that can be classified as ordinal do reflect numerical values—that is, one number can be described as greater than or less than another value—but the exact magnitude of difference cannot be ascertained. The numbers simply represent increasing or decreasing orders of magnitude. An excellent example of ordinal data is college undergraduate classifications of freshman, sophomore, junior, and senior. A student classified as a junior is higher ranked in terms of education than a sophomore, but exactly how much higher is unknown. It is possible that the sophomore in question could be as few as 3 semester hours away from being classified as a junior or even as many as 30 hours.

The third and fourth scales of measurement, *interval* and *ratio*, are quite similar in that they both have well-defined intervals of scale. This means that the difference between 2 and 3 years of age is the same as the difference between 62 and 63 years of age: The 1-year difference in both cases is identical in terms of scale interval. Interval and ratio scales differ in that ratio scales have a true zero whereas interval scales do not, where a true zero means "the absence of." Temperature, when measured in Fahrenheit or Celsius, does not have a true zero because both scales can result in negative temperatures and thus Fahrenheit and Celsius temperature readings are interval scales of measurement; temperature also can be measured with a ratio scale if one uses the Kelvin measurement. An important implication of true-zero scales is that an exact magnitude of difference can be obtained: 200°K is twice as hot as 100°K. This is not the case for 200° and 100°F or C.

SELECTING THE APPROPRIATE STATISTICAL TEST

Several introductory statistical texts present flow charts for selecting an appropriate statistical test. I do not present a flow chart because most readers have access to one or more of these tools (most of the references at the end of this chapter contain at least one flow chart). Flow charts range from a single page to many but share similar characteristics. With any flow chart, the reader must respond to a series of questions that are relevant to the specific analysis situation. The answers to these questions dictate the correct path to follow, with the end result being the recommended statistical test(s). Several statistical software packages have flow charts integrated in the program. Readers respond to questions (as in a flow chart), with the end result again being the recommended statistical test(s).

These decision tools typically ask three to four series of questions. One series of questions deals with the type of data being analyzed. Are the data continuous or discrete? Are the data nominal, ordinal, interval/ratio? Although this is the most basic question one must deal with in selecting an appropriate statistical test, I have found it to be the one that most students have difficulty with at the end of their first statistics course. Because the concept is relatively simple (compared with other statistical concepts), instructors tend not to spend a sufficient amount of time in the semester ensuring that this basic concept is fully understood.

A second series of questions deals with the group(s) being evaluated. For example, is the researcher interested in evaluating a single value from a sample by comparing it with a hypothesized population value? Alternatively, is the researcher interested in comparing values from two samples or from three or more samples? A third question (sometimes integrated with the questions regarding groups) asks, What statistic is being evaluated? For example, does the researcher want to evaluate a measure of central tendency (mean, median, mode) or a measure of variability (variance/standard deviation, semi-interquartile range)?

Finally, the researcher must address a series of questions that relate to important underlying assumptions of statistical tests. The statistical tests that have underlying assumptions are called *parametric statistical tests* and are usually the preferred methods of analysis; when these assumptions have not been met by the data, the researcher must choose an alternative test from a set of procedures called *nonparametric statistical tests.*

These underlying assumptions include such issues as the normality of data, independence of observations, and homogeneity of variance. These are the most difficult questions to answer, and the answers are rarely exact. For example, a data set may not appear exactly normal but may be "close enough." Some of these assumptions are robust to violations—that is, they may be violated to a certain degree without seriously affecting the results of the statistical analysis. Some assumptions are not robust, which means that they cannot be violated. The list of underlying assumptions is too great to present here, and readers are encouraged to consult other statistical texts to identify assumptions specific to the statistical test of interest.

DESCRIPTIVE STATISTICS

Descriptive statistics include two types. The first type of descriptive statistics provides an expanded view of the data and includes such things as frequency distribution tables and graphs. Frequency distribution tables provide a view of the data in terms of the number of events that exist for specified levels of a variable. The levels of the variable that are presented depend on the range of values. If the range of values is small, then individual levels (e.g., 54, 55, 56) may be presented. If the range is large, then values are typically grouped in intervals (e.g., 50–54, 55–59). In addition to presenting the number of events (frequency) for each level/interval, a frequency distribution table also includes the relative frequencies (percent or proportion) and the cumulative relative frequencies.

Frequency distributions can also be displayed using graphs such as histograms, bar charts, or frequency polygons. Histograms are typically used to present the frequency or relative frequency distributions for variables that are continuous. The bars in the histogram are usually connected to reflect the continuous nature of the variable values. Discrete data are usually represented using bar charts in which the bars are not connected. A frequency polygon may be used instead of a histogram, and instead of bars, a line is drawn connecting the points that would have been located at the top and center of each bar had a histogram been drawn.

It is also useful to describe the data using summary measures, which differ from the expanded view provided by frequency distribution presentations in that they provide a single value that describes the data. These summary measures describe either central tendency or variability.

Summary measures of central tendency include the mean, median, and mode. The mean is the preferred measure and is simply the average of all values. It is the preferred measure because it includes information from all the data. The median is the value that splits the data set in half, the middle value. The median is used when the data are skewed—significant numbers of events that are extremely low or high compared with the rest of the data. The mode is simply the value that occurs most often and is used primarily with nominal and ordinal data. Data sets can have more than one mode, such as when two or more values are represented by the same number of events.

Summary measures of variability include the range, the semi-interquartile range, and the standard deviation/variance. The range is the simplest measure of variability to compute and is the difference between the highest and lowest values in the data set. The semi-interquartile range uses the three values that separate the data set into quartiles (Q1, Q2, Q3); specifically, it is the value of the difference (Q3 − Q1) divided by 2. The standard deviation and variance are the preferred summary measures of variability because they use all of the information provided by the data set. A deviation (or deviation score) is the value represented by subtracting the mean (summary measure of central tendency) from a specific value of the variable under study; each individual event has its own deviation score. The standard deviation can be thought of as the typical deviation score or the average deviation score. The standard deviation is not a true average because it is computed from the square root of squared deviation scores and is not a simple average of deviation scores. The variance is simply the squared value of the standard deviation.

Choosing an appropriate measure of variability to describe a data set depends primarily on the measure of central tendency being used. When reporting the mean, the researcher should use the standard deviation/variance. If the data dictate the use of a median, the researcher should report the semi-interquartile range. The range should not be used as the only measure of variability, but it should be presented as an additional descriptor of variability along with the standard deviation/variance or semi-interquartile range.

INFERENTIAL STATISTICS

Inferential statistics are used to make decisions about statistical hypotheses. The inferential statistic that is used most often is the *t* statistic, sometimes referred to as the *t*-test. The *t* statistic is similar to the Z statistic with one exception: The Z statistic requires the researcher to know the value of the population variance. Because this value is rarely known, the *t* statistic is used instead.

Inferential statistics, such as the *t* statistic, are calculated and compared with a critical value of the *t* distribution. When the calculated *t* statistic is greater than the critical value, the null hypothesis is rejected. The critical value of the *t* distribution is determined from a table of values that correspond to the *t* distribution and depend on (1) the α level chosen (.05, .01, and so on); (2) whether a one-tail or two-tail test is being used; and (3) the degrees of freedom. Degrees of freedom (df) depend on the sample size (n) of the group(s) being tested and vary depending on whether one is comparing a single sample value (such as the sample mean) with a hypothesized population value (then $df = n - 1$), comparing two independent samples ($df = n_1 + n_2 - 2$), or comparing paired/related samples ($df = n - 1$, where $n = n_1 = n_2$). The process is the same whether one is using a *t* statistic or some other statistic: The calculated statistic is compared with a critical value, and when greater (for most statistical tests), the null hypothesis is rejected.

The *t* statistic is also used to test hypotheses other than those comparing means. It is used to test hypotheses regarding the degree of association between two variables when measured as a correlation coefficient. It is also used to test hypotheses regarding the slope of a regression line that is represented by a value known as the beta coefficient. When conducting a multiple regression analysis (more than one independent variable and hence a multidimensional slope), a *t* statistic is calculated for each individual slope.

One limitation of the *t* statistic is that it can be used only to compare two values—for example, two means, a single value (mean, correlation coefficient, beta coefficient) with a hypothesized value, and so forth. When the researcher is interested in comparing more than two values, such as the means from three or more groups, a different inferential statistic must be used. For situations in which its underlying assumptions have been met, the F statistic is preferred. The F statistic is derived by using a method known as the analysis of variance (ANOVA), which essentially evaluates differences in group means by comparing the degree of variation within each group and between the groups. The process is the same as described for the *t* statistic: The researcher must calculate the F statistic for the data set being examined and compare this value with a critical F value. The critical F value, like the critical *t* value, is also determined from a table of values describing the F distribution. Information that is needed to determine the critical F value includes the α value chosen and degrees of freedom. Because the F statistic evaluates variation from two sources, two values exist for degree of freedom. The F statistic is the ratio of the variation between the groups to the variation within each group. When the ratio is less than or equal to 1 (no difference), then the evidence suggests that most of the variability comes from within each group (as compared to between groups) and therefore the groups are not different. As the magnitude of difference between groups increases, the F statistic (ratio) also increases. Large values of the F statistic tend to suggest that differences exist between groups; how large the differences are depends on the critical value, which depends on the degrees of freedom. The two values for degrees of freedom are sometimes referred to as the *numerator* (between group variance) and *denominator* (with group variance) degrees of freedom. The numerator degrees of freedom is calculated as $(k - 1)$, where k equals the number of groups. The denominator degrees of freedom is calculated as $(N - k)$, where N equals the total number of observations across all groups $(n_1 + n_2 + n_3 + \ldots + n_k)$.

When carrying out ANOVA, it is important to understand what it means when the null hypothesis is rejected. The null hypothesis for the ANOVA essentially states that the means from all the groups are equal. When this hypothesis is rejected, the alternative hypothesis, which is now accepted, simply states that at least two of the group means are not equal. It does not mean that all groups are different. Because the researcher is more interested in determining which groups are different, additional statistical tests must be used. These tests are referred to as *post hoc comparisons*. Several post hoc comparison methods may be used—the Scheffe, Tukey, and Dunnett, to name a few—the choice of which depends on several parameters. Some post hoc comparisons tend to be more conservative than others, and some may be used only in limited situations. Most of these post hoc tests use *t* statistics, and the reader is encouraged to review other statistical texts (which provide more detail than can be given in a single chapter) when the need arises.

The chi-squared is another test statistic that is often used, particularly in the medical field. Researchers often are not interested in comparing summary values such as the mean but are more interested in evaluating the distribution of the number of events across different categories. For example, a researcher might be interested in the number of births across a 2×2 table that describes the distribution of events by two categories such as (1) preterm or otherwise and (2) mother smokes cigarettes or not. In this type of analysis situation, the researcher is interested in determining if there is a relationship between two variables, e.g., preterm birth status and maternal smoking status.

When variables are independent (not related), the distribution of the number of events that occur within each of the four cells (four combinations exist for two variables each with two levels) should be relatively equal. When variables are not independent, a disproportionate distribution of the number of events is noted across the four cells. The degree of disproportionality is determined by calculating a chi-squared statistic, which is a function of the differences between the values observed and the values that would be expected when the variables are independent. The greater the disproportion, the larger the chi-squared statistic. As with the other statistical tests, the process is the same: The chi-squared statistic is compared with a critical value that is obtained from a table that describes the distribution of chi-squared values. To determine the critical value, the researcher must know the prescribed α value and degrees of freedom. For a 2×2 table, the degrees of freedom is equal to 1. The chi-squared test of independence can also be used to test the independence of variables when the number of levels of each variable is greater than 2. For example, one could examine gestation status—preterm, term, and postterm—compared with the number of cigarettes smoked daily using the categories of 0, 1 to 10, 10 to 20, and more than 20. This would result in a 3×4 table. Degrees of freedom is determined by the equation $df = (C - 1)(R - 1)$, where C equals the number of columns and R equals the number of rows in the table.

Many other statistical tests may be used, but the ones just described are without a doubt used most often. A set of nonparametric statistical tests may be used in lieu of parametric tests, such as the *t*-test and F test, when important underlying assumptions have been violated. Each statistical test uses a similar process: The calculated test statistic is compared with a critical value. Depending on the test being used, the decision to reject or fail to reject a null hypothesis depends on which value is larger. Readers should refer to other statistical texts when choosing a statistical test and for knowing the correct decision rule.

Meta-Analysis

Research hypotheses are often formulated based on reviews of earlier studies. When reviewing other studies, it is common to find considerable disagreement. Some studies result in a rejection of the null hypothesis (statistical significance was obtained), whereas others result in a failure to reject the null hypothesis (statistical significance was not obtained). Researchers must decide from the cumulation of studies what is "truth," which is difficult to do when similar studies result in disparate findings. A simple but erroneous approach that is often used is simply to weigh the number of studies that are statistically significant against those not statistically significant. This procedure is referred to as vote counting.

The problem with vote counting is that statistical significance depends too much on sample size. Studies that have large sample sizes have a greater chance of obtaining statistical significance than those with small sample sizes. Most statistical tests are a function of two parameters. The first, as mentioned earlier, is sample size. The second parameter is the magnitude of the effect being studied, or effect size. The size of the effect is analogous to clinical significance. It is quite possible to achieve statistical significance even when clinically the effect is small. It is also possible to observe a significant clinical effect and still report a nonstatistical significance. When reviewing the literature, it is important to examine statistical significance in terms of effect size (clinical significance) and sample size.

Meta-analysis is a set of statistical techniques that allow researchers to examine the magnitude of effect across studies, thereby avoiding the pitfalls of significance tests and sample sizes. It typically incorporates an effect size statistic, which is the standardized difference of two means (the difference between the experimental and control group means divided by their pooled standard deviation); other methods of calculating effect sizes are also available. When reviewing studies, the meta-analyst calculates an effect size statistic for each study and then calculates a weighted average effect size across all studies. The average effect size is weighted by the degree of variation within each study, with studies having less variation receiving greater weight. The weighted average effect size can then be used to determine, on average, the magnitude of effect that is to be expected.

Meta-analysis can also be used to study variables that otherwise could not be studied in a single research effort. For example, geographical location of patients might be an important variable in the incidence or prevalence of a disease, but when a single study is carried out on a set of patients, geographical location is more often than not a constant. Meta-analysis would allow estimation of the relationship between geographical location and the incidence/prevalence of disease because multiple studies can be used, particularly when each study has been conducted in different geographical locations. Meta-analysis also allows identification of gaps in knowledge (what existing studies do not tell us) and can minimize the inefficient repetition of studies in which knowledge of relationships between variables is well established.

Meta-analysis has received increased attention as a statistical technique during the past decade and is a valuable tool for conducting quantitative reviews of the scientific literature for both confirming hypotheses and generating new directions for research. A wealth of literature on meta-analysis techniques is available, and readers are strongly encouraged to investigate the opportunities provided by these procedures.

In Conclusion

Carrying out a statistical analysis is a relatively simple exercise if one understands the process involved. We no longer have to calculate test statistics manually—statistical software packages do this for us. Nor do we have to determine critical values, because the software packages also provide *P* values, which reflect the probability that the observed findings are due to chance alone. When the *P* value is less than our chosen α level, we reject the null hypothesis. Because technology eliminates the drudgery of statistical analyses (and much of the error), students (with regard to statistics, most of us remain students for life) can now focus their attention on interpreting statistical results. Statistics instructors can focus on teaching the statistical process and not the statistical equations.

This chapter has not attempted to provide a detailed description of statistical tests, because this information is readily available elsewhere. Rather, what I have attempted to provide is my conceptualization of the statistical analysis process, which then enables an investigator to select appropriate statistical tests. In some situations, statistical consultants must be brought in to review statistical analyses or to help design and carry out complex procedures beyond the capabilities of the average researcher. The best researchers understand the statistical process (and can therefore apply it to various research situations) but also know the limitations of their own knowledge (and hence know when to use the services of a trained statistician).

SELECTED READINGS

Chatfield C: Problem Solving—A Statistician's Guide. Chapman & Hall, London, 1991.

Daniel DW: Biostatistics: A Foundation for Analysis in the Health Sciences, 5th ed. John Wiley & Sons, New York, 1991.

Freedman D, Pisani R, Purves R, et al: Statistics, 2nd ed. WW Norton, New York, 1991.

Glantz SA: Primer of Bio-Statistics, 3rd ed. McGraw-Hill, New York, 1992.

Hedges LV, Olkin I: Statistical Methods for Meta-Analysis. Academic Press, Orlando, 1985.

Hunter JE, Schmidt FL: Methods of Meta-Analysis, Correcting Error and Bias in Research Findings. Sage Publications, Newbury Park, CA, 1990.

Kleinbaum DG, Kupper LL, Muller KE: Applied Regression Analysis and Other Multivariable Methods, 2nd ed. PWS-KENT Publishing, Boston, 1988.

Mullen PD, Ramírez G: Information synthesis and meta-analysis. In: Ward WB, ed: Advances in Health Education and Promotion, vol 2. JAI Press, Greenwich, CT, 1987.

CHAPTER 5

PHYSICS AND METHODOLOGY OF OBSTETRICAL SONOGRAPHY

Terry J. DuBose
Larry W. Hill, MD

Sonographic Geometry and Transducer Manipulation

SONOGRAPHIC METHODS

Cybernetics

Diagnostic medical sonography is an exercise in cybernetics. The Random House *Dictionary of the English Language* (1981) defines cybernetics as "The study of human control functions and of mechanical and electric systems designed to replace them, involving the application of statistical mechanics to communication engineering." The Random House *American College Dictionary* (1959) defines cybernetics this way: "The scientific study of those methods of control and communication which are common to living organisms and machines, esp. as applied to the analysis of the operations of machines such as computers."

In sonography, the cybernetic exercise is more a process of controlling the sonographic equipment in order to extend the human senses rather than a process of controlling or replacing the senses. In a very real sense, the sonographer and the sonographic equipment become integrated in such a way that the sonographer's knowledge and mental imagery and the sonographic machine's ability to extend vision beyond the surfaces of the body allow accumulation of information about the internal organs that is not available without this integration. This integration of machine and observer is not unique to diagnostic medical sonography. It also applies to radiographic equipment and other devices. With sonography, however, an intimate relationship exists between the sonographer and the machine, requiring constant interpretation of the image and adjustment in order to optimize the information gained. With most radiographic equipment, the controls are adjusted once, before the exposure, and repeat images are considered poor practice.

Sonography requires more than normal eye-hand coordination and control. As the hand moves the transducer across or inside a patient's body, the area of interest is actually a plane that extends beyond the front of the transducer. The eye observes the area of interest on a video screen. In between the hand and eye is the sonographic machine, with its integrated computer video system of considerable sophistication. Sonography requires more than simply the eye's guiding the finger to touch an object or perform some task. The sonographic machine is within this eye-hand neural loop.

While the eye is observing the computer video, the brain is transmitting signals and requests to the hand for certain manipulations of the transducer. The mind is assimilating the information available and forming a mental image of the three-dimensional shape of the organs in front of the transducer. This bit of eye-computer-hand coordination and mental gymnastics is the essence of sonographic cybernetics.

To perform diagnostic medical sonography smoothly and quickly requires considerable experience. Learning to perform sonography is similar to learning to drive an automobile, when one must think about stepping on the brake or accelerator, giving turn signals, turning the steering wheel, watching for other autos and pedestrians, and staying off the sidewalk and on the road. At first everyone is a bit jerky. With experience and time, though, this process becomes more automatic, and after a while, a driver can do all of this without giving it much thought at all. With experience, the driver will perform the tasks and even simultaneously carry on a conversation without difficulty.

When learning diagnostic medical sonography, a student first feels much concern over controlling the equipment, selecting the correct transducer, setting the focal range, gain, and field of view, manipulating the transducer, and recording images. It is easy for a beginner to be distracted from the real objective of defining the anatomy and any pathology that may be present. However, with strong desire, time, experience, proper supervision, knowledge of acoustic physics, and a solid understanding of the three-dimensional anatomy and pathological processes, a neophyte sonographer/sonologist will be able to concentrate on the job at hand without much distraction from the equipment. It must be emphasized that this process is complex and requires experience for success. A strong desire to learn sonography is a prerequisite.

Mental Imaging

A sonographer/sonologist uses all the available information—a patient's medical history, palpation, sonographic anatomy, and sonographic artifacts—to form a mental image of the three-dimensional anatomy. This means that the first task of fetal sonography, after setting up the machine, recording the medical history, and preparing the patient, is to form a mental image of the contents of a pregnant woman's abdomen and uterus (Fig. 5–1).

Presented with the mound of flesh that is a pregnant woman's abdomen at term, the sonographer should first perform a survey scan. This initial survey allows the determination of whether the head is up (breech presentation) or down (cephalic presentation), whether the fetus is lying on its left or right side, whether it is prone or supine, and whether the spine is to the woman's left or right.

Forming this first mental image of the fetal position within the woman greatly facilitates and speeds the rest of the examination. This initial survey helps to locate specific organs as the examination continues. However, one must not forget that a fetus may change position during an examination. A fetus in the first two trimesters can move from a breech to a cephalic presentation in a very short time. During the third trimester, a fetus tends to move less as it becomes more crowded in the uterus.

The mental imaging process involves remembering the location of the gross anatomical features as the initial survey progresses. In this context, the observer's mind becomes an integral part of the cybernetic complex, which includes the eye, hand, and neural system as well as the sonographic equipment. The mental image actually serves as a memory bank and logic system that is much larger and more sophisticated than is available in any sonographic machine.

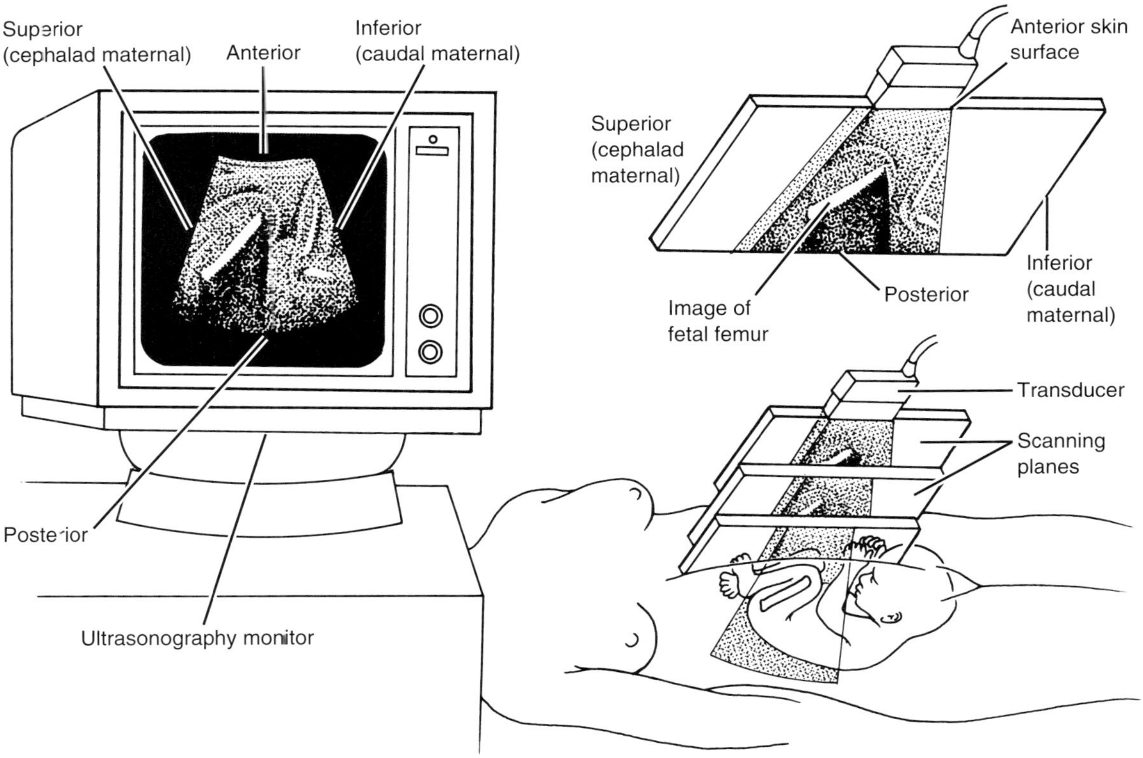

FIGURE 5–1.
Scanning plane orientation—longitudinal. The fetal femur is displayed in the field of view. Because only one section of the total fetus and uterus can be observed at a time, the transducer must be moved in order to visualize the entire anatomy. Linear structures such as the femur must be in the plane of view to be measured.

Sonographic Video Conventions

Most sonographic machines have wheels or can be carried and thus are portable. It follows that the sonographic laboratory or examination room can be arranged however a sonographer chooses. Many sonographers perform carotid Doppler examinations from a patient's head; others have the examination table to their right. For abdominal and obstetrical sonography, the most common arrangement seems to be the one in Figure 5–2.

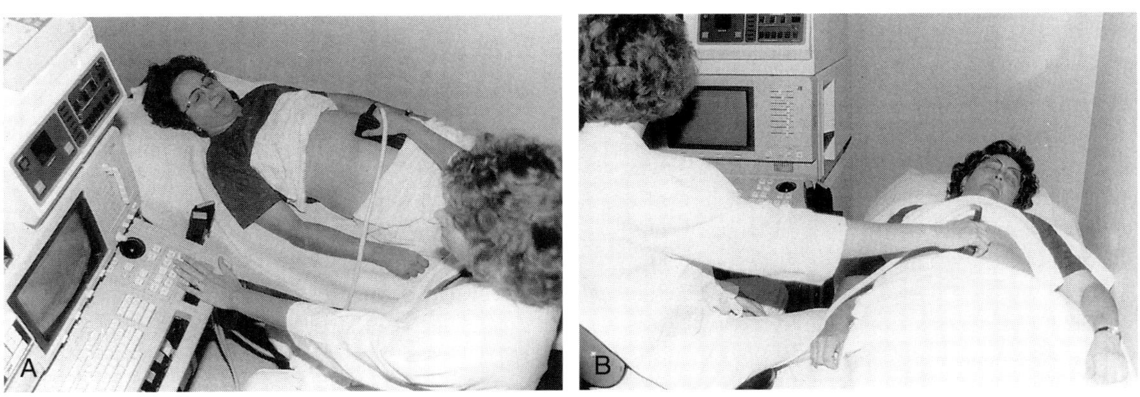

FIGURE 5–2.
The typical arrangement of the sonographic examination room. Notice that the patient's right side is on video left and her left side is on video right. It should also be noted that when the sonographer faces the patient, the patient's head is to the left and her feet are to the right. This is also the convention for the video display that is shown in Figure 5–1.

The arrangement shown in Figures 5–1 and 5–2 corresponds well with mental imaging. The patient's head is forward, or in the direction of the screen, and using the transverse field of view, the patient's right side is on the observer's video left. With this orientation, the patient's right is to the left and the patient's left is to the right for both the video and the sonographer. It also helps for the sonographer to realize that if he or she faces the patient, then the patient's head will be toward the left, just as it is in the conventional video display. This is similar to stage right and stage left versus audience right and audience left. It is also the reason why sonography can be somewhat more confusing to an observer who is standing on the other side of the patient. The patient's head is then physically on the right, which is backward to the conventional sonographic video presentation.

This discussion uses the conventions mentioned earlier for the transducer orientation. The head of the transducer is always toward a patient's head or right and is video left. The transducer toe is the end that is video right and toward a patient's feet or left.*

GEOMETRY OF TRANSDUCER MANIPULATION

To perform the initial survey and to complete the entire sonographic examination, the sonographic transducer must be manipulated over or inside a patient's body. The Austin Community College Diagnostic Medical Sonography class of 1991–1992 (see acknowledgments) developed a working vocabulary to describe these transducer manipulations. This was similar to the transvaginal transducer manipulation vocabulary proposed by Abramowicz.[1,2] A similar attempt at codifying transducer movements was made by Timor-Tritsch and Rottem.[3] Their book discusses only transvaginal sonography and three types of transducer motions: rotating, angling, and pushing-pulling. Although this systematic description is applicable to endocavity sonography, it is not comprehensive enough to describe all types of transducer manipulations, particularly transabdominal sonography.

*Toe/head terms from Pam Clayton, RDMS.

In order to develop a comprehensive vocabulary to describe the motions used with all transducers, we drew from Timor-Tritsch and Rottem's description and developed what we believe is a useful working vocabulary to describe the process. In this vocabulary, four basic motions are used in diagnostic sonography: sliding, rocking or angling, rotating, and compression. These four motions can be used singly or in combinations. This may seem obvious to an experienced sonographer/sonologist but most likely is confusing to a beginner. For the experienced, it is hoped that this vocabulary will make discussion of the sonographic process easier. For the student, it is hoped that this discussion, although perplexing at first, will facilitate an understanding of the process.

One addition to the vocabulary of the motions is a description of the direction in which the motions are occurring. Because these terms describe the movement of the transducer, which is producing a scan plane or field of view that moves with the transducer and that is related to a patient's anatomy, we tried to avoid the use of words that would be confused with commonly used anatomical terms such as lateral, transverse, longitudinal, axial, and so forth. The terms we chose to use relate to the scan plane or field of view and not a patient's anatomy. These descriptions of the motions are used in conjunction with the four motions described earlier and include *in-plane* and *cross-plane* motions. Anatomical modifiers are then used to describe the relationship of the motion to the patient—that is, some motions would be described as a *transverse in-plane slide*, *sagittal in-plane slide*, and so on (discussed later).

The following is a discussion of each of the four basic motions and the combinations of motions. The concepts are not difficult to understand, but considerable verbiage is required to describe them. However, once the vocabulary is understood, we believe that these descriptions will expedite the teaching of sonography and provide a method of discussing these concepts.

For the purpose of this discussion, it is assumed that the sonographer is using a linear array transducer. The principles are the same for sector transducers, including transvaginal; however, because of the narrow near field of view, it is slightly more difficult to explain. Also, in this discussion, it is necessary to discuss the ends of the linear array transducer. The discussion uses the foregoing conventions. The head of the transducer is always toward video left and toward a patient's head or right, and the transducer toe is toward video right and toward a patient's feet or left.

Sliding

In-Plane Sliding. In-plane sliding involves sliding the transducer without a change of the angles of the field of view. This means that the orientation of the plane does not change; it only moves along in the same plane (Fig. 5–3*A* and *B*). This maneuver is used to study the long axes of the uterus, fetal spine, or long bones of the extremities. A sonographer might begin scanning in the midsagittal plane over the lower uterine segment and slide the transducer toward the woman's head while remaining in the midsagittal plane. This would cause the urinary bladder to move slowly out of the field of view to the right of the video, whereas more cephalic anatomy would enter the field of view from video left. This type of maneuver would be referred to as a *cephalic in-plane slide*.

Because a fetus might be in a transverse lie with its head to the woman's right, it would be necessary to perform a transverse in-plane slide to examine the long axis of the fetal spine. This transverse in-plane slide could be in the direction of the woman's left or right.

A transverse in-plane slide used to examine the longitudinal fetal spine from the head to the pelvis, with the head to the woman's right, would start with the transducer on the woman's right, slowly sliding toward her left while keeping the fetal spine in the field of view. This right-to-left in-plane slide would slowly bring the long axis of the fetal lower spine into the field of view from video right as the head and upper spine would leave the field of view on video left.

The in-plane slide can be used with any orientation to a woman's body. It may be a sagittal in-plane slide from the head to foot or from the foot to head. It may be from left to right or from right to left, and it may be in a coronal approach, which would also be described as a head-to-foot or foot-to-head, coronal, in-plane slide.

Cross-Plane Sliding. The cross-plane slide is a motion that moves the field of view perpendicular to the sonographic plane (Fig. 5–3*C* and *D*). This corresponds to the directions of the lateral resolution, which is perpendicular to the transducer field of view. This motion is used to examine successive cross sections of anatomy, as in cross-sectional examination of the fetal spine. This maneuver was termed the *cross-plane slide* rather than the *lateral-plane slide* because we thought that the term *lateral* would be confused with the anatomical lateral aspect.

The cross-plane slide could be a field of view that is transverse to the woman's long axis or spine, sliding toward the woman's head or feet, providing successive, parallel, transverse fields of view. It could also be a sagittal field of view, sliding from left to right or right to left, providing successive, parallel, parasagittal fields of view.

In the foregoing example of the transverse fetal lie with the fetal head to the woman's right and fetal rump to her left, the cross-sectional examination of the fetal spine might start with a transverse view of the fetal head. The field of view is parasagittal in the woman but transverse to the fetus. By cross-plane sliding the transducer across the plane or field of view, toward the woman's left, successive cross sections of the fetal spine come into the field of view as the transducer is moved down the fetal spine.

The cross-plane slide can also be used from any orientation. It is useful for examining large volumes. This motion is often used during the initial obstetrical survey in order to see as much of the uterus and its contents as possible.

Rocking or Angling

Cross-Plane Rocking. During cross-plane rocking or angling, the transducer is kept in one place on a patient's skin and the transducer is rocked from side to side, moving the field of view in a waving or sweeping motion (Fig. 5–4*A*). In this text, the terms *rocking* and *angling* are used interchangeably.

Cross-plane rocking is very useful but is not well understood by most beginner sonog-

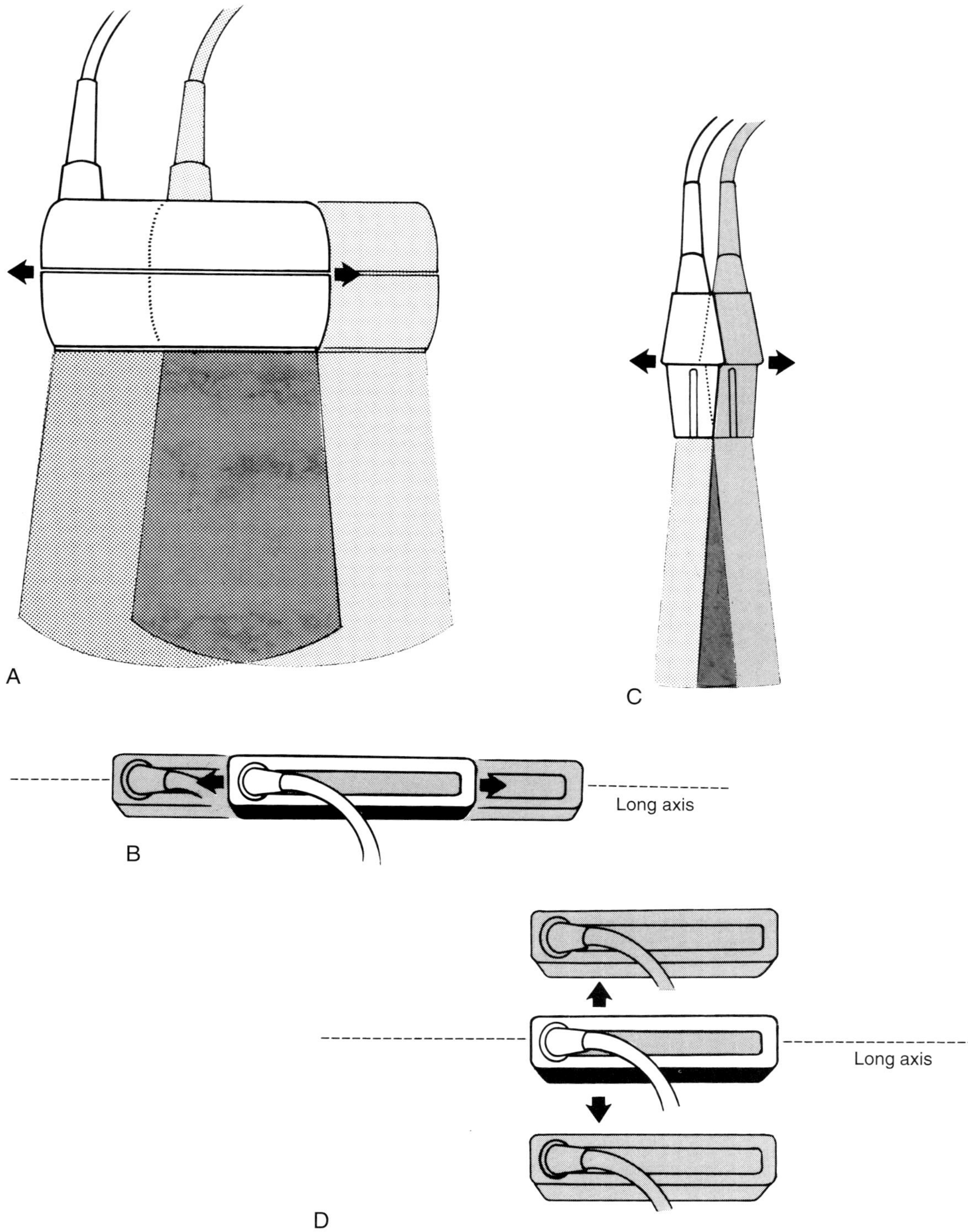

FIGURE 5–3.
Transducer sliding. *A*, The in-plane slide from the side of a linear array. The angles of the plane do not change; the transducer is only slid along in the same plane. This maneuver is effective for observing linear structures such as the fetal spine or extremities. It is also useful for bringing anatomy at the edge of the field of view into the center of the image. *B*, The same in-plane slide that is demonstrated in *A*, but this view is from the top of the linear array. *C*, Cross-plane slide from the end of a linear array transducer. This motion sweeps the field of view so that large volumes of anatomy can be quickly surveyed. *D*, The cross-plane slide from the top. This is the same motion that is being demonstrated in *C*. The cross-plane slide is used to study the fetal spine in cross section.

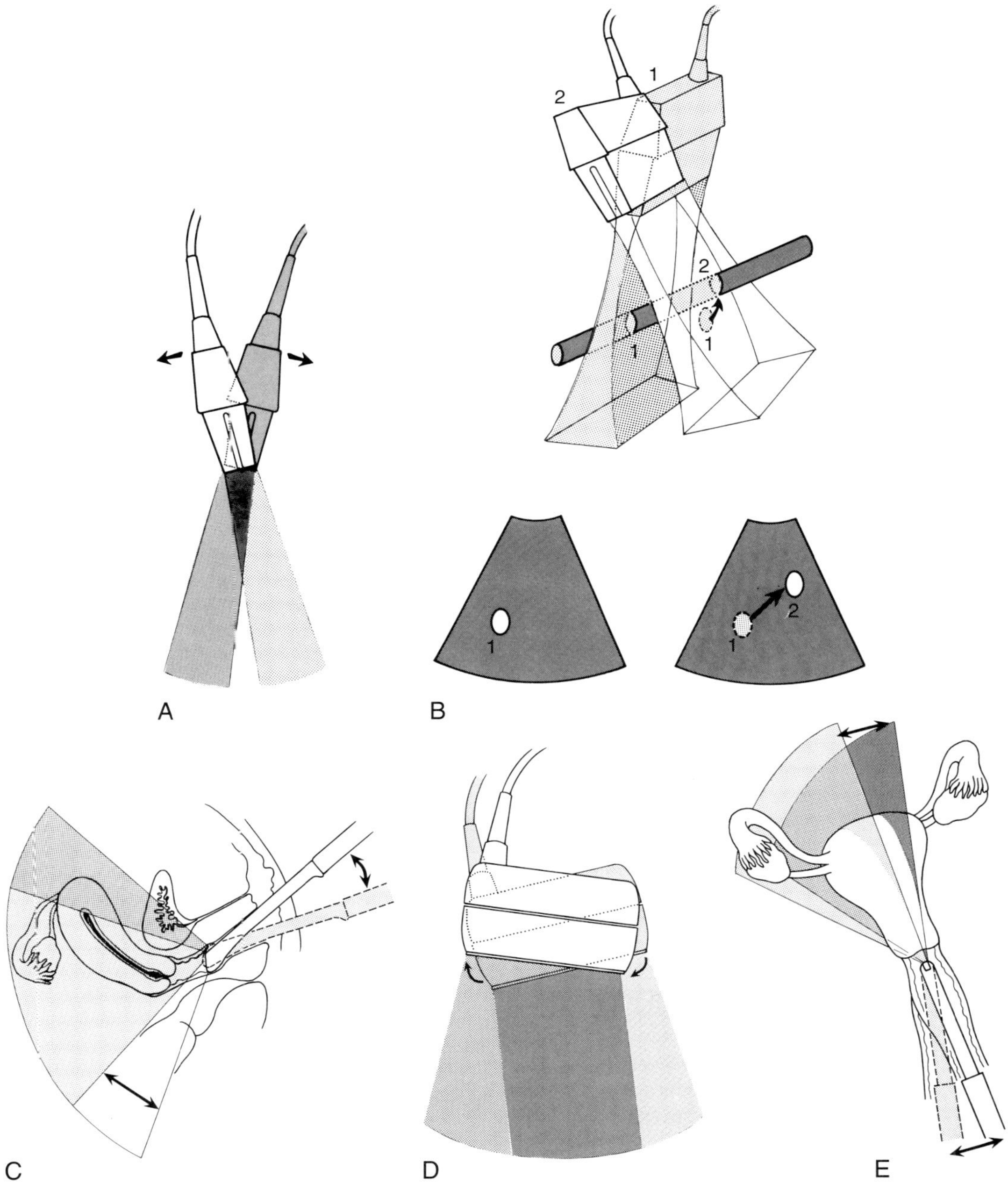

FIGURE 5–4.
A, The side-to-side rocking motion of a transducer. The transducer is not moved but is rocked in a cross-plane motion. *B*, The same cross-plane rocking as demonstrated in *A*. When a linear structure such as the femur is oblique to the plane of view, it appears as a single dot or echo. With cross-plane rocking, this echo appears to move across the field of view. The direction of the movement of the echo in the field of view is the clue that indicates in which direction the transducer must be rotated in order to line up the structure in the plane for measurements. Experienced sonographers do this without much thought. Beginners have to give it some thought and practice in order to understand the process. *C*, The transvaginal transducer handle is moved up and down in order to obtain different views in the same plane. In this drawing, sagittal views of the uterus are obtained. *D*, Transducer in-plane rocking is very similar to cross-plane rocking, except that the motion is in-plane. With this maneuver, the transducer remains on the skin at the same location and in the same plane but is angled in-plane. *E*, Endocavitary cross-plane rocking is the same as cross-plane rocking transabdominally. As the field of view is moved by this action, successive, almost parallel slices of anatomy are observed. In this drawing, successive sagittal or parasagittal images of the uterus are observed.

raphers or sonologists. It is very important in determining the orientation of linear structures. Once the orientation is determined, it is easy to rotate the field of view to visualize the long axis of the structure. This process is important for measuring the femur, humerus, or other long bones, as well as for studying the long axis of the spine.

For example, let's suppose you are attempting to measure the length of the femoral diaphysis. You have determined the lie of the fetus, followed the spine down to the pelvis, and located the femur, but it is visualized in cross section. To determine which way to rotate the transducer, use cross-plane rocking. As the transducer is rocked side to side, if the field of view is truly perpendicular to the femur, the echo that is the femur does not move much. If the field of view is slightly oblique to the femur, however, then the femoral echo appears to move toward one edge of the field of view or the other when the transducer is rocked (Fig. 5–4*B* and *E*). The direction of movement of the femoral echo is the clue to which direction to rotate the transducer to obtain the long-axis view of the femur (see the following discussion of clockwise and counterclockwise rotations). With time and experience, this method of determining the orientation of linear structures becomes more automatic; in fact, most experienced sonographers do this without realizing it.

In-Plane Rocking. Once one understands cross-plane rocking, in-plane rocking becomes self-explanatory. During transducer rocking, the transducer is not slid over a patient's skin but is kept in the same location while angling the field of view. This angling keeps the field of view in the same plane while moving the view slightly toward one edge of the field of view. This is a very simple process but difficult to explain (Fig. 5–4*C* and *D*).

In-plane rocking is often used in pelvic sonography to maintain a true midsagittal plane while angling beneath the pubic bone to view the base of a patient's bladder. In fetal sonography, in-plane rocking is used when the proper field of view of the fetal head is obtained but the interhemispheric fissure is not perpendicular to the sonographic beam. By in-plane rocking, it is possible to orient the interhemispheric fissure to obtain specular reflections with the fissure in the true horizontal.

When using a transvaginal or endocavitary transducer, in-plane rocking is used to angle the field of view in a sagittal, long-axis view of the uterus (Fig. 5–4*C*). The field of view could be moved from a sagittal plane through the uterine cervix to a view of the uterine body or fundus in the same plane.

Rotation

Clockwise and Counterclockwise Rotations. Rotation of the transducer is one of the simplest and most often used maneuvers of the transducer (Fig. 5–5*A* and *B*). The transducer is held in a single location on a patient's skin and rotated either clockwise (Fig. 5–5*A*) or counterclockwise (Fig. 5–5*B*). The rotation can be through any number of degrees. A complete 360-degree rotation would take the transducer in a complete circle, with the field of view arriving back where it was at the start. There is little use for 360-degree rotations except to untangle a twisted transducer cable. A 180-degree rotation completely reverses the field of view. A 90-degree rotation is often used to obtain two views that are perpendicular to each other. Rotations of 90 degrees or less are most often used in sonography.

One important consideration in rotating a transducer is the conventions of sonographic viewing discussed earlier. Because the transducer can be rotated in either a clockwise or counterclockwise direction, one should be sure to rotate in the direction that keeps the anatomy in the conventional orientation (i.e., the woman's right or her head on the left side of the screen and her left or foot to video right).

With a transvaginal transducer, rotation is used to move from a sagittal plane to a coronal plane or vice versa (Fig. 5–5*C*).

Compression

Compression with the transducer is occasionally used. A sonographer/sonologist should always be aware of a patient's comfort and well-being when using the compression maneuver. It has been documented that excessive compression of the fetal head may cause decelerations of the fetal heart rate.[4] Although this in and of itself may not be critical, it should not be ignored.

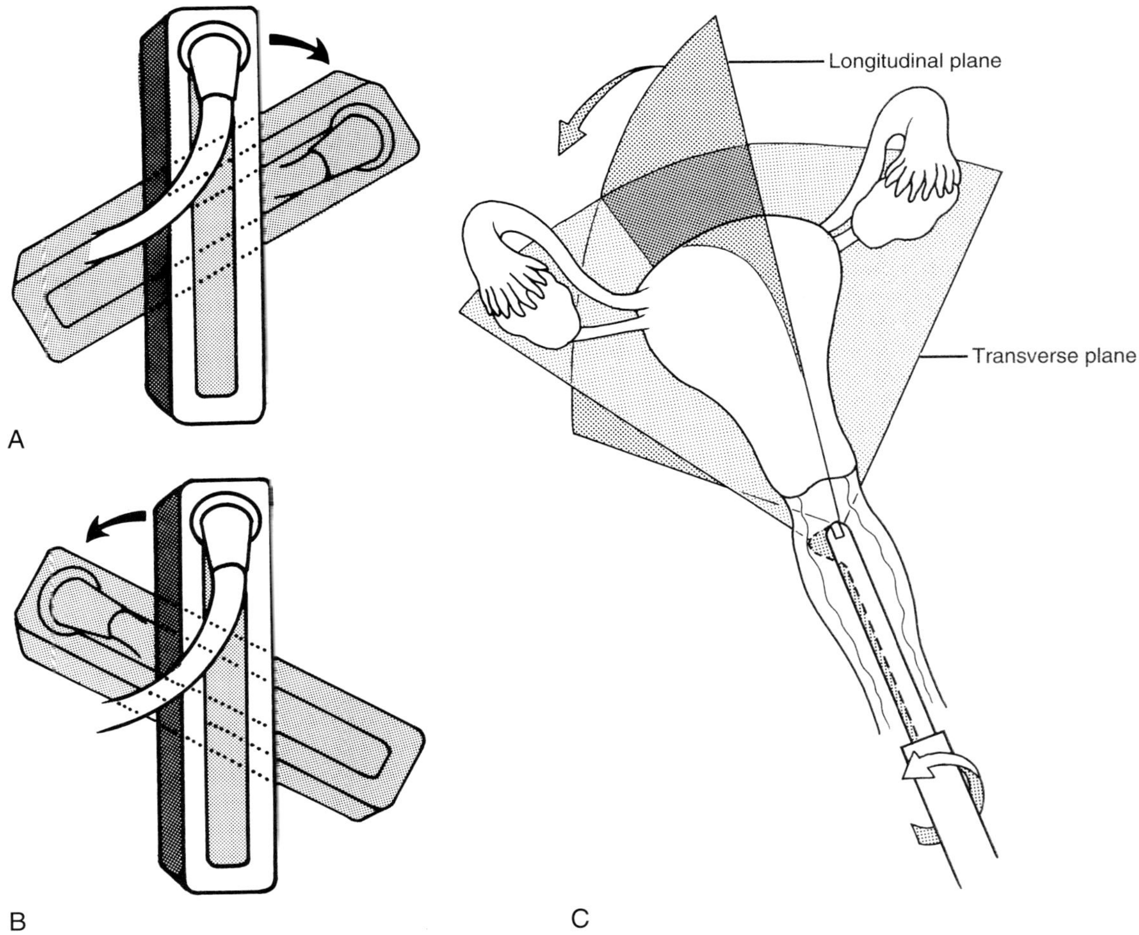

FIGURE 5–5.
A, Clockwise rotation. The center of the transducer remains at the same location on the patient's skin; only the transducer and resulting field of view are rotated. *B*, Counterclockwise rotation. Rotations are very simple and are the easiest to understand. *C*, The transvaginal transducer is rotated counterclockwise to move from a sagittal plane to a coronal plane of the right adnexa. If the transducer is rotated clockwise toward the coronal view of the left adnexa, the left and right sides of the video image have to be reversed in order to keep the conventional presentation of the left-side anatomy on the right side of the monitor.

Compression with transvaginal transducers has been called *push-pull*[3] (Fig. 5–6*A* and *B*). The terms *push* and *pull* are appropriate in transvaginal sonography, but they are less descriptive when discussing the abdominal approach. With the abdominal approach, no maneuver corresponds well to the pull of the transvaginal transducer. Although one can compress with the transducer, the absence of compression is really just normal scanning. No pulling motion is used with the abdominal approach, only normal, light abdominal scanning while keeping a good gel seal, or degrees of hardness may be used (i.e., compression scanning). Therefore, *push-pull* may be a better way of describing compression or the lack thereof with a transvaginal transducer.

Compression may be used abdominally to reposition the fetus, bowel gas, or other contents of the abdomen or uterus. Compression has also been used for elastography in the study of breast lesions,[5–7] but elastography is not fetal sonography nor the topic of this text.

Light compression is most often used to produce a good gel seal while angling the transducer. This is very useful for looking left and right at the ovaries or looking at the base of the bladder to observe the internal portion of the urethra.[8,9] The sonographer is constantly angling about the abdomen to obtain a

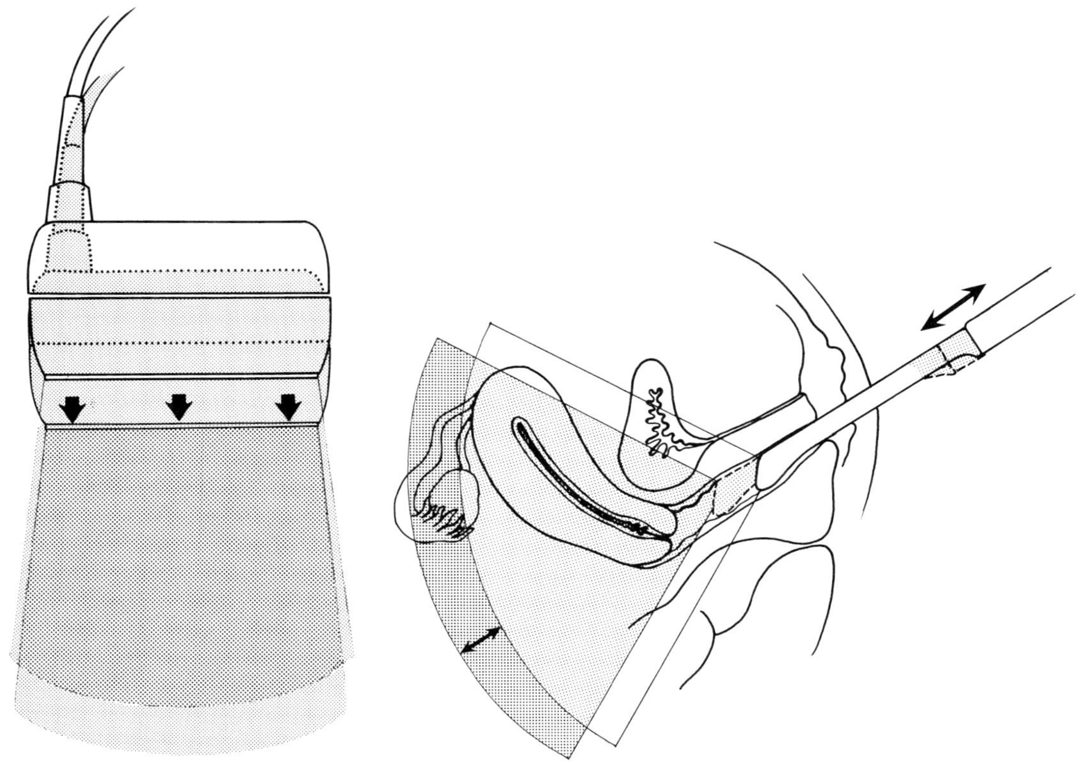

FIGURE 5–6.
A, Compression with a linear array. The same motion would be used with a sector transducer. *B,* With endocavitary or transvaginal transducers, this motion would be called pushing. These transducers can also be used with a pulling motion, which is in the opposite direction from compression. Pushing motions are used to view the deeper structures of the uterus, and pulling motions are used to retract the transducer to view the cervix.

better view of the organs. Exerting slight pressure keeps a better gel seal between a patient's skin and the transducer face. Another common reason for using compression and angling is to obtain a better sonographic view around the maternal umbilicus, which can cast a strong shadow. It is advisable not to try to scan through the maternal umbilicus.

Regardless of whether a sonographer or sonologist is pushing or compressing, he or she should always remain conscious of a patient's comfort and care. At some point, the improvement in the sonogram when compared with the pressure reaches a point of diminishing returns. Too much pressure is not a good thing, be it transducer pressure or bladder pressure.

SOLID GEOMETRY

Sonography is the study of three-dimensional human organs within the body. The field of view is a two-dimensional plane. Sonography essentially provides information about textures, shapes, locations, and sizes of organs. In cases of masses or tumors, it is hoped that sonography will allow the sonographer to determine the organ of origin or attachment.

This ability to view two-dimensional slices of three-dimensional organs calls for some mental gymnastics and mental imaging (discussed earlier). It also requires some minimal understanding of plane and solid geometry. The following is a discussion of certain basic geometric concepts, an understanding of which is helpful in comprehending fetal sonographic morphology. Some of the geometric concepts here are not used in day-to-day clinical sonography but are included for completeness and in the interest of documenting what we have learned.

It must be noted here that in 1995 working prototypes of sonographic machines and special transducers can produce a three-dimensional image. These new machines may be available commercially soon. This equipment actually takes several successive planes or slices and uses sophisticated computer graphic algorithms to display a three-dimensional image. These new three-dimensional imaging devices will assist in obtaining the proper planes for taking several measurements quickly and easily from a single anatomical volume acquisition.

For the purpose of discussion, we progress from the single dimension of linear measurements to two-dimensional measurements of circles, ellipses, and more complex shapes. After that follows a discussion of solid geometry and volumes. Although it is convenient to think of geometry in these simplistic ways, you should remain aware that for every three-dimensional volume there are infinite numbers of useful two-dimensional measures of circumference and area, as well as an infinite number of linear measurements of that volume. It is the sonographer's task to define any volume in a few accurate and understandable two-dimensional measures.

These two-dimensional measures may be linear values or circumferences. Whichever measures are used, their goal should be to document and communicate the three-dimensional size and shape of the anatomical volume of interest.

Certain formulas establish the relationships of the dimensions of circles and ellipses and are often required in sonography. Sonographers need these from time to time to calculate fetal size and age estimates from the various fetal parameter measurements and to document the organ dimensions. These are available from any basic geometry textbook. For a comprehensive book of geometric formulas and tables, *Standard Mathematical Tables* is recommended.[10]

The most useful of these formulas are gathered together in the later section titled "Geometric Formulas."

Some Generalities of Geometry

There are three main reasons for measuring a fetus. The first is to estimate the duration of the gestation, the second is to estimate the size of the fetus, and the third is to evaluate fetal growth. Growth is described as the rate of change of fetal size in time. The study and documentation of the development of the human fetus is, in many ways, the purpose of this book. This topic arises throughout the text. The mathematical concepts of fetal growth are addressed in Chapter 7, but to understand the concepts of the rate of change in fetal size, we must discuss some basic plane and solid geometry.

In general, sonographic measurements of the fetal parameters are taken using linear calipers. However, ellipse drawing functions, which are very useful and as accurate, are becoming widely available.[11] Many of the pa-rameters are simple linear measurements, such as the femoral and humeral diaphysis lengths or the diameters of the head and abdomen. Others are circular or, more often, elliptical. The fetal eyes, cysts, and some sections of the gallbladder, blood vessels, and the coronal view of the normal fetal skull are about the only perfectly round structures in a fetus that are large enough to be useful in diagnostic medical sonography. These elliptical and circular measurements are circumferences of three-dimensional structures such as the head or abdomen. Other researchers have published tables using areas of the fetal head.[12] A few have estimated fetal parameter volumes.[12–14]

The circumferences, areas, and volumes can be calculated from appropriate linear measurements. These calculations as well as the linear measurements can be read directly from the sonographic display on many modern machines.

A knowledge of the mathematical relationships of solid geometry is necessary for understanding the "why" and "how" of sonographic fetal biometry. The following formulas are commonly available in other books and are included here for completeness and the reader's convenient reference. The formulas in bold type are those in general use in diagnostic medical sonography.

Solid organs have two-dimensional planes or cross sections that can be used to describe their three-dimensional volumes or shapes. Cross sections can be transverse to the long axis of the body, called *transverse sections*, or longitudinal sections, which are often referred to as *sagittal sections* or *coronal sections*. Because both sagittal and coronal sections are in the long axis of human anatomy, this text will not use the term *longitudinal section* without explanation of the orientation. In the same fashion, the term *cross section* is often used to describe any two-dimensional section of a solid structure and other times is used to describe a true transverse section; therefore, text uses the terms *transverse*, *sagittal*, and *coronal* to describe the three sectional views of solid organs.

Another problem in discussing cross-sectional anatomy is the way in which it is referenced to a patient's body. In the case of obstetrical sonography, a patient is actually two patients, a woman and a fetus. Because a fetus can be in any position in a woman, a midline sagittal section of a pregnant woman's abdomen may be a coronal or any other section of her fetus. For this reason, in this text, the orientation terms *transverse*, *sagittal*, or *coronal* used alone refer to maternal anatomy. If the orientation is in relationship to the fetus, it is referred to as fetal, as in, The most common sonographic view for measuring the biparietal diameter (BPD) is a transverse section of the fetal head.

Plane Geometry

Linear Measurements. Plane geometry is the real business of sonography. A sonographer is constantly generating and measuring in a two-dimensional field of view. Although one must not forget that the two-dimensional field is within a three-dimensional space, one must also understand the concepts of plane geometry and a few formulas.

The basic measurement of sonography and plane geometry is a straight line, or linear dimension. The linear dimension is simple and should be understood by all. It is simply the straight distance from points A to B or from points C to D in Figure 5–7*A*. These points define the ends of a straight line; in this case, the lines are line AB and line CD. A common linear sonographic measurement is that of the femoral diaphysis, which is simply the measurement of its length from one end to the other.

Linear dimensions may also be one axis of a circle, ellipse, or more complex shapes such as a kidney or uterus. These are discussed next. The lengths of the sides of a square or rectangle are also linear dimensions, but because there are few squares or rectangles in the human body, this discussion is limited to the more biological shapes.

Linear dimensions have a unit of measurement such as inches, centimeters, or millimeters. This text uses the metric scale of measurements: meters, centimeters, or millimeters. The algebraic formulas that describe these relationships are gathered together in the "Geometric Formulas" section later.

Circles and Circumferences. Circles and circumferences are still in the purview of plane geometry but are precursors to solid geometry. A circle may be a cross section of a sphere, cylinder, cone, or ellipsoid volume. Because the sphere, cylinder, and ellipsoid are common biological forms or shapes, the circumference is an important sonographic measurement.

A circle has four commonly used dimensions (Fig. 5–7*B* and *C*), the radius, diameter, circumference, and surface area. In a perfect circle, these four measures have specific mathematical relationships.

The radius is the distance from the exact center of a circle to its edge. In Figures 5–7*B* and *C*, lines AC, CB, and CD are radii of the circle, C being the point at the center.

A diameter is two radii end to end. In these cases (Fig. 5–7*B* and *C*), the diameter is composed of lines AC plus CB, which is the line AB or the distance across the circle. A circle can have any number of radii or diameters; but all radii are equal and all diameters are equal in a perfect circle.

The circumference of a circle is the distance around its outer perimeter. The circumference of a circle is a curved line without an end. A part of the circumference is a sector of a circle and is arc shaped. In Figure 5–7*B* the arc ADB is the top half of the circumference.

The surface area of a circle is simply the square units of area that make up the area inside the circumference. The surface areas of organ cross sections have occasionally been used to evaluate organ size, but diameters, circumferences, and volumes are more commonly used.

Other Plane Geometry. Other plane geometry that is useful in fetal sonography is the relationship of the circle and the triangle. Because the true coronal plane of a normal fetal

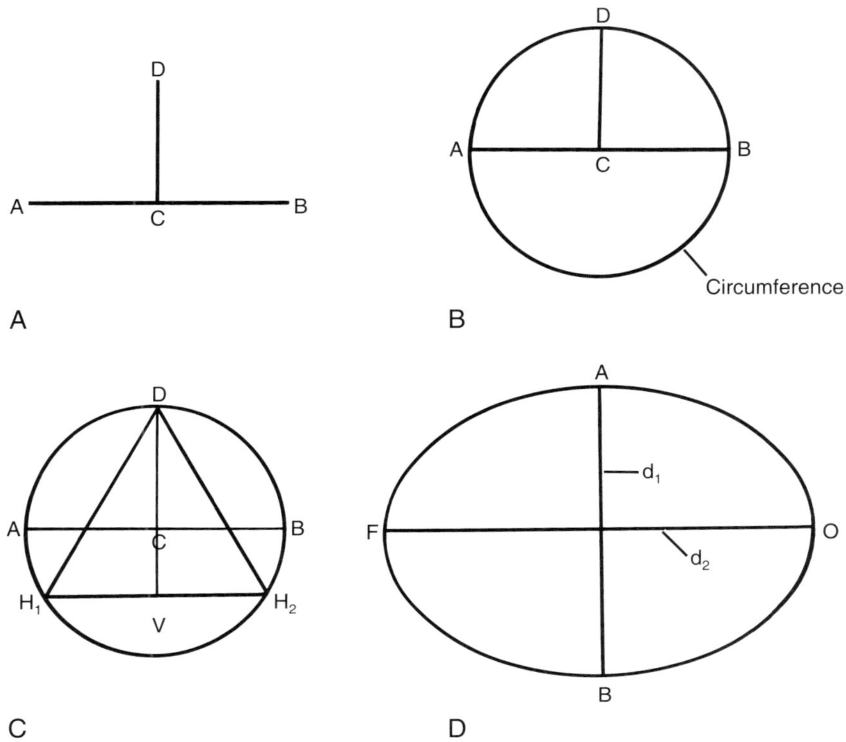

FIGURE 5–7.
A, Four lines are shown here. Line CD is perpendicular to lines AC and CB, which are end to end and form the line AB. Each line represents a different linear measurement. *B*, This perfect circle could have four different measurements to describe its size. The surface area is the square units of space that are inside the circumference, which is the curved line that defines the circle. Lines DC, AC, and CB all are radii. The two radii AC and CB form the diameter. Point C, the intersection of lines DC and AB, is the center of the circle. *C*, This illustration is similar to *B*, with the addition of a triangle (DH_1H_2), which is circumscribed by the circle. The height of the triangle is line DV. In this example, the triangle is equilateral, meaning that all sides are equal ($DH_1 = DH_2 = H_1H_2$). It is also isosceles, meaning that two sides are equal ($DH_1 = DH_2$). The diameter (AB) can be measured directly or calculated using the mensuration formula for the triangle circumference diameter (TriCD). The mensuration formula can be used to determine the circle that circumscribes any triangle, but the measured diameter (AB) will equal the TriCD only if it is in a perfect circle. The usefulness of this observation is discussed in Chapter 8. *D*, An ellipse similar to the sonographic transverse section of a fetal skull. Two perpendicular diameters (AB and FO) are shown. AB is the shortest diameter, and FO is the longest diameter for this ellipse. The formulas used to calculate the various dimensions (areas, circumferences, radii, and diameters) of ellipse shapes are derived from those of the perfect circle. See the text for discussion of these measurements.

skull is very nearly a perfect circle (see Chapter 8), the plane geometry of the coronal view can be looked at in several different ways. The specifics of the fetal cranial anatomy and measurements are discussed in Chapters 8 and 9. Let it suffice here to point out that the most common fetal sonographic measurement taken worldwide is the BPD, which is normally taken from the transverse view of the fetal cranium; however, the BPD can also be measured in the coronal view and is a diameter of the coronal circle.[13,15–19] (see Fig. 5–8*B* and *C*).

Figure 5–7*C* shows triangle H_1H_2D, which has for its sides lines DH_1 and DH_2. The base of the triangle is the line H_1H_2, and the height of the triangle is line DV. This triangle is circumscribed by the circumference of a perfect circle. A complex mensuration formula describes the relationship of any triangle and its circumscribing circumference. This mensuration formula can be found in the *CRC Standard Mathematics Tables* and is discussed later.[20] The triangle in Figure 5–7*C* is an isosceles triangle, which has equal sides. That is, the lines that form the triangle sides are equal: $H_1H_2 = DH_1 = DH_2$. The triangle is also an equilateral triangle, which means that the two sides ($DH_1 = DH_2$) are equal in length.

The formula that describes the triangle circumference (TriC) is presented later in the "Geometric Formulas" section. The TriC formula yields the circumference around any triangle. Readers who are familiar with the BPD should note that the TriC diameter, or TriCD, is equal to the BPD in normally shaped heads. In Figure 5–7*B* and *D*, the BPD is equal to the diameter AB. For those unfamiliar with the BPD, this topic is discussed in detail in Chapter 8. This formula has several algebraic steps, making it rather difficult to calculate using a hand-held calculator, and is best left to computers.

The TriCD can be useful as a substitute for the BPD when the fetal head position makes it difficult to measure the BPD or to view the full circumference of the cranium. One can usually demonstrate enough of the fetal head to measure three points in order to form a triangle. This does not have to be an equilateral or isosceles triangle; it can be any coronal triangle.

Solid Geometry

Spheres and Ellipsoids. As pointed out previously, the circle can be cross sections of spheres, ellipsoids, cones, or cylinders. Because most of the fetal organs we are concerned with are spherical or ellipsoidal volumes, this discussion is limited to sections of those.

Figures 5–8*A* and *B* show various three-dimensional sections through a sphere and ellipsoid. The planes that pass through the shapes represent planes or fields of view. Lines that intersect at the center of the volumes are the various diameters. In Figure 5–8*A*, the shape is a perfect sphere and all diameters are equal. However, Figure 5–8*B* is an ellipsoidal volume or egg shape, and two diameters are equal (D_1 and D_3). The longest axis is D_2, which runs the length of the ellipsoid.

The human brain is not a true egg shape. It is an ellipsoidal volume with an irregular surface and a relatively flat base. Figures 5–8*C* and *D* illustrates stylized brain shapes showing the similarities and dissimilarities to the true egg shape. Because it is impossible to measure all the various bumps and creases of the brain, we cannot calculate its exact volume with sonographic measurements. However, because the skull is relatively smooth and contains the brain, we can measure the dimensions of the skull. If we use consistent methods, we can obtain consistent results, even if the results are only estimates of the circumferences or volumes.

Geometric Formulas

The next two subsections contain several formulas for calculating the previous geometric measurements. Not all of the formulas presented are used often in sonography.

For formulas that are commonly used in sonography but that are derived or reduced to a simpler form, the step-by-step derivation is shown. The formulas in more common use are in bold type. These formulas can be found in the *CRC Standard Mathematical Tables*.[21]

Circles and Ellipses. In a perfect circle (see Fig. 5–7*B* and *C*), r = radius = AC, d = diameter = AB, C = center of circle, c = circumference = ADB, a = area, and pi = π = 3.14159.

Diameter

$$d = 2r$$

conversely

$$r = d/2$$

and

circumference

$$c = \pi 2r = \pi d$$

Because most fetal organs have more or less elliptical circumferences with two different diameters (see Fig. 5–7*D* for d_1 and d_2), we substitute the average diameter in the previous formula to estimate the circumference. In the example ellipse (see Fig. 5–7*D*), line AB = d_1 and FO = d_2:

$$c = \pi(d_1 + d_2)/2 = (d_1 + d_2)3.14159/2$$

therefore:

$$\mathbf{c = (d_1 + d_2)1.57}$$

This formula is the most commonly used in diagnostic medical sonography for calculat-

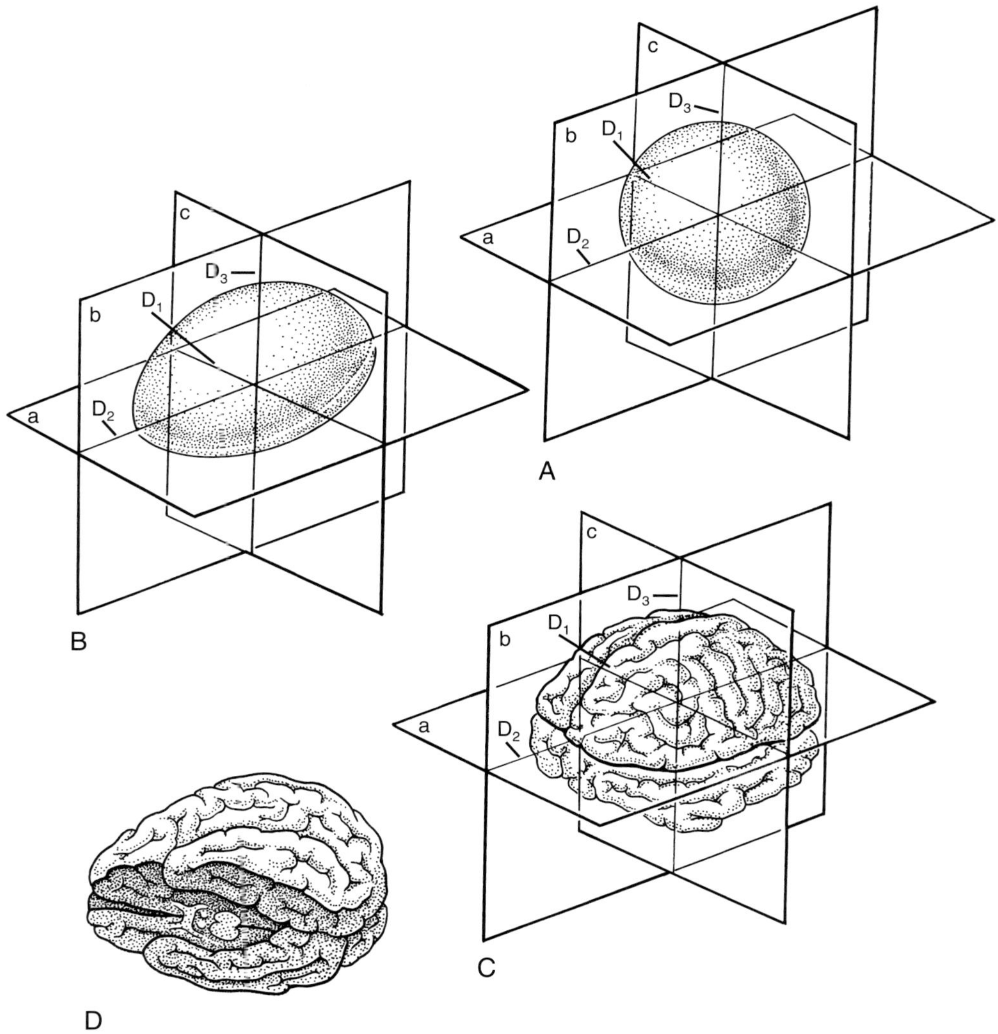

FIGURE 5–8.
The relationship of the solid geometry of the fetal cranium. Similar relationships are often used to describe the kidneys, ovaries, and other biological ellipsoidal volumes. *A*, All the calculations of the various dimensions of the cranium are based on the sphere. The text explains how these calculations are made. In this perfect sphere, all radii and diameters are equal. *B*, An ellipsoidal solid volume or mass. A perfect egg-shaped ellipsoid has two different diameters. D_2 is the long axis, and D_1 and D_3 are the short axes. If the ellipsoid has a more or less flat bottom, similar to the human brain (*C* and *D*), it has different lengths for each of the three diameters. *C*, The fetal brain and the three perpendicular planes that are used to estimate its volume. Plane a is transverse, plane b is sagittal, and plane c is coronal. The three dimensions of the fetal skull can be used to estimate the mass of the brain. *D*, The bottom of the brain is relatively flat. It is this irregular flat surface that causes the brain to have three diameters rather than two. The relatively flat surface also defines the base of the coronal triangle, which is shown in Figure 5–7*C*. This triangle would be in plane c, the coronal plane.

ing the circumference of any elliptical organ. It is used often for both the cranial[22,23] and abdominal[24] circumferences of a fetus.

One occasionally finds reference to or needs the formula for calculating the cross-sectional area of an organ. The sectional area of a circle or ellipse is not often used in sonography but is offered here in the interest of completeness.

Area

$$a = \pi r^2 = \tfrac{1}{4} d^2 \pi = d^2\ 3.14159/4$$

$$a = 0.7854\ d^2 = 0.8\ d^2$$

For an ellipse, the area is often calculated from the average of two diameters. In that case, approximate the area with the following formula:

$$a = 0.7854\ ((d_1 + d_2)/2)^2 = 0.8\ ((d_1 + d_2)/2)^2$$

The previous formulas are most often used in the plain geometry of sonography. One other formula that is interesting and useful is the circle that circumscribes a triangle. This is a complex mensuration formula that is best left to computers; it has 24 discrete mathematical operations, which make it relatively difficult to do on calculators. Here we will call this formula the TriCD. This is because the result of the formula is the diameter of the circle that circumscribes the triangle.

The basic formula for the TriCD is from the *CRC Standard Mathematical Tables*.[20,21] The original formula is for the radius (r = AC = CB) of the circumscribing circle; the diameter (d = AB) formula was derived by multiplying by 2 (see Fig. 5–7*C*):

$$r = (H_1H_2 \times DH_1 \times DH_2)/(4 \times \sqrt{(s(s - H_1H_2)(s - DH_1)(s - DH_2))})$$

$$d = 2r$$

therefore

$$d = 2(H_1H_2 \times DH_1 \times DH_2)/(4 \times \sqrt{(s(s - H_1H_2)(s - DH_1)(s - DH_2))})$$

and

$$d = AB$$

where

$$s = .5(H_1H_2 + DH_1 + DH_2)$$

and

$$\text{triangle base} = H_1H_2$$

$$\text{triangle sides} = DH_1 \text{ and } DH_2$$

The previous mensuration formula works for any triangle, its circumscribing circle, and the circle's radius or diameter. In the example (see Fig. 5–7*C*), the triangle is an equilateral triangle—all sides are equal. It is also an isosceles triangle—it has two sides equal. Although the formula works for a triangle in which all sides are unequal, the nearer the triangle is to equilateral, the smaller the error due to variations in the measurement of the sides. That is to say, if one side of the triangle is very small or short, then a slight error in measuring any side(s) produces a relatively larger error in the resulting diameter calculation.

Spheres and Ellipsoids. The volume of ellipsoids such as the gravid uterus, kidney, ovary, and other organs has been used for comparison in normal populations.[14,25] The volume of an organ increases exponentially as the diameter increases (Table 5–1 and Fig. 5–9). This means that the volume of a mass is more sensitive to changes in size than is the diameter or circumference (see Fig. 5–9).

One should remember that the units of radii, diameters, and circumferences are always linear measurements such as millimeter, centimeter, or meter. Area measurements are square units, which have a superscript 2 (i.e., square centimeters are abbreviated cm^2). Volumes, which are cubed units such as cubic centimeters, are abbreviated as cm^3 or ml.

In a perfect sphere, the formulas for the diameter, circumference, and cross-sectional area are the same as described for the circle. Because a sphere is a three-dimensional object, it has two other dimensions: The volume (V) is useful sonographically, and surface area (S) is less often used.[26]

$$V = 4/3\ \pi r^3 = 4.189\ r^3 = 1/6\ \pi d^3$$

therefore

$$V = 0.5236\ d^3$$

and

$$S = 4\ \pi r^2 = \pi d^2$$

For three-dimensional ellipsoids or egg-shaped solids, we again use variations on the previous formulas. The kidney, ovary, or, especially for the current discussion, the fetal head is not a perfect egg-shaped ellipsoidal volume. The fetal cranium actually has a symmetrically irregular, almost flat base (see Fig. 5–8*C* and *D*). Because organs are rarely per-

TABLE 5–1. FETAL HEAD MEASUREMENTS

FETAL AGE (weeks)	3-D AVERAGE DIAMETER (mm)	BPD D_1 (mm)	FOD D_2 (mm)	VCD D_3 (mm)	CIRCUMFERENCE $1.57(D_1+D_2)$ (mm)	CROSS-SECTIONAL AREA (mm to cm²) $0.008(((D_1+D_2)/2)^2)$ (cm²)	SPHERE AREA (mm to cm²) $pi((D_1+D_2+D_3)/30)^2$ (cm²)	VOLUME$_1$ (mm to ml) $0.00052\times D_1\times D_2\times D_3$ (ml)	VOLUME$_2$ (mm to ml) $0.000555\times D_1\times D_2\times D_3$ (ml)
10.1	13.6	13.6	15.8	11.5	46	1.7	5.84	1.3	1.4
15.0	29.9	29.7	34.0	25.9	100	8	28.02	17	15
20.1	46.9	45.9	59.1	35.6	165	22	39.00	50	54
25.0	61.5	61.6	78.8	44.1	220	39	118.82	111	119
30.1	74.9	77.0	98.3	49.5	275	61	176.40	195	208
35.0	87.6	86.0	108.8	68.0	306	76	241.08	331	353
40.0	97.0	102.5	120.6	68.0	350	100	295.80	437	467

This table contains the three-dimensional sonographic measurements from actual fetal skulls during five different weeks of gestation. The fetal measurements were selected using the criteria that the average of multiple fetal parameter ages were equal to the desired week (± 0.1 week) and that all three diameters had been measured. The first column is the weeks of age from the last menstrual period (LMP). The second column is the three-dimensional average of the three diameters. The next three columns are the three diameters of the skull: BPD, biparietal diameter; FOD, fronto-occipital diameter; VCD, vertical cranial diameter (all measurements are in millimeters). The remaining columns are the calculations of various other measurements from the three diameters. Sphere area is the surface area of the fetal head in cm². Volume$_1$ and volume$_2$ are volumes (in milliliters) calculated from the three diameters using two slightly different formulas, which are discussed in the text. Note that the BPD normally is equal to the three-dimensional average ($r^2=0.99$).

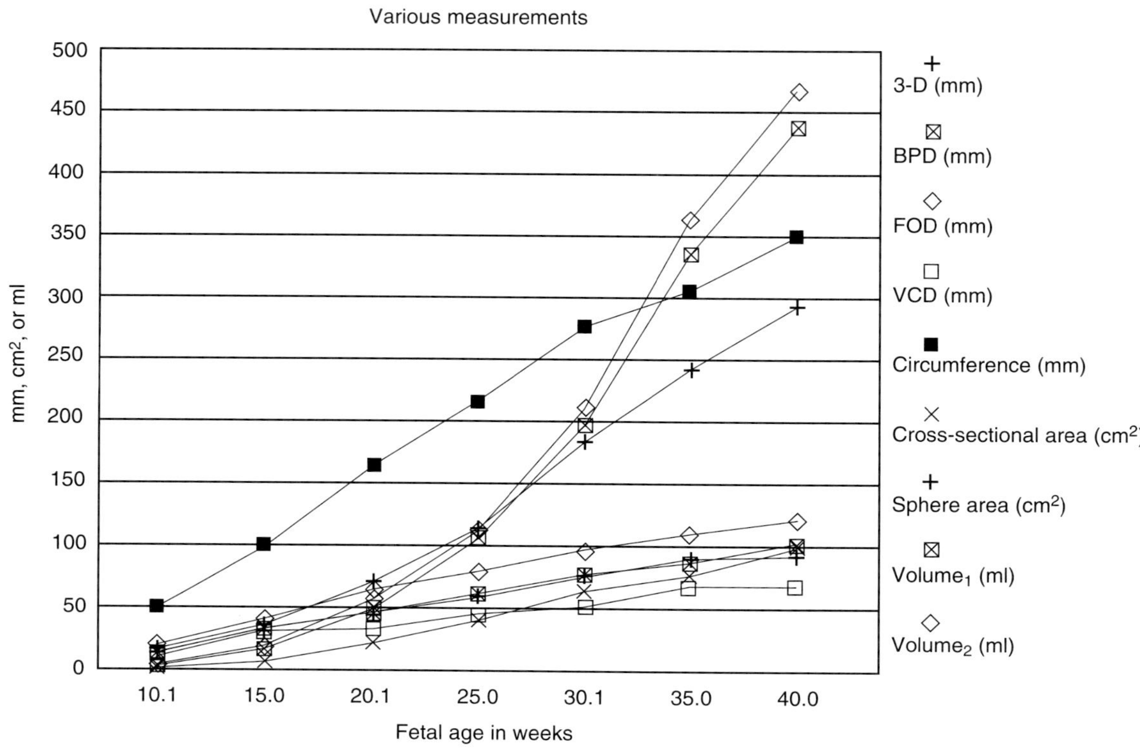

FIGURE 5–9.
A graph of the values from Table 5–1 provided to show how the various measurements change with change in size. The x-axis is time or fetal age in weeks, and the y-axis consists of measurements in millimeters, square centimeters, or milliliters. Note that the volumes have the greatest change, followed by the circumference and area. The slowest to change in time are the diameters. These measurements of the fetal skull are discussed in detail in Chapter 8. 3D, three-dimensional average of three diameters; BPD, biparietal diameter; FOD, fronto-occipital diameter; VCD, vertical cranial diameter.

fect spheres or ellipsoids but often have three different axes or diameters, we use r_1, r_2, r_3, and d_1, d_2, d_3 for the respective radii and diameters.

$$V\text{ (approximate)} = 4/3\ \pi r^3 = 4.189\ r_1 r_2 r_3$$

also

$$V\text{ (approximate)} = 4.189(d_1 d_2 d_3)/2^3 = 4.189(d_1 d_2 d_3)/8$$

therefore

$$\mathbf{V\text{ (approximate)} = 0.5236\ d_1 d_2 d_3}$$

This latter formula is the most frequently used formula for volumes in diagnostic medical sonography. It has been adapted in several variations in which the constant is rounded down[27]:

$$V\text{ (approximate)} = 0.52\ d_1 d_2 d_3$$

or

$$V\text{ (approximate)} = 0.5\ d_1 d_2 d_3$$

To convert millimeter (mm) measures to milliliter (ml) volumes, use

$$V\text{ (approximate)} = 0.00052\ d_1 d_2 d_3$$

or

$$\mathbf{V\text{ (approximate)} = 0.000555\ d_1 d_2 d_3}$$

The last formula is less often used and produces a result that is slightly larger than the standard formula.[28] This formula was derived because several researchers found that the more standard formula slightly underestimated the volume in some shapes.[29] The last formula was tested using clay models that simulated the shapes of a normal fetal skull and was found to be consistent and reliable. This is the volume formula used to construct the fetal skull volume table for fetal age (see Table 7–1), and it should be used if that table is used to estimate menstrual age.

For the surface area of an ellipsoid, the following formula is used. By dividing by 30, the average of the three diameters and conversion from millimeters to milliliters is accomplished in a single step.

$$S = \pi((d_1 + d_2 + d_3)/30)^2$$

These are most of the geometric formulas routinely used to document organ sizes by sonography, although the surface area formula is rarely used. Other formulas and mathematical constructs such as linear regressions, higher-order regressions, and mathematical rules of thumb are discussed in the text with the fetal parameter to which they are relevant.

It should be noted that all measurements do not increase in a linear fashion in time; indeed, only linear measurements increase in a near linear fashion. For each unit increase in the diameter measurement of a spherical or ellipsoidal mass, there will be a change in the rate of change for the circumference, cross-sectional area, or volume of that mass. As an example of how the diameters, circumferences, areas, and volumes change as the measurement of the diameter changes, see Table 5–1 and Figure 5–9. This table and graph are for the three-dimensional measurements of representative fetal heads at 5-week increments from 10 to 40 weeks selected from 7500 consecutive examinations quasi-randomly, with the only criteria being that the average age of multiple fetal parameters for the individual equal the representative age in weeks (±0.1 week) and that all three diameters of the fetal cranium were measured. Note that the volume increases more rapidly (exponentially), the circumference increases less rapidly, and the diameter increases the least rapidly. The faster a measurement changes in time, the more sensitive it is to change in mass. (For more on fetal head measurements, see Chapter 8.)

Sonographic Physics and Resolution

Sonographers should understand that the fields of view that are used in diagnostic medical sonography are referred to as *sections* or *planes*, as in cross section or plane of view. However, these sections or planes have thickness (Fig. 5–10*A* and *B*). Because sonograms are the results of sound waves bouncing off tissue surfaces and interfaces, the amount of clarity or sharpness of an image is determined by the shape and acoustic properties of the beam, as well as the shape and habitus of the patient. The latter aspects of acoustic imaging are discussed in the section on fetal imaging.

The shape and acoustic properties of the beam are somewhat controllable by the operator. The frequency and focus of the transducer beam are usually operator selectable. These may be controlled on the sonographic machine, or sometimes the frequency and focus are specific to a transducer. This means that a sonographer must change transducers

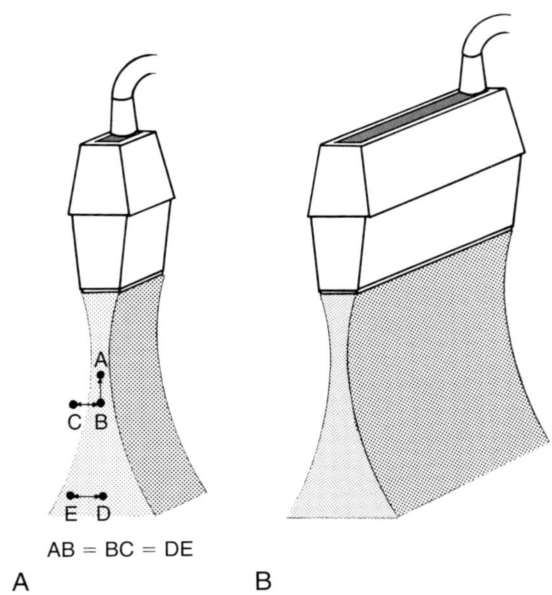

FIGURE 5–10.
A stylized drawing of the shape of sector and linear array transducer beams and the resulting fields of view. The focal range is at the location where the beam is most narrow. In this image, the distances between various points are equal: AB = BC = DE. Points C and B, and D and E are resolved with lateral resolution. Points A and B are resolved with axial resolution.

to optimize an image. We must be constantly vigilant and not accept suboptimum resolution simply because we are too lazy or unconcerned to change transducers.

The shape of the beam has three aspects that describe the plane or field of view. The depth of the field of view determines how far into a patient we can see. The depth is limited by the frequency of the transducer. Lower frequencies penetrate better and allow a greater depth of view. The length of the field of view is determined by the transducer size and shape. Some are linear and form a rectangular field of view. Other transducers are sector type and provide a field of view that is shaped like a piece of pie (see Fig. 5–10*A* and *B*). A linear array transducer, with its rectangular field of view, provides a much longer image in the near field and is usually more useful in fetal measurements, especially toward term, when a fetus is larger. The sector or wedge-shaped image may work better early in gestation, when the uterus and its contents are relatively small. All transvaginal transducers provide a sector beam shape. The width of the sector beam is a function of the beam focus and varies at different depths (see Fig. 5–10*A* and *B*).

In general, it can be said that there are two aspects of sonographic resolution: lateral and axial resolutions. These are determined by the beam shape, frequency, pulse length, and reproduction rate of those pulses. An understanding of these is necessary in a discussion of the way certain measurements of the fetal organs are taken. The following is a more specific discussion of the lateral and axial resolutions.

RESOLUTIONS

Axial Resolution

Axial resolution is directly related to the frequency of the sound, the pulse length, and the reproduction rate of those pulses that make up the sonographic beam. Shorter and frequent pulses yield the greatest axial resolution but at less depth of view. A sonographic system cannot distinguish the echoes from two different structures separated by less than the length of a single pulse (see Fig. 5–10*A*). Transducers that operate at higher frequency do not penetrate as deeply and therefore can have a higher pulse repetition period or rate.[30] This is because all frequencies of sound travel in the human body at approximately the same speed, but the higher frequencies do not penetrate as deeply; therefore, at higher frequencies, the incident sound and returning echoes have a shorter round trip. Lower frequencies can penetrate to relatively deeper structures and therefore must allow for a correspondingly longer travel time for the incident beam and returning echoes and can have longer pulse lengths and lower pulse repetition frequencies.

The tradeoff is that the deeper-penetrating low frequencies have a larger field of view but less axial resolution. The higher frequencies cannot penetrate as deeply but provide much better axial resolution. In other words, the transducer that provides the highest frequency and axial resolution and that penetrates to the depth of interest should be used.

The generally accepted wisdom for measuring in the axial beam resolution is to place the cursor at the leading edge of the echo of interest. This provides the least variation in the measurements along the beam path—that is, with axial resolution.

Lateral Resolution

Lateral resolution is related to beam width. It may be said that the wider the beam of sound is, the wider a single echo in the image appears. It can also be said that an ultrasound system cannot separate echoes that are closer together than the width of the beam. In Figure 5–10*A*, the distance between points C and B is equal to the distance between points E and D. Points C and B are near the focal range for this transducer and are resolved as two echoes. However, points E and D are in the far field, out of focus, and are not resolved as two separate echoes. A beam-width artifact tends to make echoes somewhat fuzzy.[31, 32]

When measuring in the lateral resolution or in the length of the field of view (perpendicular to beam travel), the cursors should be placed at the edge of the most definite echo observed and should not include the beam-width artifact. This makes the sonographic measurements somewhat subjective. Some variation from person to person occurs in terms of where to place the cursor in any specific measurement. This operator variation in measurements is due in large part to the limitations of the resolution of the sonographic equipment, as well as to the experience, patience, and skill of the operator.

PHYSICS OF FETAL MEASUREMENTS

It is important for sonographers to understand how axial and lateral resolution affect fetal measurements with respect to the orientation of the fetal structure in the beam or field of view. Sonographers must be aware of whether the measurement being taken is in axial resolution or lateral resolution. In general, it is true that axial resolution produces the least measurement error, whereas measurements taken transversely to the beam, using lateral resolution, show the greatest errors. A sonographer/sonologist must exercise judgment and skill when selecting the appropriate transducer, obtaining the images, and taking the measurements if the greatest accuracy is to be obtained.

Although any modern real-time transducer can be used effectively for fetal measurements, linear array transducers, with their larger near field of view, make measurements easier to obtain near term.[33] During early pregnancy, transvaginal transducers are able to approach the embryo much closer and use higher frequencies in order to provide a much clearer image.

Measurements can either be taken using electronic calipers or can be taken directly from the film. The former produce the more accurate measurement. The latter measurements, from the film, can be taken after the examination is completed using a straightedge or dividers to compare the parameter or organ of interest with the scale along the edge of the image.

In general, measurements taken with most modern sonographic machines are very accurate. Some older machines have shown a tendency to drift or change their ability to produce accurate measurements over time. To be sure a machine is accurate, a sonographer can test the equipment by using a test object such as the AIUM Standard Test Object or other acceptable sonographic phantom. If the ultrasound machine does not produce acceptably accurate measurements of the test object, then the machine should be calibrated by an authorized service person. Generally, sonographic measurement errors in the range of 1% to 2%, or 1 or 2 mm per 10 cm, can be accepted.[34] The errors are due to beam-width artifacts, transducer frequency, machine calibration, and operator cursor placement variations.[35, 36]

REFERENCES

1. American Institute of Ultrasound in Medicine (AIUM), Standards Committee: Standard Presentation and Labeling of Ultrasound Images. AIUM, Rockville, MD, 1986, pp 11–35.
2. Abramowicz, J: Standard Presentation and Labeling of Ultrasound Images. AIUM, Rockville, MD (in press).
3. Timor-Tritsch IE, Rottem S: Transvaginal Sonography, 2nd ed. Elsevier, New York, 1991, pp 64–66.
4. Mendoza GA, Almeida O, Steinfeld L: Intermittent fetal bradycardia introduced by midpregnancy fetal ultrasonographic study. Am J Obstet Gynecol 1989; 160:1038–1040.
5. Ophir J, Cespedes I, Ponnekanti H, et al: Elastography: A method for imaging the elasticity of biological tissues (abstract 0500). J Ultrasound Med 1992;11:S2.
6. Cespedes I, Ponnekanti H, Ophir J, et al: Elastography: Experimental results from phantoms and tissues (abstract 0501). J Ultrasound Med 1992;11:S2.
7. Cespedes I, Ophir J: Trade-offs from improved image resolution in elastography (abstract 0502). J Ultrasound Med 1992;11:S2.
8. Hennigan HW, DuBose TJ: Sonography of the normal female urethra. AJR 1985;145:839–841.
9. de Gonzalez EL, Cosgrove DO, Joseph AE, et al: The appearances of the female urethral sphincter. Br J Radiol 1988;61:687–690.
10. Eves H: Geometry. In: Beyer WH, ed: Standard Mathematical Tables. CRC Press, Boca Raton, FL, 1987, pp 121–133.
11. Hadlock FP, Kent WR, Loyd JL, et al: An evaluation of two methods for measuring fetal head and body circumference. J Ultrasound Med 1982;1:359–360.
12. Kurtz AB, Goldberg BB: Obstetrical Measurements in Ultrasound. Year Book Medical Publishers, Chicago, 1988, p 35.
13. DuBose TJ: Fetal biometry: Vertical calvarial diameter and calvarial volume. J Diagn Med Ultrasound 1985;1:205–217.
14. Baltarowich OH: Female pelvic organ measurements. In: Goldberg BB, Kurtz AB, eds: Atlas of Ultrasound Measurements. Year Book Medical Publishers, Chicago, 1990, pp 190–242.
15. Kurtz AB, Wapner RJ, Kurtz RJ, et al: Analysis of biparietal diameter as an accurate indicator of gestational age. J Clin Ultrasound 1980;8:319–326.
16. DuBose TJ: Assessment of fetal age and size: Techniques and criteria. In: Berman MC, ed: Obstetrics and Gynecology: Diagnostic Medical Sonography, A Guide to Clinical Practice, vol 1. JB Lippincott, Philadelphia, 1991, p 284.

17. Goldkrand JW, Kuhlman T, Fox E, et al: Coronal biparietal diameter: A reliable alternative to the traditional transverse biparietal diameter. J Ultrasound Med 1990;9:555–557.
18. Weinraub Z, Herman A, Ron-El R, et al: Measuring coronal biparietal diameters (letter). J Ultrasound Med 1991;10:486.
19. DuBose TJ: Coronal BPD revisited (letter). J Ultrasound Med 1992;11:84.
20. Hodgman CD, editor in chief: CRC Standard Mathematical Tables, 12th ed. Chemical Rubber Publishing Company, Cleveland, 1959, p 397.
21. Eves H: Geometry mensuration formulas. In: Beyer WH, ed: Standard Mathematical Tables. CRC Press, Boca Raton, FL, 1987, p 121–133.
22. Hadlock FP, Deter RL, Harrist RB, et al. Estimating fetal age: Computer assisted analysis of multiple fetal growth parameters. Radiology 1984;152:497–501.
23. Hadlock FP, Deter RL, Harrist RB, et al: Fetal head circumference: Relation to menstrual age. AJR 1982;138:649–653.
24. Hadlock FP, Deter RL, Harrist RB, et al: Fetal abdominal circumference as a predictor of menstrual age. AJR 1982;139:367–370.
25. Hricak H, Lieto RP: Sonographic determination of renal volume. Radiology 1983;148:311–312.
26. Goldberg BB, Kurtz AB: Atlas of Ultrasound Measurements. Year Book Medical Publishers, Chicago, 1990, p 277.
27. Fleischer AC, Kalemeiras GC, Entman SS: Sonographic depiction of the endometrium during normal menstrual cycles. Ultrasound Med Biol 1986; 12:271–277.
28. DuBose TJ: Assessment of fetal age and size: Techniques and criteria. In: Berman MC, ed: Obstetrics and Gynecology: Diagnostic Medical Sonography, A Guide to Clinical Practice, vol 1. JB Lippincott, Philadelphia, 1991, pp 273–299.
29. Hopman WPM, Rosenbusch G, Jansen JBMS, et al: Gallbladder contraction: Effect of fatty meals and cholecystokinin. Radiology 1985;157:37–39.
30. Kremkau FW: Diagnostic Ultrasound: Principles, Instruments, and Exercises. WB Saunders, Philadelphia, 1989, pp 50–51.
31. Sarti DA: Diagnostic Ultrasound, 2nd ed. Year Book Medical Publishers, Chicago, 1987, pp 14–15.
32. Zagzebski JA: Basic physics. In: Sabbagha RE, ed: Diagnostic Ultrasound, Applied to Obstetrics and Gynecology, 2nd ed. JB Lippincott, Philadelphia, 1987, pp 12–13.
33. Hadlock FP: Evaluation of fetal weight estimating procedures. In: Deter RL, Harrist RB, Birnholz JC, et al, eds: Quantitative Obstetrical Ultrasonography. John Wiley & Sons, New York, 1986, pp 115–117.
34. McDicken WN: Diagnostic Ultrasound: Principles and Use of Instruments, 2nd ed. John Wiley & Sons, New York, 1981, pp 31–34.
35. Zador IE, Sokol RJ, Chik L: Interobserver variability: A source of error in obstetric ultrasound. J Ultrasound Med 1988;7:245–249.
36. DuBose TJ: A simple test of excessive B scanner transducer ring. J Med Ultrasound 1983;7:169–172.

CHAPTER 6

ETHICS AND LEGAL ISSUES

INTRODUCTION

Terry J. DuBose

As a relatively new field in medical imaging, diagnostic medical sonography has been experimented with and has had limited use since the early 1950s. It was not widely used until the mid-1970s, or approximately 20 years ago at this writing. This development has come at a time that has caused sonography to be caught up in the political-legal battle over abortion. The field is also involved in its own growing pains of having to define the profession of diagnostic medical sonography legally, because it did not exist as a professional entity until the American Registry of Diagnostic Medical Sonographers (ARDMS) was incorporated in June 1975.[1] The development of this new field and the legal battle over abortion in the United States during the same time have merged to focus attention that has both increased public awareness of sonography and complicated the lives of sonographers and sonologists.

It would be easy simply to say that these issues are too complicated and out of the purview of this type of textbook. However, because these are vital issues to those who work in the field, I decided not to take the easy way out by avoiding them. I attempt to present a balanced overview of the issues and other subjects of interest to the field that are not strictly related to fetal anatomy or the methodology of diagnostic medical sonography but that do affect the day-to-day routine of the sonographic laboratory.

Three principal topics can appropriately be included here: (1) a definition of what sonographers and sonologists are; (2) the current legal status of abortion as it relates to the professions; and (3) issues such as fetal-maternal bonding. Other issues are such topics as using sonography to tell the parents the sex of the baby and how that might relate to the abortion controversy and selection of the sex of progeny. All of these in various ways are included in the larger field of ethics.

The idea of this textbook was developed during the U.S. presidential campaign of 1992. In that campaign, the issue of abortion was prominent. In thinking about abortion, I started out trying to explain the two positions, generally referred to as *pro-life* and *pro-choice*. In the extreme, pro-life is, of course, the position that abortion should be illegal, and the pro-choice position is generally in favor of a woman's right to choose between abortion or continuation of pregnancy. During the research of these opposing views, it became clear that a very distinct third position is emerging in the medical literature—that of possibly mandating abortion in certain cases. Because we now have medical technology to detect early fetal anomalies, some people are starting to question whether society can afford these abnormal individuals who will be expensive to maintain after birth and may never become productive, self-supporting adults.[2,3]

Many people question the wisdom of delivering children with birth defects and of sustaining them after birth. Regardless of the ability to correct many birth defects surgically, the surgery does not correct the genetic code that may have caused the defect. It is possible that by keeping these babies alive, we are degenerating the entire human gene pool. In the very long run, this degradation may cause a great burden on the future society and its health care system. If birth defects were to become numerous as a result of environmental effects or degradation of the gene pool, is it inconceivable that society might someday consider mandatory abortion in some cases? However, even to consider legislation to forcibly terminate certain pregnancies seems inconceivable today. Who would make such a decision? How severe would the defect have to be before such a law would come into effect? What would be the definition of birth defect? Would it be possible for the laws to be manipulated in a way that allowed genocide? Perhaps some might consider people of particular skin coloring as being defective. Could these laws be manipulated to allow the decision to abort a pregnancy to be based on the desired sex of the baby?[4–6] Clearly, this is a dangerous direction for society to take. Because of the great complexity of these questions, I decided to request help.

As a registered sonographer (ARDMS), I discuss questions related to the field as a profession. For the other ethical issues that are in many ways more complex and that affect society as a whole and not primarily from a sonographic standpoint, I invited a nonmedical, formally trained philosopher to provide some guidance for approaching these difficult questions.

William Meacham, PhD, studied philosophy at the University of Texas at Austin during the turbulent 1960s and 1970s. I met Meacham in those days at the University of Texas after my tour of duty with the U.S. Army in Vietnam. During my service, I concluded that the Vietnam War was not only a misadventure but an outright mistake, possibly criminal. Meacham was working on his degree and writing for the local counterculture newspaper, *The Rag*. He was also actively opposing the war. It was his dedication to truth, as well as his human approach, that engendered my respect. Meacham wanted to hear my questions rather than simply condemn me as a Vietnam veteran or war criminal, the mood on most campuses in those days.

Dr. Meacham offers us a thoughtful essay that we hope will help professional sonographers and sonologists think about these difficult questions. He does not give us answers; rather he provides some framework for thinking about these questions and then discusses various positions. The ultimate answers, as always, must come from the individual—yourself.

Medical-Legal Questions

The question of just what is diagnostic medical sonography is as old as the profession, which is in its infancy. How current sonographers perform their duties and how the public perceives the duties of sonographers will determine the definition of the profession in the future. The question is very important now that it has been formally submitted to several American Institute of Ultrasound in Medicine (AIUM) committees.

In common parlance, a sonologist is any individual licensed to practice medicine, more commonly known as a physician or Doctor of Medicine (MD), who is qualified to "read" sonograms and render a diagnosis from them. The term *sonographer* usually includes all nonphysician individuals who perform diagnostic medical sonographic imaging. In this text, we follow this convention. In some places, the terms *sonographer* and *sonologist* may be used alone. The term *sonologist* used alone implies a *physician*. A registered diagnostic medical sonographer (DMS) has passed the American RDMS examinations or equivalent examinations in another country. In most cases, what is said here applies to both sonographers and sonologists.

Currently debated is what exactly a DMS can do and say in the practice of diagnostic medical sonography. The center of the debate is a statement that was submitted to the AIUM Standards Committee during the 1992 meeting in San Diego: "Interpretation of ultrasound is the practice of medicine." At first glance, this seems clear and simple enough, but what does it really mean? "The practice of medicine" should have fairly clear legal definitions in most places, although the phrase becomes somewhat nebulous as related to nurses, physical therapists, nurse practitioners, physician's assistants, optometrists, psychiatric social workers, cytotechnologists, chiropractors, and many other health care professionals. Diagnostic medical sonography is a new field, and its purview is still being defined. Sonographers must jealously defend their profession if it is not to be degraded.

The foregoing statement was reworded by the Standards Committee and forwarded to the AIUM Practice Committee (1992) where it was again changed to the final form as the official AIUM policy (approved in October 1992).

> **STATEMENT ON INTERPRETATION OF ULTRASOUND EXAMINATIONS**
>
> Ultrasound studies shall be supervised and interpretations must be rendered by a physician with training and experience in the specific area of ultrasonography. Findings must be recorded and results communicated in a timely fashion to the physician responsible for care. Although a sonographer may play a critical role in extracting the information essential to deriving a diagnosis, the rendering of a final diagnosis of ultrasound studies represents the practice of medicine, and, therefore, is the responsibility of the supervising physician.

Although this statement does acknowledge that a DMS does have a role in sonography, it does not recognize that a DMS must interpret which images to record in order to portray the anatomy and pathology accurately. The official AIUM statement does not place enough emphasis on the judgment required for a DMS to make these decisions. If a DMS cannot judge whether a particular image defines the anatomy or whether a fetal measurement is accurate, then sonologists are in the position of having to scan every patient. In these times of health care reform, it is clearly not realistic for a physician to scan every patient unless more medical doctors are trained and are willing to accept less income per patient. Otherwise, this very useful diagnostic imaging modality will become less available and very costly.

At issue is the phrase "interpretation of ultrasound." Does this really mean the practice of medicine? Can any DMS imagine appearing before a court of law and being asked, "Who took these images?" "Why did you record this image and not others?" "How did you make the decision of which images to record and which images not to record?" "How do you know that this image best represented the anatomy?" Clearly, one cannot operate sonographic equipment without interpreting the images. This does not mean that a DMS should assume responsibility for issuing a diagnosis, prescribing treatment, or performing surgery.

In an article entitled "Legal Aspects of Diagnostic Sonography," the esteemed doctors A. Everette James, Jr., Albert L. Bundy, Arthur C. Fleischer, John Gore, Roger C. Sanders, and John C. Hobbins state:

> Many ultrasound examinations are performed by a technologist [*sic*] when a physician is not present, and a report is issued by a physician at a later time. The legal responsibilities are extraordinary because a necessary part of care may involve rendering an interpretation at the time the study is performed, especially if real-time instrumentation is used. This differs from the relative roles of technologists and physicians in other imaging disciplines. The technologist-Sonographer is acting as the 'agent' of the physician and anything of consequence that the Sonographer does in the course of normal activity (scope of employment) is the ultimate responsibility of the physician. If the technologist [*sic*] renders an incorrect diagnosis and issues an erroneous preliminary report, this remains the ultimate responsibility of the physician.[7]

Should DMSs be constrained in their profession because some untrained people are using the equipment? Far worse, should DMSs be constrained because some medical doctors have not had proper training in the field? Does having a Doctor of Medicine degree mean that one automatically knows how to interpret a sonogram? Of course not, yet the American Medical Association, American College of Radiology, American College of Obstetricians and Gynecologists, and other organizations are only recently requiring documentation that their members who use sonographic equipment diagnostically have proper training.

Under the "respondeat superior" or "captain of the ship" doctrine,[7] a physician who hires and communicates clearly with a trained DMS is probably on fairly safe ground. However, if a physician untrained in sonography hires an untrained person to perform sonography or hires a DMS but does not communicate clearly with him or her, then that physician probably has considerable legal exposure.

This important issue deserves much consideration. The results of the debate will ultimately define the profession of diagnostic medical sonography and sonology. If it is decided that DMSs are blind and stupid and that only medical doctors can do scanning, then health care will be less available and more expensive. It will also do mortal damage to an interesting and challenging profession that can provide excellent diagnostic information more quickly, economically, and with wider availability than can some of the other diagnostic modalities developed during the past 20 years.

Another consideration of the respondeat superior doctrine is that of malpractice. As long as DMSs are acting within the scope of their profession, they are under the ultimate responsibility of the physician, as pointed out earlier. DMSs should thus be safe from direct malpractice suits; however, in terms of law suits, almost anyone can be named.[8]

If a DMS's actions are beyond or outside the normal practice of diagnostic medical sonography, however, then they will be outside the legal definition of the practice of sonography. This means that if DMSs do anything that would not normally be a part of an examination, they are at risk. For example, if a patient is sexually molested in the course of a sonographic transvaginal examination, then any legal action against that DMS would be considered under the laws governing assault and battery and the DMS would not be protected under malpractice law or insurance. The definition of what constitutes sexual molestation is determined by the courts. It goes without saying that DMSs should be very prudent and professional in all examination activities, not just transvaginal examinations. It would also be prudent to caution that for many intimate and invasive procedures, a DMS may require a chaperone for the protection of all parties concerned.

The safest way for a DMS to proceed is always to keep in mind the Code of Professional Conduct of the Society of Diagnostic Medical Sonographers[9]:

1. Sonographers shall act in the best interest of the patient.
2. Sonographers shall provide sonographic services with compassion, respect for human dignity, honesty, and integrity.
3. Sonographers shall respect the patient's right to privacy, safeguarding confidential information within the constraints of the law.
4. Sonographers shall maintain competence in their field.
5. Sonographers shall assume responsibility for their actions.

ETHICAL SONOGRAPHY

William Meacham, PhD

This chapter outlines a philosophical approach to ethics in general and then applies that approach to certain ethical dilemmas in fetal sonography. The approach is teleological and humanistic, although it denies no religion. Practical advice about selected ethical issues is given.

The practice of fetal sonography touches issues of life and death, love and obligation, knowledge and power—indeed, the very fabric of human existence. It is not surprising that these issues arouse strong feelings and opinions. What's important from a philosophical point of view is not that one avoid strong opinion but that one be able to back up one's opinion with careful reasoning. In this chapter, I chart a course of reasoning from certain ethical principles and assumptions about the nature of human beings to practical advice and admonitions about the issues at hand.

This chapter is meant to give an illustration of how to think about these issues, not to tell readers what to think. If you merely believe what I say—even though I think it's correct and that good consequences will come from following my advice—you will not have thought it through for yourself. When someone else offers a different plausible argument, you will not have a strong foundation for judging between the two. Instead of merely believing what I say, think for yourself.

Principles of Ethics

Before one makes ethical judgments about fetal sonography—indeed about any subject—one needs to have some understanding of the principles on which those judgments are made. If you think something is good or bad, right or wrong, why do you think so? On what basis is it reasonable to make these ethical judgments?

The practice of the philosophy of ethics is the attempt to think carefully about ethical issues with a view to deciding how to live one's life. The idea is to base your actions on rational thought. It consists of two parts, often called *normative ethics* and *metaethics*. (Professional ethics, the consensus in the profession about what constitutes appropriate behavior, is a subset of normative ethics.)

The goal of normative ethics is to figure out what to do, beginning by defining broadly applicable maxims or rules for conduct and then making specific decisions in response to particular circumstances. Normative ethics reasons from general principles to decisions about what to do in specific cases.

What follows is an example of normative ethics. Suppose your ethical principle is that it is always wrong to tell a lie, and you find a wallet full of money and an identification card. You could return the wallet and keep the money, saying you found it empty, but that would be a lie. Therefore, despite the allure of material gain, you return the wallet and the money. Given a strong commitment to the principle, the course of action is clear.

What do you do, however, if ethical principles conflict? Suppose you are living in Holland during World War II and Germany has invaded your country. An ethical principle is that it is good to protect people from harm, so you hide a family of Jews in your house. The Nazis come looking for them and ask if you are harboring any fugitives. You now have two ethical principles in conflict. Shall you tell the truth or protect the Jews? This is a metaethical issue.

Metaethics (*meta* means "beyond" in Greek) is the attempt to figure out what the general principles are in the first place. It asks what the most fundamental ethical principles are, how we can find out what they are and how it makes sense to think about them, and what it really means to speak in ethical terms. It is much more nebulous than normative ethics, because if you ask what are good ethical principles to live by (instead of simply what to do in a certain case), you are already begging the question. What do you mean by good? How do you decide what's good? Maybe instead of asking what's good you should ask what's right. But why should you, and what's the difference between good and right? And what do you mean by *should*, anyway?

Regretfully, I cannot answer all these questions in this short space. I can only describe some of the major issues and give an overview of the landscape, so to speak. This will put my normative ethical stance in perspective so you will have a basis for thinking about it.

Teleological Ethics

Normative ethical principles fall into two basic categories, teleological and deontological. Teleology, from a Greek word meaning "end" or "goal," speaks in terms of good and bad. Deontology, from a Greek word meaning "duty," speaks more often in terms of right and wrong. Teleology justifies an act on the basis of its consequences. If an act has useful or beneficial results, it's good, and if it doesn't, it's not. Deontology justifies one's actions on the basis of some quality or characteristic of the act itself, regardless of its consequences. Often this characteristic is its conformance to a rule. (This is oversimplified but serves to define the difference in broad terms.)

Without trying to justify my reasons, I'll just state that I'm in the teleological camp. In my view, to say that something is good is to say that it is good for something, that it has some use or value, that it is or can be instrumental for accomplishing some purpose. By way of analogy, you might ask (philosophers like to do things like this), Is a hammer good? Well, a hammer is neither good nor bad in and of itself. The question has no meaning unless you ask, Good for what? A hammer is good for driving nails and might be good for propping open a window, but it's not much good for stirring soup and certainly not for painting a picture. A better way of stating the question would be, What good is a hammer?

The ethical dimension arises when you extend this way of thinking to issues of human behavior in broad terms. It is certainly reasonable to ask, Is it good to tell the truth? Teleologically, we can rephrase the question and ask, What good is telling the truth? or What is truthfulness good for? It's good in most cases because it promotes harmony, trust, and cooperation between people. It helps us all acquire accurate knowledge of reality, which in turn enables us to act effectively and master our environment. In some cases, however, it might not be good. Most of us (indeed, all of us who are thinking clearly) would agree that telling the truth to Nazi soldiers would be a bad idea. We ask, then, not just whether it's good to tell the truth but when it's good to tell the truth.

Just as good is defined in relation to an end, the value of the end is defined in relation to another end. For instance, a hammer is good for driving nails. What good is driving nails? Driving nails is good for, among other things, building houses. Why build houses? To have shelter and warmth. Why is it good to have shelter and warmth? Because they sustain human life. Why is sustaining human life good? Because—and here is a critical point, to which we'll return shortly—it enables us to function appropriately and well, to do what we are good for.

This chain of goods and ends stretches in both directions from wherever we arbitrarily start looking. A hammer is good for driving nails. That's what it does; its function is to drive nails. So what is good for the hammer? Whatever enables it to serve its purpose or to perform its function. It's not good to leave it out in the rain; it is good to handle it carefully, swing it accurately with grace and force, and put it away safely.

The teleological model, incidentally, is one well suited for thinking about medical issues. One is healthy when all the parts of one's being are functioning well and in harmony, each organ and subsystem doing its job to support other subsystems and in turn being nourished and supported by them. Disease arises when a malfunction occurs, perhaps caused by environmental stress or an invading organism. When some element in our being is not performing its function well, our health is impaired.

The point of all this is that it gives us an important wedge to pry open the hard questions of ethics. Questions such as whether it would be good to take sonograms routinely in every pregnancy or only when an abnormality is suspected, or how best to make use of the knowledge gained from sonography, become answerable when we put them into a human context. Sonography is not good or bad in itself; it and the uses to which it is put are good or bad in relation to human beings. We must ask what's good for us in general and what's good for the particular people in the particular circumstances in which the questions arise.

Human Nature

What's good for human beings is whatever enables us to function well, to do elegantly and efficiently the things that are uniquely ours to do. The next question, then, is what these things are. What are our fundamental qualities as human beings?

First and foremost, we are intelligent. We are the most intelligent beings we know of. By "intelligent," I mean that we have the ability to think rapidly and accurately and to come up with an exact, appropriate response to every situation. Part of our intelligence consists in our ability to know, to be fully conscious of and understand, the universe surrounding us to whatever level of precision we need or desire.

Second, we are loving and cooperative. Humans are social beings; as babies we would die in isolation, and as children and adults we thrive in the company of others like us. We are inherently connected with other people, indeed the entire world. Our natural way of feeling about each other is love, and our natural way of interacting with each other is to cooperate to accomplish our chosen goals.

Third, we have great personal power and the ability to decide at any moment how to approach life and what actions to take. By "power," I mean simply the ability to get things done, to accomplish what we have decided to do. Our fundamental nature is to say to life's challenges, I can and I will.

Finally, we are inherently enthusiastic and zestful about life. The natural way for us to feel is vibrantly alive. We take great delight in enjoying and mastering our environment.

These things may not seem obviously true. Many of us do not act this way. The reason we don't, in brief, is that we have been hurt, physically and especially emotionally. Emotional hurts that have not been healed impair our ability to think clearly, love and cooperate with each other, act powerfully, and enjoy life. Luckily, there are ways to heal our hurts and regain our true nature, but that discussion is beyond the scope of this chapter.*

I'm not going to try to justify these assumptions about human nature, just as I did not justify my preference for teleological ethics. Selected readings at the end of this chapter provide more information about this theory of human nature. For the purposes of this chapter, I ask only that you observe how certain things fall into place when fundamental principles are assumed. The philosophical point is that if these things are true, then certain ethical conclusions follow. In real life, of course, the point is for you to verify these things for yourself.

Before we go on, I want to point out an important principle that follows from these assumptions. Human beings are intrinsically valuable. We are valuable to ourselves and other human beings. We possess, as far as we know, the most complicated intelligence and the greatest capacity for mastery of the environment of any organism that exists. It has been said that the only thing sufficiently complex to engage the human intelligence for a long time is another human intelligence. Any action or attitude that ignores or diminishes anyone's value is bad. It harms not only that person but the person taking the action or holding the attitude. Because we are all connected, any harm done to a person harms the person doing it as well.

*These assertions come out of the theory and practice of re-evaluation counseling, which explains not only what people are really like but also why people act in ways contrary to their true nature and how they can stop doing so and recover their true intelligence, power, and zest. You can find out more about re-evaluation counseling by writing to Re-Evaluation Counseling Headquarters, 719 Second Avenue North, Seattle, WA 98109.

Applying Teleological Ethics

Having determined some basic principles, we can now move to normative ethics, the process of deciding what to do in specific cases. At this level, the teleological principles focus on weighing risks and benefits. When deciding what to do, we want to know what good and what harm each choice might produce. To determine this, we need to examine the potential consequences of our actions. It is also useful to formulate general rules for behavior so we don't have to spend a lot of time thinking about each action we take. On an individual level, these are called *maxims* or *rules for conduct*. On a societal level, they are called *policies* and are codified in laws and regulations.

In the absence of perfect foresight, we have to make educated guesses about the consequences of our actions or our maxims and policies. I don't mean to disparage the process. Intelligence, our foremost human trait, consists in assessing the probability of something happening in the future based on our experience of the past and present. The important thing in such an assessment is to fully account for all the risks and all the potential benefits for all the people involved. In specific cases, we are trying to determine what is good for specific people. The first thing to ask, then, is, Who is affected?

Those affected by decisions about abortion include a woman, her fetus, the sonographer, the physician, other family members, and society as a whole. You may question my including the fetus in this list, because it may seem to beg the question. Whether a fetus is a full human being is an issue fraught with controversy. There can be no doubt, however, that a fetus is a potential human being and that the farther advanced the pregnancy, the fuller that potential is. For the purpose of examining abortion issues, we need to take the needs of the fetus into account. Indeed, one of the main purposes of sonography is to determine whether the fetus needs special treatment of any sort.

In what follows, then, I consider a number of issues currently before the sonographic community and attempt to reason about them on the basis of the principles stated above.

Routine Screening

The issue of whether sonograms should be taken as a routine part of prenatal care was addressed in 1984 by the National Institutes of Health, whose Consensus Panel decided to recommend against the practice. The benefit of sonographic screening is that it gives increased knowledge about the state of the fetus. Is it alive and healthy? What is its age? Are any abnormalities detectable? Because it is the nature of human beings to investigate and master our world, it would seem appropriate to extend that knowledge through sonography. But what if doing so could cause harm to someone, particularly to a fetus? The Consensus Panel was not convinced that the safety of the procedure had been sufficiently proved, although it could find no evidence of harm.

There can be no doubt about the benefits of sonography when there are complications in a pregnancy. Determining the age of a fetus can be of great benefit in deciding when to induce labor. Some fetal abnormalities, detectable through sonography, can be corrected in utero. However, do the benefits of increased knowledge about the state of a fetus in which abnormalities are not suspected outweigh the risks?

The potential ill effects of sonography are usually considered to be damage to the fetus, such as destruction of tissue, abnormal cell development, or production of abnormal chemical reactions. Diagnostic levels of ultrasound produce minute amounts of heat, but these have never been demonstrated to be harmful. They also produce cavitation, small bubbles of gas in the tissue. The effect of these bubbles, whether benign, harmful, or indifferent, has not been determined. Other considerations include the shortage of adequately trained sonographers and lack of knowledge on the part of some physicians. Inaccurate scans and misdiagnoses are certainly risks to be considered. In addition, we must consider the possibility of delayed effects, as exemplified by those caused by diethylstilbestrol, once thought to be safe for routine use.

There are more subtle risks, not easily quantified. One is the increasing mechanization of pregnancy, the increasing reliance on technology as a way of knowing as opposed to the age-old wisdom of women and midwives. Sonography is, at least to some minimal degree, invasive. Its increasing routine use suggests that pregnancy is increasingly being viewed as an illness or problem that needs medical attention, instead of a healthy, normal process.

An important aspect of fetal sonography is the psychological effect on the mother. Unfortunately, the evidence is mostly anecdotal. Viewing the fetus on a sonographic screen is quite a different experience from feeling the growth of a living being in one's womb. Does the former tend to distance a woman from the experience of her own body? The latter, no doubt, makes use of an intuitive knowledge that has evolved through eons and has proved efficacious in by far the majority of cases.

Much anecdotal evidence suggests that viewing the sonographic image tends to increase maternal-infant bonding. In fact, in our highly technological society, in which people are removed from the cycles of nature in a way that our forebears were not, seeing an image on the sonographic screen may be a mode of perception well suited to our time. We must also ask, however, whether there is an equal if not greater risk that such a technological mode of perception may inhibit a mother's attunement to the state of the incipient person inside her. Related considerations apply to the sonographer and the physician. Reliance on electronic techniques may lead to atrophy of less high-technology but perhaps more important skills such as physical and emotional contact and empathy with one's patient.

Such a development would be debilitating not only to the mother but to the practitioner as well. Anything that cuts us off from one of our essential human traits, our connectedness as human beings, cannot be good for us.

All this may be a moot point. There appears to be a growing trend toward the routine use of sonography despite the recommendations of official bodies. However, this trend undercuts another essential human trait, our ability to choose. If a woman is not given a clear opportunity to choose fetal sonography, if a sonogram is presented as a routine part of prenatal care without any alternatives being considered, then she is being treated as less than fully human. A woman needs to be allowed, indeed encouraged, to make an informed choice in the matter, as with all matters pertaining to her health. This means asking what information the sonographic scan could provide that is not available through other means such as a stethoscope or palpation. It means asking whether the information gained through the scan would affect prenatal care and how. If the information gained through the scan has little probability of altering the prenatal care—as would be the case in a routine, noncomplicated pregnancy—then the scan would not be useful and should be avoided.

One reason that the Consensus Panel advised against routine sonography was the issue of its cost-effectiveness. Sonography is expensive. When no abnormality is suspected, it was believed that the cost did not justify the potential benefits. Interestingly, in England and other countries where medical care is seen as a right and not a commodity, official bodies have come to the opposite conclusion, that routine screening is cheaper than dealing with undetected medical problems later. If the cost to the patient were reduced, one of the drawbacks to routine screening would be of less importance.

In the end it comes down to a matter of choice. In the absence of suspected abnormalities, the choice should be given to a woman, in consultation with her physician and immediate family, because to be able to choose and decide is fundamental to our humanness.

Quality of Feedback During the Examination

Regardless of whether fetal sonography is performed as part of routine prenatal care or only in selected circumstances, there appears to be little doubt about the benefit of appropriate feedback to the woman during the examination. A number of studies (Cox et al, 1987; Field et al, 1985) have revealed that showing the woman the image and giving her a running commentary about it are good for both her and her fetus. Giving lots of feedback reduces maternal anxiety and produces more pleasant emotional experiences than hiding the image and giving only a summary after the examination. The babies whose mothers had received plentiful feedback in these studies were born with fewer complications, had greater birth weight, and were less irritable after birth than those whose mothers had received only summary information.

This outcome is to be expected. We are curious and intelligent beings. It is our nature to want to know what's going on around us. Satisfying this curiosity fulfills our nature; restricting information frustrates it, resulting in more anxiety and stress.

The Sonographer as Diagnostician

How much should a sonographer tell a patient? Sonographers are, by and large, not licensed physicians and are not qualified to make medical diagnoses. However, they must have enough knowledge to know whether a scan is satisfactory or not and will certainly have acquired a working recognition of normal anatomy and the various abnormalities.

The benefits of sharing information with a patient and her family are numerous. Doing so is rewarding; it increases recognition of one's connectedness with them as human beings. It also mitigates the potential ill effects of relying on electronic techniques instead of human intuition, as discussed earlier. Sharing knowledge treats a woman as a person and not merely an object to be scanned.

The risk, of course, is that not being a fully qualified physician, a sonographer may give inaccurate information. To many physicians, this is of paramount concern. The patient is under the doctor's care, and the sonographer is the doctor's agent, carrying out a specific investigative procedure. As such, the sonographer should give no interpretation of the results of the investigation at all, say these physicians.

At this writing, there is conflict about this area, and the issue is before the Standards Committee of the AIUM. The conflict is whether interpretation of sonographic images should be considered the practice of medicine. If so, in a strict sense it would mean that only Doctors of Medicine could interpret the images and that sonographers should say nothing.

Dr. Ken Taylor, of Yale University, addressed this question in the November/December 1982 issue of the Society of Diagnostic Medical Sonographers Newsletter. His own words are clear and concise:

> There is a very important difference between sonographers and other imaging technologists. Other technologists may reject an image because of sub-optimal technical quality, but the sonographer usually rejects over 95% of the scans because they do not provide the diagnosis. The sonographer must make the diagnosis and be able to interpret the scan to document the presence of any abnormalities. This is the unique responsibility of the sonographer.

To say that only Doctors of Medicine may interpret sonographic images not only is contrary to current practice, but it ends up denying the humanity of the sonographer. It cuts off personal contact with a patient and forbids the natural recognition and expression of our connectedness as humans. Such a result is harmful and thus, within our framework of ethics and assumptions about human nature, bad; it harms both the person being denied and the one denying. It treats the sonographer as merely a tool, and this is as bad as treating a woman as merely an object.

One reason for so much controversy may be the economics involved. We live in a society in which medical care is treated as a commodity, available to those with the means to pay and restricted for those without. The effect of a policy restricting interpretation to physicians would probably be an increase in the cost of sonographic health care, because doctors are more costly than sonographers. The best long-term solution may be a restructuring of the way health care is provided in our society.

In the meantime, there is no clear answer. Certainly it would be well to treat both the sonographer and the woman with respect and delight. To forbid sonographers to make any comments about anatomy seems much too harsh. Besides, it would probably be unworkable. Sonographers will communicate their judgment nonverbally in any case. On the other hand, it is important that medical advice and interpretation of pathology be the responsibility of the physician in charge, if only because he or she has had more training in diagnosis and treatment. At the very least, anything that a sonographer says should be accompanied by a disclaimer that this procedure does not give all the relevant information. This is primarily an issue between the sonographer and the physician.

It is unfortunate that sonographers and physicians see themselves, at times, as adversaries. The best approach would be to view each other as partners, each bringing a particular expertise to the task of providing good medical care for women and their unborn infants.

Involvement of Family and Friends

How many people should be in the room viewing the image? In some areas, it has become common to allow family members and friends to accompany the patient. This can be of great benefit to all concerned. It can produce increased bonding between other members of the family and the infant. It can promote a feeling of community and connectedness among family members and the woman. In cases in which some abnormality is suspected, it can be of great help to a woman to have a trusted friend there with her to lend emotional support. If the fetus is healthy, it allows a woman to share her joy.

The principal objection to this practice seems to come from certain sonographers. Having a lot of people around may be distracting and may produce a less than optimal scan. Also, it may be emotionally distressing to the sonographer if abnormalities are detected when many people are present. There is certainly the possibility that worry and stress may be magnified if the scan detects anything out of the ordinary. In addition, the more people who are around, the more pressure there is for the sonographer to make interpretations that may verge on medical diagnosis.

Many sonographers welcome family and friends. It seems clear that their presence is a recognition of our being connected to each other as humans. For this reason, I believe it would be wise to encourage the practice. What is important, however, is to respect and balance the wishes of all concerned. Guidelines that are agreeable to all parties, including especially the sonographer, should be adopted. We would do well to respect sonographers' intelligence in determining how best to do their job.

Abortion

Sonography is not an abortive procedure. It only gives information about the state of a fetus; it does not abort a fetus. Based on sonographic information, people can and do make decisions about whether to abort a fetus or continue a pregnancy. Two ethical questions arise here, both related. The larger question is under what circumstances, if any, is it appropriate or useful to abort. The more restricted question is how sonographers are to relate to the issue and how best to use the information gained from sonographic scanning.

The larger question is really twofold, because we must ask it not only for the individual but also for the society. The individual must ask herself whether in a particular case it would be better to abort or not. She must think about what circumstances would influence her to decide to abort or to continue the pregnancy. For society, we must think about policy in general. What rules and laws does it make sense to establish to govern the choices that individuals make? Under what circumstances would it be wise to allow abortion or to encourage it or to forbid it?

The larger question has to be answered first because it determines the framework within which to answer the more restricted question. If, for instance, abortion is seen as universally bad and to be condemned, sonographic data are in at least one sense irrelevant to the question (although certainly not irrelevant to the care of a woman and fetus). In this view, no matter what abnormalities are found, one should never abort a fetus. The only relevance might be to use the sonographic image as a way to remind a woman that her fetus is in fact a human being and thereby to dissuade her from aborting. If however, the question of whether to abort is seen as one that must be answered for each specific case and that there is no universal answer, then sonographic data become quite relevant indeed.

The issues surrounding abortion are emotionally loaded and full of controversy. The debate is usually framed as one of pro-life versus pro-choice. The pro-life side, at its extreme, claims that a fetus is a human being from the moment of conception and that therefore abortion is murder. The pro-choice side claims that any restriction on abortion amounts to subjugation of women, which is cruel and unjust. Philosophically, the arguments on both sides range from appeals to unquestioned authority all the way to reasoned examination of consequences.

What makes the debate so fierce is that each side feels compelled to deny the validity of the other's position. Extreme pro-choice proponents deny the humanity of the unborn in order to avoid feeling the pain of severing the connection with that life. Extreme pro-life advocates deny women's dignity and freedom and take refuge in stark, black-and-white moralism in order to avoid feeling the debasement of the person to whom they would deny the freedom of choice. We all want to avoid the discomfort of recognizing some validity in the other side's view. We want to avoid not only the intellectual discomfort of cognitive dissonance but the very real emotional pain of recognizing with empathy the other's anguish.

The fact is that both sides have validity. What makes the issue so hard is the conflict between two goods, two aspects of our human nature. One is our connectedness with each other as humans, and the other is our freedom of choice. There is no doubt that a fetus is an incipient human being. The closer a fetus is to term, the more fully human it is, but even in the early stages of pregnancy we have a human connection with it, and it pains us to deny that connection and to terminate it. However, we also have the freedom to choose how to live and the power to direct our own life. To deny anyone that choice is to diminish their humanity. What's needed is a position that recognizes the value of all aspects of our essential humanity.*

ABORTION AND SOCIAL POLICY

Using the teleological approach to ethics, we look at the consequences of each of the two positions. We concentrate on the question of social policy because individual circumstances are so varied that it is hard to make generalizations that would be applicable to each individual. The generalizations that we can make apply to social policy. What, then, are the risks and benefits of a societal policy allowing abortion and of a policy forbidding it?

Let's consider the pro-life position first. In some ways, forbidding abortion might be beneficial. To do so would certainly provide an opportunity for more people to know children's innate joy of life and exuberance. It would, if not force, at least encourage people to recognize the inherent value of human life. Who knows what great genius or talent it would save from premature oblivion?

There are also ways in which great harm would be done by forbidding women's right to choose abortion. Many pregnant women, poor and underprivileged, are not ready for motherhood and are not able to provide a nurturing environment for their baby. To force them to bear a child would be to condemn them and their children to a life of poverty and misery. In fact, many pregnant women of whatever social class are not emotionally prepared for motherhood. To force an unwanted child on a woman is to cause both of them considerable grief.

To forbid abortions would not prevent

*To frame the debate as pro-life versus pro-choice overlooks a third alternative. There are those, still a minority at present, who say that in some cases abortion should be mandatory. What if sonographic screening (or any other prenatal procedure) finds an incurable defect? What if this defect would cause the incipient person's life not to be worth living? What if it would be terribly expensive for the family and society to keep the person alive after birth? In that case, perhaps the woman should be forced to abort to spare the child the pain of a terrible life and to reduce costs.

We can quickly dispose of this position. To make abortion mandatory in certain instances is to deny both a woman's freedom of choice and our human ties with each other. Who is to say that a life will not be worth living? This position denies both our connection with each other as humans and our innate capacity to make decisions and govern our own lives.

them; it would only subject many women to the dangers of illegal and medically risky procedures. Such a policy would also contribute to the population explosion, which threatens to engulf the whole planet in conflict and suffering. Furthermore, we must not forget that the consequences of denying the full humanity of women have been hideous. Hundreds of thousands of women died brutally during the campaigns against witchcraft during the Middle Ages and as recently as the 1700s. These campaigns were largely directed against women's traditional medicine, based on herbs and other folk remedies, and against a religion that honored and valued women's place in the order of things.

In thinking of the consequences of forbidding all abortions, one can imagine that many women's lives would be enriched by love for their children, despite their initial reluctance to give birth. One can also imagine that many women's lives would be made miserable by being forced into motherhood, ready or not. The problem with imagining these scenarios is that we must also imagine their social context. The social context in the United States at present is, by and large, not helpful for parents or children, despite much talk about family values. Parents do a vitally important job for society, raising the next generation of citizens, but they are given little aid and assistance. It is a huge job to take care of a young person, and most parents are expected to do it alone. Given the present state of affairs, a social policy outlawing abortion would, I think, only contribute to the oppression of parents. Such a policy would have entirely different consequences in a society that gave ample help and encouragement, including financial assistance, to all parents. If social policy guaranteed a loving, nurturing environment for all children, especially those whose biological parents were unable or unwilling to care for them, then a prohibition on abortion would make more sense.

What, then, of the other side, the pro-choice position? The positive consequences of allowing abortion would be, in many ways, the inverse of the negative consequences of forbidding it. Women could, if they chose, be free of the burdens of parenthood for which they were not ready. Many lives would be saved by performing abortions under medically sound conditions. The population explosion would be dampened. Most important, this would be a step toward guaranteeing women the right to participate in society as fully valued persons. There is a Chinese saying, "Women hold up half the sky." We need women's full participation to solve the many problems confronting us. To deny their right to choose would be to relegate them to the status of second-class citizens.

The pro-choice position also poses dangers. Abortion does terminate a potential life. That is a great loss, not only to the prospective mother but to all of us. It can cause emotional pain, and if the pain is not dealt with, it can be brutalizing. By that, I mean very precisely that it tends to reduce us to the level of animals, of brutes, denying our connection to each other as human beings. This consequence is not so obvious as a poverty-stricken single mother with a huge family, but it is real nonetheless and may have even more disturbing consequences. If we deny our connection to unborn humans, we tend to become numb to our connection with born humans as well, leading to lives of isolation, cynicism, and despair and patterns of abuse of ourselves and others.

To be comprehensive, we need also to consider the effects of abortion on prospective fathers. Circumstances vary greatly, of course. In some cases, the prospective father may not even be known; in others, he is known very well. A man may want to have nothing to do with a child and may welcome abortion, or he may feel a deep bond with the prospective child and find abortion a terrifying alternative. Clearly, when a man has an interest in knowing and nurturing a child after birth, it would be well to take his feelings into account. Not to do so would be hurtful to him. Whether his feelings should prevail if a woman wants to abort is a question impossible to answer in general. It is not at all clear how to formulate a good social policy in this area.

The problem, again, is that we must look at the situation in a social context, or else we miss a vital part of the picture. In present-day Western society, in which commercial considerations carry great weight, people's true needs for connection and closeness are not fulfilled. Instead, we are encouraged to look for satisfaction in acquiring things and to produce and buy more and more material goods. The freedom to abort a fetus in such a context becomes much like the freedom to cut off a wart or throw out last year's wardrobe. An incipient human life is taken as a mere inconvenience. This concept is profoundly alien to our true nature, which is to take delight in all forms of humanity and to feel and to express our closeness with other people in all dimensions of our lives. As such, it is profoundly hurtful. Were we to live in a society that valued human beings as unique and awesome expressions of the creativity of our universe, abortion would take on a very different dimension. I suspect that it would be viewed as the occasion for great sorrow and would be voluntarily avoided as much as possible.

ABORTION AND THE FETUS

In all this weighing of pros and cons, benefits and risks, we have left out an important consideration. We've been discussing the possible consequences of abortion to pregnant women and to society, but what of the consequences to the fetus? What damage is done, and what potential good may come of a decision to abort as far as the fetus is concerned? Unfortunately, this is an area of which we can say nothing with any certainty. It depends on one's theological view of the nature of human beings before birth, and theology is not easily susceptible to verification.

One view might hold that abortion is a disaster for the fetus because it leaves the soul forever in purgatory. Sinful, because by nature all humans are sinful, and not allowed the chance to experience life and become redeemed, the aborted soul would have no chance of attaining salvation. Another theology might say that the aborted soul would simply go back into the pool of preborn souls and await another chance at incarnation. In this view, abortion is no disaster at all. Another view might be that abortion has no consequence for preborn humans because the soul is not human until birth, so the very concept of preborn human is self-contradictory. An eddy of energy that might have become human simply merges back into the universal plasma. Yet another view might be that the Great Spirit experiences reality through all avenues and that the pain of separation is felt through the fetus as well as through the pregnant woman, although perhaps less coherently. We have no way of judging with objectivity which, if any, of these views is correct.

Nor can one argue for the quality of life that might have been lived. Two problems arise here. One is that we cannot predict with certainty the quality of any one life. If allowed to be born and to live, would a person live a life of extraordinary satisfaction and accomplishment or a life of nearly unbearable degradation and despair, or, like most of us, a life somewhere in between? There's no way to know, although external circumstances like the social and economic milieu influence the probabilities.

The other problem is metaethical. It is sometimes argued that being alive is simply better than not being alive and that therefore abortion is always worse than the alternative (unless, perhaps, it is known that the fetus is nonviable). This view argues that it is better to be born into a life of abuse and abject misery than not to be born at all, that life of any sort is better than no life. The problem with this argument is the definition of "better." Better for whom? Better for what? The teleological view says that what's good for human beings is whatever enables us to function well, to do elegantly and efficiently the things that are uniquely ours to do. Within the context of being alive, we can say with certainty that some things are better than others, for instance that health is better than disease. From what point of view, however, can we say that being alive itself is better than not being alive? Is a chipmunk better than a chunk of rock? The problem with this argument is that it oversteps the boundaries of meaning, using words like "good" and "better" in contexts in which they are not meaningful.

ABORTION—NO EASY ANSWER

The point of view of the fetus offers no clear conclusion. The consequences to pregnant women and to society are mixed. The score card is not all pluses for one position and minuses for the other. I think it is safe to say that nobody really likes abortion, even those who insist that a woman's freedom of choice must be paramount, or if someone does, that is an indication that they are estranged from their humanity to an extreme degree. The ideal situation, of course, would be one in which no unwanted pregnancies occurred.

In order to work toward that ideal, it does not make sense to thwart anyone's thinking and creativity, which is the effect of denying one her freedom of choice. I think that this is the ultimate consideration that tips the balance in favor of freedom of choice and against forbidding abortion. Those who oppose abortion would do well to ally themselves with the many pro-choice people who find abortion itself repugnant. Working together to provide a better social context for all people would be a better way, in the long run, of avoiding abortion than legislating against freedom of choice.

ABORTION AND SONOGRAPHERS

Apart from social policy and apart from whether it would be helpful for any particular individual to abort her fetus, there are a number of issues that affect sonographers. Would it be helpful for a sonographer to be told that a woman is contemplating abortion? If a sonographer does not want to aid abortion, does it make sense to force him or her to perform a scan? If a woman is contemplating abortion, is it wise to show her the image if she does not ask to see it? What of the attitude and behavior of the sonographer? What is the most helpful way for the sonographers to behave when abortion is a possibility?

There is no doubt that sonographic data are quite relevant to the question, given the current social context in which freedom of choice is still, by and large, social policy. When abortion is being considered, sonographic scans are often performed to detect the age and size of the fetus; this information enables a physician to choose the appropriate procedure. If a scan shows a fetus to be nonviable or to have severe defects such as anencephaly, it would tend to weigh in favor of abortion. If a scan shows the fetus to be viable and normal, then the potential bonding effect of seeing the image might tend to influence a woman against abortion. For sonographers who have strong feelings about the issue, the effect on them must be considered as well as the effect on the woman.

First of all, it seems only fair to tell a sonographer when a woman is considering abortion. Not to do so relegates the sonographer to the status of a functionary, not a participant in a full human sense. It is demeaning to be treated as a mere instrument, without any say in the matter at hand, even though that is all too often the status of workers today.

Given an informed sonographer, what is the best course of action for both the sonographer and the woman if abortion is a possibility? The question is most acute when the sonographer is opposed to abortion. If the sonographer is in favor of freedom of choice, then the most helpful attitude is one of providing information in order to help a woman make an informed decision. If the sonographer is opposed to abortion, however, then he or she may not wish to provide information that might lead a woman to choose it or a physician to perform it. On the other hand, a sonographer might want to insist that a woman view the image in order to convince her that a human life is at stake, not just a mass of tissue. This is a case in which it is hard to make any kind of generalization, because so much depends on the individuals in the situation. How strong are the sonographer's feelings about the issue? Has the woman made up her mind? If so, how firm is her decision? How much information does she want to be given?

Given an overall preference for freedom of choice, as stated earlier, probably the most helpful attitude for a woman is to provide her the information she requests and not force information on her that she does not request. There is no obvious benefit, however, in forcing a sonographer to act contrary to his or her moral convictions. It could be quite distressing for a sonographer to participate in a way that violates deeply held beliefs, and it would be best for a sonographer not to do so.

In any case, there is a relationship—perhaps brief but real nonetheless—between the sonographer and the pregnant woman. Mutual respect and consideration are appropriate, and this would preclude both forcing the sonographer's opinions on the woman and forcing the sonographer to violate his or her integrity.

Conclusion

This chapter has outlined a way of thinking about ethics and has applied that way of thinking to a number of ethical issues facing sonographers today. The conclusions may seem quite reasonable to you, or they may seem absolutely outrageous. In either case, I hope they have stimulated you to think. I have approached the issues philosophically. The word *philosophy* comes from two Greek words meaning "the love of wisdom." Wisdom is not attained by glossing over the issues nor by merely accepting whatever conventional opinions you have come to hold. Wisdom is attained by carefully thinking for yourself. What do you think about these issues, and why?

REFERENCES

1. ARDMS Executive Office: History of the ARDMS. In: The American Registry of Diagnostic Medical Sonographers: Directory and Information Booklet, 1991; ARDMS, Cincinnati, OH, 1991, p 4.
2. Robertson JA: Legal and ethical issues arising from the new genetics. J Reprod Med 1992;37:521–524.
3. Post SG, Botkin JR, Whitehouse P: Selective abortion for familial Alzheimer disease? Obstet Gynecol 1992; 79:794–798.
4. Hobbins JC: Determination of fetal sex in early pregnancy. N Engl J Med 1983;309:979–980.
5. Evans MI, Durgan A, Bottoms SF, et al: Attitudes of the ethics of abortion, sex selection, and selective pregnancy termination among health care professionals, ethicists, and clergy likely to encounter such situations. Am J Obstet Gynecol 1991;164:1092–1099.
6. Stephens JD: Sex selection and early pregnancy fetal sex determination: Ethics and personal freedom of choice (letter). Am J Obstet Gynecol 1992;166: 1024–1025.
7. James AE, Bundy AL, Fleischer AC, et al: Legal aspects of diagnostic sonography. Semin Ultrasound CT MR. 1985;6:209.
8. Gill K: Legal liability and sonography: An update. J Diagn Med Sonogr 1992;8:93–96.
9. SDMS Code of Conduct. Society of Diagnostic Medical Sonographers, Dallas, TX.

SELECTED READING

Bar-Yam, NB: The trouble with ultrasound. Mothering Magazine 1990;57:73–77. Argues strongly against routine sonographic screening and suggests great caution in any case.

Berman MC, ed: Diagnostic Medical Sonography, vol I: Obstetrics and Gynecology. JB Lippincott, New York, 1991. Contains several chapters listing ethical and controversial issues in sonography.

Boyce WD, Jensen LC: Moral Reasoning: A Psychological-Philosophical Integration. The University of Nebraska Press, Lincoln, NE, 1978. This work provides a good overview of various ethical theories, including the teleological and the deontological schools.

Cox DN, Wittman BK, Hess M, Ross AG, Lind J, Lindahl S: The psychological impact of diagnostic ultrasound. J Obstet Gynecol 1987;70:673–676. Mothers given high feedback during ultrasound examination had less anxiety and more positive emotional experiences than those given low feedback.

DiIanni D: Ultrasound. Mothering Magazine 1982; 24:27–29. Overview of sonography for the lay audience.

Doyle ET: Window on the womb. RT Image Magazine 1992; July 27:4–6. The story of a sonographer's attempt to make fetal images widely available to dissuade women from choosing abortion.

Field T, Sandberg D, Quetel TA, Garcia R, Rosario M: Effects of ultrasound feedback on pregnancy anxiety, fetal activity, and neonatal outcome. J Obstet Gynecol 1985;66:525–528. This study shows that video and verbal feedback during ultrasound examinations reduces anxiety and results in better neonatal outcome.

Jackins H: The Human Side of Human Beings, The Theory of Re-Evaluation Counseling. Rational Island Publishers, Seattle, 1965. This and other works by Jackins describe human nature as intelligent, loving, cooperative, powerful, decisive, and zestful.

Jackins H. A Proposed Revision of the Postulates of Re-Evaluation Counseling. Start Over Every Morning. Rational Island Publishers, Seattle, 1989, pp 23–25.

Salam C: How sound is ultrasound? Mothering Magazine 1985;34:73–75. Reports on the 1984 findings of the National Institutes of Health recommending against routine sonographic screening.

Taylor K: Society of Diagnostic Medical Sonographers Newsletter (letter to the editor). Nov/Dec, 1982, p 2.

Versenyi L: Socratic Humanism. Yale University Press, New Haven, 1963. Scholarly but readable exposition of Socratic teleological ethics.

SECTION II

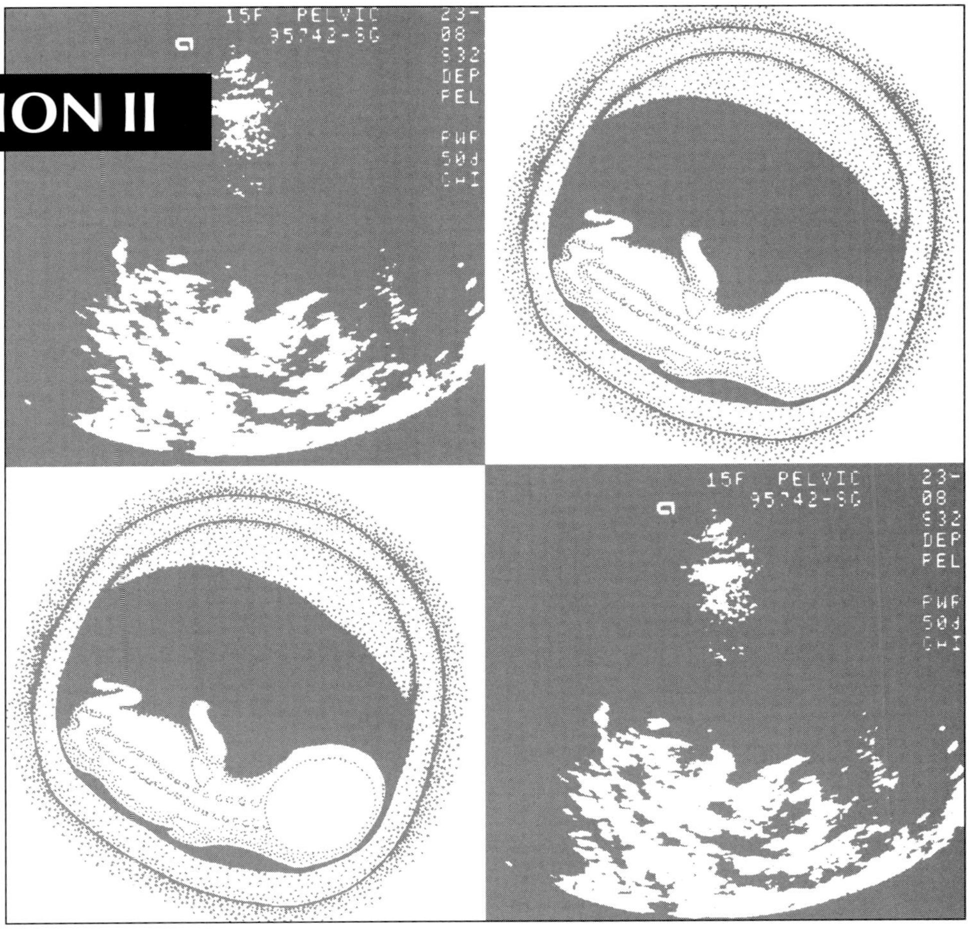

Fetal Anatomy by Organ/System

CHAPTER 7

SIZE/AGE ANALYSIS

Terry J. DuBose

This chapter is about estimating embryofetal age and size. In general, three statistical tools are used for predicting fetal age or size using sonographic measurements. The table or graph relating to age currently appears to be the most commonly used. The formula, or regression formula, that uses fetal measurements to predict age is actually the most common but is less visible because it is usually hidden inside computer software. One other common tool is the ratio that is used to compare relative sizes of one parameter with another.

A new method that is gaining acceptance for evaluating fetal size, age, and proportionality is the age range analysis (ARA).[1-7] This process requires converting all fetal parameters' measurements to their equivalent ages. The parameter age then represents the relative size in time—that is, the fourth dimension of the parameter.[4,7] The ARA is an extension of Hadlock and associates' multiple fetal parameters average age method (MFP AA).[8,9] This method has been proved to be the most accurate estimator of age.

Although a sonographer does not have to know how to calculate a regression analysis in order to use a table, a graph, or even the resulting formula that was developed by the analysis, it is necessary to have some understanding of this process. This understanding helps in selecting the appropriate statistical tool for fetal assessment and judging the relative accuracy of the assessment results. It is also necessary to qualify on the American Registry of Diagnostic Medical Sonographers examinations as well as other specialty boards.

The 1980s was an amazing decade for fetal sonography. During that decade, real-time sonography became the standard modality, color Doppler was introduced, and intracavitary transducers became available for general clinical practice. These new tools, in those 10 years, probably have given us more information about the development of the human fetus than had been available during the rest of human history.

In particular, as a result of high-resolution real-time sonography, the number of fetal parameter growth rates that were documented greatly increased. Before 1980, about the only parameters for estimating fetal age and size that had been studied were the crown-rump length (CRL)[10] and biparietal diameter (BPD).[11] The gestational sac diameter (GSD)[12] and uterine volume[13] were also used, but they were found to be somewhat less accurate.[14,15] Although other parameters such as head circumference and abdominal circumference (AC) were studied before 1980,[16] it was Hadlock and associates' work in the early 1980s that brought them into common use,[17,18] along with research by others on the femoral length (FemL) and humeral length (HumL)[19,20] and the binocular[21] and cerebellar widths.[22]

The fetal kidneys,[23] liver,[24] spine,[3] feet,[25] ulna and radius, tibia and fibula,[26] and soft tissues at various places on the fetus were also measured.[27-29] More obscure and esoteric fetal measurements were also documented, such as the clavicular[30] and mandibular[31] lengths. Other measurements that were documented in that active decade but were rarely used were the cranial volume (CV), coronal head circumference (CHC), and three-dimensional BPD correction (3-D BPD).

With all these various parameter measurements available, the reader may wonder how many parameter measurements are necessary for accurate fetal size or age estimations. That is the topic of this chapter. There is no simple answer to the question. It depends on how much accuracy is needed, how much time is available, how skillful and knowledgeable the sonographer/sonologist is, what the fetal position is, and how normal the fetus appears.

Another question that arises is which parameters should be used for estimating fetal age and which should be used for fetal size. Here again there is not a simple answer; indeed, the same parameters are often used for estimating both the size and the age of a fetus. Thus is opened the very real possibility of establishing the dates of the pregnancy using the fetal parameters and then assuming that the fetus is normal for that age when it is actually small for its time in gestation. The later Tale of Two Babies illustrates this problem.

A discussion of these fetal parameters requires some statistical background. For this reason, this chapter should be read in conjunction with Chapter 4, even though this chapter does not strictly follow classical statistical methodology. Some understanding of the meaning of *means* and *normal distribution* and a few statistical tests is necessary. This should not be too complex for anyone who can understand the concept that heavier babies tend to have fatter or larger abdomens or that as pregnancies progress, fetal bones normally grow longer.

The earliest and most basic method for studying fetal growth was by constructing a table or graph from the measurements of a group of normal fetuses. Table 7–1 is one type of table for estimating fetal age from multiple fetal parameters, and Table 7–2 is another form of a table for estimating age from a single parameter. The latter is the more common. Figure 7–1 includes XY graphs compiled from Table 7–1. These graphs and Table 7–1 show how rapidly a parameter changes with time, and the data in the graphs are known as *growth curves.*

One of the most useful of the parameters to be studied in this way is the BPD (see Table 7–2). Figure 7–2*A* is a dating curve for the BPD using a random selection of data, and Figure 7–2*B* is a growth curve for the same data. It would appear logical that either of these curves could be used interchangeably to date a pregnancy (dating curve) or to determine if the BPD is the appropriate size for the age of the fetus (growth curve); however, they are not precisely interchangeable—close, but not exact. See the later regression analysis discussion for an explanation about why this is true.

From fetal data, we can also perform regression analysis on the data to construct formulas that allow us to use fetal parameter measurements in the resulting formulas to estimate fetal age. These formulas may be relatively simple linear regressions or quite complex higher-order polynomials, which are best left to computers for solutions. An infinite number of formulas can be used to describe the growth of any single parameter. These various formulas are more or less accurate when compared with one another. Some may exhibit more accuracy at one time in pregnancy and others at another time in pregnancy.

Thus, basically three tools are available for estimating the age of a fetus from sonographic measurements: the table, the graph, and the regression formula. These same three tools can be used to estimate fetal size, with the additional tool of ratios to compare the relative size of one parameter with that of another. Although a large number of different regression formulas may be used to describe a single parameter, in this discussion we treat them as one method or tool. The tricky part is determining which formula to use so that the process is not too complicated yet has good

Text continued on page 102

TABLE 7–1. FETAL AGE AND AGE RANGE ANALYSIS—BASIC BABY II

AGE	E/FHR	GSD	CRL	BPD	3-D BPD	FOD	VCD	CV	THC	CHC	CERB	BiOD	FSL	FemL	HumL	ADA	AC	LNMP	MFP AA	AGE	AA	RANGE
41				100	96	123	66	482	349	260			74	79	70	120	376	39.7	40.75	41		
40				97	96	119	70	451	339	264	43	60	73	77	67	118	371	38.0	39.84	40		
39				95	93	116	66	421	330	252	44	58	71	76	67	116	365	38.5	38.78	39		
38				93	91	116	66	397	328	249	47	60	69	73	65	114	359	36.1	37.94	38		
37				91	90	113	65	376	320	244	51	59	67	73	63	110	342	38.0	36.99	47		
36				89	88	111	64	351	314	240	46	59	65	71	62	103	325	35.4	36.00	36		
35				87	86	109	63	329	307	234	40	57	63	68	60	99	310	35.2	34.96	35		
34				85	84	106	62	307	299	230	38	55	61	66	58	95	299	35.0	34.02	34		
33				83	82	104	60	289	294	224	40	52	59	64	56	92	289	33.2	33.04	33		
32				80	80	101	58	260	285	217	38	51	56	62	55	89	281	32.2	31.99	32		
31				78	78	98	57	243	277	212	36	50	54	59	53	85	268	30.2	31.02	31		
30				75	75	95	55	220	268	205	35	48	52	57	51	81	253	30.2	29.99	30		
29				73	73	93	55	204	260	200	33	46	49	55	50	77	243	30.1	29.00	29		
28				71	71	89	52	181	251	192	32	46	47	53	48	74	231	28.3	28.00	28		
27				68	68	86	51	166	242	187	30	44	45	50	46	71	221	26.4	27.04	27		
26				65	66	83	49	146	233	178	28	43	43	48	44	68	212	26.7	26.01	26		
25				62	63	79	47	127	221	171	27	41	41	46	43	65	205	26.3	25.01	25		
24				59	60	76	45	110	211	163	25	40	39	43	40	61	191	23.4	24.00	24		
23				56	56	71	42	93	199	154	24	38	37	40	38	58	181	23.8	23.00	23		
22				53	53	67	40	78	188	146	22	36	34	37	36	54	170	22.4	22.00	22		
21				49	50	62	38	65	175	137	21	34	32	35	34	51	160	21.1	21.02	21		
20				46	47	59	35	54	165	129	19	32	30	32	31	47	149	20.7	20.02	20		
19			130	44	44	55	33	44	155	121	19	30	28	29	29	44	138	19.5	19.05	19		
18			121	40	40	50	31	35	142	112	18	28	25	26	26	40	126	18.6	17.99	18		
17		115	113	37	37	46	29	28	131	104	17	25	22	23	23	36	113	16.7	17.03	17		
16		112	104	34	34	42	25	20	118	93	15	23	20	20	20	33	103	16.6	16.02	16		
15		104	92	30	30	37	23	14	105	83	14	21	17	16	16	29	91	15.4	15.01	15		
14	150	93	83	27	26	33	20	10	93	73	12	17	15	13	13	25	78	14.8	14.01	14		
13	152	80	71	23	23	28	17	6	81	63	10	15	13	10	10	21	68	15.0	13.01	13		
12	159	76	58	20	20	24	14	3.8	69	54		13	11	7	7	18	57	12.1	12.02	12		
11	163	63	46	16	17	20	13	2.4	56	46		13		6	5	15	48	12.4	11.00	11		
10	167	53	37	13	13	17	9	1.2	42	46		9		4	4	13	40	12.0	9.99	10		
9	173	46	25	11	11	13	8	0.7	31	30						10	30	10.4	9.01	9		

Table continued on following page

TABLE 7–1. **FETAL AGE AND AGE RANGE ANALYSIS—BASIC BABY II *(Continued)***

AGE	E/FHR	GSD	CRL	BPD	3-D BPD	FOD	VCD	CV	THC	CHC	CERB	BiOD	FSL	FemL	HumL	ADA	AC	LNMP	MFP AA	AGE	AA	RANGE
8	165	35	17	7	7	9	5	0.2	19	19						7	22	10.2	8.01	8		
7	142	26	10	5														9.2	7.00	7		
6	114	18	5															8.0	6.01	6		
5	98	11	2															6.7	4.94	5		
4		5																6.2	4.01	4		

Age range analysis summary:	LNMP	AA
Growth interval:	Weeks	Weeks
Last exam #n		
−First exam		
Difference:		

Instructions

To perform age range analysis (ARA) for each examination:

Take measurements and calculate values for each parameter using the formulas below. Circle the table values, determine each parameter age, and average all parameter ages; interpolate for more accuracy. Enter the examination average age in tenths of weeks under AA. Subtract the examination's smallest parameter age from the largest and enter the difference under RANGE.

ARA: The range of ages should not be more than 20% (±10% = ±2 SD) of the average age. Single parameters should not be more than ± 10% from the average age. To determine the relative location of any parameter in the time-series distribution, use the following formula:

$$(\text{Parameter age} - \text{AA})/(\text{AA} \times 0.05) = \text{location in standard deviations (SD)}$$

$$(\_\_\_\_\_ - \_\_\_\_\_)/(\_\_\_\_\_ \times 0.05) = \_\_\_\_\_\text{SD}$$

For growth intervals in serial studies:

Take measurements and calculate values for each parameter, and determine average age for each examination. Place the mother's reported LNMP in weeks and average for each examination in the blanks at the bottom of the table. Subtract the LNMP and average ages of the first (dating) examination from the last (comparative) examination (LMP_n and AA_n).

Interpretation: If the $LNMP_n - LNMP_1$ and $AA_n - AA_1$ differences (time intervals) are approximately equal, then appropriate growth has occurred. In general, the difference between the LNMP and AA time intervals should not be greater than 10% of the fetal age. If the LNMP difference is greater than the AA difference, then less growth than expected has occurred (possible intrauterine growth restriction). If the LNMP difference is less than the AA difference, then accelerated growth has occurred.

CALCULATIONS

Circumferences may be calculated from two diameters: circumference = $(d_1 + d_2) \times 1.57$

Cranial volume is calculated from three diameters: CV = FOD × BPD × VCD × 0.000555

Acronym	Description	Measurement or Calculation	Unit
E/FHR	Heart rate	M-mode {age < 9.2 LMP weeks = ((EHR × .3) + 6)/7}	B/M
GSD	Gestational	Largest diameter of chorionic cavity	mm
CRL	Crown-rump length	Top of head to rump; do not include legs	mm
BPD	Biparietal diameter	Leading edge to leading edge (outer to inner)	mm
3-D BPD	3-D BPD correction	Average (FOD + BPD + VCD)/3 = BPD	mm
FOD	Fronto-occipital diameter	Middle of frontal to middle of occipital bones	mm
VCD	Vertical cranial diameter	Middle of cranial vertex to middle of hippocampal base line	mm
CV	Cranial volume	Use CV calculation above, mm diameters for CV in milliliters	ml
THC	Transverse head circumference	THC = (FOD + BPD) × 1.57	mm
CHC	Coronal head circumference	CHC = (VCD + BPD) × 1.57	mm
CERB	Cerebellar transverse diameter	Transverse cerebellar diameter	mm
BiOD	Binocular diameter	Distance between outer edges of the ocular globes	mm
FSL	Fractional spine length	Seven complete thoracolumbar vertebral bodies and spaces	mm
FemL	Femur length	Length of femoral diaphysis	mm
HumL	Humerus length	Length of humeral diaphysis	mm
ADA	Abdominal diameter average	Average of transverse (TAD) and AP (AAD) abdominal diameters	mm
AC	Abdominal circumference	AC = (TAD + AAD) × 1.57	mm
LNMP	Last normal menstrual period	Mean of mothers' reported LNMPs for this population	week
Average	Average age	Mean of all exam AAs for each week (± 0.25 week)	week
Age	Age in weeks	Age on day 1 of week	week
AA	Average age in LMP weeks	Blank for average of parameter ages for current exam	week
Range	Range of ages	Subtract smallest parameter age from largest parameter age	week

This table facilitates manual calculation of the multiple fetal parameter and age range analysis. This is possibly the largest number of parameters ever measured in a single population and correlated with age, then compiled into a table of human fetal development. It was developed during a period of 10 years (1984–1994), and the population includes more than 10,000 sets of fetal measurements and observations. Use of these analyses produces results similar to those produced by computer software shown in Figures 7–15A and B, 7–18, and 7–20.

TABLE 7–2. COMPOSITE BIPARIETAL DIAMETERS*

MILLIMETERS	WEEKS WITH VARIATION	MILLIMETERS	WEEKS WITH VARIATION
20	12.0	60	22.3 to 25.5
21	12.0	61	22.6 to 25.8
22	12.2 to 13.2	62	23.1 to 26.1
23	12.4 to 13.6	63	23.4 to 26.4
24	12.6 to 13.8	64	23.8 to 26.8
25	12.9 to 14.1	65	24.1 to 27.1
26	13.1 to 14.3	66	24.5 to 27.5
27	13.4 to 14.6	67	25.0 to 27.8
28	13.6 to 15.0	68	25.3 to 28.1
29	13.9 to 15.2	69	25.8 to 28.4
30	14.1 to 15.5	70	26.3 to 28.7
31	14.3 to 15.9	71	26.7 to 29.1
32	14.5 to 16.1	72	27.2 to 29.4
33	14.7 to 16.5	73	27.6 to 29.8
34	15.0 to 16.8	74	28.1 to 30.1
5	15.2 to 17.2	75	28.5 to 30.5
36	15.4 to 17.4	76	29.0 to 31.0
37	15.6 to 17.8	77	29.2 to 31.4
38	15.9 to 18.1	78	29.6 to 32.0
39	16.1 to 18.5	79	29.9 to 32.5
40	16.4 to 18.8	80	30.2 to 33.0
41	16.5 to 19.3	81	30.7 to 33.5
42	16.6 to 19.8	82	31.2 to 34.0
43	16.8 to 20.2	83	31.5 to 34.5
44	16.9 to 20.7	84	31.9 to 35.1
45	17.0 to 21.2	85	32.3 to 35.7
46	17.4 to 21.4	86	32.8 to 36.2
47	17.8 to 21.6	87	33.4 to 36.6
48	18.2 to 21.8	88	33.9 to 37.1
49	18.6 to 22.0	89	34.6 to 37.6
50	19.0 to 22.2	90	35.1 to 38.1
51	19.3 to 22.5	91	35.9 to 38.5
52	19.5 to 22.9	92	36.7 to 38.9
53	19.8 to 23.2	93	37.3 to 39.3
54	20.1 to 23.7	94	37.9 to 40.1
55	20.4 to 24.0	95	38.5 to 40.9
56	20.7 to 24.3	96	39.1 to 41.5
57	21.1 to 24.5	97	39.9 to 42.1
58	21.5 to 24.9	98	40.5 to 43.1
59	21.9 to 25.1		

*Recommended biparietal diameter to gestational age based on the calculated weighted least-mean-squares-fit equation and 90% variation of the 17 studies.

Kurtz and colleagues' original BPD table compiled from 17 BPD charts developed worldwide. BPD to age in weeks for 90% variation. This table requires leading-edge to leading-edge BPD measurements.

From Kurtz AB, Wapner RJ, Kurtz RJ, et al: Analysis of biparietal diameter as an accurate indicator of gestational age. J Clin Ultrasound 1980;8:319–326.

FIGURE 7–1.
Growth curves for fetal cranial and body parameters from Table 7–1. Gestational sac diameter (GSD) is not a true fetal parameter, and heart rate (E/FHR) is not a parameter measurement in the common sense of morphology. Note the differences in rates of change between volume, circumferences, and linear measurements.

A, Data from the fetal cranium, except for the E/FHR. CHC, coronal head circumference; FOD, fronto-occipital diameter; 3-D BPD, three-dimensional biparietal diameter correction; VCD, vertical cranial diameter; BiOD, binocular diameter; cerebellum, transverse cerebellar diameter. The labels for the BiOD (diamonds) and cerebellum (dashes) are slightly below their corresponding curves. CV, cranial volume; THC, transverse head circumference.

B, Growth curves for the body parameters. AC, abdominal circumference; ADA, abdominal diameter average; CRL, crown-rump length; FemL, femur length; FSL, fractional spine length; HumL, humerus length.

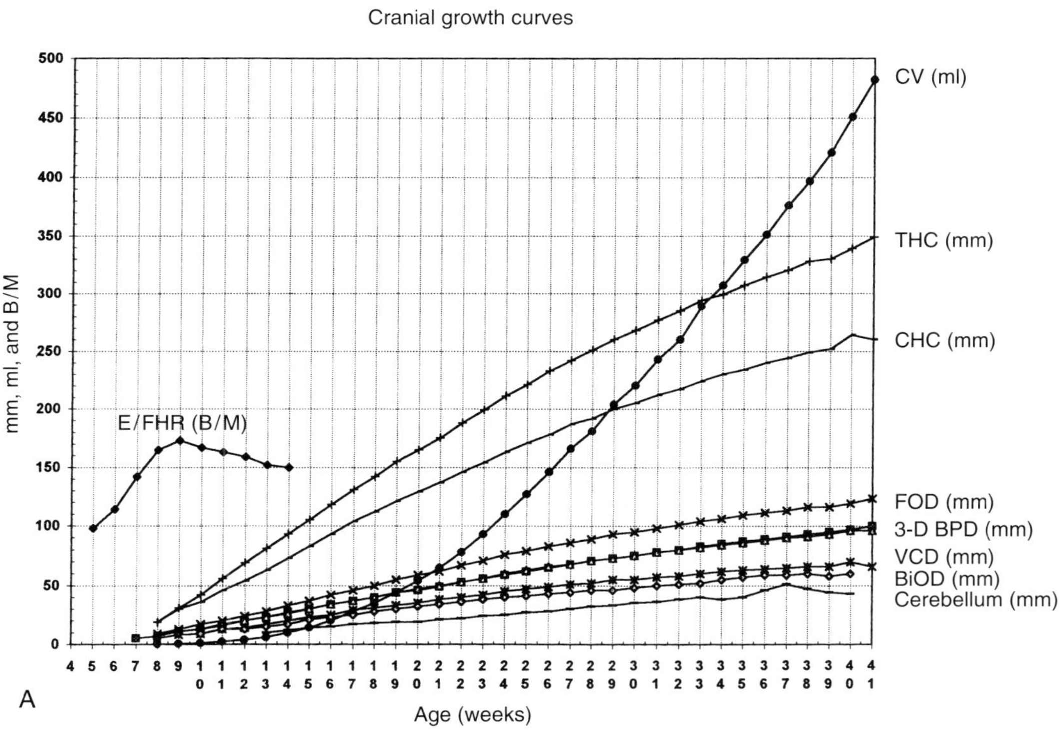

Cranial growth curves
mm, ml, and B/M
Age (weeks)
CV (ml)
THC (mm)
CHC (mm)
E/FHR (B/M)
FOD (mm)
3-D BPD (mm)
VCD (mm)
BiOD (mm)
Cerebellum (mm)
A

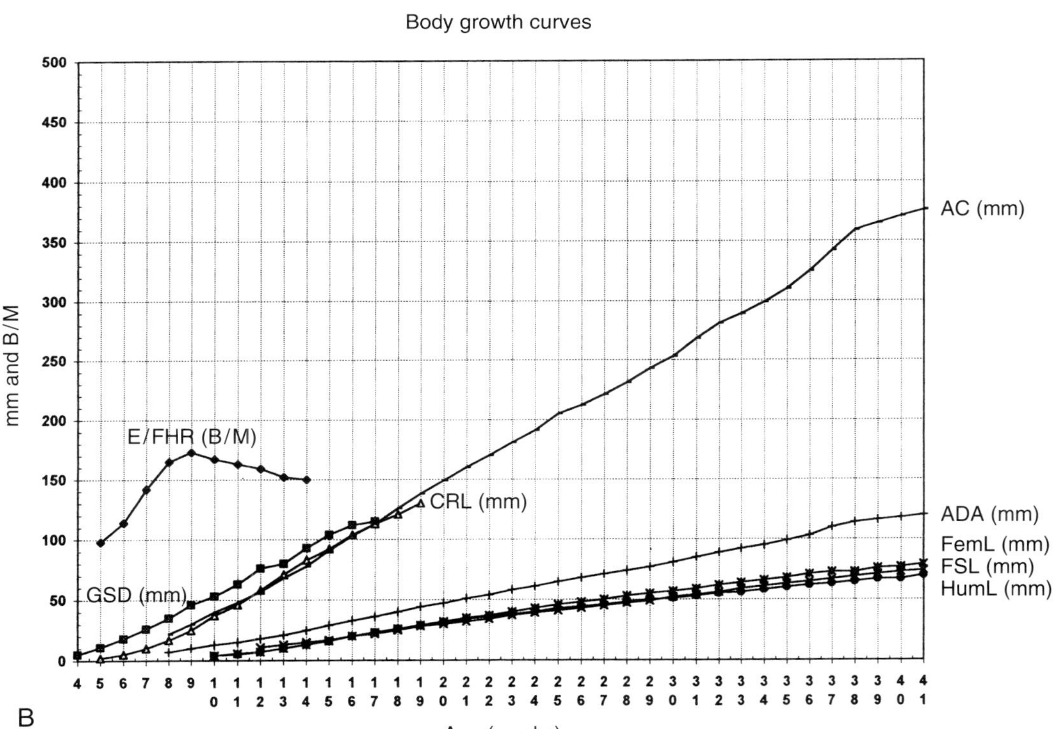

Body growth curves
mm and B/M
Age (weeks)
AC (mm)
E/FHR (B/M)
CRL (mm)
GSD (mm)
ADA (mm)
FemL (mm)
FSL (mm)
HumL (mm)
B

FIGURE 7–1.

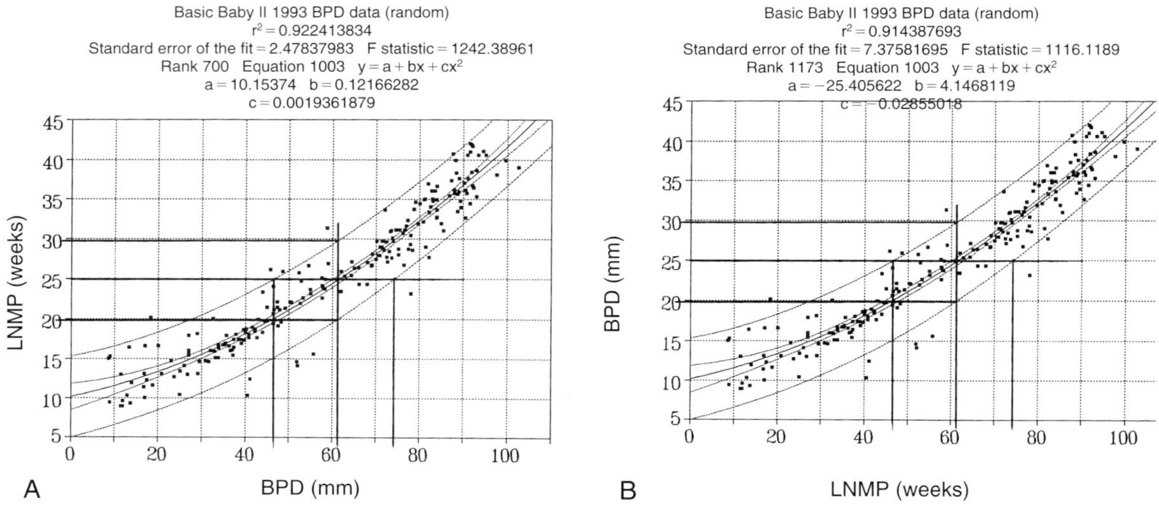

FIGURE 7–2.
Dating and growth curves. Both *A* and *B* are generated from the same data set. This example can be used to show why growth curves should not be used for dating a pregnancy. Results can be checked by using other BPDs and LNMPs in the equations at the top of the figures. In *A*, the BPD is a dating curve and is the independent variable (x-axis) and the LNMP is the dependent variable (y-axis). A BPD of 61.6 mm predicted an age of exactly 25 weeks. In *B*, a growth curve, the LNMP is the independent variable and the BPD is the dependent. An LNMP of 25 weeks predicts a BPD of 60.4 mm.

accuracy.[32] As mentioned earlier, many formulas, tables, and graphs have been published by various researchers for the more commonly measured fetal parameters, and some of these are more accurate than others.

The following discussion begins with tables, formulas, curves, and a family of formulas for estimating fetal age using personal computer spreadsheets. Next follows a look at ratios for fetal parameter proportionality and weight estimations. The chapter ends with a new method of assessing fetal age, parameter proportionality, and fetal weight. This new method, ARA, was first proposed and presented at the 1988 World Federation for Ultrasound in Medicine and Biology (WFUMB) meeting, jointly sponsored in Washington, D.C., by the WFUMB, the American Institute of Ultrasound in Medicine, and the Society of Diagnostic Medical Sonographers.[1]

Embryofetal Age

LAST MENSTRUAL PERIOD

The date of the last normal menstrual period (LNMP) is the most common method for estimating the expected delivery date for a fetus. This date is most likely used because in ancient times the cessation of menses was the only date with which pregnancy could be linked. Although pregnancies are dated from the LNMP, the LNMP is really the end of the last fertility period. As it is described in *Williams Obstetrics*, "menstruation must be viewed, in a physiological sense, as the end-result of fertility failure, whether chosen or naturally occurring."[33] The menstrual cycle is variable from woman to woman and from cycle to cycle. Stress and anxiety may alter the length of the cycle.[34–41] Some bleeding may be associated with implantation of the blastocyst and is often mistaken for a menstrual period. Another problem is that many women simply do not keep a calendar of menses or sexual activities. The fetal age as determined by the LNMP may be referred to as the *gestational age*.[34]

Normally, a woman ovulates 2 weeks (14 days) after the start of her LNMP, and conception usually takes place within 2 or 3 days after ovulation. Normal human gestation is 38 weeks; therefore, the birth day is expected to be 40 weeks after the LNMP. The problem here is that we are discussing normality, and almost no one is absolutely normal. Some women do not have 28-day menstrual cycles; therefore, they may not ovulate precisely 14 days after their LNMP. Sperm may live for 2 or 3 days, and after fertilization, the fertile oocyte (egg) must travel down the fallopian tube to the implantation site in the uterus. All tubes are not the same length, thus introducing another variable.[42] Figure 7–3 is a BPD dating curve in which the BPD (in millimeters) is the independent variable (x-axis), the fetal ages are determined in weeks from the woman's LNMP, and the MFP AAs are the dependent variables (y-axis). This figure illustrates the greater variability of the LNMP.

At the other end of pregnancy are more variables. As stated earlier, normal human gestation is 38 weeks. Adding the 2 weeks between the LNMP and ovulation, a normal duration of pregnancy from the LNMP is said to be 40 weeks, or 280 days. However, all women do not carry a pregnancy for exactly the same amount of time. Various degrees of prematurity and postmaturity are common. According to *Williams Obstetrics*,[43,44] a delivery can normally occur from 266 days to 299 days after the LNMP, with a mean of 281 days. This calculates in weeks to be 38 to 42.5 weeks, with a mean of 40 weeks after the LNMP. Today, with modern medicine, premature infants may be kept alive after only 26 weeks' gestation.[45] It is this variability in the length of pregnancies that makes exact prediction of the end of pregnancy difficult.

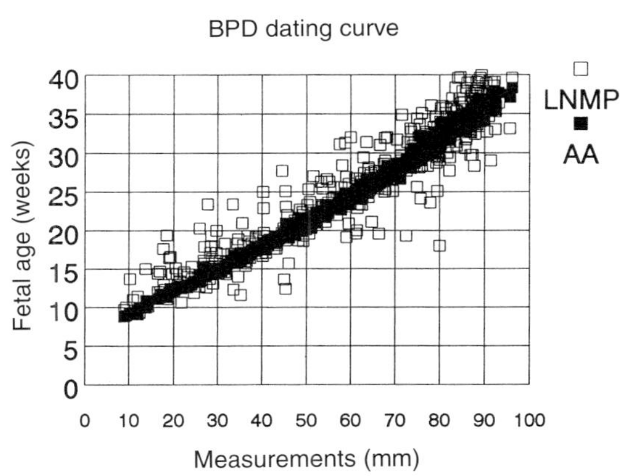

FIGURE 7–3.
A dating curve with the LNMP and the average age of multiple fetal parameters (open squares) in weeks as the dependent variable. The LNMP exhibits much more variability than the average age (AA, solid squares).

Naegele's rule is often used to estimate the birth date of a fetus: "It is customary to estimate the expected date of delivery by adding 7 days to the date of the first day of the last normal menstrual period and counting back 3 months."[44] This rule gives the day of the month in which delivery is expected, but this date will be no more accurate than the LNMP date on which it is based.

Diagnostic medical sonography has given more precision to the dating of pregnancies. This precision is achieved by using fetal measurements to estimate the duration of the pregnancy. Different dates are now used to discuss pregnancy, and they may or may not have the same meaning. A woman's reported LNMP is often used to estimate gestational age, although ovulatory age or fertilization age usually refers to the date of conception.[45] Because of the inherent variability of the LNMP date and of the following time of conception, other methods have been used to date pregnancies.[46] One method that seems very valid but has been questioned used ovulation dates as determined in fertility studies to construct a fetal CRL dating chart.[4,47] Serum levels of beta-human chorionic gonadotropin (hCG),[48–50] follicular puncture plus 14 days in in vitro fertilization studies,[51] the day of insemination, gamete intrafallopian transfer (GIFT), and the day of intercourse in couples who had isolated midcycle sexual activity and who kept basal body temperature charts or who monitored urine for the luteinizing hormone surge[52] all have been used to date pregnancies in sonographic research. Some have even used dates from fetal measurements to establish the timing of other fetal parameters in the same population.[53]

For purposes of simplicity, this chapter uses the following conventions for discussing the dates of pregnancies or fetal ages. The LNMP is used *only* for the date reported by a woman as the first day of her last menstrual period. The *last menstrual period* (LMP) refers to dates established by other means, such as sonographic fetal measurements, beta-hCG levels, MFP AA, GIFT dates, and others, and is given in equivalent menstrual weeks. The conceptual age is used when the date of conception is established or calculated. It normally starts 2 weeks after the LMP.

The use of sonographic measurements to establish the LMP does not mean that the LNMP was normal, even if these measurements coincidentally match. It also does not mean that the birth date will be normal. In fact, because some fetuses are smaller or larger than normal at the same time in gestation, fetal size is not always precise in estimating the dates of individual pregnancies. Sonographic dates from large populations are more precise, but a normal human pregnancy has many variables. In all probability, prediction of exact dates for an individual pregnancy is not possible in every case.

TABLES, GRAPHS, AND REGRESSIONS

Methods

Population

Throughout this chapter, sonographic fetal measurement data are used to generate original tables, graphs, and formulas and for examples. The data are from a population of 10,336 consecutive obstetrical examinations performed during the decade of 1984 to 1993. Each examination was referred by the patient's primary care obstetrician to one of four outpatient diagnostic imaging laboratories in Austin, Texas. In the 1990 census, the Austin Metropolitan Statistical Area was 9.2% black, 0.4% Native American, 2.4% Asian and Pacific, 20.5% Hispanic, and 67.5% white and others. Of this population, 87.8% of the examinations recorded a beating heart and 82.2% reported a LNMP. Of the examinations in which a heart rate was recorded, no significant difference (analysis of variance [ANOVA], $P > 0.05$) was found in the mean age by LNMP (21.72 weeks) and the mean MFP AA (21.47). The variance for the LNMP and the MFP AA was significantly different (F test, $P < 0.05$). This was expected because the large majority of patients are referred to these laboratories for uncertain LNMP dates. The 1993 subset (n = 2728) contains parameters that were not included in the early years of the study, and a random selection of 300 from that year is used for some analyses. There was no significant difference in the MFP AAs or LNMPs for the year (1993) or the random selection ($P > 0.01$).

Because these data are from a population referred for medical reasons, a statistical bias is possible. However, because of the size of the population and the fact that these laboratories have a good reputation for dating pregnancies and the vast majority were referred for dating, most were considered normal pregnancies. In addition, most high-risk cases are referred to perinatology laboratories in the same geographic areas; therefore, any bias in the study population or random samples from it should be minimal.

In a test population of 925 consecutive sonographic examinations, follow-up was obtained by stamped return-addressed postcards requesting birthing information. The cards were given to the women at the time of their examinations (1985–1986). Of these, 489 cards (52.9%) were returned. In these 489 pregnancies, there were three sets (0.6%) of twins (one set miscarried at 22 LMP weeks), one Rh incompatibility, one amniotic band (which did not involve the normal baby), one case of maternal preeclampsia, one spontaneous abortion at 23 LMP weeks (reason unknown), and only one baby (0.2%) with congenital defects (cleft palate and intestinal blockage). These incidents tend to be lower than those reported by others.[54–56] However, it is easy to imagine that in an informal, voluntary follow-up study such as this, parents disappointed in the outcome of a pregnancy might not respond. From this study, the population appears normal; and informal and limited as it may be, it shows no direct evidence that the current study population is abnormal.

Equipment and Staff

All sonographic measurements were made using real-time sonography and electronic calipers. Heart rates were determined by M-mode. Sector, linear, and transvaginal transducers were used as required by the time in gestation. Measurements obtained are listed in Table 7–1. Fetal skull measurements were taken as described in Chapter 8. The BPD was leading edge to leading edge (outer to inner); fronto-occipital diameter

(FOD) was midfrontal to midoccipital bones. Long bone measurements are of the echogenic diaphysis (see Chapter 15), and abdominal diameters and circumferences are to the outer skin edge at the level of the confluence of the umbilical and the hepatic veins (see Chapter 14).

These sonographic examinations were performed by more than 15 sonographers (1993 data by 12 sonographers, 11 certified by the American Registry of Diagnostic Medical Sonography and 1 eligible) or students under their direct supervision in the four laboratories using seven different sonographic machines, at any given time, from five different manufacturers (six Acuson, six General Electric, one Phillips, one ATL, and one Diasonic). All measurements were entered into fetal size/age analysis software at the time of the examination.[2] Analysis found no statistically significant differences between observers, laboratories, or machines (see Chapter 8 for more discussion of the statistical population and methods).

The sonographers were requested to rate the difficulty of obtaining selected fetal sonographic measurements and observations. Each sonographer rated each item on a scale from 0 to 10, with 0 being the easiest to obtain and 10 the most difficult. The results were coded into a spreadsheet for analysis. Because the sonographers had overall ratings that were higher or lower, the scores were adjusted so that the mean score for each sonographer was 5. The sonographers' experience in obstetrics ranged from ½ year to 18 years; the mean was 7 ½ years. Figure 7–4 shows the results of this study. No relationship was found between the sonographers' experience and their mean scores ($r^2 = 0.167$).

Regression Tables, Graphs, and Formulas

Multiple Fetal Parameters Average Age. Table 7–1 is not like most fetal age dating tables. It was not constructed from regression formulas. It is designed to calculate MFP AA and perform ARA of fetal proportionality. The table was developed during a period of 10 years. The first version (1984–1985) included

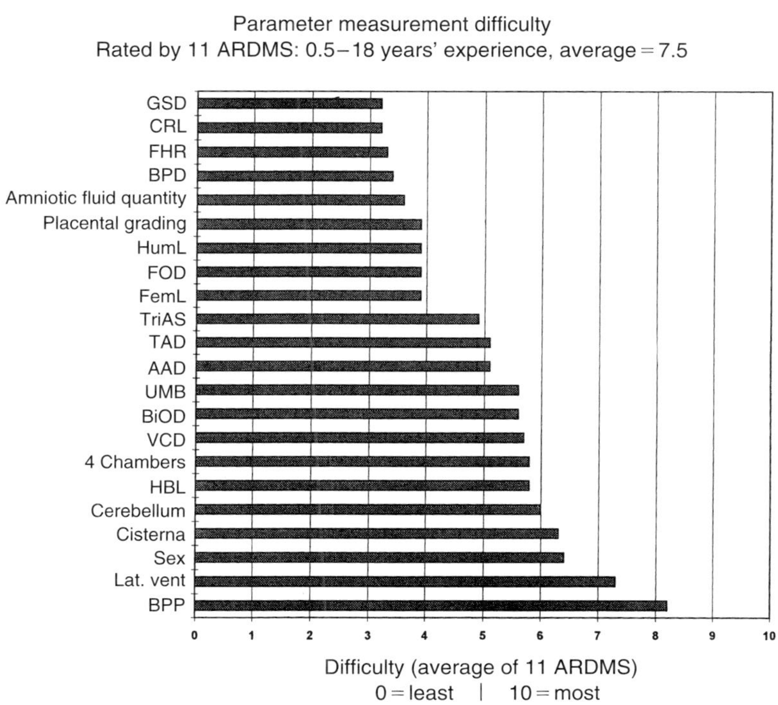

FIGURE 7–4.
Eleven sonographers were requested to rate selected fetal parameter measurements and observations according to difficulty, from 0 (easiest) to 10 (most difficult). Each sonographer's ratings were adjusted so their mean rating was 5, and ratings for each parameter were then averaged. GSD, gestational sac diameter; CRL, crown-rump length; FHR, M-mode heart rate for embryos and fetuses; BPD, biparietal diameter; HumL, humerus length; FOD, fronto-occipital diameter; FemL, femur length; TriAS, coronal triangle side measurement; TAD, transverse abdominal diameter; AAD, anteroposterior abdominal diameter; UMB, count of umbilical cord vessels; BiOD, outer binocular distance; VCD, vertical cranial diameter; 4 chambers, visualization of a four-chamber heart; HBL, hippocampal base line; cerebellum, transverse cerebellar measurement; cisterna, measurement of the cisterna magna; sex, determination of fetal sex; lat. vent, measurement of the tranverse cerebral ventricle antrum; BPP, biophysical profile scoring; ARDMS, American Registry of Diagnostic Medical Sonographers.

fewer parameters: the GSD, CRL, BPD, transverse head circumference (THC), FemL, and AC. The original ages were determined by recording the measurements by hand and using established look-up tables to determine ages.[6, 10, 12, 27, 57] In 1986, the table was computerized[2] and several other measurements were added; the weekly mean ages were determined using the MFP AA from the earlier table. This process of updating the table was repeated at 1- to 2-year intervals as data were added. This final table is based on the data from 2728 examinations performed in 1993; the demographic data are the same as those for the larger 1984–1993 population. The table was constructed using a locally weighted scatterplot smoother (LOWESS).[58] The LOWESS technique is described later.

In Table 7–1, the MFP AA column (next to last) lists the averages of all individual MFP AAs for each week (±0.25); the two age weeks columns (first and last for easier comparison with parameters) are the rounded equivalent MFP AA LMP weeks. The LNMP weeks column is the weekly mean LNMP for the cases and is included for comparison purposes only. The other columns represent the mean parameter measurement for each week, except the embryofetal heart rate (E/FHR), which is not a true parameter measurement in the common sense. The last two columns are for calculations of individual MFP AAs using the table and the ARA. These calculations and the interpretations are discussed later under Age Range Analysis. Figure 7–1 shows XY plots from this table. The cranial and body parameters were plotted separately for simplicity.

Table 7–1 can be used to estimate the MFP AA for any number of the fetal parameters that the sonographer chooses. This table was ordered with ascending ages so that smaller ages are below the larger for easier subtraction in growth series analysis. It produces very accurate age estimates, and the ARA (discussed later) is an easy way of observing fetal proportionality.

The following is a discussion of selected individual parameters for estimating fetal age. These are parameters that are commonly used and have been proved through research and replication by others. Other parameters may also be used to estimate fetal age.

Regression Formulas. Regression formulas are used to predict one value from one or more other values, such as the BPD measurement to predict fetal age. An infinite number of regression formulas can be used to estimate a variable such as the fetal age or weight. These may be as simple as a linear relationship, which takes the following form:

$$y = a + bx$$

where y is being predicted and is the dependent variable, x is the known measurement or independent variable, a is the intercept constant of the line on the y-axis, and b is the slope constant of the line or how the units of y change for each change in the x units.

Table 7–3 has several formulas for estimating embryonic age from the embryonic heart rate (EHR). The first four formulas for predicting the age from the EHR are simple linear regressions.

Higher-order regressions may involve multiple x_n variables, logarithms, exponentials, square roots, or powers of any of these. Many formulas that have been published in the sonographic literature produce valid results for nonlinear or curvilinear relationships. Some are so complex that they are virtually useless in most clinical settings without a computer to perform the analysis. Many of these formulas can be used realistically only with a computer, and even with a computer they can be difficult to interpret and use.[59–61] In fact, fetal assessment is becoming so complex that I suggest that all sonographers become familiar with personal computers, spreadsheets, databases, and other forms of software.

Because fetal parameters rarely have linear relationships with age (time), a higher-order regression is often used. It may take the following form:

$$y = a + bx + cx^n$$

where a, b, and c are constants; y and x are the dependent and independent variables, re-

TABLE 7–3. EMBRYONIC HEART RATE AND AGE

When age is less than 9.2 LMP weeks:	
Age (days) Regression	±2 SD (days)
$LMP = EHR \times 0.285 + 8.18$	±8 days
$C\ age = EHR \times 0.285 - 5.82$	±8 days
$LMP = EHR \times 0.3 + 6$	±8 days
$C\ age = EHR \times 0.3 - 8$	±8 days
To estimate appropriate EHR from age:	±2 SD (B/M)
When age is less than 9.2 LMP weeks:	
$EHR = ((LMP \times 7) - 8.18)/0.285$	±24 B/M
When age is less than 8.0 LMP weeks (CRL < 16 mm):	
$EHR = (CRL \times 6) + 80$	±24 B/M
Throughout pregnancy:	
$E/FHR = 140 + (20 \times (LMP - 7)) \times LMP^{(-0.11 \times (LMP - 7))}$	±24 B/M
Lower threshold (EHRt = 2.5 percentile)	Before CRL = 27 mm
$EHRt = -6 + (-7.2 \times CRL) + (0.2 \times CRL^2) + (65.5 \times \sqrt{CRL})$	EHR should be > EHRt before 9.2 LMP weeks

The top four formulas may be used to calculate age from the embryonic heart rate (EHR) before 9.2 MFP AA weeks. The lower formulas predict the appropriate heart rate from the crown-rump length (CRL) or LMP. The formula to predict the heart rate throughout pregnancy was developed in collaboration with James Meiss, PhD, Applied Mathematics, University of Colorado, Boulder, CO.

The last formula defines the normal EHR lower threshold (EHRt). The EHR should be greater than the EHRt during the embryonic period. See Figure 13–4.

C age, conceptual age; E/FHR, embryofetal heart rate.

spectively; and x^n is "to the power of," often a square or cube of x.

This is a common form of regression equation for curvilinear data. When using curves generated from regression formulas, it is important to remain conscious of which variable is the independent (what is known independently of other information) and which is the dependent (what is predicted). Although intuition may tell us that it does not matter, the truth is that it does matter. They produce results that may be close, depending on the shape of the curves, the distribution of the data, and the equations, but the results are not the best if the dependent variable is used to predict the independent variable. Figure 7–2 shows curves plotted from formulas derived from the exact same data. Figure 7–2*A* has the BPD as the independent variable (x-axis), and Figure 7–2*B* has the LNMP as the independent variable. It can be observed in Figure 7–2*A* that a BPD of 61.21 mm predicts an LNMP of 25 weeks, whereas in Figure 7–2*B* an LNMP of 25 weeks predicts a BPD of 60.42 mm. This can be tested by inserting your own data into these formulas, which are given at the top of the figure.

One such formula for estimating the fetal age (LMP) from the THC was published by Hadlock and associates[62]:

$$LMP = 8.8 + 0.55(THC) + 0.00028(THC)^3$$

This formula was produced by Hadlock and colleagues using outer perimeter measurements of the fetal calvarium. This formula does not produce the same age from the THC as shown in Table 7–1 because that THC was calculated using the more standard leading-edge to leading-edge BPDs and midedge FODs. If the THC is calculated using a leading-edge to leading-edge BPD, then the previous formula underestimates the age because the leading-edge perimeter is smaller than the outer perimeter (see Chapter 8). The reader should be aware that almost all modern sonographic formulas, tables, or graphs produce fairly valid estimates of age, size, or weight of a fetus, as long as the measurements are taken in the same way that the researcher constructed the original model.

This chapter presents a family of formulas for estimating fetal ages from various fetal parameters. All of these formulas have the same form; only the constants and the independent variables change. The basic formula used here is

$$y = a + bx^2 + c\sqrt{x}$$

This regression model was developed using a curve-fitting software program called Tablecurve v3.10.[63] This version of the program compares XY data with more than 5000 formulas and allows the user to select the most appropriate formula. The model selected here produced a good coefficient of determination ($r^2 > 0.93$) for all parameters and did not require the use of logarithms, exponentials, or mathematical manipulation beyond squares and square roots. Thus, this family of formulas is easy for handheld calculators as well as computers. Table 7–4*A* gives the constants and r^2 for the means and 95% confidence limits for selected fetal parameters. The descriptive statistics for the parameter age residuals as a percentage of the MFP AA are in Table 7–4*B*. The standard error, standard deviation (SD), and sample variance provide an indication of the relative accuracy of each parameter as a predictor of age; the smaller these numbers, the better the predictor.

After each parameter's curve functions were determined using Tablecurve on the entire 1993 population (n = 2730), the tests for the means and variances were performed on a random sample of 300 from a different and larger population (n = 4486) using MicroSoft Excel.[64] No statistical difference was found in the MFP AA and the predicted means for any parameter ($P \leq 0.05$) except for the BPD, CRL, and GSD, and no significant differences were noted in the variances for any parameter. The significant difference in the MFP AA and predicted CRL ages was surprising at first. However, with study I realized that during early pregnancy, the MFP AA is most often an average of only the CRL and GSD ages; thus, the large variation of the GSD has an effect on the comparative statistics of the CRL ages. Later in pregnancy, as many as 11 fetal parameters are used to calculate the MFP AA; therefore any single parameter has a relatively small influence on the AA.

Table 7–4*A* is sorted by descending correlation, r^2. These formulas produce results similar to those found in Table 7–1. The parameters not included in Table 7–4*A* are those not in the Basic Baby II database. The use of this family of formulas in a spreadsheet allows quick replication of the formulas for analysis of large numbers of parameters and populations.

Voodoo Statistics. Statistical gurus probably consider this discussion "voodoo statistics." Less fastidious sonographers may consider it hair splitting; after all, how much accuracy in fetal sonography is required? Most women do not know the exact day or night they conceived, and the length of menstrual cycles varies. Pregnancy dating is confused even more because of the wide range of time for which different women carry a pregnancy. So what's the difference in a few days or a week or two?

To respond to the latter issue, it is true that predicting the exact date of a normal labor and delivery is nearly impossible or is at least an educated gamble. However, the rate of increase in the size of a fetus is a reliable indicator of its state of health. A diabetic woman's fetus may gain weight too fast and have difficulty in delivery; hydrops fetalis and other problems are also possible. In twin gestations, one or both twins may increase in size too slowly and require close monitoring to determine the optimum time and method for delivery. For these kinds of questions, all possible accuracy is advisable.

Voodoo statistics are a bit more difficult to explain. A difficulty in contemporary fetal growth statistical analysis is that most studies have used the LNMP to date pregnancy. This is because statistical analysis requires an established variable, the independent variable, as a starting point. As anyone who has gotten this far in this book should know, the LNMP is not a very accurate date. The accuracy for dates of most sonographic fetal parameters is better than the LNMP in a large population, and the LNMP's variability enters into the estimates of both size and age.

Some studies also exclude women who have used birth control pills during the 3 months before conception. Our studies followed this convention throughout the 1993 period. Using the LNMP as the independent variable or standard of comparison increases the resulting variance of studies of both size and age. The problems of knowing the LNMP were discussed in some detail previously. We are left with the problem of how to date a pregnancy. Hadlock and associates

TABLE 7–4A. FETAL AGE FORMULA: LMP in weeks = $a + bx^2 + c\sqrt{x}$

PARAMETER	CONSTANTS (for Means) a	b	c	CONSTANTS (for 95% confidence limits) Lower 2.5% a	b	c	CONSTANTS (for 95% confidence limits) Upper 97.5% a	b	c	r^2	FIT STANDARD ERROR	$P(T< t)$ *t*-TEST OF TWO SAMPLES FOR MEANS	$P(F< f)$ F TEST OF TWO SAMPLES FOR VARIANCES
3-D BPD	4.4	0.00213349	1.57536934	4.04	0.00209381	1.50966617	4.74	0.00217316	1.64107252	0.9960	0.4687	0.14	0.46
THC	3.6	0.00015868	0.92953421	3.31	0.00015584	0.89973167	3.89	0.00016151	0.95933674	0.9958	0.5173	0.47	0.47
CV	9.8	0.00000465	1.35447232	9.74	0.00000310	1.34147996	9.94	0.00000620	1.36746468	0.9946	0.5468	0.18	0.47
CHC	4.2	0.00028812	0.96326673	3.87	0.00028323	0.92666650	4.51	0.00029300	0.99986696	0.9943	0.5641	0.60	0.48
BPD	2.8	0.00188671	1.90632612	2.60	0.00185684	1.86024635	3.07	0.00191658	1.95240589	0.9941	0.6226	0.24	0.49
FOD	3.6	0.00124242	1.57583012	3.24	0.00121544	1.51613440	3.93	0.00126941	1.63552584	0.9895	0.8142	0.04	0.42
FemL	6.4	0.00261293	1.97660168	6.06	0.00253464	1.89750207	6.76	0.00269121	2.05570189	0.9874	0.8576	0.73	0.49
AC	−0.86	0.00007100	1.61736800	−1.3	0.00006698	1.57281943	−0.4	0.00007524	1.66191657	0.9867	0.9045	0.85	0.48
CRL	4.1	0.00020798	0.94113212	3.98	0.00018974	0.91737871	4.18	0.00022621	0.96488552	0.9856	0.3728	0.04	0.34
HumL	7.6	0.00421714	1.54223731	7.27	0.00412985	1.46633875	7.91	0.00430443	1.61813587	0.9854	0.9173	0.57	0.46
BiOD	5.7	0.00574911	1.53632784	4.81	0.00551719	1.34070851	6.51	0.00598103	1.73194718	0.9814	0.8354	0.01	0.44
HBL	2.2	0.00226570	2.03424006	1.51	0.00217778	1.90192928	2.88	0.00235361	2.16655084	0.9748	1.1784	0.79	0.40
VCD	4.3	0.00402084	1.79972236	3.57	0.00386092	1.63303022	5.10	0.00418077	1.96641449	0.9671	1.3515	0.08	0.37
GSD	1.7	0.00029895	1.00590423	1.50	0.00025895	0.96523084	1.86	0.00033895	1.04657762	0.9620	0.4248	0.00	0.42
FSL	−2.6	0.00114576	4.07831501	−7.61	0.00006072	2.97132910	2.32	0.00223080	5.18530093	0.9476	1.7067	N/A	N/A
CERB	−11.5	−0.00108777	7.24715288	−13.22	−0.00184139	6.80790864	−9.87	−0.00033415	7.68639711	0.9328	1.3307	0.30	0.29

This table presents a family of formulas that have the same form. To use this formula, substitute the parameter measurement for x and the corresponding constants a, b, and c in the appropriate places. The upper and lower 95 percentile confidence limits are predicted by using the appropriate constants a, b, and c. The last four columns are the results of statistical analysis of the coefficient of determination (r^2), the standard error, and significance of differences from the multiple fetal parameter average age for the means and variances. The table is sorted in descending order for r^2. This family of equations was produced using curve-fitting software and resulted in Figures 7–5, 7–6, and 7–7.

3-D BPD, three-dimensional biparietal diameter correction; THC, transverse head circumference; CV, cranial volume; CHC, coronal head circumference; BPD, biparietal diameter; FOD, fronto-occipital diameter; FemL, femur length; AC, abdominal circumference; CRL, crown-rump length; HumL, humerus length; BiOD, outer binocular distance; HBL, hippocampal base line; VCD, vertical cranial diameter; GSD, gestational sac diameter; FSL, fractional spine length; CERB, transverse cerebellar diameter.

TABLE 7–4*B*. DESCRIPTIVE STATISTICS: RESIDUAL AGES/AVERAGE AGE OF MULTIPLE FETAL PARAMETERS

	LNMP AA	GSD AA	CRL AA	EHR AA	CV AA	3-D AA	THC AA	BPD AA	CHC AA	TriCD AA	BiOD AA	CERB AA	FemL AA	HumL AA	AC AA
Mean	0.0704	−0.0109	0.0079	−0.0049	−0.0076	−0.0022	−0.0034	−0.0028	−0.0099	−0.0121	−0.0119	0.0024	0.0018	0.0084	0.0106
Standard error	0.0120	0.0145	0.0068	0.0054	0.0011	0.0011	0.0011	0.0018	0.0015	0.0018	0.0029	0.0032	0.0023	0.0024	0.0020
Median	0.0200	−0.0100	0.0100	0.0000	−0.0100	0.0000	0.0000	0.0000	−0.0100	0.0100	−0.0200	0.0000	0.0000	0.0000	0.0100
Mode	−0.0200	−0.0400	−0.0400	0.0000	0.0000	0.0000	0.0000	0.0000	0.0000	0.0200	−0.0200	−0.0100	0.0000	0.0000	0.0200
Standard deviation	0.1918	0.1188	0.0592	0.0371	0.0176	0.0173	0.0176	0.0282	0.0235	0.0282	0.0350	0.0326	0.0362	0.0369	0.0315
Sample variance	0.0368	0.0141	0.0035	0.0014	0.0003	0.0003	0.0003	0.0008	0.0006	0.0008	0.0012	0.0011	0.0013	0.0014	0.0010
Kurtosis	7.7467	0.7767	2.2916	1.1264	−0.1492	−0.0281	0.0815	1.0920	0.2161	0.8814	3.8148	1.1663	0.5331	0.2193	−0.2835
Skewness	2.2345	0.1142	−0.6220	0.2748	0.1938	0.2907	0.2668	0.1664	−0.0316	−0.0475	0.9901	0.4299	0.3501	0.3006	0.1418
Range	1.550	0.660	0.370	0.180	0.090	0.090	0.100	0.190	0.130	0.190	0.250	0.200	0.210	0.220	0.170
Minimum	−0.410	−0.280	−0.230	−0.090	−0.050	−0.040	−0.050	−0.090	−0.070	−0.070	−0.080	−0.080	−0.080	−0.090	−0.060
Maximum	1.140	0.380	0.140	0.090	0.040	0.050	0.050	0.100	0.060	0.120	0.170	0.120	0.130	0.130	0.110
Sum	17.94	−0.73	0.60	−0.23	−0.178	−0.51	−0.84	−0.72	−2.31	2.83	−1.79	0.25	0.44	2.03	2.58
Count	255	67	76	47	234	234	247	254	234	234	150	106	242	241	244
Confidence level (95.0%)	0.0235	0.0284	0.0133	0.0106	0.0023	0.0022	0.0022	0.0035	0.0030	0.0036	0.0056	0.0062	0.0046	0.0047	0.0039

Descriptive statistics for the residuals of the above formulas (Table 7–4*A*) based on 300 random sets of fetal measurements. The fractional spine length is not included because it is not routinely measured and is not in the Basic Baby II database. In this table, the degree of accuracy for the prediction of fetal age is best gleaned from the standard errors, standard deviations, and sample variances. The smaller that these three numbers are, the more accurate the age estimates. Residual ratios = parameter age − AA/AA.

GSD, gestational sac diameter; CRL, crown-rump length; EHR, embryonic heart rate; CV, cranial volume; 3-D, three-dimensional biparietal diameter correction; THC, transverse head circumference; BPD, biparietal diameter; CHC, coronal head circumference; TriCD, triangle circumference diameter; BiOD, outer binocular distance; CERB, transverse cerebellar diameter; FemL, femur length; HumL, humerus length; AC, abdominal circumference.

have demonstrated that the MFP AA can predict the dates of a pregnancy better than any single parameter used alone.[8,9] However, when one is testing the accuracy of a new fetal parameter such as the 3-D BPD correction, it is usually unacceptable statistically or a bit voodooish to use the MFP AA to establish the dates for the study when some of the 3-D head measurements are included in the MFP. That is, the BPD and THC would not normally be used to estimate the fetal age as well as to calculate the 3-D parameters, using both in the dependent and independent variables. There is a very logical reason why this is normally unacceptable. If a fetus is smaller or larger than normal, the use of parameters from that fetus in both the dependent and independent variables tends to influence the normal results toward that fetus's size or age.

Voodoo statistics are exactly what we have used here, however. The MFP AAs were used to construct dating charts from the size of individual parameters. There are five reasons for believing that this method will produce valid results:

1. In the current study population, most of the patients were referred for sonography specifically because of a question about the dates of the LNMP and pregnancy. Thus, the LNMPs in this population are not valid and tended to be overestimated (see Fig. 7–3 and Table 7–4*B*). Using a *t*-test for paired two-sample means, a significant difference was found in the means (1993 data with LNMPS, n = 1677, $P < 0.05$, $r^2 = 0.93$). This is in conflict with the fifth reason, following, because of the pairing of the LNMPs and corresponding AAs here.
2. It is believed that the vast majority of these fetuses are no different from the cross section of the population of Austin, Texas. The fetal measurements were contributed by four different laboratories scattered across the city. They represent all economic and educational levels of the society and include Medicaid, HMO, insured, and self-pay patients.
3. The use of a relatively large number of fetal parameters from a large number of examinations that were performed by at least 12 different sonographers provides protection against systematic observer bias.
4. Because of some variation in the length of menstrual cycles from woman to woman and some variation in the exact day of conception after the start of the menstrual cycle, as well as variation in the time of implantation,[51] an inherent variability is introduced into the dating charts and graphs that are constructed using LNMP dates. Using established fetal parameter charts from peer-reviewed publications to construct new parameter age charts should provide valid results in a large population, with less variation than the LNMP.
5. Using ANOVA (Excel), no statistical difference was found between the overall mean LNMPs and the MFP AAs in this population (1993 data with LNMPs, n = 1677, $P > 0.05$, $r^2 = 0.93$).

The problem of variability in dating a pregnancy is emphasized by the different dating methods that have been used in sonographic research. The LNMP is by far the most common date used and is one of the most valid dates available if it is remembered that "Education regarding the necessity for accurate menstrual records has fundamental value for those couples pursuing a pregnancy."[65] Because of the inherent variability of the LNMP date and of the following time of conception, other methods have been used to date pregnancies, as described earlier. Some have even used dates from fetal measurements to establish the timing of other fetal parameters in the same population,[53] similar to the voodooish method we are proposing to use here. It obviously would be worthwhile to find an accurate method for dating pregnancies and estimating normal variation.

This study uses MFP AA to investigate the growth of the individual fetal parameters from the same population. There is a precedent for this, as shown earlier.[53] In addition, Hadlock's MFP AA has been proved to be the most accurate indicator of size/age.[8,9,66,67] Hadlock and colleagues used four parameters—the BPD, FemL, and head and abdominal circumferences—to calculate the MFP. In our study, more parameters were used, as appropriate to the time in the pregnancies. Thus, the effects of the study parameter on the MFP AA should be minimized. As many as 10 fetal parameters plus the GSD were measured and averaged for the current MFP AA.

One advantage of using the MFP AA to study individual parameters is that it allows a view of fetal proportionality that does not include the variability inherent in the LNMP, ovulation, and implantation dates discussed earlier. A much better observation of the variability in fetal parameter proportions in time is thus possible. Figure 7–3 demonstrates the difference in variability by using the BPD to predict age using the LNMP and MFP AA as the dependent variables.

Individual Parameter Ages

First Trimester

GESTATIONAL SAC DIAMETER AND HUMAN CHORIONIC GONADOTROPIN. The sonographic diameters of the chorionic cavity or gestational sac have been in use as an estimator of pregnancy dates since the late 1960s.[12] Although the GSD is not a true fetal parameter, it is the diameter of the chorionic cavity, which contains the amnion and embryo. It is often used in combination with the fetal CRL to estimate fetal age and well-being. Some researchers have found that GSDs that are inappropriately small for fetal age are predictive of first-trimester spontaneous abortion.[68]

The mean GSD (three perpendicular diameters) can be observed, using transvaginal sonography, by the early 4th LNMP week,[69] and the GSD grows linearly at about 1.1 mm per day from the 5th to the 11th LMP weeks. GSD growth less than 0.6 mm per day is abnormal during this period.[70] Nyberg and colleagues' study also found that the embryo should be observed by the time the GSD reaches 25 mm (see Chapter 16 for more discussion of this topic).

The gestational sac can be quite variable in its shape and therefore in its date estimates. The chorionic cavity (GSD) conforms to abnormal uterine shapes, fibroids, or other external pressures. For this reason, I have tended not to use the GSD measurements if the CRL is measurable. Thus, this measurement is most useful during only a short window of time from the 4th to the 6th week. During this period, a fetus is rapidly changing.

The quantitative serum hCG assay is a useful method for determining when the GSD should be observable, even in women whose LNMP history may be irregular or unavailable. Some researchers have used hCG quantities of 1800 mIU/ml (Second International Standard) as a threshold at which the chorionic cavity can be observed by transabdominal sonography. Using transvaginal transducers, this threshold may be dropped to as low as 500 mIU/ml, and Filly recommends a more conservative 1000 mIU/ml.[69] If the hCG reaches these threshold levels and an intrauterine GSD is not found, an ectopic pregnancy must be considered.

Table 7–5, a composite table for the first trimester, correlates the GSD, CRL, E/FHR, and hCG with age by LMP and conceptual age in both days and weeks. The hCG in this table is a derived composite from different publications.[4, 8, 71–74]

Because the shape of the GSD can be so variable—hourglass, teardrop, or more bizarre shapes—it is often difficult to determine where to measure the diameters; therefore, Table 7–2 allows for the average of the two largest perpendicular diameters from a single image or the average of three perpendicular diameters (3-D mean).[12] If the chorionic cavity is normally shaped, both methods produce similar estimates of age, and the two-diameter method is easier and faster. If the cavity is not normally shaped, both methods are quite variable in their results. The GSD estimates the dates of a pregnancy to approximately ±10% of the age; for example, at 6 LMP weeks, 95% of the population is within ±0.6 of a week (4.2 days) of the mean.

Figure 7–5*A* is a GSD dating curve. This curve can be used to estimate the dates of pregnancy in LMP weeks from the average of the two largest GSDs (in millimeters).

CROWN-RUMP LENGTH. The CRL is the single most accurate estimator of embryofetal ages of all sonographic parameters in the first trimester. This is because the CRL is a relatively large parameter at any given time in pregnancy, and it grows rapidly. Early in the fifth LMP week, the embryonic disk or pole can be identified by the flicker of the embryonic heartbeat (EHR).[75, 76]

After the first trimester, a fetus begins to move (flex and extend) more. The CRL then becomes less accurate, although it remains a good estimator of age until it is too large for

TABLE 7–5. **FIRST-TRIMESTER AGE TABLE**

AGE (DAYS)		AGE (WEEKS)		hCG MEAN	CRL	EHR	FHR	CHORIONIC CAVITY	
LMP	C age	LMP	C age	(mIU/ml)	(mm)	(B/M)	(B/M)	(3-D MEAN) GSD (mm)	(2-D MEAN) GSD (mm)
26	12	3.7	1.7	100					
29	15	4.1	2.1	233					4
32	18	4.6	2.6	533		84			0
33	19	4.6	2.6	2,796		89			10
35	21	5.0	3.0	4,151	1	94		10	12
38	24	5.4	3.4	4,794	2	105		13	15
41	27	5.9	3.9	6,429	3	115		16	17
40	26	5.7	3.7	7,510	5	121		18	19
44	30	6.3	4.3	10,117	6	126		19	20
47	33	6.7	4.7	13,397	8	136		22	24
50	36	7.1	5.1	21,526	10	147		25	27
53	39	7.6	5.6	39,164	14	157		28	31
55	41	7.9	5.9	56,211	15	163		30	33
56	42	8.0	6.0	75,000	16	168		31	34
59	45	8.4	6.4		22	178		34	39
62	48	8.9	6.9		26	189		37	44
65	51	9.3	7.3		28		180	40	48
68	54	9.7	7.7		29		173	43	54
71	57	10.1	8.1		32		168	46	57
74	60	10.6	8.6		37		167	49	62
77	63	11.0	9.0		45		166	52	68
80	66	11.4	9.4		46		164	55	74
83	69	11.9	9.9		52		162	58	79
86	72	12.3	10.3		57		160	60	82
89	75	12.7	10.7		63		158		88
92	78	13.1	11.1		68		155		89

This table can be used to compare various embryo/fetal parameters with age by days and weeks. Conceptual age (C age) = LMP −14 days. The 3-D mean GSDs are the average of three perpendicular diameters of the chorionic sac, and the 2-D mean GSDs are the average of the two greatest diameters from a single image. The human chorionic gonadotropin (hCG) (Second International Standard) values are a composite of five published tables.[100–104] CRL, crown-rump length; EHR, embryonic heart rate; FHR, fetal heart rate; GSD, gestational sac diameter.

the sonographic field of view, assuming that the image is captured with the fetus in extension.

The CRL is measured as the greatest dimension of the embryonic disk or pole, not including the legs or yolk sac. The fetal legs usually are not observed until the 10th week or later (see Chapter 18 for representative images in early pregnancy). Figure 7–5*B* is a dating curve for the CRL and can be used to estimate the equivalent LMP dates for the pregnancy. In the population studied in 1993, the ages estimated using the CRL were within ±7.3% (±2 SD) of the mean age. Both Table 7–1 and Table 7–5 may be used to estimate ages from CRL measurements. These tables show close agreement with recent publications.[46]

EMBRYONIC HEART RATE. The EHR is one of the newest parameters for estimating embryonic age. The first regression to predict the appropriate E/FHR was published by Fine and colleagues in 1988.[77] My colleagues and I also suggested that the EHR correlated with age in 1988[78] and published a regression in 1989.[79–81] These formulas are among the most simple of any used to estimate dates of a pregnancy (see Table 7–3).

The EHR appears to be sensitive to the condition of the embryo. In our 1993 population, six embryos had heart rates that were below the 2.5 percentile before the CRL was 25 mm. Follow-up on these six found one continued normally, one was unavailable for follow-up, and four ended in first-trimester spontaneous abortion (see Fig. 12–4). This is a probability of 67% to 83% that a pregnancy will fail if the EHR is inappropriately low in the embryonic period. The formula for this time-series thresh-

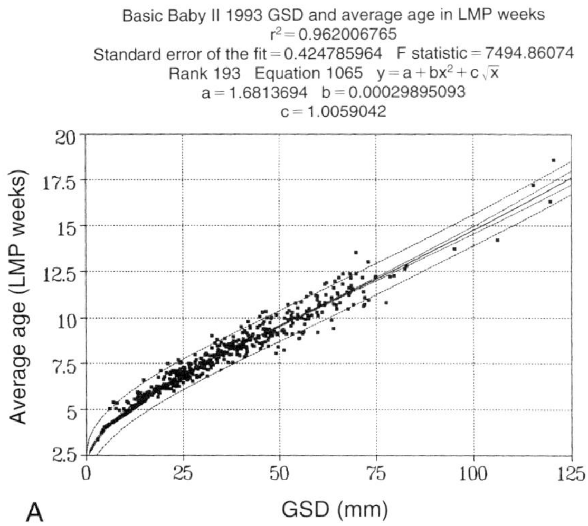

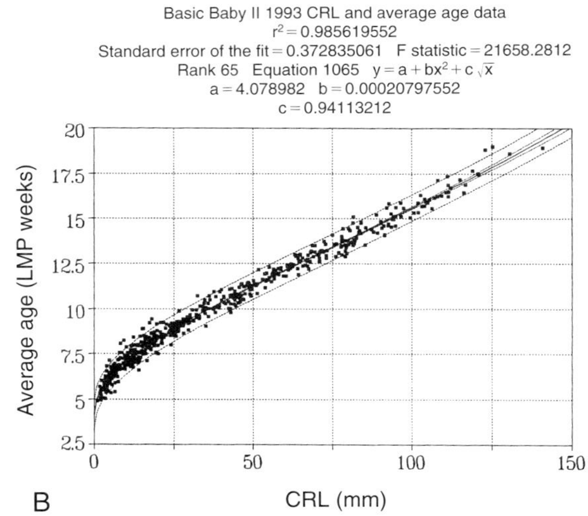

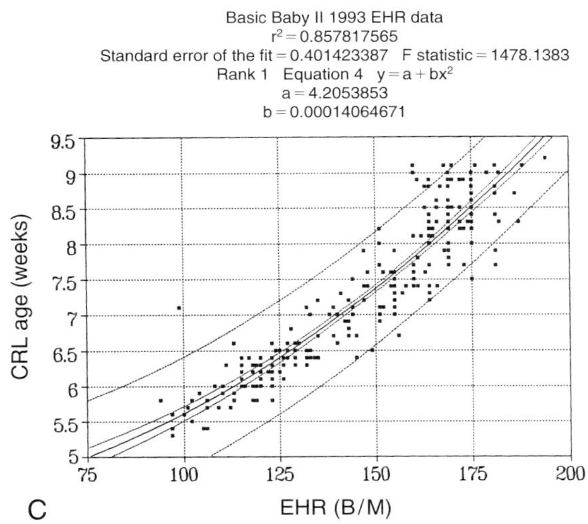

FIGURE 7–5.
Dating curves for use in the first trimester. In *A* and *B*, the dependent variable (y-axis) is the average age of multiple fetal parameters. In *C*, the y-axis is the crown-rump length (CRL) age in LMP weeks. GSD, two greatest diameters of the gestational sac (chorionic cavity); EHR, embryonic heart rate by M-mode measurement before 9.2 LMP weeks.

old is shown in Table 7–3 (see Chapter 12 for detailed discussion of the E/FHR).

The EHR should always be measured using M-mode imaging with automatic electronic caliper calculation of the rate. For greatest accuracy, use a fast M-mode trace speed to spread out the beat-to-beat interval for easy measurements. The EHR may reach rates as high as 190 to 200 beats/minute during the early ninth LMP week. This rate is impossible to count accurately while watching a sonographic monitor.

Figure 7–5C is a dating curve for the EHR. Tables 7–1 and 7–5 also contain heart rate dating data. These can be used to estimate the dates of pregnancy. The EHR estimates of the age in ±2 SD of the population were ±8 days or ±1.2 weeks. EHR ages that are more than −8 days below an embryo's corresponding age by CRL may be indicative of danger of embryonic demise. A simple formula for predicting the embryonic age from the EHR follows:

$$\text{Age in days} = \text{EHR} \times 0.3 + 6$$
$$(\pm 8 \text{ days}, \pm 2 \text{ SD})$$

The EHR and CRL can be used in combination in a linear regression to estimate age. The following two-variable regression formula was found to have no significant difference in the means or variances with the ages estimated by EHR, CRL, or MFP AA (ANOVA, $P > 0.05$, n = 251 random). This formula is valid only before the ninth LMP week and predicts the fetal age to ±4.3 days (±2 SD), $r^2 = 0.91$.

$$\text{LMP age} = 4.9 + (1.2 \times \text{CRL}) + (0.006 \times \text{EHR})$$

Fetal Head

BIPARIETAL DIAMETER AND THREE-DIMENSIONAL BIPARIETAL DIAMETER CORRECTION. The BPD of the head was one of the first fetal sonographic measurements. It is also one of the easiest and most accurate, if the head is normally shaped. The topic of head shape and 3-D geometry is addressed in detail in Chapter 8, and cranial and neural anatomy in Chapter 9. It is appropriate to cover the basics here.

In 1980, Kurtz and associates published a composite BPD chart from 17 different studies published worldwide. This remarkable publication produced a table that the authors believed to be valid for 90% of the world's recorded variations for the BPD. Table 7–2 was the result of this historical research. Note that the table does not include the mean age but only the weeks' variation. They stated, "It is our belief that one gestational age does not accurately represent a single biparietal diameter measurement."[82] This is true, of course: Variations in head shape and molding can give a range of sizes to the BPD at any given age. This concept is the basis of the 3-D BPD correction and ARA (discussed later). In subsequent publications, Kurtz and colleagues did publish a mean for this table; however, the associated regression formula has the age as the independent variable and predicts the BPD in centimeters.[83]

The plane used to measure the BPD is the standard transverse plane through the midthalamus and extending front to back along the longest skull diameter, the FOD. The BPD is measured from leading edge to leading edge, sometimes referred to as outer to inner edges. Here the FOD is measured from the middle of the frontal bone to the middle of the occipital bone echoes. The transverse cephalic index (TCI) is the ratio of the BPD to the FOD and should be between 0.7 and 0.9, with a mean of approximately 0.8 (TCI = BPD/THC = 0.80, ±0.1).[84]

In the coronal view, a normally shaped fetal skull appears as a perfect circle (see Figs. 8–2 to 8–6). If this view of the skull is circular and the TCI is normal, the BPD is a very reliable estimator of fetal age. However, if the head does not appear normal in either the transverse or coronal planes, the use of the 3-D BPD correction is recommended.[85] The 3-D BPD correction is the average of the three diameters of the fetal calvarium (3-D BPD = [BPD + FOD + VCD]/3), where VCD is the vertical cranial diameter (see Chapter 8 for detailed discussion of how to take this new measurement).

Once these three diameters of the skull are mastered, Table 7–1 can be used to estimate the fetal age from the 3-D BPD or CV (CV = 0.000555 × FOD × BPD × VCD).[83, 84, 86–88] The 3-D BPD correction produces more accurate estimates of age regardless of the shape of the fetal head. It can also be used as a more accurate substitute for the standard BPD in tables and formulas to estimate fetal weight. Figure 7–6 shows growth curves for the various cranial parameters mentioned here and described in Chapter 8.

In our random sample of 300, the residuals of the parameter ages from the AA as a percentage of the AA were as follows (±2 SD): BPD = ±4.9%, 3-D BPD = ±2.8%, and CV = ±2.9%. This percentage is relatively consistent throughout pregnancy and represents the distribution of the parameter.

HEAD CIRCUMFERENCES. The fetal THC has been more commonly known as simply the head circumference. However, because we discuss 3-D geometry of the skull, it is necessary to discuss both the THC and the CHC (see Chapter 8 for a detailed discussion of 3-D fetal head geometry).

Both the THC and the CHC are calculated using the standard formula for an ellipse:

$$\text{Ellipse circumference} = 1.57\,(d_1 + d_2)$$

where d_1 and d_2 are the two perpendicular diameters of the skull. For the THC, these two diameters are the BPD and FOD; for the CHC, they are the BPD and VCD.

The CHC is not a true coronal circumference but is approximately 0.84 (±0.05, 2 SD) of the true coronal circumference observed. This is because the VCD is not a diameter of the coronal circle but is the height of the coronal triangle. The reason I have called this calculation the CHC is because it is calculated using the same formula as the THC. The circle that circumscribes the coronal triangle is the true coronal circumference, but it is found with a menstruation formula that is best left to computers (see Chapter 8 for details).

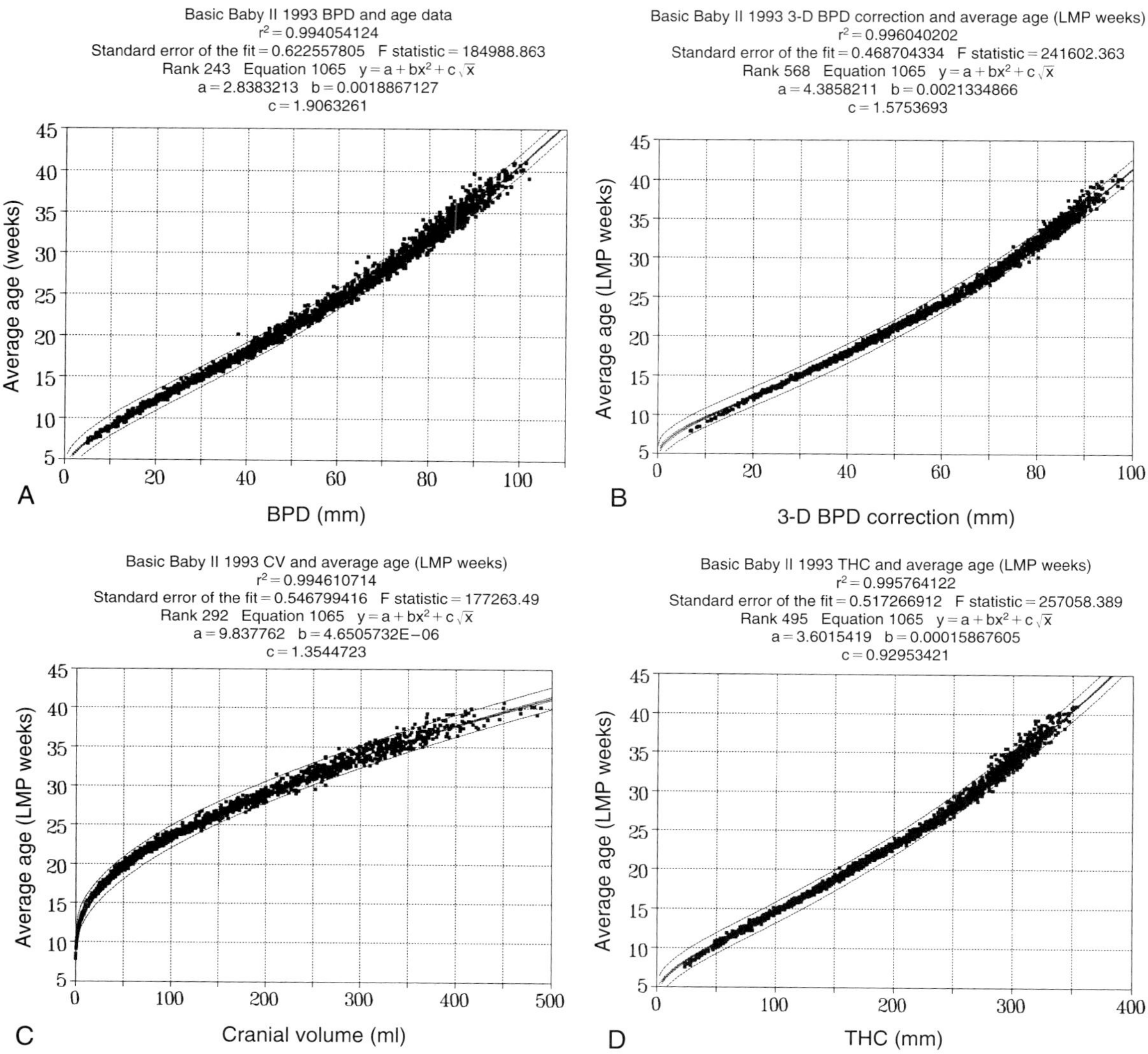

FIGURE 7–6.
Graphs representing a large number of fetal head parameters. (See Chapters 8 and 9 for a description of the specific measurements and anatomy.) In each graph, the dependent variable (y-axis) is the average age of multiple fetal parameters in weeks. These were calculated using a family of equations with the same form on a random sample of 300 cases (see Table 7–4*A*). Table 7–4*B* gives the descriptive statistics for the random sample of each parameter. The data are from all cases evaluated in 1993, for a total of 2728 cases in which each measurement was attempted as appropriate to the stage of pregnancy. Examples: *A*, biparietal diameter (BPD) = 2216; *B*, 3-D BPD = 1924; *D*, transverse head circumference (THC) = 2190; *I*, outer binocular distance (BiOD) = 935.

Figure 7–6*D* and *E* shows growth curves for the THC and CHC; they are also found in Table 7–1. These are reliable estimators of fetal age if the head is normally shaped. The residual percentage of the MFP AA (±2 SD) for the THC was ±2.9% and was 4.0% for the CHC. If the outer perimeter THC is measured, Hadlock and colleagues' table is recommended (Table 7–6). Do not use this table for THCs calculated from leading-edge BPDs as discussed earlier.

Fetal Body

LONG BONES. The bones of the fetal extremities are good estimators of age and growth. They do have the disadvantage of a larger variation than the cranial parameters (see the later ARA discussion).

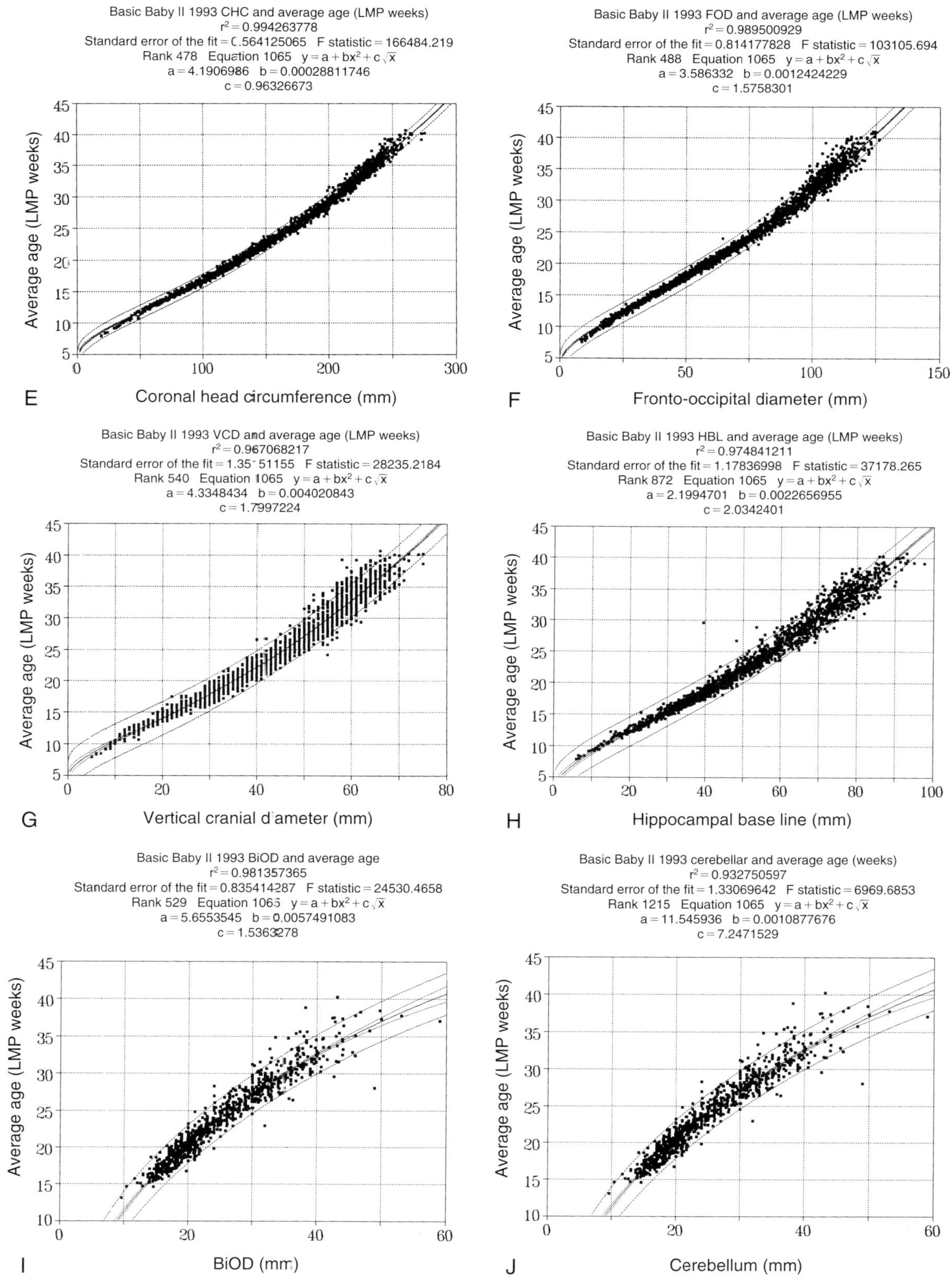

FIGURE 7–6 *Continued*

TABLE 7–6. **PREDICTED MENSTRUAL AGE FOR HEAD CIRCUMFERENCE**

HEAD CIRCUMFERENCE (cm)	MENSTRUAL AGE (WEEKS)	HEAD CIRCUMFERENCE (cm)	MENSTRUAL AGE (WEEKS)
8.0	13.4	22.5	24.4
8.5	13.7	23.0	24.9
9.0	14.0	23.5	25.4
9.5	14.3	24.0	25.9
10.0	14.6	24.5	26.4
10.5	15.0	25.0	26.9
11.0	15.3	25.5	27.5
11.5	15.6	26.0	28.0
12.0	15.9	26.5	28.1
12.5	16.3	27.0	29.2
13.0	16.6	27.5	29.8
13.5	17.0	28.0	30.3
14.0	17.3	28.5	31.0
14.5	17.7	29.0	31.6
15.0	18.1	29.5	32.2
15.5	18.4	30.0	32.8
16.0	18.8	30.5	33.5
16.5	19.2	31.0	34.2
17.0	19.6	31.5	34.9
17.5	20.0	32.0	35.5
18.0	20.4	32.5	36.3
18.5	20.8	33.0	37.0
19.0	21.2	33.5	37.7
19.5	21.6	34.0	38.5
20.0	22.1	34.5	39.2
20.5	22.5	35.0	40.0
21.0	23.0	35.5	40.8
21.5	23.4	36.0	41.6
22.0	23.9		

Note: Menstrual age = 8.8 + 0.55 (head circumference) + 2.8×10^{-4} (head circumference)^3; r^2 = 97.9%; 1 SD = 1.18 weeks.

This table was published for the prediction of fetal age from outer perimeter transverse head circumferences (THCs). This table should not be used for THCs calculated using leading-edge to leading-edge biparietal diameter measurements.

From Hadlock FP, Deter RL, Harrist RB, et al: Fetal head circumference: Relation to menstrual age. AJR 1992;138:651.

The FemL and HumL are particularly reliable parameters for measurements because the femur and humerus are attached on either side of the fetal trunk and thus are relatively easy to locate. The more distal long bones, the ulna and radius of the forearm and the tibia and fibula of the leg, can be more difficult because of their greater range of motion and locations in the uterus.

Caution should be taken to determine which bone is being measured. If a fetus has its elbow flexed, with its hand near its face, the ulna and radius will be approximately parallel to the humerus. An inexperienced or rushed sonographer may be confused by this arrangement. The same caution applies to the femur and lower leg if the knee is tightly flexed. With experience, it is not difficult to locate the fetal head, trunk, spine, and pelvis and then slide the field of view to the shoulder or hip to follow the extremity. With this method, a sonographer builds a mental image of the fetal lie within the uterus and the relative location of its parts. Beginning each obstetrical examination in this way expedites the measurements because the operator has some idea of the relative location of each parameter. This cybernetic aspect of sonography is discussed at length in Chapter 5.

Fetal sonographic measurements of the long

bones are of the bone diaphyses, the calcified portion of the shafts. The heads and distal condyles of the humerus and femur do not completely calcify until after birth and appear as hypoechoic areas until near term. An accepted convention in the field of diagnostic sonography is to refer to the diaphysis measurement by the name of the bone, although it is not the true length of the entire bone. The measurements also do not include artifactual echoes such as the distal femoral point[89] or the proximal humeral point, which are echoes from the near surfaces of the cartilaginous material beyond the ends of the diaphyses (see Chapter 15 for example images of the long bones and discussion of the anatomy and artifacts).

The femur and humerus are normally of a similar length until about the 20th LMP week, and the humerus may be longer. The femur is more often longer after that week and is normally longer after the 25th week. However, because of the relatively large normal variations in the body and extremities, this relationship is not a hard-and-fast rule. Either femur or humerus may be longer before the 25th LMP week. Some developmental anomalies of the extremities do not manifest until the 25th week (see Chapter 15 for more discussion of this topic).

Figure 7–7 includes dating curves for the femoral and humeral lengths. Fetal age estimates from these bones may also be made using Tables 7–1 and 7–7. In the random sample of 300 used here, the FemL and HumL were found to have a distribution of the ratios of the residuals to the AA of ±6.0% and ±7.0%, respectively, that is, (FemL weeks −AA)/AA = residual percentage of the AA. The later ARA discussion explains this method of describing fetal parameter proportionality. One of the best long bone dating tables is that of Jeanty and associates (Table 7–7).

ABDOMINAL CIRCUMFERENCE. The AC has been a commonly used fetal parameter measurement since 1979.[90–92] The AC is measured at a well-documented level, transverse and perpendicular to the fetal spine at the level where the umbilical vein joins the portal venous system. The correct AC measurement plane is described with illustrative images in Chapter 14, and in Section III at various ages (Table 7–8).

The AC can be used to estimate fetal age; however, because the AC is affected by both fetal fat and liver size, it can produce markedly variable results. Relatively fat fetuses have relatively large ACs, and conversely, thin fetuses tend to have smaller ACs. The AC is a better indicator of fetal growth and size than age. The AC is a factor in most regression formulas for estimating fetal weight. Many disease factors can affect the AC and liver size.[93] Any time the AC approaches +2 SD above the fetal cranial size/age, it is suggested that the liver be measured and compared with charts for normal sizes. Maternal or gestational diabetes can also cause a fetus to have an increased AC. See Chapter 14.

For the foregoing reasons, the AC may not be the best estimator of fetal age. However, the AC age can be useful in the ARA for assessing proportionality and relative size. Tables 7–1 and 7–8 and Figure 7–7*C* can be used to evaluate AC measurements. I found the AC residuals ([AC weeks − AA]/AA) to be ±5.5% (±2 SD) of the MFP AA using Table 7–1 for the AC age (LMP weeks) estimate.

Shepard and colleagues' version of Warsof and associates' table for estimating fetal weight has been popular since its publication in 1982.[94, 95] These and other methods for estimating fetal weight are discussed later.

FRACTIONAL SPINE LENGTH. The fractional spine length (FSL) is not often used for estimating fetal age. However, when the fetal back is turned toward the transducer or when the extremities or other parameters are abnormal or difficult to observe, the FSL may be very useful.[3, 96]

The FSL measurement is obtained from images of the long axis containing at least seven thoracolumbar vertebral bodies and spaces. Table 7–1 lists the FSL in millimeters for estimating fetal age. The major caution is to be sure to include seven full bodies and spaces and not exclude one space by measuring from the edge of one vertebral body to the end of the seventh, thus excluding one space at the end (see Chapter 9 for a discussion of this measurement and the anatomy associated with the FSL, as well as regression formulas for evaluating the FSL). Figure 7–7*D* is a dating curve for the FSL.

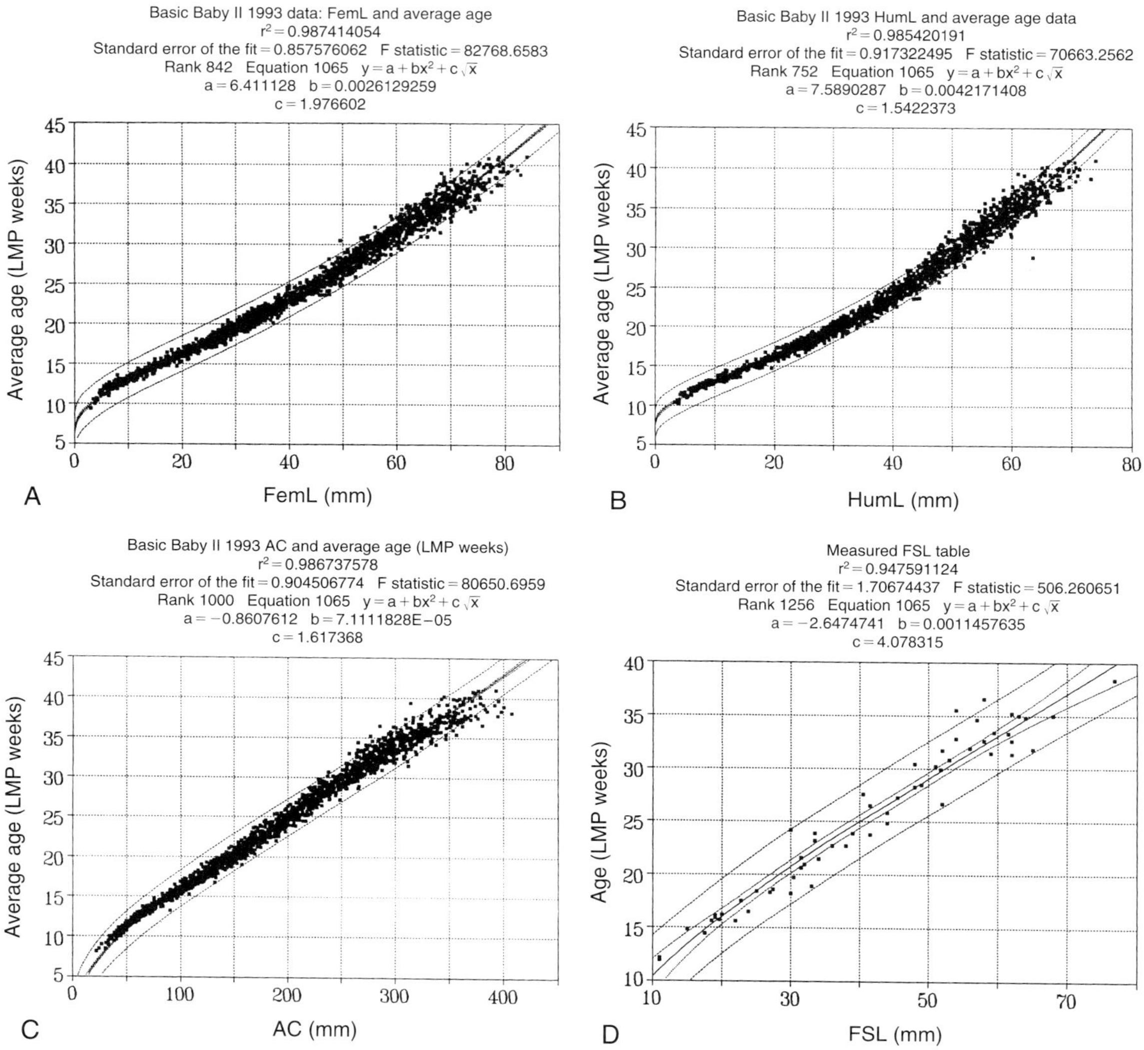

FIGURE 7–7.
Dating curves for four fetal body parameters. The femur length (*A*, FemL), humerus length (*B*, HumL), and abdominal circumference (*C*, AC) are from the same population as used for Figure 7–6. The fractional spine length (*D*, FSL) was from a small random test sample. (See Chapter 15 for FemL and HumL measurement techniques; see Chapter 14 for abdominal measurement and Chapter 9 for the FSL.)

Ratios

The generally accepted wisdom is that ratios are the best method for evaluating the proportions of a fetus. Ratios, which may also be called an index, have no units because they cancel out algebraically. Percentages are ratios multiplied by 100 and expressing the numerator as a percentage of the denominator. Ratios are sensitive to changes in the relative size of two parameters. However, because the various parameters of the fetal body usually grow at differing rates, a table or graph must be used to determine if any particular ratio is appropriate at a particular time in the pregnancy (Fig. 7–8). Another consideration for the use of ratios is to evaluate proportions.[97] When a particular ratio is abnormal, the observer must decide if the numerator or the denominator of the ratio is the abnormal parameter.

TABLE 7–7. GESTATIONAL AGES AS OBTAINED FROM THE LONG BONES (IN WEEKS + DAYS)

BONE LENGTH (mm)	FEMUR PERCENTILE			HUMERUS PERCENTILE			ULNA PERCENTILE			TIBIA PERCENTILE		
	5th	50th	95th	5th	50th	95th	5th	50th	95th	5th	50th	95th
10	10 + 3	12 + 4	14 + 6	9 + 6	12 + 4	15 + 2	10 + 1	13 + 1	16 + 1	10 + 4	13 + 3	16 + 2
11	10 + 5	12 + 6	15 + 1	10 + 1	12 + 6	15 + 4	10 + 4	13 + 4	16 + 4	10 + 6	13 + 5	16 + 4
12	11 + 1	13 + 2	15 + 4	10 + 3	13 + 1	15 + 6	10 + 6	13 + 6	16 + 6	11 + 1	14 + 1	17
13	11 + 3	13 + 4	15 + 6	10 + 6	13 + 4	16 + 1	11 + 1	14 + 1	17 + 2	11 + 4	14 + 3	17 + 2
14	11 + 5	13 + 6	16 + 1	11 + 1	13 + 6	16 + 4	11 + 4	14 + 4	17 + 5	11 + 6	14 + 6	17 + 5
15	12	14 + 1	16 + 3	11 + 3	14 + 1	16 + 6	11 + 6	15	18	12 + 1	15 + 1	18
16	12 + 3	14 + 4	16 + 6	11 + 6	14 + 4	17 + 2	12 + 2	15 + 3	18 + 3	12 + 4	15 + 4	18 + 3
17	12 + 5	14 + 6	17 + 1	12 + 1	14 + 6	17 + 4	12 + 5	15 + 5	18 + 6	13	15 + 6	18 + 6
18	13	15 + 1	17 + 3	12 + 4	15 + 1	18	13 + 1	16 + 1	19 + 1	13 + 2	16 + 1	19 + 1
19	13 + 3	15 + 4	17 + 6	12 + 6	15 + 4	18 + 2	13 + 4	16 + 4	19 + 4	13 + 5	16 + 4	19 + 4
20	13 + 5	15 + 6	18 + 1	13 + 1	15 + 6	18 + 5	13 + 6	16 + 6	20	14 + 1	17	19 + 6
21	14 + 1	16 + 2	18 + 4	13 + 4	16 + 2	19 + 1	14 + 2	17 + 2	20 + 3	14 + 4	17 + 3	20 + 2
22	14 + 3	16 + 4	18 + 6	13 + 6	16 + 5	19 + 3	14 + 5	17 + 5	20 + 6	14 + 6	17 + 6	20 + 5
23	14 + 5	16 + 6	19 + 1	14 + 2	17 + 1	19 + 6	15 + 1	18 + 1	21 + 1	15 + 1	18 + 1	21 + 1
24	15 + 1	17 + 2	19 + 4	14 + 5	17 + 3	20 + 1	15 + 4	18 + 4	21 + 4	15 + 4	18 + 4	21 + 3
25	15 + 3	17 + 4	19 + 6	15 + 1	17 + 6	20 + 4	16	19	22 + 1	16	18 + 6	21 + 6
26	15 + 6	18	20 + 1	15 + 4	18 + 1	21	16 + 3	19 + 3	22 + 4	16 + 3	19 + 2	22 + 1
27	16 + 1	18 + 2	20 + 4	15 + 6	18 + 4	21 + 3	16 + 6	19 + 6	22 + 6	16 + 6	19 + 5	22 + 4
28	16 + 4	18 + 5	20 + 6	16 + 2	19	21 + 6	17 + 2	20 + 2	23 + 3	17 + 1	20 + 1	23
29	16 + 6	19	21 + 1	16 + 5	19 + 3	22 + 1	17 + 5	20 + 8	23 + 6	17 + 4	20 + 4	23 + 4
30	17 + 1	19 + 3	21 + 4	17 + 1	19 + 6	22 + 4	18 + 1	21 + 1	24 + 2	18 + 1	21	23 + 6
31	17 + 4	19 + 6	22	17 + 4	20 + 2	23	18 + 4	21 + 5	24 + 6	18 + 4	21 + 3	24 + 2
32	17 + 6	20 + 1	22 + 2	18	20 + 5	23 + 4	19 + 1	22 + 1	25 + 1	18 + 6	21 + 6	24 + 5
33	18 + 2	20 + 4	22 + 5	18 + 3	21 + 1	23 + 6	19 + 4	22 + 5	25 + 5	19 + 2	22 + 1	25 + 1
34	18 + 5	20 + 6	23 + 1	18 + 6	21 + 4	24 + 2	20 + 1	23 + 1	26 + 1	19 + 5	22 + 4	25 + 4
35	19	21 + 1	23 + 3	19 + 2	22	24 + 6	20 + 4	23 + 5	26 + 5	20 + 1	23 + 1	26
36	19 + 3	21 + 4	23 + 6	19 + 5	22 + 4	25 + 1	21 + 1	24 + 1	27 + 1	20 + 4	23 + 4	26 + 3
37	19 + 6	22	24 + 1	20 + 1	22 + 6	25 + 5	21 + 4	24 + 4	27 + 5	21	23 + 6	26 + 6
38	20 + 1	22 + 3	24 + 4	20 + 4	23 + 3	26 + 1	22 + 1	25 + 1	28 + 1	21 + 4	24 + 3	27 + 2
39	20 + 4	22 + 5	24 + 6	21 + 1	23 + 6	26 + 4	22 + 4	25 + 4	28 + 5	21 + 6	24 + 6	27 + 5
40	20 + 6	23 + 1	25 + 2	21 + 4	24 + 2	27 + 1	23 + 1	26 + 1	29 + 1	22 + 3	25 + 2	28 + 1
41	21 + 2	23 + 4	25 + 5	22	24 + 6	27 + 4	23 + 4	26 + 5	29 + 5	22 + 6	25 + 5	28 + 4
42	21 + 5	23 + 6	26 + 1	22 + 4	25 + 2	28	24 + 1	27 + 1	30 + 2	23 + 2	26 + 1	29 + 1
43	22 + 1	24 + 2	26 + 4	23	25 + 5	28 + 4	24 + 5	27 + 5	30 + 6	23 + 5	26 + 4	29 + 4
44	22 + 4	24 + 5	26 + 6	23 + 4	26 + 1	29	25 + 1	28 + 2	31 + 2	24 + 1	27 + 1	30

Table continued on following page

TABLE 7–7. **GESTATIONAL AGES AS OBTAINED FROM THE LONG BONES (IN WEEKS + DAYS)** ***(Continued)***

BONE LENGTH	FEMUR PERCENTILE			HUMERUS PERCENTILE			ULNA PERCENTILE			TIBIA PERCENTILE		
(mm)	5th	50th	95th	5th	50th	95th	5th	50th	95th	5th	50th	95th
45	22 + 6	25	27 + 1	24	26 + 5	29 + 4	25 + 6	28 + 6	31 + 6	24 + 4	27 + 4	30 + 4
46	23 + 1	25 + 3	27 + 4	24 + 4	27 + 1	30	26 + 2	29 + 3	32 + 3	25 + 1	28	30 + 6
47	23 + 4	25 + 6	28	25	27 + 5	30 + 4	26 + 6	29 + 6	33	25 + 4	28 + 4	31 + 3
48	24	26 + 1	28 + 3	25 + 4	28 + 1	31	27 + 3	30 + 4	33 + 4	26 + 1	29	31 + 6
49	24 + 3	26 + 4	28 + 6	26	28 + 6	31 + 4	28	31 + 1	34 + 1	26 + 4	29 + 3	32 + 2
50	24 + 6	27	29 + 1	26 + 4	29 + 2	32	28 + 4	31 + 4	34 + 5	27	29 + 6	32 + 6
51	25 + 1	27 + 3	29 + 4	27 + 1	29 + 6	32 + 4	29 + 1	32 + 1	35 + 2	27 + 4	30 + 3	33 + 2
52	25 + 4	27 + 6	30	27 + 4	30 + 2	33 + 1	29 + 5	32 + 6	35 + 6	28	30 + 6	33 + 6
53	26	28 + 1	30 + 3	28 + 1	30 + 6	33 + 4	30 + 2	33 + 3	36 + 3	28 + 4	31 + 3	34 + 2
54	26 + 3	28 + 4	30 + 6	28 + 5	31 + 3	34 + 1	30 + 6	34	37	29	31 + 6	34 + 6
55	26 + 6	29 + 1	31 + 2	29 + 1	32	34 + 5	31 + 4	34 + 4	37 + 5	29 + 4	32 + 3	35 + 2
56	27 + 2	29 + 4	31 + 5	29 + 6	32 + 4	35 + 2	32 + 1	35 + 1	38 + 2	30	32 + 6	35 + 6
57	27 + 5	29 + 6	32 + 1	30 + 2	33 + 1	35 + 6	32 + 6	35 + 6	38 + 6	30 + 4	33 + 3	36 + 2
58	28 + 1	30 + 2	32 + 4	30 + 6	33 + 4	36 + 3	33 + 3	36 + 3	39 + 4	31	33 + 6	36 + 6
59	28 + 4	30 + 5	32 + 6	31 + 3	34 + 1	36 + 6	34	37 + 1	40 + 1	31 + 4	34 + 3	37 + 2
60	28 + 6	31 + 1	33 + 2	32	34 + 6	37 + 4	34 + 4	37 + 5	40 + 6	32	34 + 6	37 + 6
61	29 + 3	31 + 4	33 + 6	32 + 4	35 + 2	38 + 1	35 + 2	38 + 2	41 + 3	32 + 4	35 + 3	38 + 2
62	29 + 6	32	34 + 1	33 + 1	35 + 6	38 + 5	35 + 6	39	42	33	35 + 6	38 + 6
63	30 + 1	32 + 3	34 + 4	33 + 6	36 + 4	39 + 2	36 + 4	39 + 4	42 + 5	33 + 4	36 + 4	39 + 3
64	30 + 5	32 + 6	35 + 1	34 + 3	37 + 1	39 + 6	37 + 1	40 + 2	43 + 2	34 + 1	37	39 + 6
65	31 + 1	33 + 2	35 + 4	35	37 + 5	40 + 4				34 + 4	37 + 4	40 + 3
66	31 + 4	33 + 5	35 + 6	35 + 4	38 + 2	41 + 1				35 + 1	38	41
67	32	34 + 1	36 + 3	36 + 1	38 + 6	41 + 5				35 + 5	38 + 4	41 + 4
68	32 + 3	34 + 4	36 + 6	36 + 6	39 + 4	42 + 2				36 + 1	39 + 1	42
69	32 + 6	35	37 + 1	37 + 3	40 + 1	42 + 6				36 + 6	39 + 5	42 + 4
70	33 + 2	35 + 4	37 + 5									
71	33 + 5	35 + 6	38 + 1									
72	34 + 1	36 + 3	38 + 4									
73	34 + 4	36 + 6	39									
74	35 + 1	37 + 2	39 + 4									
75	35 + 4	37 + 5	39 + 6									
76	36	38 + 1	40 + 3									
77	36 + 3	38 + 4	40 + 6									
78	36 + 6	39 + 1	41 + 2									
79	37 + 2	39 + 4	41 + 5									
80	37 + 6	40	42 + 1									

A well-known table for estimating fetal age from the long bones of the extremities.
From Jeanty P, Rodesch F, Delbeke D, et al: Estimation of gestational age from measurements of fetal long bones. J Ultrasound Med 1984;3:76–77.

TABLE 7–8. **PREDICTED MENSTRUAL AGE FOR ABDOMINAL CIRCUMFERENCE VALUES**

ABDOMINAL CIRCUMFERENCE (cm)	MENSTRUAL AGE (WEEKS)	ABDOMINAL CIRCUMFERENCE (cm)	MENSTRUAL AGE (WEEKS)
11.0	15.6	23.5	27.7
10.5	16.1	24.0	28.2
11.0	16.5	24.5	28.7
11.5	16.9	25.0	29.2
12.0	17.3	25.5	29.7
12.5	17.8	26.0	30.1
13.0	18.2	26.5	30.6
13.5	18.6	27.0	31.1
14.0	19.1	27.5	31.6
14.5	19.5	28.0	32.1
15.0	20.0	28.5	32.6
15.5	20.4	29.0	33.1
16.0	20.8	29.5	33.6
16.5	21.3	30.0	34.1
17.0	21.7	30.5	34.6
17.5	22.2	31.0	35.1
18.0	22.6	31.5	35.6
18.5	23.1	32.0	36.1
19.0	23.6	32.5	36.6
19.5	24.0	33.0	37.1
20.0	24.5	33.5	37.6
20.5	24.9	34.0	38.1
21.0	25.4	34.5	38.7
21.5	25.9	35.0	39.2
22.0	26.3	35.5	39.7
22.5	26.8	36.0	40.2
23.0	27.3	36.5	40.8

Note: MA = 7.6070 + 0.7645 (AC) + 0.00393 $(AC)^2$; r^2 = 97.8%; 1 SD = 1.2 weeks.
Use the standard abdominal circumference measurement to estimate fetal age.
From Hadlock FP, Deter RL, Harrist RB, et al: Fetal abdominal circumference as a predictor of menstrual age. AJR 1982;139:369.

Ratio = numerator/demonominator
Percentage = 100 (numerator/denominator)

To illustrate, if a ratio is found to be abnormally large for the fetal age, then it must be determined if the numerator is too large, if the denominator is too small, or if both are only moderately large and small, respectively. If the ratio is too small, the conditions of this illustration are reversed. In either case, it may be difficult to determine which of the two parameters is the one causing the ratio to appear abnormal. It is also possible that both numerator and denominator may be abnormal in the same direction, both too large or both too small, resulting in what appears to be a normal ratio. Because of these problems, I prefer the ARA (discussed later) for the assessment of fetal proportions.

The ratio that is most often used in fetal sonography is the Campbell and Thomas head/abdomen (H/A) circumference ratio.[115] This is the ratio of the THC divided by the AC. Here we refer to it as the THC/AC ratio (see Fig. 7–8*A*). This ratio works very well for assessment of relative fetal weight because fat fetuses have fat abdomens but not fat heads. The skull is normal in most cases. (Note that the THC includes only the skull and not the scalp, which may be affected by fat content.) As the AC becomes smaller compared with the THC, the H/A ratio becomes larger, and vise versa. Thus, the H/A ratio is inversely related to the AC size.

Because I believe that this inverse relationship of H/A ratio and AC is not descriptive or intuitive, the reverse ratio is also given here

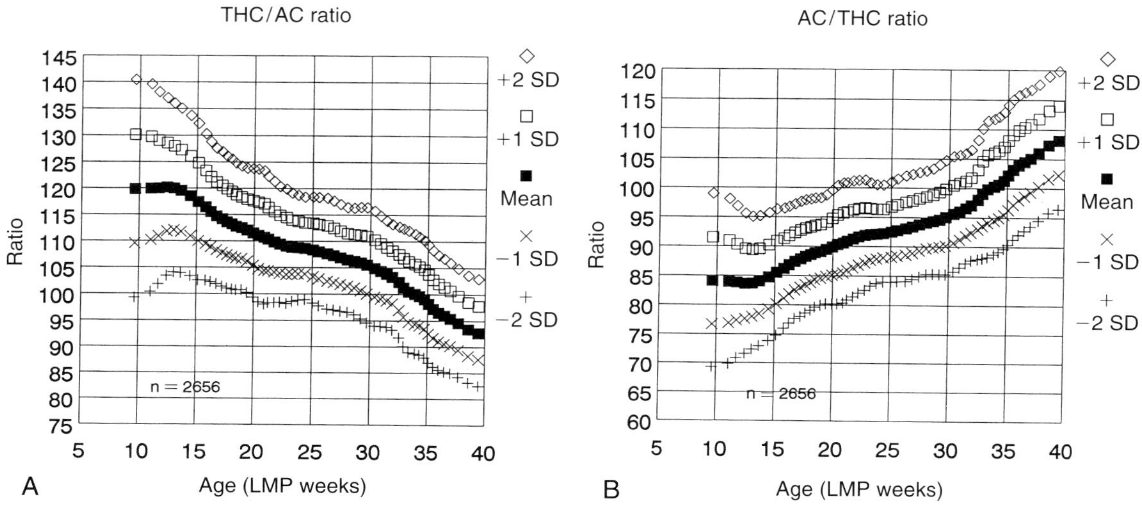

FIGURE 7–8.
Ratios of the transverse head circumference (THC) and abdominal circumference (AC). *A,* With the THC/AC ratio, as the fetal abdomen enlarges, the ratio becomes smaller. Also, as fetal age increases, the ratio becomes smaller. *B,* The inverse ratio from the same data. With this ratio (AC/THC), as the fetal abdomen gets larger, the ratio is larger, and as the fetal age increases, the ratio also increases.

(AC/THC) (see Fig. 7–8*B*). This AC/THC ratio is in more agreement with the statistical convention for indexes, in which "the ratios of one anatomic variable [are] divided by a larger, so called standard one."[97] I consider the head to be the standard with which the AC is compared because the head is more consistent in size and growth. With this ratio, relatively fat fetuses have relatively larger ratios and thin fetuses have smaller ratios. In addition, the ratio increases as a fetus grows, rather than getting smaller as fetal size increases. This seems to be more intuitive and descriptive of fetal growth.

The two graphs in Figure 7–8 were developed from the same data set (n = 2656, 1993 data). Figure 7–8*A* produces results similar to the original H/A ratio. In both graphs, the mean ratios are in a 1:1 relationship at about 34 LMP weeks. These graphs were constructed using the standard AC measurement and the THC calculated from leading-edge to leading-edge BPDs and mid-to-mid FODs (see Chapter 8). The LOWESS technique was used to calculate both the moving average or mean and the moving standard deviations for these graphs.

Ratios can be a powerful method of comparing two parameters, as long as one of the parameters can be determined to be normal, as stated earlier. For this reason, several other ratios are presented here in graphic form, which the reader may find useful and interesting. The most useful parameters are those that remain constant through some period, thus making them easier to remember. Ratios of the cranium are constant throughout the second and third trimesters (see Chapter 8). Many ratios become relatively constant after midpregnancy.

Figure 7–9 shows the two ratios for the 3-D BPD and the average of the two abdominal di-

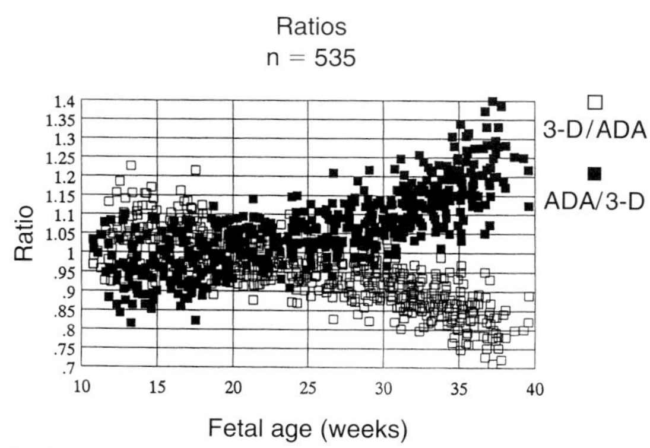

FIGURE 7–9.
The average diameter of the abdomen (ADA) compared with the average of the three diameters of the cranium (3-D = (FOD + BPD + VCD)/3). These ratios can be used in a manner similar to those in Figure 7–8, if the head is not normally shaped.

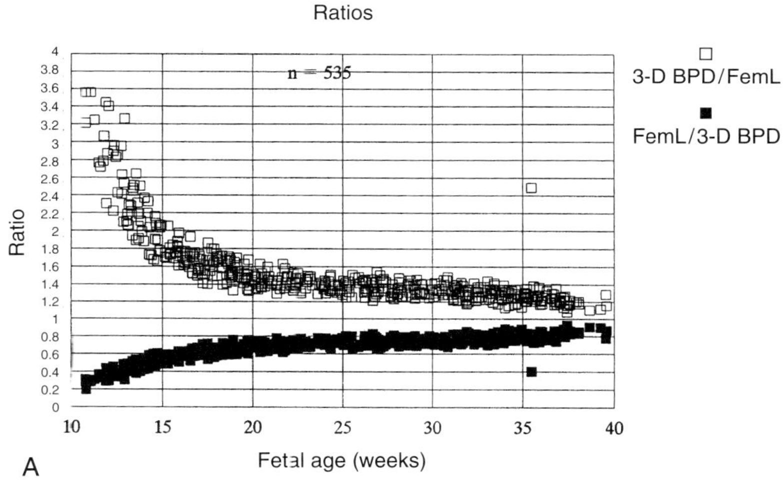

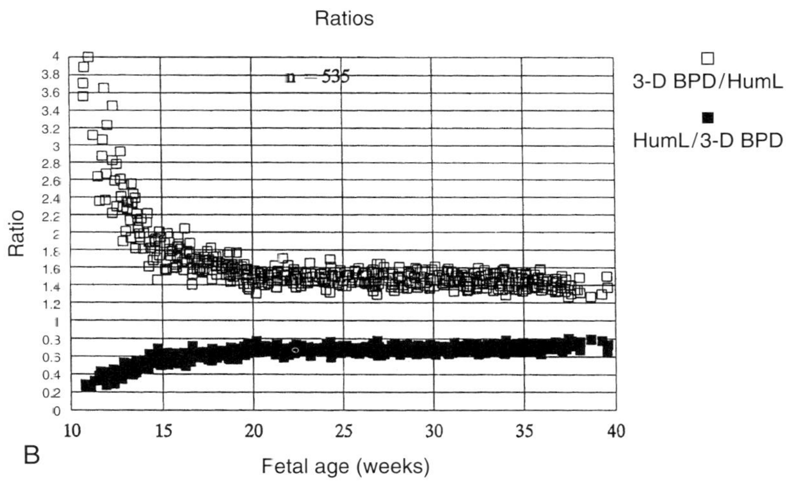

FIGURE 7–10. The length of the femur (FemL, *A*) and humerus (HumL, *B*) is compared with the three-dimensional biparietal diameter (3-D BPD) in ratios. These can be used to determine if the FemL and HumL are appropriate compared with the head size at a given time in pregnancy.

ameters used to calculate the AC. This ratio compares the average of linear measurements of the head and abdomen. It can be used in a way similar to the AC/THC or THC/AC.

Figure 7–10 shows the ratios of the 3-D BPD and the FemL and HumL. These are most useful to evaluate the normalcy of the long bones. A simple BPD can be substituted for the 3-D if the fetal head shape is confirmed to be normal. The HumL/3-D BPD is constant after midpregnancy (HumL/3-D = 0.69, ±0.08, 2 SD).

Figure 7–11 shows the ratios of the abdominal diameter average (ADA), FemL, and HumL. The femoral ratios are the most constant after 20 LMP weeks. The mean AD/FemL ratio is 1.45, ±0.19 (±2 SD). The FemL/AD mean is also constant at 0.69, ±0.09.

As useful as ratios are for comparing two measurements, they are complex to interpret if one is not sure of which measurement may be abnormal. When three or more parameters have varying degrees of abnormality, the situation is even worse. As the number of parameters increases, the number of ratios required to evaluate them, one to each of the others, becomes exponentially larger and more confusing. For this reason, I encourage the reader to develop an understanding of ARA. ARA is a type of multivariate analysis[98] for looking at the fourth dimension (size in time) of several fetal parameters in a time-series symbolic histogram. This description makes the ARA sound much more complicated than it really is. It allows instant visual assessment of total fetal proportionality.

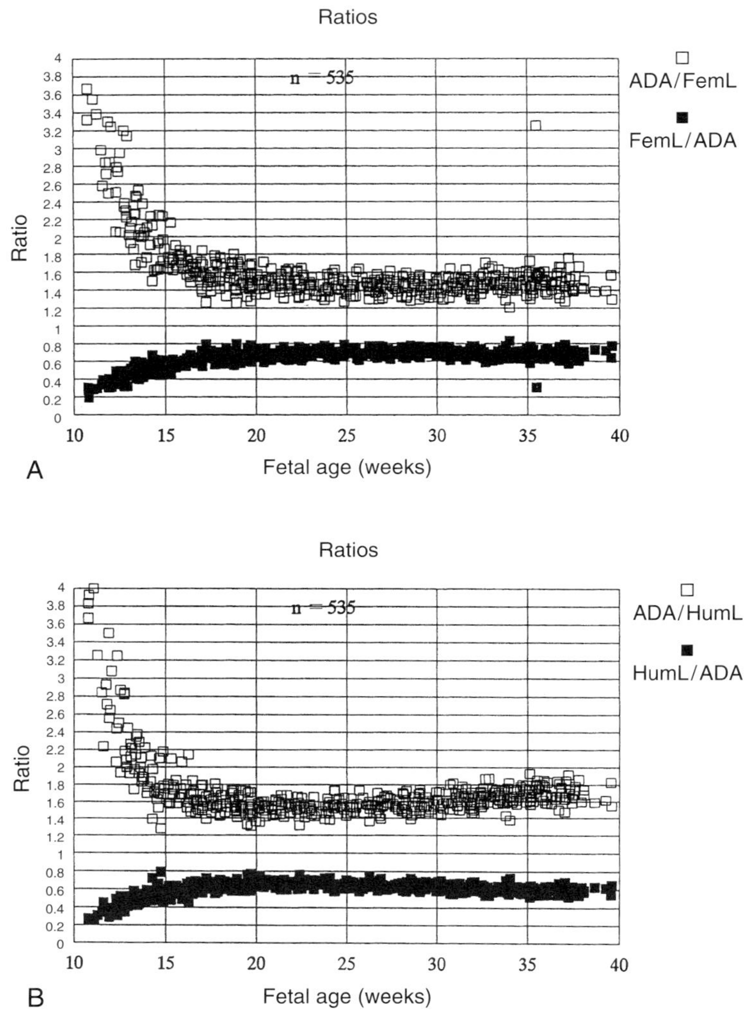

FIGURE 7–11.
The linear measurements of the average abdominal diameter (ADA) are compared with the measurements of the femur (FemL) and humerus (HumL).

Weight Estimation

Fetal weight is one of the most important and most often sought parameters of fetal growth. Extremes in fetal weight are associated with poor perinatal outcomes.[99] For this reason, reliable estimates of fetal weight can be valuable in the management of pregnancy.

Many studies have addressed sonographic estimation of weight. Several tables have been published. Kurtz and Goldberg's reference manual of 1988 for sonographic obstetrical measurements listed 95 references on fetal weight alone,[92] and more have been published since then. One of the best known is Shepard and colleagues' variation of Warsof's table (Table 7–9).[94, 95] It should be noted here that the regression formula published in association with the table in Shepard and colleagues' original article has two different typographical errors that produce inaccurate results.[100, 101] Unfortunately, these typographical errors have been perpetuated by almost every reference to that article since its publication. One letter to the journal pointing out one of the typos overlooked the second error.[101] The formula is printed correctly at the top of Table II of the article but incorrectly on the first page and in the more obvious location at the top of the table used for weight estimates. This commonly used table estimates weight based on the BPD and AC measurements. The following is the *correct* Shepard's formula:

$$\text{Log}_{10}(\text{BW}) = -1.7492 + 0.166(\text{BPD}) + 0.046(\text{AC}) - 2.646(\text{AC} \times \text{BPD})/1000$$

where $\log_{10}$ is the base 10 logarithm, BW is weight in grams, and all measurements (BPD and AC) are in centimeters.

However, this formula is not very useful as it stands. Who wants the logarithm of the weight as a result? What is needed is the formula to produce the weight in grams. The following formula is one that works in the FrameWork IV[102] computer spreadsheet and produces the same results given in Shepard and colleagues' table. Some spreadsheet formulas use functions that are written differently, and the function for the logarithm might be, for example: @ln(n), @log(n), ln(n), or log(n). Refer to your specific software manuals for formula syntax details.

```
Weight in grams = @INT((@EXP(−1.7492+
        0.166*(BPD)+0.046*(AC)−
            2.646*(BPD*AC)/1000)^@LN(10))*1000)
```

where @INT rounds the result to an integer, @LN gives the natural logarithm, @EXP is the exponent that is the inverse of @LN, the * is computerese for multiply, and the ^ means "raise to the power of." All measurements for this formula are in centimeters. Division and multiplication by 1000 have to do with multiplying centimeters and the resulting decimal points and are necessary for accurate results.

Other researchers use the FemL and AC or some other combination of parameters.[103, 104] Both of these references contain similar tables for estimating the fetal weight from the FemL and AC. Hadlock and colleagues' table is reproduced here (Table 7–10). The difficulty with fetal weight tables is that if more than two parameters are used, the table becomes voluminous. Even Shepard and colleagues' table is several pages long using just two parameters. For this reason, many researchers publish only regression formulas, many of which require a computer for reasonable computations.

The combination of three variables has been thought to be more accurate than two variables in the estimation of fetal weight. In 1984, Hadlock and associates published a weight formula that included the THC, AC, and FemL.[103] This research compared seven regression equations and found that the three-parameter model was as accurate as the four-parameter model, which included the BPD in addition to the THC, AC, and FemL. The three- and four-regression models were more accurate than models using only one or two parameters. The rationale stated by Hadlock and colleagues for the inclusion of the FemL was that "The improved weight estimates obtained with models including the femur are based on the fact that femur length is related linearly to crown-heel length.[105] Jordaan[106] has demonstrated that values of crown-heel length at the extremes of normal may cause significant errors in fetal weight estimates based on models which include only head and abdomen measurements." As stated earlier, three or more parameter weight tables would be extremely long; therefore, the following formula is recommended for use with computer spreadsheets for estimations.

$$\text{Log}_{10}\,\text{BW} = 1.5662 - 0.0108(\text{THC}) + 0.0468(\text{AC}) + 0.171(\text{FemL}) + 0.00034(\text{THC})^2 - 0.003685(\text{AC} \times \text{FemL})$$

where $\log_{10}$ is the base 10 logarithm, BW is weight in grams, and parameter measurements are in centimeters.

The following weight estimation formula is a spreadsheet version of the foregoing Hadlock's formula for the THC, AC, and FemL in millimeters. This formula was derived using measurements of the outer perimeter of the calvaria. If the leading-edge to leading-edge BPD and midedge FOD measurements are used for the THC, then 3% is added to the measurement. If centimeters are used, do not multiply the parameters by 0.1. The other computer syntax is as explained under Shepard's formula.

```
Weight in grams =
  @INT((@EXP(1.5662−.0108*(THC*.1)+
    .0468*(AC*.1)+.171*(FemL*.1)+.00034*
      ((THC*.1)^2)−.003685*((AC*.1)*
                    (FemL*.1)))^@LN(10)))
```

Hadlock and colleagues also published a useful table (see Table 7–11) and formula for estimating the normal weight from the fetal age.[107] This formula assumes that the age used in the equation is an accurate age. If the

Text continued on page 139

TABLE 7–9. **ESTIMATED FETAL WEIGHTS:**
LOG_{10} (BIRTH WEIGHT) = −1.7492 + 0.166(BPD) + 0.046(AC) −2.646 (AC × BPD)/1000

BIPARIETAL DIAMETERS	ABDOMINAL CIRCUMFERENCES											
	15.5	**16.0**	**16.5**	**17.0**	**17.5**	**18.0**	**18.5**	**19.0**	**19.5**	**20.0**	**20.5**	**21.0**
3.1	224	234	244	255	267	279	291	304	318	332	346	362
3.2	231	241	251	263	274	286	299	312	326	340	355	371
3.3	237	248	259	270	282	294	307	321	335	349	365	381
3.4	244	255	266	278	290	302	316	329	344	359	374	391
3.5	251	262	274	285	298	311	324	338	353	368	384	401
3.6	259	270	281	294	306	319	333	347	362	378	394	411
3.7	266	278	290	302	315	328	342	357	372	388	404	422
3.8	274	286	298	310	324	337	352	366	382	398	415	432
3.9	282	294	306	319	333	347	361	376	392	409	426	444
4.0	290	303	315	328	342	356	371	386	403	419	437	455
4.1	299	311	324	338	352	366	381	397	413	430	448	467
4.2	308	320	333	347	361	376	392	408	424	442	460	479
4.3	317	330	343	357	371	387	402	419	436	453	472	491
4.4	326	339	353	367	382	397	413	430	447	465	484	504
4.5	335	349	363	377	393	408	425	442	459	478	497	517
4.6	345	359	373	388	404	420	436	454	472	490	510	530
4.7	355	369	384	399	415	431	448	466	484	503	523	544
4.8	366	380	395	410	426	443	460	478	497	517	537	558
4.9	376	391	406	422	438	455	473	491	510	530	551	572
5.0	387	402	418	434	451	468	486	505	524	544	565	587
5.1	399	414	430	446	463	481	499	518	538	559	580	602
5.2	410	426	442	459	476	494	513	532	552	573	595	618
5.3	422	438	455	472	489	508	527	547	567	589	611	634
5.4	435	451	468	485	503	522	541	561	582	604	627	650
5.5	447	464	481	499	517	536	556	577	598	620	643	667
5.6	461	477	495	513	532	551	571	592	614	636	660	684
5.7	474	491	509	527	547	566	587	608	630	653	677	701
5.8	488	505	524	542	562	582	603	625	647	670	695	719
5.9	502	520	539	558	578	598	619	642	664	688	713	738
6.0	517	535	554	573	594	615	636	659	682	706	731	757
6.1	532	550	570	590	610	632	654	677	700	725	750	777
6.2	547	566	586	606	627	649	672	695	719	744	770	797
6.3	563	583	603	624	645	667	690	714	738	764	790	817
6.4	580	600	620	641	663	686	709	733	758	784	811	838

BIPARIETAL DIAMETERS	ABDOMINAL CIRCUMFERENCES												
	15.5	16.0	16.5	17.0	17.5	18.0	18.5	19.0	19.5	20.0	20.5	21.0	
6.5	597	617	638	659	682	705	728	753	778	805	832	860	
6.6	614	635	656	678	701	724	748	773	799	826	853	882	
6.7	632	653	675	697	720	744	769	794	820	848	876	905	
6.8	651	672	694	717	740	765	790	816	842	870	898	928	
6.9	670	691	714	737	761	786	811	838	865	893	922	952	
7.0	689	711	734	758	782	807	833	860	888	916	946	976	
7.1	709	732	755	779	804	830	856	883	912	941	971	1002	
7.2	730	763	777	801	827	853	880	907	936	965	996	1027	
7.3	751	775	799	824	850	876	904	932	961	991	1022	1054	
7.4	773	797	822	847	874	901	928	957	987	1017	1049	1081	
7.5	796	820	845	871	898	925	954	983	1013	1044	1076	1109	
7.6	819	844	870	896	923	951	980	1009	1040	1072	1104	1137	
7.7	843	868	894	921	949	977	1007	1037	1068	1100	1133	1167	
7.8	868	894	920	947	975	1004	1034	1065	1096	1129	1162	1197	
7.9	893	919	946	974	1003	1032	1062	1094	1126	1159	1193	1228	
8.0	919	946	973	1002	1031	1061	1091	1123	1156	1189	1224	1259	
8.1	946	973	1001	1030	1060	1090	1121	1153	1187	1221	1256	1292	
8.2	974	1001	1030	1059	1089	1120	1152	1185	1218	1253	1288	1325	
8.3	1002	1030	1059	1089	1120	1151	1183	1217	1251	1286	1322	1359	
8.4	1032	1060	1090	1120	1151	1183	1216	1249	1284	1320	1356	1394	
8.5	1062	1091	1121	1151	1183	1216	1249	1283	1318	1355	1392	1430	
8.6	1093	1122	1153	1184	1216	1249	1283	1318	1354	1390	1428	1467	
8.7	1125	1155	1186	1218	1250	1284	1318	1353	1390	1427	1465	1505	
8.8	1157	1188	1220	1252	1285	1319	1354	1390	1427	1465	1504	1543	
8.9	1191	1222	1254	1287	1321	1356	1391	1428	1465	1503	1543	1583	
9.0	1226	1258	1290	1324	1358	1393	1429	1456	1504	1543	1583	1624	
9.1	1262	1294	1327	1361	1396	1432	1468	1506	1544	1584	1624	1666	
9.2	1299	1332	1365	1400	1435	1471	1508	1546	1586	1626	1667	1709	
9.3	1337	1370	1404	1439	1475	1512	1550	1588	1628	1668	1710	1753	
9.4	1376	1410	1444	1480	1516	1554	1592	1631	1671	1712	1755	1798	
9.5	1416	1450	1486	1522	1559	1597	1635	1675	1716	1758	1800	1844	
9.6	1457	1492	1528	1565	1602	1641	1680	1720	1762	1804	1847	1892	
9.7	1500	1535	1572	1609	1547	1686	1726	1767	1809	1852	1895	1940	
9.8	1544	1580	1617	1654	1693	1733	1773	1815	1857	1900	1945	1990	
9.9	1589	1625	1663	1701	1740	1781	1822	1864	1907	1951	1996	2042	
10.0	1635	1672	1710	1749	1789	1830	1871	1914	1958	2002	2048	2094	

Table continued on following page

TABLE 7–9. **ESTIMATED FETAL WEIGHTS:**
LOG_{10} (BIRTH WEIGHT) = −1.7492 + 0.166(BPD) + 0.046(AC) −2.646 (AC × BPD)/1000 *(Continued)*

BIPARIETAL	ABDOMINAL CIRCUMFERENCES												
DIAMETERS	21.5	22.0	22.5	23.0	23.5	24.0	24.5	25.0	25.5	26.0	26.5	27.0	27.5
3.1	378	395	412	431	450	470	491	513	536	559	584	610	638
3.2	388	405	423	441	461	481	502	525	548	572	597	624	651
3.3	397	415	433	452	472	493	514	537	560	585	611	638	666
3.4	408	425	444	463	483	504	526	549	573	598	624	652	680
3.5	418	436	455	475	495	517	539	562	587	612	638	666	695
3.6	429	447	466	486	507	529	552	575	600	626	653	681	710
3.7	440	458	478	498	519	542	565	589	614	640	667	696	725
3.8	451	470	490	510	532	554	578	602	628	654	682	711	741
3.9	462	482	502	523	545	568	592	616	642	669	697	727	757
4.0	474	494	514	536	558	581	606	631	657	684	713	743	773
4.1	486	506	527	549	572	595	620	645	672	700	729	759	790
4.2	498	519	540	562	585	609	634	660	688	716	745	776	807
4.3	511	532	554	576	600	624	649	676	703	732	762	793	825
4.4	524	545	567	590	614	639	665	692	719	749	779	810	843
4.5	538	559	581	605	629	654	680	708	736	765	796	828	861
4.6	551	573	596	620	644	670	696	724	753	783	814	846	880
4.7	565	588	611	635	660	686	713	741	770	801	832	865	899
4.8	580	602	626	650	676	702	730	758	788	819	851	884	919
4.9	594	617	641	666	692	719	747	776	806	837	870	903	938
5.0	610	633	657	683	709	736	765	794	824	856	889	923	959
5.1	625	649	674	699	726	754	783	812	843	876	909	944	980
5.2	641	665	690	717	744	772	801	831	863	895	929	964	1001
5.3	657	682	708	734	762	790	820	851	883	916	950	986	1023
5.4	674	699	725	752	780	809	839	870	903	936	971	1007	1045
5.5	691	717	743	771	799	828	859	891	924	958	993	1030	1068
5.6	709	735	762	789	818	848	879	911	945	979	1015	1052	1091
5.7	727	753	780	809	838	869	900	933	966	1001	1038	1075	1114
5.8	745	772	800	829	858	889	921	954	989	1024	1061	1099	1139
5.9	764	792	820	849	879	911	943	977	1011	1047	1085	1123	1163
6.0	784	811	840	870	900	932	965	999	1035	1071	1109	1148	1189
6.1	804	832	861	891	922	955	988	1023	1058	1095	1134	1173	1214
6.2	824	853	882	913	945	977	1011	1046	1083	1120	1159	1199	1241
6.3	845	874	904	935	967	1001	1035	1071	1107	1145	1185	1226	1268
6.4	867	896	927	958	991	1025	1059	1096	1133	1171	1211	1253	1295

BIPARIETAL DIAMETERS	ABDOMINAL CIRCUMFERENCES 21.5	22.0	22.5	23.0	23.5	24.0	24.5	25.0	25.5	26.0	26.5	27.0	27.5
6.5	889	919	950	982	1015	1049	1084	1121	1159	1198	1238	1280	1323
6.6	911	942	973	1006	1039	1074	1110	1147	1185	1225	1266	1308	1352
6.7	935	965	997	1030	1065	1100	1136	1174	1213	1253	1294	1337	1381
6.8	958	990	1022	1056	1090	1126	1163	1201	1241	1281	1323	1367	1411
6.9	983	1015	1048	1082	1117	1153	1190	1229	1269	1310	1353	1397	1442
7.0	1008	1040	1074	1108	1144	1181	1219	1258	1298	1340	1383	1427	1473
7.1	1033	1066	1100	1135	1171	1209	1247	1298	1328	1370	1414	1459	1505
7.2	1060	1093	1128	1163	1200	1238	1277	1317	1358	1401	1445	1491	1538
7.3	1087	1121	1156	1192	1229	1267	1307	1348	1390	1433	1478	1524	1571
7.4	1114	1149	1184	1221	1259	1297	1338	1379	1421	1465	1511	1557	1605
7.5	1143	1178	1214	1251	1289	1328	1369	1411	1454	1499	1544	1592	1640
7.6	1172	1207	1244	1281	1320	1360	1401	1444	1487	1533	1579	1627	1676
7.7	1202	1238	1275	1313	1352	1393	1434	1477	1522	1567	1614	1663	1712
7.8	1232	1269	1306	1345	1385	1426	1468	1512	1557	1603	1650	1699	1749
7.9	1264	1301	1339	1378	1418	1460	1503	1547	1592	1639	1687	1737	1787
8.0	1296	1333	1372	1412	1453	1495	1538	1583	1629	1676	1725	1775	1826
8.1	1329	1367	1406	1446	1488	1531	1575	1620	1666	1714	1763	1814	1866
8.2	1363	1401	1441	1482	1524	1567	1612	1657	1704	1753	1803	1854	1906
8.3	1397	1436	1477	1518	1561	1605	1650	1696	1744	1793	1843	1895	1948
8.4	1433	1473	1513	1555	1599	1643	1689	1735	1784	1833	1884	1936	1990
8.5	1469	1510	1551	1594	1637	1682	1728	1776	1825	1875	1926	1979	2033
8.6	1507	1548	1589	1633	1677	1722	1769	1817	1866	1917	1969	2022	2077
8.7	1545	1586	1629	1673	1717	1764	1811	1859	1909	1960	2013	2067	2122
8.8	1584	1626	1669	1714	1759	1806	1854	1903	1953	2005	2058	2113	2169
8.9	1625	1667	1711	1756	1802	1849	1897	1947	1998	2050	2104	2159	2216
9.0	1666	1709	1753	1799	1845	1893	1942	1992	2044	2097	2151	2207	2264
9.1	1708	1752	1797	1843	1890	1938	1988	2039	2091	2144	2199	2255	2313
9.2	1752	1796	1841	1888	1936	1984	2035	2086	2139	2193	2248	2305	2363
9.3	1796	1841	1887	1934	1982	2032	2083	2135	2188	2242	2298	2356	2414
9.4	1842	1887	1934	1982	2030	2080	2132	2184	2238	2293	2350	2407	2467
9.5	1889	1935	1982	2030	2080	2130	2182	2235	2289	2345	2402	2460	2520
9.6	1937	1984	2031	2080	2130	2181	2233	2287	2342	2398	2456	2515	2575
9.7	1986	2033	2082	2131	2181	2233	2286	2340	2396	2452	2510	2570	2631
9.8	2037	2085	2133	2183	2234	2286	2340	2395	2451	2508	2567	2627	2688
9.9	2089	2137	2186	2237	2288	2341	2395	2450	2507	2565	2624	2684	2746
10.0	2142	2191	2241	2292	2344	2397	2452	2507	2564	2623	2682	2743	2806

Table continued on following page

TABLE 7–9. **ESTIMATED FETAL WEIGHTS:**
LOG_{10} (BIRTH WEIGHT) = −1.7492 + 0.166(BPD) + 0.046(AC) −2.646 (AC × BPD)/1000 ***(Continued)***

BIPARIETAL DIAMETERS	ABDOMINAL CIRCUMFERENCES											
	28.0	**28.5**	**29.0**	**29.5**	**30.0**	**30.5**	**31.0**	**31.5**	**32.0**	**32.5**	**33.0**	**33.5**
3.1	666	696	726	759	793	828	865	903	943	985	1029	1075
3.2	680	710	742	774	809	844	882	921	961	1004	1048	1094
3.3	695	725	757	790	825	861	899	938	979	1022	1067	1114
3.4	710	740	773	806	841	878	916	956	998	1041	1087	1134
3.5	725	756	789	823	858	896	934	975	1017	1061	1107	1154
3.6	740	772	805	840	876	913	953	993	1036	1080	1127	1175
3.7	756	788	822	857	893	931	971	1012	1056	1101	1147	1196
3.8	772	805	839	874	911	950	990	1032	1076	1121	1168	1218
3.9	789	822	856	892	930	969	1009	1052	1096	1142	1190	1240
4.0	806	839	874	911	949	988	1029	1072	1117	1163	1212	1262
4.1	828	857	892	929	968	1008	1049	1093	1138	1185	1234	1285
4.2	841	875	911	948	987	1028	1070	1114	1159	1207	1256	1308
4.3	859	893	930	968	1007	1048	1091	1135	1181	1229	1279	1331
4.4	877	912	949	987	1027	1069	1112	1157	1204	1252	1303	1355
4.5	896	932	969	1008	1048	1090	1134	1179	1226	1275	1326	1380
4.6	915	951	989	1028	1069	1112	1156	1202	1249	1299	1351	1404
4.7	934	971	1010	1049	1091	1134	1178	1225	1273	1323	1375	1430
4.8	954	992	1031	1071	1113	1156	1201	1248	1297	1348	1401	1455
4.9	975	1013	1052	1093	1135	1179	1225	1272	1322	1373	1426	1482
5.0	996	1034	1074	1115	1158	1203	1249	1297	1347	1399	1452	1508
5.1	1017	1056	1096	1138	1181	1226	1273	1322	1372	1425	1479	1535
5.2	1039	1078	1119	1161	1205	1251	1298	1347	1398	1451	1506	1563
5.3	1061	1101	1142	1185	1229	1276	1323	1373	1425	1478	1533	1591
5.4	1084	1124	1166	1209	1254	1301	1349	1399	1452	1506	1562	1620
5.5	1107	1148	1190	1234	1279	1327	1376	1426	1479	1534	1590	1649
5.6	1131	1172	1215	1259	1305	1353	1402	1454	1507	1562	1619	1678
5.7	1155	1197	1240	1285	1332	1380	1430	1482	1535	1591	1649	1709
5.8	1180	1222	1266	1311	1358	1407	1458	1510	1564	1621	1679	1739
5.9	1205	1248	1292	1338	1386	1435	1486	1539	1594	1651	1710	1770
6.0	1231	1274	1319	1366	1414	1464	1515	1569	1624	1682	1741	1802
6.1	1247	1301	1346	1393	1442	1493	1545	1599	1655	1713	1773	1835
6.2	1284	1328	1374	1422	1471	1522	1575	1630	1686	1745	1805	1868
6.3	1311	1356	1403	1451	1501	1552	1606	1661	1718	1777	1838	1901
6.4	1339	1385	1432	1481	1531	1583	1637	1693	1751	1810	1872	1935

BIPARIETAL DIAMETERS	ABDOMINAL CIRCUMFERENCES											
	28.0	28.5	29.0	29.5	30.0	30.5	31.0	31.5	32.0	32.5	33.0	33.5
6.5	1368	1414	1462	1511	1562	1615	1669	1725	1784	1844	1906	1970
6.6	1397	1444	1492	1542	1594	1647	1702	1759	1817	1878	1941	2006
6.7	1428	1474	1523	1574	1626	1679	1735	1792	1852	1913	1976	2042
6.8	1458	1505	1555	1606	1658	1713	1769	1827	1887	1949	2012	2078
6.9	1489	1537	1587	1639	1692	1747	1803	1862	1922	1985	2049	2116
7.0	1521	1570	1620	1672	1726	1781	1839	1898	1959	2022	2087	2154
7.1	1553	1603	1654	1706	1761	1817	1875	1934	1996	2059	2125	2193
7.2	1586	1636	1688	1741	1796	1853	1911	1971	2044	2098	2164	2232
7.3	1620	1671	1723	1777	1832	1890	1948	2009	2072	2137	2203	2272
7.4	1655	1706	1759	1813	1869	1927	1987	2048	2111	2176	2244	2313
7.5	1690	1742	1795	1850	1907	1965	2025	2087	2151	2217	2265	2354
7.6	1727	1779	1833	1888	1945	2004	2065	2127	2192	2258	2326	2397
7.7	1764	1816	1871	1927	1985	2044	2105	2168	2233	2300	2369	2440
7.8	1801	1855	1910	1966	2025	2085	2146	2210	2275	2343	2412	2484
7.9	1840	1894	1949	2006	2065	2126	2188	2252	2318	2386	2456	2528
8.0	1879	1934	1990	2048	2107	2168	2231	2296	2362	2431	2501	2574
8.1	1919	1975	2031	2089	2149	2211	2275	2340	2407	2476	2547	2620
8.2	1960	2016	2073	2132	2193	2255	2319	2385	2462	2522	2594	2667
8.3	2002	2059	2116	2176	2237	2300	2364	2431	2499	2569	2641	2715
8.4	2045	2102	2160	2220	2282	2345	2410	2477	2546	2617	2689	2764
8.5	2089	2146	2205	2266	2328	2392	2457	2525	2594	2665	2739	2814
8.6	2134	2192	2251	2312	2375	2439	2505	2573	2643	2715	2789	2864
8.7	2179	2238	2298	2359	2423	2488	2554	2623	2693	2765	2840	2916
8.8	2226	2285	2346	2408	2472	2537	2604	2673	2744	2817	2892	2968
8.9	2274	2333	2394	2457	2521	2587	2655	2725	2796	2869	2944	3021
9.0	2322	2382	2444	2507	2572	2639	2707	2777	2849	2923	2998	3076
9.1	2372	2433	2495	2559	2624	2691	2760	2830	2903	2977	3053	3131
9.2	2423	2484	2547	2611	2677	2744	2814	2885	2958	3032	3109	3187
9.3	2475	2536	2599	2664	2731	2799	2869	2940	3014	3089	3166	3245
9.4	2527	2590	2653	2719	2786	2854	2925	2997	3070	3146	3224	3303
9.5	2582	2644	2709	2774	2842	2911	2982	3054	3129	3205	3283	3362
9.6	2637	2700	2765	2831	2899	2969	3040	3113	3188	3264	3343	3423
9.7	2693	2757	2822	2889	2958	3028	3099	3173	3248	3325	3404	3484
9.8	2751	2815	2881	2948	3017	3088	3160	3234	3309	3387	3466	3547
9.9	2810	2874	2941	3009	3078	3149	3222	3296	3372	3450	3529	3611
10.0	2870	2935	3002	3070	3140	3211	3285	3359	3436	3514	3594	3676

Table continued on following page

TABLE 7–9. ESTIMATED FETAL WEIGHTS: LOG_{10} (BIRTH WEIGHT) = −1.7492 + 0.166(BPD) + 0.046(AC) −2.646 (AC × BPD)/1000 *(Continued)*

BIPARIETAL DIAMETERS	ABDOMINAL CIRCUMFERENCES												
	34.0	34.5	35.0	35.5	36.0	36.5	37.0	37.5	38.0	38.5	39.0	39.5	40.0
3.1	1123	1173	1225	1279	1336	1396	1458	1523	1591	1661	1735	1812	1893
3.2	1143	1193	1246	1301	1358	1418	1481	1546	1615	1686	1761	1838	1920
3.3	1163	1214	1267	1323	1381	1441	1504	1570	1639	1711	1786	1865	1946
3.4	1183	1235	1289	1345	1403	1464	1528	1595	1664	1737	1812	1891	1973
3.5	1204	1256	1311	1367	1426	1488	1552	1619	1689	1762	1839	1918	2001
3.6	1226	1278	1333	1390	1450	1512	1577	1645	1715	1789	1865	1945	2029
3.7	1247	1300	1356	1413	1474	1536	1602	1670	1741	1815	1893	1973	2057
3.8	1269	1323	1379	1437	1498	1561	1627	1696	1768	1842	1920	2001	2086
3.9	1292	1346	1402	1461	1523	1586	1653	1722	1794	1870	1948	2030	2115
4.0	1315	1369	1426	1486	1548	1612	1679	1749	1822	1898	1977	2059	2145
4.1	1338	1393	1451	1511	1573	1638	1706	1776	1849	1926	2005	2088	2174
4.2	1361	1417	1475	1536	1599	1664	1733	1804	1878	1954	2035	2118	2205
4.3	1385	1442	1500	1562	1625	1691	1760	1832	1906	1984	2064	2148	2236
4.4	1410	1467	1526	1588	1652	1718	1788	1860	1935	2013	2094	2179	2267
4.5	1435	1492	1552	1614	1679	1746	1816	1889	1964	2043	2125	2210	2298
4.6	1460	1518	1579	1641	1706	1774	1845	1918	1994	2073	2156	2241	2330
4.7	1486	1545	1605	1669	1734	1803	1874	1948	2024	2104	2187	2273	2363
4.8	1512	1571	1633	1697	1763	1832	1904	1978	2055	2136	2219	2306	2396
4.9	1539	1599	1661	1725	1792	1861	1934	2009	2086	2167	2251	2339	2429
5.0	1566	1626	1689	1754	1821	1891	1964	2040	2118	2200	2284	2372	2463
5.1	1594	1655	1718	1783	1851	1922	1995	2071	2150	2232	2317	2406	2498
5.2	1622	1683	1747	1813	1882	1953	2027	2103	2183	2266	2351	2440	2532
5.3	1651	1713	1777	1843	1913	1984	2059	2136	2216	2299	2386	2475	2568
5.4	1680	1742	1807	1874	1944	2016	2091	2169	2250	2333	2420	2510	2604
5.5	1710	1773	1838	1906	1976	2049	2124	2203	2284	2368	2456	2546	2640
5.6	1740	1803	1869	1938	2008	2082	2158	2237	2319	2403	2491	2582	2677
5.7	1770	1835	1901	1970	2041	2115	2192	2272	2354	2439	2528	2619	2714
5.8	1802	1866	1934	2003	2075	2150	2227	2307	2390	2475	2564	2657	2752
5.9	1834	1899	1966	2037	2109	2184	2262	2342	2426	2512	2602	2694	2790
6.0	1866	1932	2000	2071	2144	2219	2298	2379	2463	2550	2640	2733	2829
6.1	1899	1965	2034	2105	2179	2255	2334	2416	2500	2588	2678	2772	2869
6.2	1932	1999	2069	2140	2215	2291	2371	2453	2538	2626	2717	2811	2909
6.3	1967	2034	2104	2176	2251	2328	2408	2491	2577	2665	2757	2851	2949
6.4	2001	2069	2140	2213	2288	2366	2446	2530	2616	2705	2797	2892	2991

BIPARIETAL DIAMETERS	ABDOMINAL CIRCUMFERENCES												
	34.0	**34.5**	**35.0**	**35.5**	**36.0**	**36.5**	**37.0**	**37.5**	**38.0**	**38.5**	**39.0**	**39.5**	**40.0**
6.5	2037	2105	2176	2250	2326	2404	2485	2569	2656	2745	2838	2933	3032
6.6	2073	2142	2213	2287	2364	2443	2524	2609	2696	2786	2879	2975	3075
6.7	2109	2179	2251	2326	2403	2482	2564	2649	2737	2827	2921	3018	3117
6.8	2147	2217	2290	2365	2442	2522	2605	2690	2778	2869	2964	3061	3161
6.9	2184	2255	2329	2404	2482	2563	2646	2732	2821	2912	3007	3104	3205
7.0	2223	2295	2368	2444	2523	2604	2688	2774	2863	2955	3050	3149	3250
7.1	2262	2334	2409	2485	2564	2646	2730	2817	2907	2999	3095	3193	3295
7.2	2302	2375	2450	2527	2607	2689	2773	2861	2951	3044	3140	3239	3341
7.3	2343	2416	2491	2569	2649	2732	2817	2905	2996	3089	3186	3285	3388
7.4	2384	2458	2534	2612	2693	2776	2862	2950	3041	3135	3232	3332	3435
7.5	2426	2501	2577	2656	2737	2821	2907	2996	3088	3182	3279	3380	3483
7.6	2469	2544	2621	2700	2782	2866	2953	3042	3134	3229	3327	3428	3531
7.7	2513	2588	2666	2746	2828	2912	3000	3090	3182	3277	3376	3477	3581
7.8	2557	2633	2711	2792	2874	2959	3047	3137	3230	3326	3425	3526	3631
7.9	2603	2679	2757	2838	2921	3007	3095	3186	3279	3376	3475	3576	3681
8.0	2649	2725	2804	2886	2969	3056	3144	3235	3329	3426	3525	3627	3733
8.1	2695	2773	2852	2934	3018	3105	3194	3286	3380	3477	3577	3679	3785
8.2	2743	2821	2901	2983	3068	3155	3244	3336	3431	3529	3629	3732	3838
8.3	2791	2870	2950	3033	3118	3206	3296	3388	3483	3581	3682	3785	3891
8.4	2841	2920	3001	3084	3169	3257	3348	3441	3536	3634	3735	3839	3945
8.5	2891	2970	3052	3135	3221	3310	3401	3494	3590	3688	3790	3894	4000
8.6	2942	3022	3104	3188	3274	3363	3454	3548	3644	3743	3845	3949	4056
8.7	2994	3074	3157	3241	3328	3417	3509	3603	3700	3799	3901	4005	4113
8.8	3047	3128	3210	3295	3383	3472	3565	3659	3756	3855	3958	4063	4170
8.9	3101	3182	3265	3351	3438	3528	3621	3716	3813	3913	4015	4120	4228
9.0	3155	3237	3321	3407	3495	3585	3678	3773	3871	3971	4074	4179	4287
9.1	3211	3293	3377	3464	3552	3643	3736	3832	3930	4030	4133	4239	4347
9.2	3268	3350	3435	3522	3611	3702	3795	3891	3989	4090	4193	4299	4408
9.3	3326	3409	3494	3581	3670	3761	3855	3951	4050	4151	4254	4361	4469
9.4	3384	3468	3553	3641	3738	3822	3916	4013	4111	4213	4316	4423	4532
9.5	3444	3528	3614	3701	3791	3884	3978	4075	4174	4275	4379	4486	4595
9.6	3505	3589	3675	3763	3854	3946	4041	4138	4237	4339	4443	4550	4659
9.7	3567	3651	3738	3826	3917	4010	4105	4202	4302	4404	4508	4615	4724
9.8	3630	3715	3802	3890	3981	4074	4170	4267	4367	4469	4573	4680	4790
9.9	3694	3779	3866	3956	4047	4140	4236	4333	4433	4536	4640	4747	4857
10.0	3759	3845	3932	4022	4113	4207	4303	4400	4501	4603	4708	4815	4924

SD = ±106.0 g/kg of birth weight.
Shepard and colleagues' variation of Warsof's table for estimating the fetal weight from the biparietal diameter and abdominal circumference in centimeters.
From Shepard MJ, Richards VA, Berkowitz RL, et al: An evaluation of two equations for predicting fetal weight by ultrasound. Am J Obstet Gynecol 1982;147:47–54.

TABLE 7–10. **ESTIMATES OF FETAL WEIGHT (IN GRAMS) BASED ON ABDOMINAL CIRCUMFERENCE AND FEMUR LENGTH**

FEMUR LENGTH (cm)	ABDOMINAL CIRCUMFERENCE (cm)																				
	20.0	**20.5**	**21.0**	**21.5**	**22.0**	**22.5**	**23.0**	**23.5**	**24.0**	**24.5**	**25.0**	**25.5**	**26.0**	**26.5**	**27.0**	**27.5**	**28.0**	**28.5**	**29.0**	**29.5**	**30.0**
4.0	663	691	720	751	783	816	851	887	925	964	1006	1048	1093	1139	1188	1239	1291	1346	1403	1463	1525
4.1	680	709	738	769	802	836	871	907	946	986	1027	1070	1115	1162	1211	1262	1315	1371	1429	1489	1551
4.2	697	726	757	788	821	855	891	928	967	1007	1049	1093	1138	1186	1235	1287	1340	1396	1454	1515	1578
4.3	715	745	776	808	841	875	912	949	988	1029	1071	1116	1162	1209	1259	1311	1365	1422	1480	1541	1605
4.4	734	764	795	827	861	896	933	971	1010	1051	1094	1139	1185	1234	1284	1336	1391	1448	1507	1568	1632
4.5	753	783	815	847	882	917	954	993	1033	1074	1118	1163	1210	1259	1309	1362	1417	1474	1534	1596	1660
4.6	772	803	835	868	903	939	976	1015	1056	1098	1142	1187	1235	1284	1335	1388	1444	1501	1561	1623	1688
4.7	792	823	856	889	924	961	999	1038	1079	1122	1166	1212	1260	1310	1361	1415	1471	1529	1589	1652	1717
4.8	812	844	877	911	947	984	1022	1062	1103	1146	1191	1237	1286	1336	1388	1442	1498	1557	1618	1681	1746
4.9	833	865	899	933	969	1007	1046	1086	1128	1171	1216	1263	1312	1363	1415	1470	1527	1585	1647	1710	1776
5.0	855	887	921	956	993	1031	1070	1111	1153	1197	1243	1290	1339	1390	1443	1498	1555	1615	1676	1740	1806
5.1	877	910	944	980	1016	1055	1095	1136	1179	1223	1269	1317	1367	1418	1471	1527	1584	1644	1706	1770	1837
5.2	899	933	967	1004	1041	1080	1120	1162	1205	1250	1296	1344	1395	1447	1500	1556	1614	1674	1737	1801	1868
5.3	922	956	992	1028	1066	1105	1146	1188	1232	1277	1324	1373	1423	1476	1530	1586	1645	1705	1768	1833	1900
5.4	946	981	1016	1053	1091	1131	1172	1215	1259	1305	1352	1401	1452	1505	1560	1617	1675	1736	1799	1865	1933
5.5	971	1005	1041	1079	1118	1158	1199	1242	1287	1333	1381	1431	1482	1535	1591	1648	1707	1768	1832	1897	1966
5.6	995	1031	1067	1105	1144	1185	1227	1271	1316	1362	1411	1461	1513	1566	1622	1679	1739	1801	1864	1931	1999
5.7	1021	1057	1094	1132	1172	1213	1255	1299	1345	1392	1441	1491	1544	1598	1654	1712	1772	1834	1898	1964	2033
5.8	1047	1084	1121	1160	1200	1242	1285	1329	1375	1422	1472	1523	1575	1630	1686	1744	1805	1867	1932	1999	2068
5.9	1074	1111	1149	1188	1229	1271	1314	1359	1406	1454	1503	1555	1608	1663	1719	1778	1839	1902	1966	2034	2103
6.0	1102	1139	1178	1217	1258	1301	1345	1390	1437	1485	1535	1587	1641	1696	1753	1812	1873	1936	2002	2069	2139
6.1	1130	1168	1207	1247	1289	1331	1376	1421	1469	1518	1568	1620	1674	1730	1788	1847	1908	1972	2038	2105	2175
6.2	1160	1198	1237	1278	1319	1363	1408	1454	1501	1551	1602	1654	1709	1765	1823	1882	1944	2008	2074	2142	2212
6.3	1189	1228	1268	1309	1351	1395	1440	1487	1535	1585	1636	1689	1744	1800	1858	1919	1981	2045	2111	2180	2250
6.4	1220	1259	1299	1341	1384	1428	1473	1520	1569	1619	1671	1724	1779	1836	1895	1956	2018	2082	2149	2218	2289
6.5	1251	1291	1332	1373	1417	1461	1507	1555	1604	1655	1707	1760	1816	1873	1932	1993	2056	2121	2188	2256	2328
6.6	1284	1324	1365	1407	1451	1496	1542	1590	1640	1691	1743	1797	1853	1911	1970	2031	2094	2160	2227	2296	2367
6.7	1317	1357	1399	1441	1486	1531	1578	1626	1676	1728	1780	1835	1891	1949	2009	2070	2134	2199	2267	2336	2408
6.8	1351	1391	1433	1477	1521	1567	1615	1663	1713	1765	1819	1873	1930	1988	2048	2110	2174	2240	2307	2377	2449
6.9	1385	1427	1469	1513	1558	1604	1652	1701	1752	1804	1857	1913	1970	2028	2089	2151	2215	2281	2348	2418	2490
7.0	1421	1463	1506	1550	1595	1642	1690	1740	1791	1843	1897	1953	2010	2069	2130	2192	2256	2322	2391	2461	2533
7.1	1458	1500	1543	1588	1633	1681	1729	1779	1830	1883	1938	1994	2051	2110	2171	2234	2299	2365	2433	2504	2576
7.2	1495	1538	1581	1626	1673	1720	1769	1819	1871	1924	1979	2035	2093	2153	2214	2277	2342	2408	2477	2547	2620
7.3	1534	1577	1621	1666	1713	1761	1810	1861	1913	1966	2021	2078	2136	2196	2258	2321	2386	2453	2521	2592	2665
7.4	1573	1616	1661	1707	1754	1802	1852	1903	1955	2009	2065	2122	2180	2240	2302	2365	2431	2498	2566	2637	2710
7.5	1614	1657	1702	1749	1796	1845	1895	1946	1999	2053	2109	2166	2225	2285	2347	2411	2476	2543	2612	2683	2756

7.6	1655	1699	1745	1791	1839	1888	1939	1990	2043	2098	2154	2211	2270	2331	2393	2457	2523	2590	2659	2730	2803
7.7	1698	1742	1788	1835	1883	1933	1983	2035	2089	2144	2200	2258	2317	2378	2440	2504	2570	2638	2707	2778	2851
7.8	1741	1786	1833	1880	1928	1978	2029	2082	2135	2191	2247	2305	2365	2426	2488	2553	2618	2686	2755	2827	2899
7.9	1786	1832	1878	1926	1975	2025	2076	2129	2183	2238	2295	2353	2413	2474	2537	2602	2668	2735	2805	2876	2949
8.0	1832	1878	1925	1973	2022	2073	2124	2177	2232	2287	2344	2403	2463	2524	2587	2652	2718	2785	2855	2926	2999
8.1	1879	1926	1973	2021	2071	2121	2173	2227	2281	2337	2394	2453	2513	2575	2638	2702	2769	2837	2906	2977	3050
8.2	1928	1974	2022	2070	2120	2171	2224	2277	2332	2388	2446	2504	2565	2626	2690	2754	2821	2889	2958	3029	3102
8.3	1978	2024	2072	2121	2171	2223	2275	2329	2384	2440	2498	2557	2617	2679	2743	2807	2874	2942	3011	3082	3155

FEMUR LENGTH (cm)	**30.5**	**31.0**	**31.5**	**32.0**	**32.5**	**33.0**	**33.5**	**34.0**	**34.5**	**35.0**	**35.5**	**36.0**	**36.5**	**37.0**	**37.5**	**38.0**	**38.5**	**39.0**	**39.5**	**40.0**
4.0	1590	1658	1729	1802	1879	1959	2042	2129	2220	2314	2413	2515	2622	2734	2850	2972	3098	3230	3367	3511
4.1	1617	1685	1756	1830	1907	1987	2071	2158	2249	2344	2442	2545	2652	2764	2880	3002	3128	3260	3397	3540
4.2	1644	1712	1783	1858	1935	2016	2100	2187	2279	2373	2472	2575	2683	2794	2911	3032	3159	3290	3427	3570
4.3	1671	1740	1812	1886	1964	2045	2129	2217	2308	2404	2503	2606	2713	2825	2942	3063	3189	3321	3458	3600
4.4	1699	1768	1840	1915	1993	2075	2159	2247	2339	2434	2533	2637	2744	2856	2973	3094	3220	3352	3488	3630
4.5	1727	1797	1869	1944	2023	2105	2189	2278	2370	2465	2565	2668	2776	2888	3004	3125	3251	3383	3519	3661
4.6	1756	1826	1898	1974	2053	2135	2220	2309	2401	2497	2596	2700	2807	2919	3036	3157	3283	3414	3550	3692
4.7	1785	1855	1928	2004	2084	2166	2251	2340	2432	2528	2628	2732	2840	2952	3068	3189	3315	3446	3582	3723
4.8	1814	1885	1959	2035	2115	2197	2283	2372	2464	2560	2660	2764	2872	2984	3100	3221	3347	3478	3613	3754
4.9	1845	1916	1990	2066	2146	2229	2315	2404	2497	2593	2693	2797	2905	3017	3133	3254	3380	3510	3645	3786
5.0	1875	1947	2021	2098	2178	2261	2347	2437	2530	2626	2726	2830	2938	3050	3166	3287	3412	3542	3677	3818
5.1	1906	1978	2053	2130	2210	2294	2380	2470	2563	2659	2760	2864	2972	3084	3200	3320	3445	3575	3710	3850
5.2	1938	2010	2085	2163	2243	2327	2413	2503	2597	2693	2794	2898	3006	3117	3234	3354	3479	3608	3743	3882
5.3	1970	2043	2118	2196	2277	2360	2447	2537	2631	2728	2828	2932	3040	3152	3268	3388	3513	3642	3776	3915
5.4	2003	2076	2151	2229	2311	2395	2482	2572	2665	2762	2863	2967	3075	3186	3302	3422	3547	3676	3809	3948
5.5	2036	2109	2185	2264	2345	2429	2516	2607	2700	2797	2898	3002	3110	3221	3337	3457	3581	3710	3843	3981
5.6	2070	2143	2220	2298	2380	2464	2552	2642	2736	2833	2933	3038	3145	3257	3372	3492	3616	3744	3877	4015
5.7	2104	2178	2254	2333	2415	2500	2587	2678	2772	2869	2970	3074	3181	3293	3408	3527	3651	3779	3911	4048
5.8	2139	2213	2290	2369	2451	2536	2624	2714	2808	2905	3006	3110	3218	3329	3444	3563	3686	3814	3946	4082
5.9	2175	2249	2326	2405	2488	2573	2660	2751	2845	2942	3043	3147	3254	3366	3480	3599	3722	3849	3981	4117
6.0	2211	2286	2363	2442	2525	2610	2698	2789	2883	2980	3080	3184	3292	3403	3517	3636	3758	3885	4016	4151
6.1	2248	2323	2400	2480	2562	2647	2736	2827	2921	3018	3118	3222	3329	3440	3554	3673	3795	3921	4052	4186
6.2	2285	2360	2438	2518	2600	2686	2774	2865	2959	3056	3157	3260	3367	3478	3592	3710	3832	3957	4087	4222
6.3	2323	2398	2476	2556	2639	2725	2813	2904	2998	3095	3195	3299	3406	3516	3630	3747	3869	3994	4124	4257
6.4	2362	2437	2515	2595	2678	2764	2852	2943	3037	3134	3235	3338	3445	3555	3668	3785	3906	4031	4160	4293
6.5	2401	2477	2555	2635	2718	2804	2892	2983	3077	3174	3274	3378	3484	3594	3707	3824	3944	4069	4197	4329
6.6	2441	2517	2595	2675	2759	2844	2933	3024	3118	3215	3315	3418	3524	3633	3746	3863	3983	4106	4234	4366
6.7	2481	2557	2636	2716	2800	2885	2974	3065	3159	3256	3355	3458	3564	3673	3786	3902	4021	4144	4271	4402
6.8	2523	2599	2677	2758	2841	2927	3016	3107	3200	3297	3397	3499	3605	3714	3826	3941	2060	4183	4309	4439
6.9	2564	2641	2719	2800	2884	2969	3058	3149	3242	3339	3438	3541	3646	3754	3866	3981	4100	4222	4347	4477

Table continued on following page

TABLE 7–10. ESTIMATES OF FETAL WEIGHT (IN GRAMS) BASED ON ABDOMINAL CIRCUMFERENCE AND FEMUR LENGTH *(Continued)*

FEMUR LENGTH (cm)	ABDOMINAL CIRCUMFERENCE (cm)																			
	30.5	31.0	31.5	32.0	32.5	33.0	33.5	34.0	34.5	35.0	35.5	36.0	36.5	37.0	37.5	38.0	38.5	39.0	39.5	40.0
7.0	2607	2683	2762	2843	2927	3012	3101	3192	3285	3381	3481	3583	3688	3796	3907	4022	4140	4261	4386	4514
7.1	2650	2727	2806	2887	2970	3056	3144	3235	3328	3424	3523	3625	3730	3838	3948	4062	4180	4300	4425	4552
7.2	2694	2771	2850	2931	3014	3100	3188	3279	3372	3468	3567	3668	3772	3880	3990	4104	4220	4340	4464	4591
7.3	2739	2816	2895	2976	3059	3145	3233	3323	3416	3512	3610	3712	3816	3922	4032	4145	4261	4381	4503	4629
7.4	2785	2861	2940	3021	3105	3190	3278	3369	3461	3557	3655	3756	3859	3966	4075	4187	4303	4421	4543	4668
7.5	2831	2908	2987	3068	3151	3236	3324	3414	3507	3602	3700	3800	3903	4009	4118	4230	4344	4462	4583	4708
7.6	2878	2955	3034	3115	3198	3283	3371	3461	3553	3648	3745	3845	3948	4053	4161	4272	4387	4504	4624	4747
7.7	2926	3003	3081	3162	3245	3331	3418	3508	3600	3694	3791	3891	3993	4098	4205	4316	4429	4545	4665	4787
7.8	2974	3051	3130	3211	3294	3379	3466	3555	3647	3741	3838	3937	4039	4143	4250	4360	4472	4588	4706	4827
7.9	3024	3100	3179	3260	3343	3427	3514	3604	3695	3789	3885	3984	4085	4188	4295	4404	4515	4630	4748	4868
8.0	3074	3151	3229	3310	3392	3477	3564	3653	3744	3837	3933	4031	4131	4234	4340	4448	4559	4673	4790	4909
8.1	3125	3202	3280	3360	3443	3527	3614	3702	3793	3886	3981	4079	4179	4281	4386	4493	4604	4716	4832	4950
8.2	3177	3253	3332	3412	3494	3578	3664	3752	3843	3935	4030	4127	4226	4328	4432	4539	4648	4760	4875	4992
8.3	3230	3306	3384	3464	3546	3630	3716	3803	3893	3985	4080	4176	4275	4376	4479	4585	4693	4804	4918	5034

This table can be used to estimate the fetal weight in grams from the femur length and abdominal circumference.
From Hadlock FP, Harrist RB, Carpenter RJ, et al: Sonographic estimation of fetal weight based on AC and FemL. Radiology 1984;150:535–540.

TABLE 7–11. **IN UTERO FETAL WEIGHT STANDARDS AT ULTRASONOGRAPHY**

MENSTRUAL WEEK	PERCENTILES (g)				
	3rd	10th	50th	90th	97th
10	26	29	35	41	44
11	34	37	45	53	56
12	43	48	58	68	73
13	55	61	73	85	91
14	70	77	93	109	116
15	88	97	117	137	146
16	110	121	146	171	183
17	136	150	181	212	226
18	167	185	223	261	279
19	205	227	273	319	341
20	248	275	331	387	414
21	299	331	399	467	499
22	359	398	478	559	598
23	426	471	568	665	710
24	503	556	670	784	838
25	589	652	785	918	981
26	685	758	913	1068	1141
27	791	876	1055	1234	1319
28	908	1004	1210	1416	1513
29	1034	1145	1379	1613	1724
30	1169	1294	1559	1824	1956
31	1313	1453	1751	2049	2189
32	1465	1621	1953	2285	2441
33	1622	1794	2162	2530	2703
34	1783	1973	2377	2781	2971
35	1946	2154	2595	3036	3244
36	2110	2335	2813	3291	3516
37	2271	2513	3028	3543	3785
38	2427	2686	3236	3786	4045
39	2576	2851	3435	4019	4294
40	2714	3004	3619	4234	4524

Normal weights and percentiles by menstrual ages. This table can be used to compare the estimated fetal weight to the normal distributions.

From Hadlock FP, Harrist RB, Martinez-Poyer J: In utero analysis of fetal growth: A sonographic weight standard. Radiology 1991;181:129–133.

age is too small (early) or too large, the weights will be in error in the same direction, too small or large. This formula is accurate in normal fetuses:

$$\text{Log(n) weight (g)} = 0.578 + 0.332\,(\text{MA}) - 0.00354\,(\text{MA})^2$$

where log(n) is the natural logarithm, MA is the age in LMP weeks, and g is grams.

The spreadsheet version of this formula is

Weight (g) = @EXP (.578+ .332*MA−.00354*MA^2)

where the computer syntax is @EXP is the exponential of the natural logarithm, * means multiply, ^ means raise to the power of (^2 = to square), and MA is age in LMP weeks. Consult your software manual for possible variations in this syntax.

Logarithms and exponentiation are more difficult to perform with hand-held calculators; thus, these calculations are less useful in some clinical settings. Because of this difficulty, I have "reverse engineered" weight estimates to derive a formula based on a fetal volume function that is a little easier to use. This was done by using Hadlock and colleagues' sonographic weight standard formula to estimate the fetal weights from the MFP AA for a random sample of 217 normal fetuses and then applying curve-fitting software to fetal data for volumetric functions for the 3-D, FemL, HumL, and abdominal diameter average. After an acceptable equation was selected, the results were tested against the three previous estimates (Hadlock's age to weight and FemL, AC and THC weight and Shepard's BPD and AC weight) using the random sample. Of this sample, 217 fetuses had all the required measurements after the 14th LMP week. Using ANOVA, no significant difference was found in the mean weight estimates for any of the four formulas ($P = 0.989$, n = 217). Using a *t*-test for paired two-sample means between Hadlock's weight standard and the volume function estimate found no significant difference between them ($P = 0.938$, n = 217). Cross-correlation was performed, and all were found to have good correlations ($r > 0.9899$) (Table 7–12).

The resulting equation is based on volumetric functions of the fetal head and trunk. These functions are not true volumes but only consistent methods of representing the change in mass. The formula requires four steps but can be performed using a hand-held calculator or computer spreadsheet. All measurements are in millimeters, and weight estimates are thus produced in grams.

The first step is to calculate the head volume function (head Vf or HVf) based on the 3-D BPD. The BPD can be used if the head shape is normal. The formula is that of a sphere using the 3-D BPD or simple BPD (measurements in millimeters):

$$\text{Spherical volume} = (1/6)\ \text{pi}\ D^3$$

therefore

$$\text{Head Vf} = \text{HVf} = 0.0005236\ (\text{3-D BPD})^3$$

The second step is to calculate the trunk volume function (trunk Vf or TVf). This function is calculated as a volume of a cylinder using the sum of the FemL and HumL (mm) as the height and the abdomen as the cross-sectional area of the cylinder. The TVf is calculated as follows:

$$\text{Cylindrical volume} = \text{pi}\ (r^2)\ \text{height}$$

therefore

$$\text{Trunk Vf} = \text{TVf} = (0.0007854(\text{TAD})(\text{AAD}))\ (\text{FemL} + \text{HumL})$$

where pi = 3.14159.

The third step produces a volume function (Vf) by adding the HVf and TVf:

$$\text{Vf} = \text{HVf} + \text{TVf}$$

The fourth and final step is to substitute the previous function (Vf) into the weight estimation equation:

$$\text{Weight (g)} = 125 + 0.1139^{*}\text{Vf}^{*}\sqrt{\text{Vf}} - 0.00173^{*}\text{Vf}^2$$

Syntax is as earlier (* = multiply).

TABLE 7–12. **FETAL WEIGHT FORMULAS' CORRELATION MATRIX**

CORRELATION MATRIX	HADLOCK WEIGHT STANDARD	DuBOSE (3-D, ADA, FemL, HumL)	SHEPARD (BPD and AC)	HADLOCK (THC, FemL, AC)
Hadlock weight standard	1.0000			
DuBose (3-D, ADA, FemL, HumL)	0.9952	1.0000		
Shepard (BPD and AC)	0.9912	0.9909	1.0000	
Hadlock (THC, FemL, AC)	0.9899	0.9943	0.9948	1.0000

The correlation matrix for four fetal weight estimation formulas. The first column is the correlation with Hadlock's fetal weight standard estimated from age. The other columns are correlations for formulas that use various fetal parameters to estimate the fetal weight. The DuBose formula uses the three-dimensional head with the femur length (FemL), humerus length (HumL), and abdominal diameter average (ADA) in a fetal volume function (Vf = HVf + TVf). The Shepard regression uses the biparietal diameter (BPD) and abdominal circumference (AC). The Hadlock weight estimation uses the transverse head circumference (THC), FemL, and AC. The formulas are given and discussed in the Weight Estimation section of this chapter.

Fetal weight estimation is important but not always easy. It is hoped that this discussion will add more light than heat to the subject. At the same time, I hope that readers will become familiar with a computer spreadsheet, which is simply an electronic accounting sheet of rows and columns for performing mathematical computations. Many good ones are available. You are cautioned always to test any formula before using it clinically. As pointed out earlier, typographical errors may occur in the original publication or in your own entry of the formulas, and the syntax of your software may be somewhat different from that shown here. The more complex the formulas, the more likely these kinds of errors are to occur. Always keep your software manuals close at hand—and use them. You cannot absorb spreadsheet syntax by osmosis.

Age Range Analysis

LOWESS

Table 7–1 was not established using regression analysis but with a modification of trend analysis called locally weighted scatterplot smoother, or LOWESS.[58] The LOWESS technique was performed using a spreadsheet. The first time the LOWESS was performed, the data were sorted by the MFP AAs using Hadlock and colleagues' four parameters—the BPD, THC, AC, and FemL—which is analogous to the independent variable in regression analysis. Once this sorting was performed, the parameter measurements about a selected point or age were averaged for the measurement of record for that week. The LOWESS smoothing function was chosen to be ±0.25 weeks around this point. This was done for each week of the pregnancy.

The final table (see Table 7–1) was constructed by reading the entire 1993 database using weekly sorting criteria of the exact week ±0.25 week (±1.75 days). To use week 25 as an example, all parameter measurements, the LNMP, and the MFP AA were read into a spreadsheet for all pregnancies that met the criteria of having a fetal heart rate (FHR > 0) and an MFP AA greater than 24.75 and less than 25.25 weeks. This sorting on the 25th week identified 37 cases that met the criteria. The averages of all weeks from the 4th to the 41st week were sorted in this way and produced a mean of 29.5 cases per week. This process is a variation on moving average time-series analysis[108] or LOWESS.[58]

The advantage of using the LOWESS over regression analysis to establish a table such as Table 7–1 is that the regression formulas may eliminate subtle variations in normal growth, turning them into smoother curves. Cleveland went so far as to state, "Statistical scientists call this a regression curve, a misnomer since there is nothing regressive about it at all."[58] The LOWESS technique minimizes the obliteration of these subtle variations. The drawback of the LOWESS is that it requires very large populations for valid results.

AGE RANGE ANALYSIS

MFP AA is known to be a more accurate estimator of fetal age than are single parameters used alone. It was first suggested in 1981 by Bovicelli and colleagues that the averaged ages of the CRL and BPD improved on the estimation of fetal age early in gestation.[9, 66] In 1983, Hadlock and his students demonstrated that an average of MFP ages derived from four parameters (BPD, THC, AC, and FemL) was more accurate throughout pregnancy.[8, 9] This was confirmed through replication by Ott in 1985.[67]

The rationale for this averaging methodology is that all fetuses have different proportions and no single parameter is always a perfect indicator of fetal age. Averaging several parameter ages together minimizes the effects of differing fetal proportions and any possible errors in parameter measurements.

Inherent in the MFP AA is the idea of the range of ages, or ARA. Although the MFP AA yields a more accurate estimate of gestational age, it does not answer the question of how dispersed are the various parameter ages of individual fetuses in a normal population. We first raised this question soon after Hadlock and colleagues published their original research.[1, 8, 9] The purpose of this section is to describe the distribution of human fetal parameter ages in a large population.

After the MFP age range (maximum − minimum parameter ages) was calculated for each fetus in the population, it became clear that the ranges and the distribution of age estimates within these ranges are very sensitive to extreme fetal disproportions.[109] This is because the range is calculated by subtracting the minimum fetal age from the maximum fetal age for the various parameters, and any fetal parameter that is disproportionately small or large results in an age range that is extreme for that gestational age. The equivalent fetal ages were found to be approximately normally distributed about the mean age (i.e., MFP AA). By plotting the equivalent fetal ages for MFPs in a symbolic histogram of ages, our group found it was possible to view the relative proportions for all the parameters for an individual fetus at a glance.

To illustrate the relative variability of single parameters and their relationship to the MFP AA, Figure 7–12 was constructed. In this figure, the bar graph histograms for the THC, BPD, AC, and FemL are shown. These histograms were constructed by reading the fetal parameter ages into a spreadsheet using the criteria that the MFP AA for that fetus equaled a specific week ±0.1 week. The MFP AA weeks read were 18 for the FemL, 20 for the BPD and THC, and 22 for the AC. In this view, the fetal age is not considered the true age for any single parameter but the equivalent parameter growth expressed as a function of time. This can be referred to as the size age or sonographic age (SA). Compared with the four histograms are the distributions of parameter ages from three different research groups, the FemL

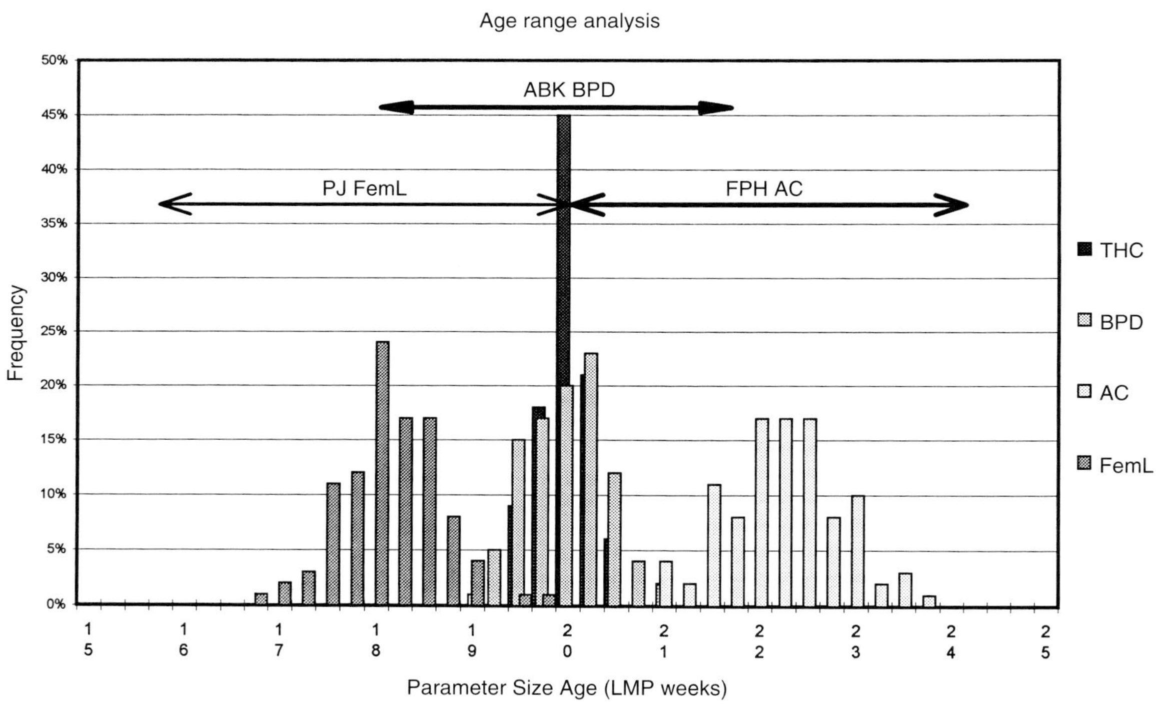

FIGURE 7–12.
A graphic representation of the principle of age range analysis (ARA) at 20 weeks.

The bar histograms are from 10,000 + cases from which each parameter age was sorted for specific multiple fetal parameter average ages (MFP AAs). The transverse head circumference (THC) and biparietal diameter (BPD) ages are from cases with MFP AAs between 19.9 and 20.1 weeks. The femur ages (FemL) are from cases with MFP AAs between 17.9 and 18.1 weeks. The abdominal circumference (AC) ages are from cases with MFP AAs between 21.9 and 22.1 weeks. The x-axis is age from the parameter's size.

The two-headed arrows represent the normal distribution of ages reported by three different researchers. ABK BPD is the A.B. Kurtz BPD distribution at 20 weeks. The PJ FemL is the P. Jeanty FemL distribution at 18 weeks. The FPH AC is the F.P. Hadlock AC distribution at 22 weeks.

Notice that all of these distributions come together or overlap at approximately 20 weeks. This means that a fetus at 20 MFP AA weeks could have a FemL age of 18 weeks, an AC age of 22 weeks, and a BPD and THC age of 20 weeks and still be relatively normal. This is the fundamental principle of the ARA.

from Jeanty and colleagues,[110] the BPD from Kurtz and associates,[82] and the AC from Hadlock and coworkers.[57] Note that in all parameters, the distributions overlap at 20 weeks. This illustrates that a single fetus may have a FemL that is the equivalent of 18 weeks, a BPD and THC at 20 weeks, and an AC at 22 weeks, for an MFP AA of 20 weeks. It would be absurd to assume that the AC was conceived 4 weeks before the femur, yet that is how many discuss parameter ages. It is more logical to assume that the true fetal age is at the MFP AA, with the FemL and AC under the extreme tails of the distribution. We found that the parameter age range distribution for all parameters is approximately ±5.0% (±1 SD) of the fetal age or ±10% for 2 SD.

Having realized that the equivalent fetal ages can be used to represent the relative sizes of the fetal parameters, I was able to develop a modified Z formula. This ARA Z formula is based on the Z function of the standard deviation[111] of the distribution for fetal age range. This formula can be used to determine the relative location of any fetal parameter in a normal distribution of MFP ages. Rather than using the fetal head to abdominal ratio that compares only those two parameters, the ARA allows comparison of the parameter age with the mean of MFP ages. The ARA Z score, expressed in standard deviations, shows the location of the parameter in the normal distribution.

The following ARA Z formula can be used to calculate the location of an individual parameter in the normal distribution of parameter ages around the average age:

$$\text{Location in ARA distribution (SD)} = ((\text{PSA} - \text{age})/(\text{age} \times 0.05))$$

where PSA is parameter of interest sonographic age in weeks and age is best actual age available in weeks.

It should be noted that the age in this formula is the most accurate menstrual age available, usually the MFP AA, or age of another parameter age such as 3-D BPD or head circumference. For this formula to yield meaningful results, the age used must be assumed to be accurate. For this reason, the reported LNMP may not be the best age estimate unless it was confirmed by an earlier sonographic examination. The best age for the study of fetal proportionality is the MFP average, assuming there is no symmetrical intrauterine growth retardation or restriction (IUGR), which is also a limitation in the use of ratios for comparison. If IUGR is suspected, a second examination a few weeks later is required to determine if the expected SA increase occurred. This determination is made by comparing the time interval between examinations and the fetal SA intervals. In theory, the growth of the fetal SA between two examinations should be equal to the actual time interval between the examinations.

These findings are similar to research data published by Hadlock and others, in which the variability of the CRL, THC, and FemL was found to be ±8% of the predicted age.[4–7] I have chosen to use ±10% of the predicted age because it is conservative, gives the advantage to the fetus, and is easy to calculate.

Another way to visualize this phenomenon is to plot the residuals of parameters minus the MFP AA against the fetal age. This presents the relative sizes of the parameters as a function of time, the fourth dimension. Figure 7–13 shows the distributions of the residual ages for three representative head (Fig. 7–13*A*) and body (Fig. 7–13*B*) parameters. The relative differences in the distributions are greater for body parameters than for cranial parameters; both increase with time. The distributions for the cranial parameters are approximately 3% to 5% of the age, whereas the body parameter residuals are approximately 7% to 10% of the age. The body parameters thus are approximately twice as variable as those of the head. The black dots in Figure 7–13 are LOWESS ±2 SD of the residuals. Each dot represents the residuals for 30 fetuses (±15 residuals) around each sorted MFP AA. It can be observed that the head exhibits a greater increase in variability (±2 SD) after approximately 29 weeks. This (and Fig. 7–8) may be the first time the LOWESS technique has been used for the representation of standard deviations. This might be called a moving standard deviation or LOWESS SD.

In Figure 7–14*A* and 7–14*B*, the residuals are presented as percentages of the MFP AA (residual % = (parameter age − AA)/AA). This treatment normalizes the residuals by

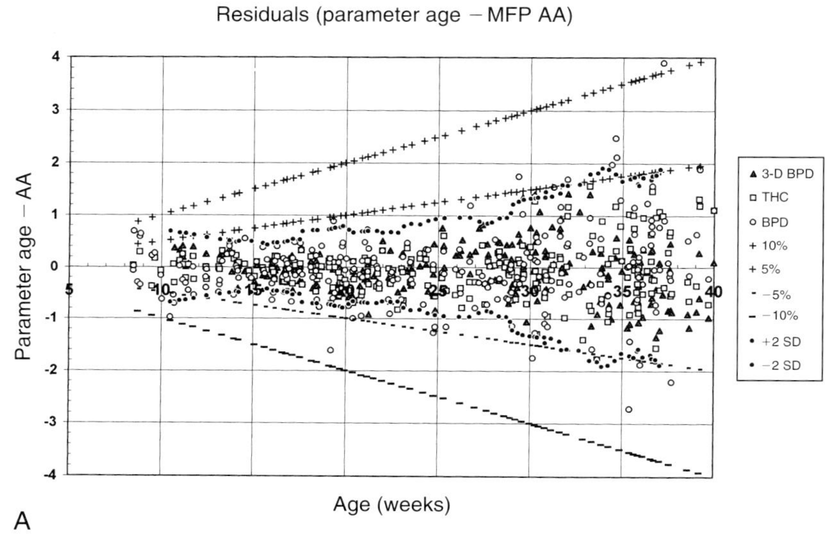

A

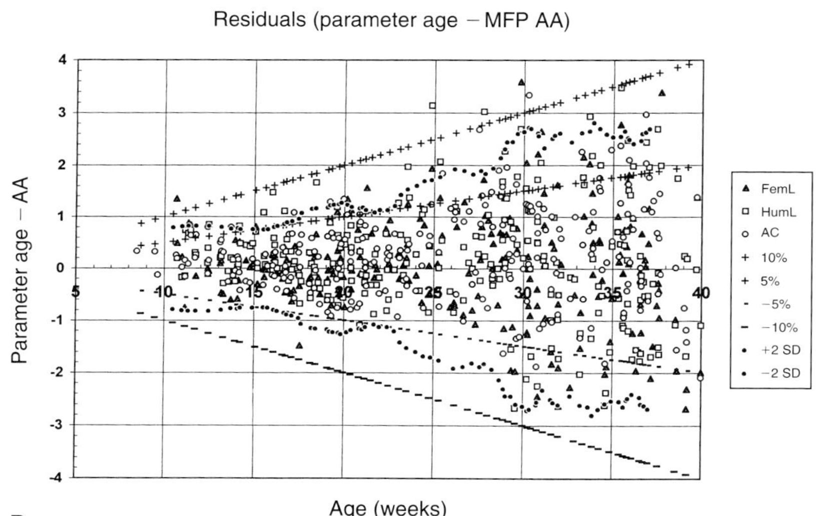

B

FIGURE 7–13.
Two scatterplots showing the residuals of the specific fetal parameter ages minus the multiple fetal parameter average age (MFP AA). The straight-line plots of the + and − are for ±5% and 10% of the MFP AA. The solid round dots are moving 2 standard deviations (±2 SD) for groups of 30 fetuses categorized by age. These graphs clearly show the increasing variation in the size of the parameters in time.

A, The residuals for three cranial parameter ages, the three-dimensional biparietal diameter (3-D BPD), transverse head circumference (THC), and BPD. Notice that cranial parameters remain between the ±5% lines except for the BPD, which has a few outliers. The ±2 SD dots also remain between and approximately parallel to the 5% lines until about 33 to 34 weeks, at which time head molding becomes influential.

B, The residuals for three body parameter ages. The fetal body parameters have a larger variation and resulting residuals than the fetal head. The ±2 SD dots remain between the 5% and 10% lines. There is a noticeable increase in the 2 SD for the body parameters after midpregnancy. FemL, femur length; HumL, humerus length; AC, abdominal circumference.

removing the influence of time. Again, this confirms the relative distributions of the head at approximately 3% to 5% and the body parameters at approximately 7% to 10% throughout pregnancy.

Since 1986, we have used a dedicated database/spreadsheet program for fetal size and age assessment (Basic Baby II).[2] This software allows accumulation of fetal measurements and observations; calculates estimated

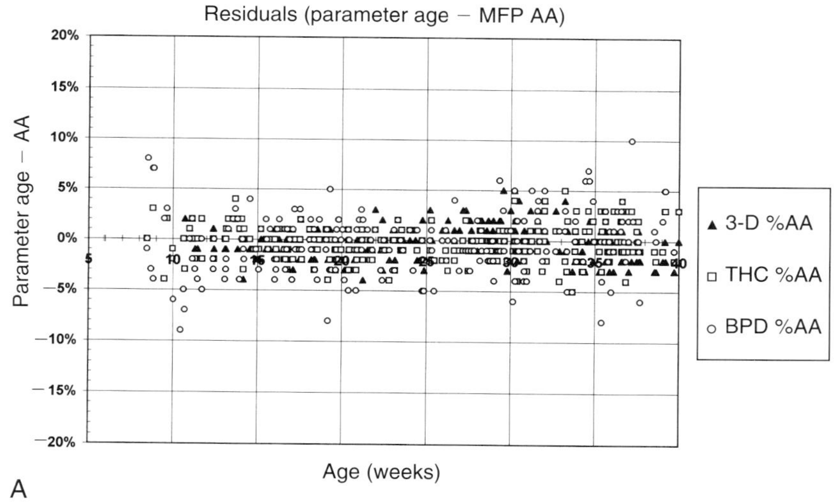

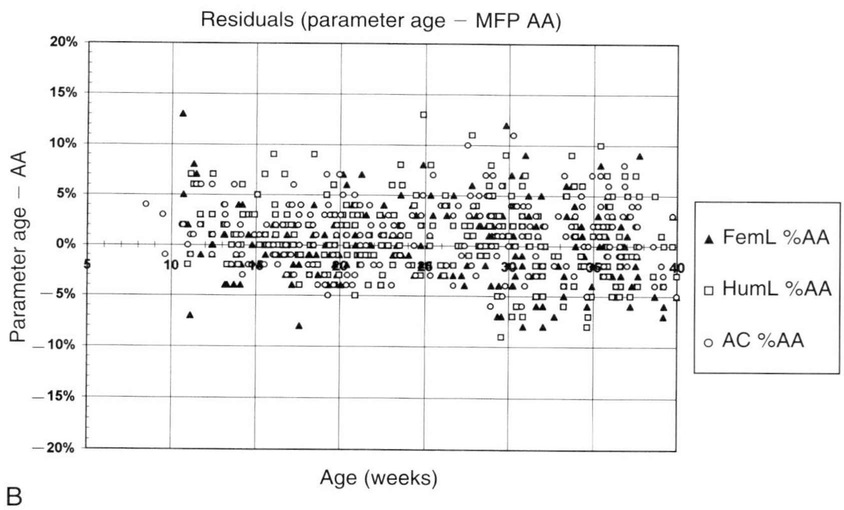

FIGURE 7–14.
These graphs are for the same data as in Figure 7–13. Here the specific parameter age residuals are shown as a percentage of the MFP AA (percentage = [parameter age − MFP AA/MFP AA]). The fetal head residual percentages remain inside the 5% line for the most part, again except for the BPD, which is the most variable (*A*). The body residual percentages extend out closer to the 10% line (*B*).

parameter ages, weight, and the relative location of each parameter in a normal distribution using the ARA Z formula; and summarizes the MFP AA as well as the average ages for the brain (cranium) and body parameters. Figure 7–15 shows two printouts for fetuses of approximately the same LNMP ages and for whom birthing feedback was obtained.

Figure 7–15*A* is the analysis for a normal-appearing fetus having all parameters within ±1.0 SD of the MFP AA, which was 26.5 LMP weeks, and the LNMP age was 26.6 weeks. Across the bottom of the printout is the time-series symbolic histogram, which has a relatively normal bell curve with slightly negative (left) skewness. A normal girl delivered on 4/8/1986 was at 39.9 weeks by LNMP and 39.8 weeks by MFP AA. Her weight was 3227 g (7.1 lb), and her length was 50.8 cm (20 in). This weight was only 356 g less than a normal of 3583 according to Hadlock and colleagues' formula for weight standards (see Table 7–11).[107]

Figure 7–15*B* represents a fetus at approximately 27 LNMP weeks with all parameter ages within ±2 SD of the MFP AA. Both the

```
EXAM DATE:    1  6  86                          EXAM# = 1  By: TD   BB#: 1115
PT:                                             AGE:     PT.#
DR.:                                            LMP = (M) =  7  4  85 = 26.6 Wks
==================================| BASIC BABY  (c) |==================================
Probable Sex F   BPD/FOD =0.78                   Fetal Heart = 171 B/M
    HistoG  Calc    WEEK +/-SD
BPD   =(B)= 67 mm.= 26.5  0.0          SUMMARY:     AVE.WKS RANGE n   SD    MIN  MAX
THC   =(T)=239 mm.= 26.7  0.2          ALL AGE   (A) 26.5    1.3  8  0.5   25.7 27.0
CHC   =(C)=188 mm.= 27.0  0.4          BRAIN AGE(b) 26.7    0.5  5  0.2   26.5 27.0
CV    =(V)=168 cc.= 26.9  0.3          BODY AGE     26.0    1.0  3 -0.3   25.7 26.7
TriCD=(>)= 67 mm.= 26.6  0.1             (b)=EDC (MM DD)= 4  8 (40 LMP WKS.Term)
HumL =(H)= 44 mm.= 25.8 -0.5                SHEPARD.WT.(Ba)  =  950 Gm.+- 190 Gm.
FemL =(F)= 47 mm.= 25.7 -0.6                HADLOCK.WT.(Fa)  =  911 Gm.+- 182 Gm.
AC   =(a)=218 mm.= 26.7  0.1                HADLOCK.WT.(TFa) =  898 Gm.+- 135 Gm.

                                                     B
                                                     >
                                                     TC
                                                    FHaV
M=A=b=(@)___________________________________|  |     @    |  |_______________________
MENSTRUAL WKS> 1   1   1   1   1   2   2   2    2↑  2   3   3   3   3   3   4   4
2  4   6   8   0   2   4   6   8   0   2   4    6↑  8   0   2   4   6   8   0   2
                                            ↑   MFP   ↑
                                            ↑    AA   ↑
__________________________________________-2SD______+2SD____________________________
```

A

```
EXAM DATE:   11  7  84                          EXAM# = 1  By: TD   BB#: 207
PT:                                             AGE:     PT.#
DR.:                                            LMP = (M) =  5  3  84 = 26.9 Wks
==================================| BASIC BABY  (c) |==================================
Probable Sex F   BPD/FOD =0.78                   Fetal Heart = 152 B/M
    HistoG  Calc    WEEK +/-SD         SUMMARY:     AVE.WKS RANGE n   SD    MIN  MAX
BPD   =(B)= 69 mm.= 27.2  0.1          ALL AGE   (A) 27.1    3.7  7  1.4   25.0 28.7
THC   =(T)=248 mm.= 27.7  0.4          BRAIN AGE(b) 28.0    1.5  4  0.7   27.2 28.7
CHC   =(C)=199 mm.= 28.7  1.2          BODY AGE     25.9    2.8  3 -0.9   25.0 27.8
CV    =(V)=195 cc.= 28.4  0.9            (b)=EDC (MM DD)= 1  30 (40 LMP WKS.Term)
HumL =(H)= 42 mm.= 25.0 -1.6                SHEPARD.WT.(Ba)  =  909 Gm.+- 182 Gm.
FemL =(F)= 52 mm.= 27.8  0.5                HADLOCK.WT.(Fa)  =  918 Gm.+- 184 Gm.
AC   =(a)=203 mm.= 25.0 -1.6                HADLOCK.WT.(TFa) =  923 Gm.+- 138 Gm.

                                              H      C
LMP=ALL AGE=(*)______________________________a____BTFV_____________________________
____________________________________________|   |  * b   |_________________________
MENSTRUAL WKS> 1   1   1   1   1   2   2   2    2 ↑ 2    3   3   3   3   3   4   4
2  4   6   8   0   2   4   6   8   0   2   4    6 ↑ 8    0   2   4   6   8   0   2
                                            ↑    MFP     ↑
                                            ↑     AA     ↑
__________________________________________-2SD_______+2SD__________________________
```

B

FIGURE 7–15.

Computer screen printouts from the Basic Baby II software for two different fetuses in the last half of the 26th LNMP week. The top of each printout contains identifying patient information, most of which has been removed, except for the reported LMP date (M). Below the heading on the left of the screen are the various parameters used for the multiple fetal parameter average age (MFP AA). The characters in parentheses after the abbreviations for each parameter are the symbols used in the time-series histogram at the bottom of each screen. These symbolic characters are followed by the actual parameter measurement. Next is the age determined from the Basic Baby II look-up table (see Table 7–1) interpolated to the nearest 0.1 week, and after that are the ±SD locations of each parameter in the normal distribution. On the right side of the screen is the summary of the average ages. The all age (A) is the MFP AA, and brain age (b) is the average age of the cranial parameters, and the body age is the average of the FemL, HumL, and AC ages. The range is the difference of the maximum and minimum ages in each of the above averages (all, brain, and body); n is the number of parameters in each of the averages; the SD is the one-tailed SD for the ranges; and the min and max are the minimum and maximum of parameter ages used in each average. Across the bottom of the screens is the time-series symbolic histogram showing the relative location of each parameter in the distribution by its character (symbol). The numerals representing the menstrual weeks are stacked vertically; each character occupies one-half week (±0.25 week). Below the menstrual weeks, arrows have been added to locate the mean (MFP AA) and ±2 SD of the normal distribution (±10% age). In this case, the ±2 SD age range analysis is for all parameters; the brain range ±2 SD is approximately half the value.

A, A normal female fetus at 26.6 LNMP weeks; the MFP AA is 26.5 weeks. The LNMP = MFP AA = brain age (M = A = b = @) to within ±0.25 week. The vertical lines in the time series represent the approximate location of ±2 SD (outer lines) and ±1 SD (inner lines) with the mean (MFP AA = @) in the center. This fetus delivered at 39.8 LMP weeks, weighed 3255 g (7.16 lb), and was 51 cm (20 in) long—a normal baby.

B, A female fetus with intrauterine growth restriction (IUGR). The LNMP is 26.9 weeks, the MFP AA (all age) is 27.1, the brain age is 28.0, and the body age is 25.9 average weeks. The MFP AA is within 0.25 week of the reported LNMP. The ARA symbolic histogram is bimodal, with a peak at 25.0 weeks (HumL = H and AC = a) and another peak at approximately 28.0 weeks. It is interesting that this is not classic asymmetrical IUGR because the FemL is relatively large whereas the AC and HumL are smaller. This fetus delivered at 40 LMP weeks weighing 2586 g (5.7 lb) and was 45.7 cm (18 in) long—a small baby.

HumL and AC ages are at −1.6 SD using the ARA Z formula. All other parameters were within ±1 SD of the MFP AA. Notice how easy it is to assess visually the location of the HumL and AC ages ("H" and "a" in the symbolic histogram) in a normal distribution, just inside the −2 SD marker. This histogram is actually bimodal—that is, it has two peaks. This fetus was delivered by cesarean section at 40.0 weeks by both LNMP and MFP AA. The birth weight was 2586 g (5.7 lb), and the length was 45.7 cm (18 in). Both weight and length were less than normal, and the weight was well below the third percentile for a 40-week delivery according to Hadlock and colleagues' standard. However, at the time of the examination (27 weeks), the FemL was actually at + 0.5 SD. This examination was in 1984, before the use of Doppler.

This case (see Fig. 7–15*B*) points out the complexity of fetal size and age assessment. One or two parameters or even four may not give a complete picture. Although none of the parameters measured could be considered abnormal because all were within ±2 SD, it must be remembered that a single study does not show growth. Growth analysis requires two or more studies. IUGR tends to be progressive, and if the AC is approaching −2 SD in the second trimester, then that AC age may be below −2 SD near term. This is not a hard-and-fast rule, because other processes may affect the AC by causing liver enlargement (see A Tale of Two Babies, later, for another complex example of this problem including liver enlargement).

Using quality control statistics to study various numbers of parameters in groups, it was found that at any given fetal age, one can expect smaller ranges of ages as fewer numbers of parameters are used to determine the MFP AA and ranges.[112] In the previous formula, 0.05 is the rounded Z function from Table 7–13. A factor of 0.05 is a conservative estimate of ±1 SD and has been tested to work for as many as 11 parameters. Table 7–13 shows the Z factors when using various numbers of parameters. These factors can be used if more accuracy is required; however, the more conservative Z factor of 0.05 is recommended and is easier to calculate. The 95th percentile for the range for MFPs in this table is 15% of the average age, or approximately ±7.5% (not including the GSD). This is similar to Hadlock and others' findings, in which the variability of the CRL, THC, and FemL was found to be ±8% of the predicted age.[4–7] I have chosen to use ±10% of the predicted age because it is conservative (approximately ±3 SD),

TABLE 7–13. **AGE RANGE ANALYSIS Z FACTOR TABLE**

NUMBER OF PARAMETERS IN CASES	AVERAGE AGE PER NUMBER OF MFPs	MEDIAN AGE PER NUMBER OF MFPs	RANGE UPPER LIMIT FACTOR AS % OF ESTIMATED AGE (95th PERCENTILE)	VARIABILITY AS % OF ESTIMATED AGE (± 2 SD)	ARA FORMULA Z FACTOR (± 1 SD)
2	7.5	7.3	11%	6%	0.03
3	9.2	8.6	16%	8%	0.04
4	11.8	9.7	14%	7%	0.04
5	20.3	12.4	14%	7%	0.04
11	13.1	13.0	—	—	—
10	14.4	14.9	13%	7%	0.03
6	20.9	19.6	16%	8%	0.04
8	23.2	21.9	15%	8%	0.04
9	26.2	26.7	15%	8%	0.04
7	26.4	28.8	16%	8%	0.04
Mean range upper limit factor			15%	8%	0.04
Conservative ARA upper limit factor			20%	10%	0.05

The age range analysis (ARA) upper limits for range and Z formula factors. The values were calculated using all parameters except the gestational sac diameter (GSD). The first column shows the number of parameters measured in the case groups used to calculate the upper limit factors. The second and third columns show the average age and median ages for each group. The table is sorted in descending order according to the median ages. The fourth column shows the ARA (range) upper limit factors as a percentage of the age; these are the maximum age ranges for a normal population. The fifth column is the normal distribution (± 2 SD) of age range as a percentage of the age. The last column lists the Z factors that are used in the ARA Z formula to predict the relative proportions of parameters. The row for 11 parameters included the GSD and has no factor for the group of 11 fetal parameters because the GSD is not a fetal parameter and was excluded.

It should be noted that the group of 10 parameters has the smallest range upper limit factor, 13%. This is the reverse of the conventional wisdom that more parameters should result in increasing ranges. However, in the case of fetal sonography, the only cases in which 10 parameters were measured included the crown-rump lengths as well as all other parameters. This means that all the cases that include 10 parameters were early in pregnancy, when individualization of proportions has the least effect on the range. Earlier in gestation, the range for larger numbers of parameter ages is smaller than it is later in pregnancy, even though fewer parameters may be used later.

gives the advantage to the fetus, and is easy to calculate. Similarly, I recommend a clinical application of 0.20 × age as a conservative indicator for the maximum age range as a test for fetal disproportion.

The use of larger numbers of parameters in the MFP average gives more statistical power to the results. However, to be clinically practical, calculation of larger numbers of MFP ages makes the use of a computer advantageous owing to the time and error rates in the manual calculation of circumferential and volumetric equivalent ages.

Fetal size and age assessment is a complex issue and deserves more study. A single study does not suffice. True fetal growth analysis requires an early dating sonogram followed by a second for growth evaluation. All the fetal parameters available with all possible accuracy are necessary for a thorough evaluation. When any abnormalities are suspected, Doppler, close observation (biophysical profile), and follow-up studies to monitor growth are advised. Computers must come into common use for these complex analyses.

We have found that if as many as 11 fetal parameters are used for the ARA, the residual range will be just less than ±10% of the MFP AA (including the GSD, which is not a true fetal parameter). This way of thinking about parameter sizes is what led our group to develop the ARA Z formula for locations in the normal distribution.

The greatest strength of the ARA method is its ability to compare a single fetus in serial growth studies or to compare one fetus with its sibling(s) in multiple gestations. The following are discussions of serial studies of two fetuses (not twins) that were small for dates late in gestation. Discussed next is a set of twins with a slightly different growth pattern. Although it seems that no two pregnancies follow exactly the same pattern of growth, within limits that are compatible with life, it is hoped that these case studies provide some concept of the ARA method of growth comparison.

A Tale of Two Babies

They are the best of babies, they were worrisome as fetuses, they were the same, they were different, there were abundant data, there weren't enough data, the data were precise, the data were confusing—in short, the fetuses were like all fetuses except that they were not growing as rapidly as expected. Thus, for the present period, before birth, the data had to be accepted, for good or for evil, in the superlative degree of comparison only.

We shall call these two fetuses Dos and Tres because two studies are used to evaluate Dos and three for Tres. (Tres actually had eight examinations, but only three are considered here. The mother worked in a nuclear medicine department throughout her pregnancy and was concerned.) Both women were primiparous, one at 27 years old (Dos) and one at 32 (Tres); in good health; and without complications at the first examination. Dos had examinations at 23.3 and 38.3 LNMP weeks. Tres had examinations at 9.6, 20.4, and 37.9 LNMP weeks. At the initial examination of Dos, there was only 0.8 week's difference between the LNMP of 23.3 weeks and the MFP AA of 22.5 weeks (< 5 days or 3.0% of the LNMP). For the initial examination of Tres, the difference was only 0.5 week between the LNMP of 9.6 and 9.1 AA weeks (< 4 days, 5.2% of the LNMP). Both of these AA discrepancies are small and well within acceptable limits (±2 SD) for comparison with the reported LNMP, and it is believed that the mothers' menstrual histories were accurate.

Figure 7–16 shows two symbolic time-series histograms for Dos; the time series at the top is from the first examination. This type of graphic representation of fetal analysis was discussed earlier. Each symbol (character) represents the age of an individual parameter in a histogram. Using ARA with the LNMP as the comparative variable, the MFP AA was trailing by only −0.8 SD at 23.3 LNMP weeks. By 38.3 LNMP weeks, however, the MFP AA for Dos was at −2.3 SD, or −4.4 weeks less than the LNMP. In addition, this last examination found low-normal amniotic fluid quantities and reduced, sluggish fetal motions. The FHR was reactive, and the biophysical profile score was 6. High-resistance flow was found in the umbilical artery and aorta, and low resistance was found in the middle cerebral artery. Figure 7–17 shows the ratios for these Doppler findings (see Chapters 13 and 16 for more discussion of fetal Doppler). Dos appeared to be in trou-

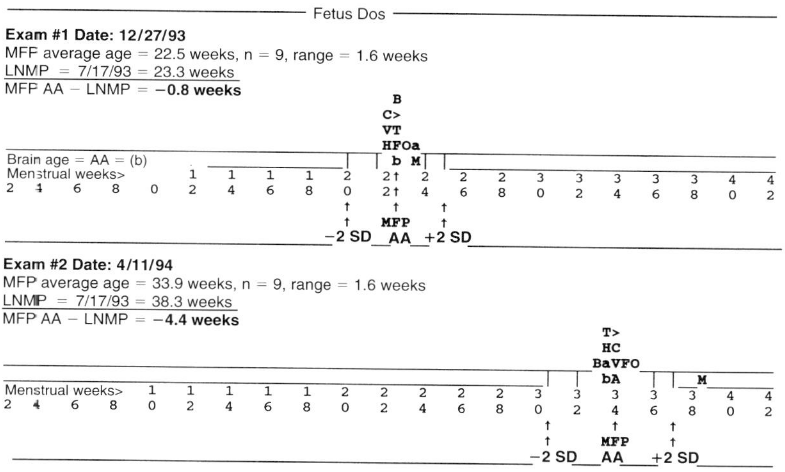

FIGURE 7–16.
Two time-series symbolic histograms for fetus Dos. The top time series is from the first examination (23.3 LNMP weeks), and the bottom one is from the last examination (38.3 LNMP weeks). Notice that in the first examination, the brain age (b) is equal to the MFP AA, and they both trail the LNMP age (M) by 0.8 week. By the second examination, the LNMP age is 38.3 weeks and both the brain age (b) and MFP AA (A) are trailing by more than 4 weeks. This progressive lagging of the fetal parameter ages is typical of intrauterine growth restriction. At the second examination, the fetus scored a six on the biophysical profile and exhibited mild oligohydramnios.

ble; however, a confounding issue was that the AC was only −0.2 SD below the MFP AA by the ARA Z formula and the AC/THC ratio was in a normal range for age (AC/THC = 290/296 = 0.98). It is possible that in some cases of IUGR, other processes may cause enlargement of the liver, thereby producing what would appear to be a normal abdomen-to-head ratio. Figure 7–18 shows the complete Basic Baby II analysis for the last examination for fetus Dos.

Delivery of Dos was induced 5 days after the last sonographic examination, and a 2045-g (4 lb, 8 oz) boy, 45 cm (17 ¾ in) long, was delivered. He was hypoglycemic. Hypoglycemia has been observed in IUGR owing to uteroplacental vascular insufficiency.[113]

Fetus Tres exhibited normal growth until after midpregnancy. Figure 7–19 shows three time-series histograms for Tres. The top histogram is the earliest examination shown. Notice the very tall, narrow (leptokurtic) bell curve for this 9.6-week symbolic histogram. Most of the symbols form a single vertical stack of characters at the mean of this narrow distribution. This is a common shape of the symbolic bell curve in the normal first trimester. In this distribution, the symbolic

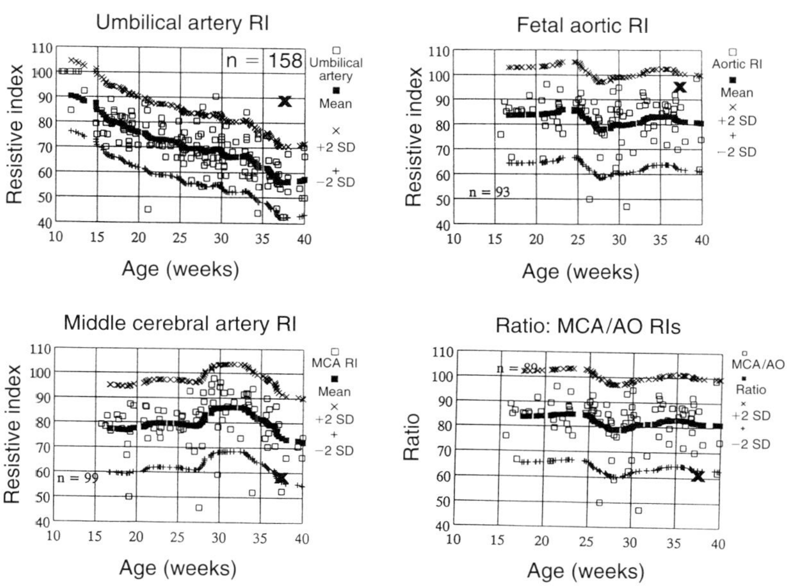

FIGURE 7–17.
Doppler analysis for fetus Dos. The resistive indexes (RIs) for an umbilical artery, two fetal arteries, and a ratio of two RIs taken at the second examination (38.3 LNMP weeks) of fetus Dos. The umbilical artery RI (X) was high at 0.87. The aortic (AO) RI was also somewhat high at 0.95, and the middle cerebral artery (MCA) RI was low at 0.58. The MCA/AO ratio was also low at 0.61. The high AO RI and low MCA RI are indicative of intrauterine growth restriction with uteroplacental vascular insufficiency (high umbilical artery RI).

```
EXAM DATE:   4  11  94                          EXAM# = 2  By: PM    BB#: 348
PT: FETUS DOS                                   AGE: 27    PT.#
DR.:                                            LNMP = (M) =  7  17  93 = 38.3 Wks
==================================| BASIC BABY  (c) |==================================
Probable Sex ?   BPD/FOD =0.78          Fetal Heart = 126 B/M
COMMENTS: FUNDAL LT SIDE PLACENTA CEPHALIC PRESENTATION
    HistoG  Calc    WEEK +/-SD         SUMMARY:      AVE.WKS RANGE n   SD      MIN  MAX
BPD   =(B)= 82 mm.= 32.9 -0.6          ALL AGE   (A) 33.9     1.9  9  0.6     32.9 34.8
THC   =(T)=296 mm.= 33.3 -0.3          BRAIN AGE(b)  33.7     1.3  5 -0.1     32.9 34.2
CHC   =(C)=231 mm.= 34.1  0.1          BODY AGE      33.8     0.8  3 -0.0     33.5 34.3
CV    =(V)=316 cc.= 34.1  0.2            (b)=EDC (MM DD)= 5   24 (40 LMP WKS.Term)
TriCD=(>)= 85 mm.= 34.2  0.2               SHEPARD.WT.(Ba)   =  2092 Gm.+- 418 Gm.
BiOcD=(O)= 55 mm.= 34.8  0.5               HADLOCK.WT.(Fa)   =  2256 Gm.+- 451 Gm.
HumL =(H)= 58 mm.= 33.5 -0.2               HADLOCK.WT.(TFa)  =  2217 Gm.+- 333 Gm.
FemL =(F)= 67 mm.= 34.3  0.3
AC    =(a)=290 mm.= 33.5 -0.2       AMNIOTIC FLUID=LOW NORMAL.
                                    PLACENTAL GRADE = 3               T>
                                    UMB.VESSELS = 3 parts.            HC
                                                                      BaVFO
______________________________________________________________| |   bA   | |__M_______
MENSTRUAL WKS> 1   1   1   1   1   2   2   2   2   2   3   3   3   3   3   4   4
2  4   6   8   0   2   4   6   8   0   2   4   6   8   0   2   4   6   8   0   2
```

FIGURE 7–18. A Basic Baby II computer printout for the final examination of fetus Dos (see Fig. 7–15 for an explanation of the parts of the screen). The ±SD locations are relative to the mean MFP AA and not relative to the LNMP. Notice that the LNMP (M), which is the true fetal age, is outside the +2 SD for the range of MFPs at this time. Also, the fetus appears normally proportioned, with all parameter ages within ±1 SD of the MFP AA. The foregoing Doppler study suggests head-sparing intrauterine growth restriction; however, the parameter sizes do not conform to this definition.

characters nearest the mean are in a single vertical column and are within ±0.25 of a week of the MFP AA. The two symbols (G and E) under the tails of the bell curve are within ±0.5 of a week of the mean.

By 20.4 LNMP weeks, Tres's MFP AA was 20.6 weeks or actually 0.2 week ahead of the LNMP. This would indicate approximately 0.7 week more growth than anticipated based on the first examination. By the last examination, at 37.9 LNMP weeks, the MFP AA (n = nine parameters) for Tres was only 35.9 weeks or 2.0 weeks' less growth than expected (−1.06 SD). This reduced growth was 5.2% of the LNMP, which is half of the 10% threshold proscribed as the limit of normal in the earlier Z formula. This is believed to represent a normal fetus that was small for gestational age.[113] Figure 7–20 shows the complete Basic Baby II biometric analysis for the last examination for fetus Tres.[2]

In September 1994, on a flight home from the Society of Diagnostic Medical Sonographers' annual conference, I sat next to a young mother and her infant. I had a three-ring binder containing sonographic images

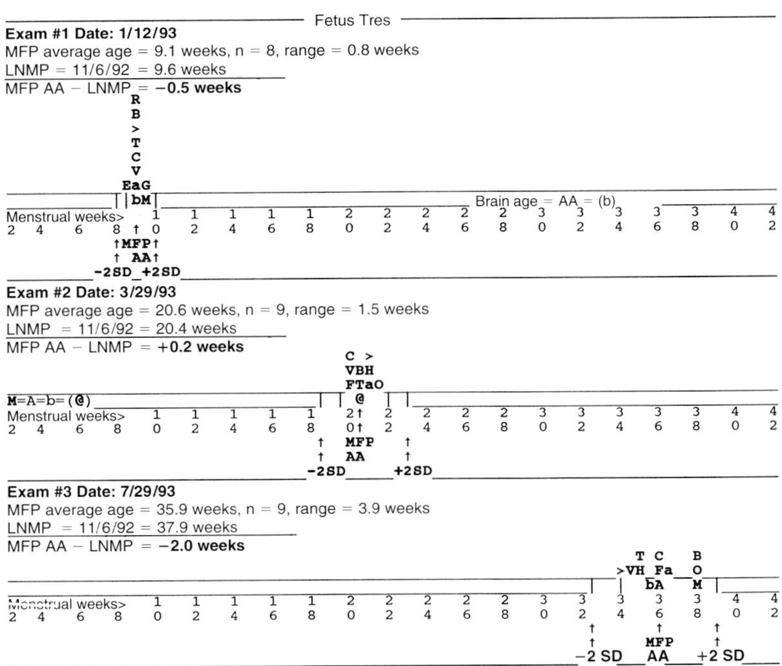

FIGURE 7–19. These three time-series histograms for fetus Tres are similar to the two shown for Dos in Figure 7–16. The earliest examination shown is at the top, and the last is at the bottom. The first examination exhibits very close correlation with most parameter symbols stacked above and near (−0.5 week) the LNMP (M). The second examination shows more dispersion of the parameters, but the MFP AA and brain age are still equal to the LNMP age (M = A = b = @). In the final examination, the parameters are even more dispersed but are still within the ±2 SD markers (vertical lines). The fetal parameter ages are now trailing the LNMP age, but not by more than 2 SD.

```
EXAM DATE:    7   29   93                         EXAM# = 8   By: TD    BB#: 233
PT: FETUS TRES                                    AGE: 33    PT.#ARA
DR.:                                              LNMP = (M) =   11   6   92 = 37.9 Wks
════════════════════════════════════════╡ BASIC BABY   (c) ╞════════════════════════════
Probable Sex ?   BPD/FOD =0.91              Fetal Heart = 135 B/M     & chambers = 4
    HistoG  Calc    WEEK +/-SD
BPD   =(B)= 93 mm.= 38.1  1.3          SUMMARY:     AVE.WKS RANGE n    SD     MIN  MAX
THC   =(T)=306 mm.= 35.0 -0.5          ALL AGE   (A) 35.9     3.9  9  1.1     34.2 38.1
CHC   =(C)=240 mm.= 35.8 -0.0          BRAIN AGE(b) 35.5      3.9  5 -0.2     34.2 38.1
CV    =(V)=321 cc.= 34.4 -0.8          BODY AGE      35.8     1.6  3 -0.0     35.0 36.6
TriCD=(>)= 85 mm.= 34.2 -0.9             (b)=EDC (MM DD)= 8   29 (40 LMP WKS.Term)
BiOcD=(O)= 59 mm.= 37.9  1.1                SHEPARD.WT.(Ba)   =  3175 Gm.+- 635 Gm.
HumL  =(H)= 61 mm.= 35.0 -0.5               HADLOCK.WT.(Fa)   =  3050 Gm.+- 610 Gm.
FemL  =(F)= 71 mm.= 35.8 -0.0               HADLOCK.WT.(TFa)  =  2924 Gm.+- 439 Gm.
AC    =(a)=331 mm.= 36.6  0.4
                         AMNIOTIC FLUID=NORMAL.
                         PLACENTAL GRADE = 3
                         UMB.VESSELS = 3 parts.                          T C   B
_________________________________________________________________>VH_Fa__O_______
______________________________________________________________|  |  bA   M |_______
MENSTRUAL WKS> 1    1    1    1    1    2    2    2    2    2    3    3    3    3    3    4    4
2   4    6    8    0    2    4    6    8    0    2    4    6    8    0    2    4    6    8    0    2
```

FIGURE 7–20. The final full Basic Baby II printout for fetus Tres at 37.9 LNMP weeks. All parameters are within ±1.3 SD of the MFP AA, and most trail the LNMP by less than −2 SD. The BPD (B) leads the MFP AA; thus, brachycephaly is suggested (TCI = 0.91). The TriCD (>) age trails the MFP AA by −0.9 SD; thus, some degree of platycephaly is suggested. This is a common configuration of head molding near term. Tres delivered as small for gestational age but otherwise normal and healthy.

and a chapter manuscript that I was editing for this book. After a while, the mother tapped my arm and said, "I know you. You did the sonograms of my boy." With some discussion, I realized that this was fetus Dos, about whom we had been concerned. He was just over 2 months old, small, but with no outward signs of disease.

Fetus Tres is now just over 1 year old and is also doing very well. His birth (8/9/93) was at 39.4 weeks after the LNMP (11/6/92). He weighed 3125 g (6 lb, 14 oz) and was 50.8 cm (20 in) long. His Apgar scores were 8 and 9, and labor lasted 3 hours.

It is hoped that this tale of Dos and Tres will help the reader with the thought process that is involved in fetal growth analysis. It is not always simple. This comparison process is similar for multiple gestations, which are briefly discussed later.

Radar Chart

Another interesting way of looking at fetal proportionality is the radar plot or chart. Figure 7–21 shows radar plots for fetuses Dos and Tres. These charts were plotted with Excel (MicroSoft Corp.). I do not find it as easy to observe relative parameter proportions with the radar chart as with the time-series symbolic histograms, but some may find these useful.

In these radar charts, each parameter is plotted along one radius, and lines connect the various parameters from the same examination. The corresponding LNMP for each examination was plotted on every radius and forms a regular polygon of 11 sides (undecagon), almost a perfect circle. For both fetuses, the examinations near 20 weeks have parameter age radar plots (PA1 for Dos and PA2 for Tres), which are near or superimposed on the LNMP plots (LNMP 1 and LNMP 2, respectively). The parameters for Dos at term (PA2), however, are obviously inside (smaller than) the undecagonal plot of LNMP 2 (Fig. 7–21*A*).

Fetus Tres near term, on the other hand, has parameter ages (PA3) that are much closer to the LNMP plot (LNMP 3). The BPD actually exceeds the LNMP slightly, and the outer binocular distance is approximately equal to it. Compare these radar charts with the previous symbolic time-series histogram and see which gives you a better feel for the fetal parameter proportionality.

Multiple Gestations

In cases of multiple gestations, not only does the process of comparison involve time-series growth studies, but the fetuses are also compared with one another. Although the fetuses often exhibit growth discrepancies, the discrepancies between the fetuses should not increase by very much as pregnancy progresses. The analysis of growth for multiple gestation is very similar to that for singletons, but there are more parameters to measure by a factor of the number of fetuses. The pres-

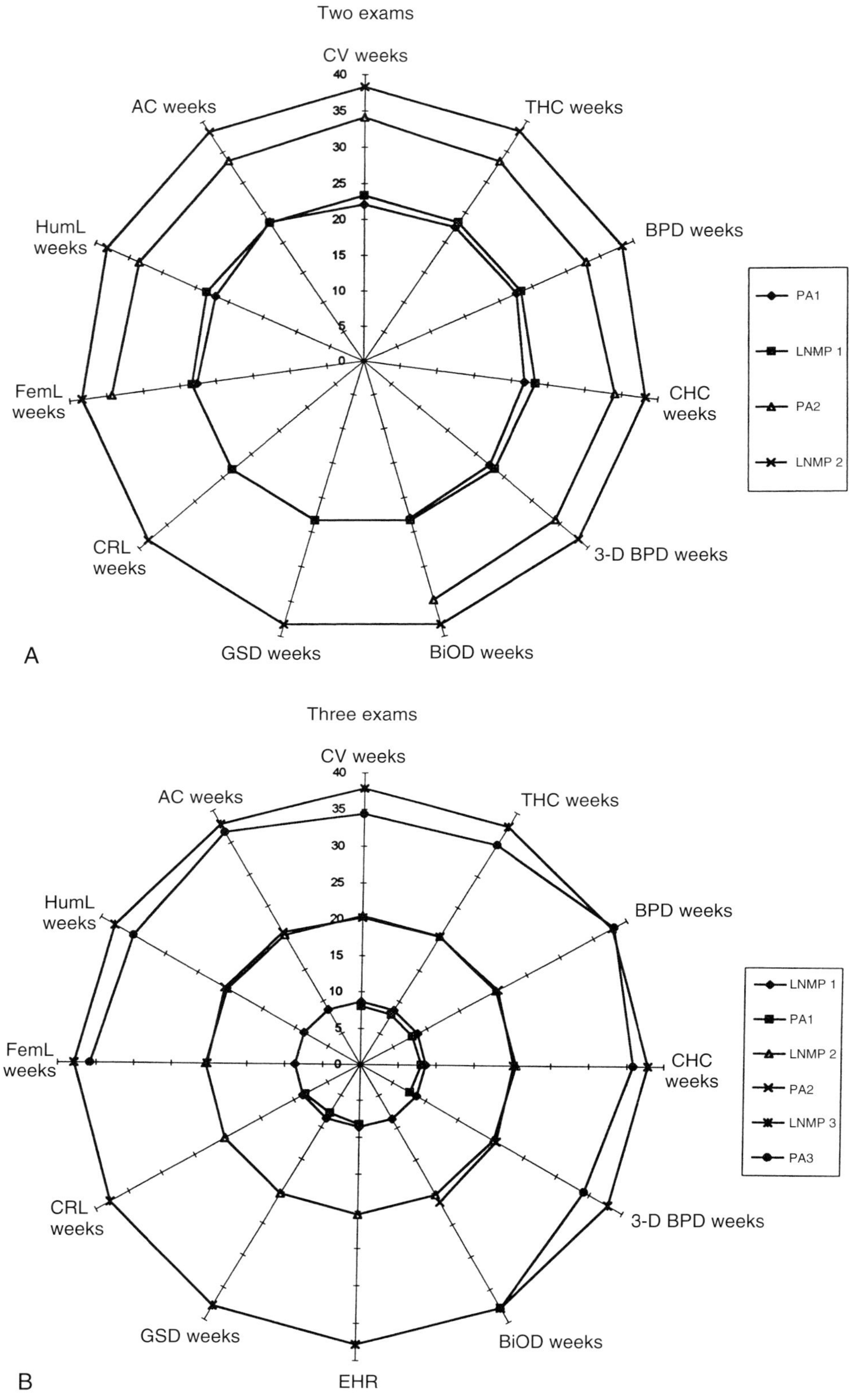

FIGURE 7–21.
These two graphics are for the two examinations from fetus Dos and the three examinations from fetus Tres. A radar plot has each parameter age plotted (PAn) along one arm or radius of the 360 degrees. In these, the LNMP ages are plotted (LNMPn) on every radius for easy comparison. The LNMP plots form a regular polygon with 11 sides (undecagon). The number (n) after the PA and LNMP represents the examination being plotted. The reader is encouraged to compare these radar plots with Figures 7–16 and 7–19, which show the same information, respectively. Note how all the parameter plots (PA2) are inside the LNMP 2 plots for fetus Dos.

ence of a membrane and its thickness are important factors, as is whether there is one or more placentas. Amniotic fluid quantities and the umbilical cord should also be evaluated (see Chapter 16 for more discussion). The following is a discussion of an interesting case to give the reader some idea of multiple gestation analysis.

Twin fetuses had a 1-week discrepancy in both the CRL and EHR ages at the very early first examination (5.9 LNMP weeks). Let's refer to these embryos as A and B. The larger, embryo A, was 10 mm long (CRL), which evaluated to 7.1 LMP weeks. The EHR was 134 beats/minute by M-mode, which evaluated to 6.6 weeks. The CRL for embryo B was 6 mm, which evaluated to 6.4 LMP weeks, and the EHR was 117 beats/minute, or 5.9 weeks. These MFP AAs placed the two fetuses at 1.2 and 0.5 weeks in advance of the LNMP age, respectively. These two twins remained approximately 1 week apart in growth until an examination at 27.9 weeks, which found a 2-week discrepancy.

Because of our concern for possible twin-to-twin transfusion and our acute interest in fetal growth, the supervising physician offered free follow-up examinations. Four were performed before a spontaneous delivery at 34 LNMP weeks.

The second examination, at 9.6 LNMP weeks, found fetus A to be 1.1 week in advance of the LNMP age, whereas B was only 0.3 week ahead. The second MFP AA was established on the basis of six parameter measurements. By the third examination, at 16.6 LNMP weeks, A was 1.8 week ahead and B was 1.1 week ahead of the LNMP age. The third-examination ages were based on the MFP AA for 10 parameters. The twins were actually slightly larger than we would have expected at that time.

The fourth sonographic examination was at 23.6 LNMP weeks. Fetus A measured 25.8 weeks by MFP AA, or 2.2 weeks in advance of the LNMP age. Fetus B was 24.8 weeks by MFP AA, or 1.2 week ahead of the LNMP age.

Sonographic examinations by a high-risk perinatal center found results similar to ours for these twins at 10 and 15.9 LNMP weeks. By 27.9 LNMP weeks, there was 2 weeks' discrepant growth, and at 34.3 LNMP weeks, there was approximately 4 weeks' discrepant growth. The smaller twin, B, remained an appropriate size for LNMP age throughout gestation, whereas twin A exhibited advancing growth during the last half of the pregnancy. This increasing discrepancy in size may be evidence of some degree of twin-to-twin transfusion, although the case does not fit the classic scenario of severe twin transfusion syndrome.[114]

Except for the size discrepancy, the twins appeared perfectly normal at all sonographic examinations. The mother gave us permission to obtain her medical records for the birth and follow-up. Twin A weighed 2700 g and had Apgar scores of 8 and 9. Twin B weighed 1955 g and had Apgar scores of 7 and 9. These weights are at the extremes of normal for the 34th week, according to Hadlock and colleagues' weight standards (see Table 7–11).

Pathology did report a "roughly discoid twin placenta which is approximately 25 × 20 × 4 cm and which has attached glistening gray-pink fetal membranes which are fused in the center of the fetal surface to form a thin, translucent partition." There were "vascular channels from side 'A' across the membranous partition onto the fetal surface of side 'B'." It is also noteworthy that the umbilical cords were quite different. Umbilical cord A was inserted 5.5 cm from the nearest placental margin and was twice the diameter of cord B. Cord B had a velamentous insertion at the other side of the placenta. The pathology report concluded, "third trimester diamniotic, monochorionic twin placenta with attached trivascular umbilical cords (two)."

The mother informed us that the smaller twin had some respiratory illness during the first 6 months, but the larger, twin A, had no problems. Both were faring well at their first birthday.

Some interesting questions are posed by this case. How early does twin-to-twin transfusion syndrome affect an embryo? Is it possible that the early 1-week growth discrepancy was due to a difference in implantation times? Could the progressively increasing discrepancies in the last half of the pregnancy be due to some degree of transfusion? The fact that the twins were identical and monochorionic would be evidence against different implantation times.

Clearly we have much to learn about human development. Sonography offers a far better way of studying this topic than we have ever had.

ACKNOWLEDGMENT

I want to particularly thank G. G. Mezaraups, M.D.; R. N. Snider, M.D.; L. Johnson, Ph.D.; Frederick Haynes, M.S.Stat.; L. W. Hill, M.D.; D. H. Nichols, M.D.; E. K. Poole, M.D.; Linda Porter, R.D.M.S., R.V.T; and the rest of the Austin Radiological Association sonographic staff for their questions, discussion, and tolerance and for using the ARA method.

REFERENCES

1. DuBose TJ, Poole E, Butschek C, et al: Range of multiple fetal parameters. Official Proceedings: 1988 World Federation for Ultrasound in Medicine and Biology. J Ultrasound Med 1988;7:S205–206.
2. DuBose TJ: Basic Baby II: Obstetrical Software (BBII). Mind's Eye Imaging, 811 West 31st Street, Austin, TX 78705-2109, copyright 1986–1994.
3. DuBose TJ: Assessment of fetal age and size: Techniques and criteria. In: Berman MC, ed: Diagnostic Medical Sonography: A Guide to Clinical Practice. JB Lippincott, Philadelphia, 1991, pp 280–281.
4. Hadlock FP, Shah YP, Kanon DJ, et al: Fetal crown-rump length: Reevaluation of relation to menstrual age (5–18 weeks) with high-resolution real-time US. Radiology 1992;182:501–505.
5. Vintzileos AM, Neckles S, Campbell WA, et al: Fetal liver ultrasound measurements in isoimmunized pregnancies. Obstet Gynecol 1986;68:162–167.
6. Goldberg BB, Kurtz AB: Atlas of Ultrasound Measurements. Year Book Medical Publishers, Chicago, 1990, p 326.
7. Callen PW: Ultrasound in Obstetrics and Gynecology, 3rd ed. WB Saunders, Philadelphia, 1993, p 719.
8. Hadlock FP, Deter RL, Harrist RB, et al: Computer-assisted analysis of fetal age in the third trimester using multiple growth parameters. J Clin Ultrasound 1983;11:313–316.
9. Hadlock FP, Deter RL, Harrist RB, et al: Estimating fetal age: Computer-assisted analysis of multiple fetal growth parameters. Radiology 1984;152:497–501.
10. Robinson HP, Flemming JEE: A critical evaluation of sonar crown-rump length measurements. Br J Obstet Gynaecol 1975;82:702–710.
11. Durkan JP, Russo GL: Ultrasonic fetal cephalometry: Accuracy, limitations, and applications. Obstet Gynecol 1966;27:399–403.
12. Hellman LF, Kobayashi M, Fillisti L, et al: Growth and development of the human fetus prior to the 20th week of gestation. Am J Obstet Gynecol 1969;103:784–800.
13. Phillips JF, Goodwin DW, Thomason SB, et al: The volume of the uterus in normal and abnormal pregnancy. J Clin Ultrasound 1976;5:107–110.
14. Kurtz AB, Goldberg BB: Gestational sac. In: Kurtz AB, Goldberg BB, eds: Obstetrical Measurements in Ultrasound: A Reference Manual. Year Book Medical Publishers, Chicago, 1988, p 3.
15. Kurtz AB, Goldberg BB: Uterine measurements. In: Kurtz AB, Goldberg BB, eds: Obstetrical Measurements in Ultrasound: A Reference Manual. Year Book Medical Publishers, Chicago, 1988, pp 181–182.
16. Gairdner D: Ultrasonic fetal cephalometry. Br Med J 1972;3:585.
17. Hadlock FP, Deter RL, Carpenter RJ, et al: Estimating fetal age: Effect of head shape on the BPD. AJR 1981;137:83–85.
18. Deter RL, Harrist RB, Hadlock FP, et al: Fetal head and abdominal circumferences: I. Evaluation of measurement errors. J Clin Ultrasound 1982;10:357–363.
19. Queenan JT, O'Brien GD, Campbell S: Ultrasound measurement of fetal limb bones. Am J Obstet Gynecol 1980;138:297–302.
20. O'Brien GD, Queenan JT, Campbell S: Assessment of gestational age in the second trimester by real-time ultrasound measurement of the femur length. Am J Obstet Gynecol 1981;139:540–545.
21. Jeanty P, Cantraine F, Cousaert E, et al: The binocular distance: A new way to estimate fetal age. J Ultrasound Med 1982;3:241–243.
22. McLeary RD, Kuhns LR, Barr M: Ultrasonography of the fetal cerebellum. Radiology 1984;151:439–442.
23. Lawson TL, Foley WD, Berland LL, et al: Ultrasonic evaluation of fetal kidneys: Analysis of normal size and frequency of visualization as related to stage of pregnancy. Radiology 1981;138:153–156.
24. Vintzileos AM, Campbell WA, Storlazzi E, et al: Fetal liver ultrasound measurements in isoimmunized pregnancies. Obstet Gynecol 1985;66:477–480.
25. Mercer BM, Sklar S, Shariatmadar A, et al: Fetal foot length as a predictor of gestational age. Am J Obstet Gynecol 1987;156:350–355.
26. Jeanty P, Rodesch F, Delbeke D, et al: Estimation of gestational age from measurements of fetal long bones. J Ultrasound Med 1984;3:76–77.
27. Benacerraf BR, Frigoletto FD, Laboda LA: Sonographic diagnosis of Down syndrome in the second trimester. Am J Obstet Gynecol 1985;153:49–52.
28. Vintzileos AM, Neckles S, Campbell WA, et al: Ultrasound fetal thigh-calf circumferences and gestational age-independent fetal ratios in normal pregnancy. J Ultrasound Med 1985;4:287–292.
29. Jeanty P, Romero R, Hobbins JC: Fetal limb volume: A new parameter to assess fetal growth and nutrition. J Ultrasound Med 1985;4:273–282.
30. Yarkoni S, Schmidt W, Jeanty P, et al: Clavicular measurement: A new biometric parameter for fetal evaluation. J Ultrasound Med 1985;4:467–470.
31. Otto C, Platt LD: The fetal mandible measurement: An objective determination of fetal jaw size. Ultrasound Obstet Gynecol 1991;1:12–17.
32. Altman DG, Chitty LS: Design and analysis of studies to derive charts of fetal size: Opinion. Ultrasound Obstet Gynecol 1993;3:378–384.
33. Cunningham FG, MacDonald PC, Gant NF, eds: Williams Obstetrics, 18th ed. Appleton & Lange, Norwalk, CT, 1989, p 7.
34. Speroff L, Glass RH, Kase NG: Clinical Gynecologic Endocrinology and Infertility, 3rd ed. Williams & Wilkins, Baltimore, 1983, pp 231–232, 285–287.
35. Clewell WH: Control of uterine circulation. In: Friedman EA, Noah ML, Work BA, eds: Uterine

Physiology: Proceedings of a Brook Lodge Workshop. PSG Publishing, Littleton, MA, 1979, pp 33–51.
36. Markee JE: Rhythmic uterine vascular changes. Am J Physiol 1932;100:32.
37. Resnik R: The endocrine regulation of uterine blood flow in the nonpregnant uterus: A review. Am J Obstet Gynecol 1981;140:151–156.
38. Markee JE: Menstruation in intra-ocular endometrial transplants in the rhesus monkey. Embryology 1940; 28:221.
39. Lantta M, Karkkainen J, Lehtovirta P: Progesterone and estradiol receptors in the cytosol of the human uterine artery. Am J Obstet Gynecol 1983;147:627–633.
40. Willson JR, Carringron ER, Ledger WJ: Obstetrics and Gynecology. CV Mosby, St Louis, 1983, pp 68–69.
41. DuBose TJ, Hill LW, Cunyus JA, et al: Sonography of menstrual changes in arcuate uterine blood vessel diameters. J Cardiovasc Ultrasonogr 1985;4: 243–251.
42. Waldroup LW: Sonographic anatomy of the female pelvis. In: Berman MC, ed: Diagnostic Medical Sonography: Obstetrics and Gynecology, vol I. JB Lippincott, Philadelphia, 1991, p 54.
43. Eastman NJ, Hellman LM, eds: Williams Obstetrics, 12th ed. Appleton-Century-Crofts, New York, 1961, pp 221–224.
44. Cunningham FG, MacDonald PC, Gant NF, eds: Williams Obstetrics, 18th ed. Appleton & Lange, Norwalk, CT, 1989, p 258.
45. McClure BG, Dornan JC: Fetal lung maturation. Fetal Med Rev 1989;1:223–234.
46. Wisser J, Drischedl P, Krone S: Estimation of gestational age by transvaginal sonographic measurement of greatest embryonic length in dated human embryos. Ultrasound Obstet Gynecol 1994;4: 457–462.
47. MacGregor SN, Tamura RK, Sabbagha RE, et al: Underestimation of gestational age by conventional crown-rump length dating curves. Obstet Gynecol 1987;70:344–348.
48. Peisner DB, Timor-Tritsch IE: The discriminatory zone of b-hCG for vaginal probes. J Clin Ultrasound 1990;18:280–285.
49. Sabbagha RE: Ultrasound: Applied to Obstetrics and Gynecology, 2nd ed. JB Lippincott, Philadelphia, 1987, p 470.
50. Shapiro BS, Escobar M, Makuch R, et al: A model-based prediction for transvaginal ultrasonographic identification of early intrauterine pregnancy. Am J Obstet Gynecol 1992;166:1495–1500.
51 van Heeswijk M, Nijhuis JG, Hollanders HMG: Fetal heart rate in early pregnancy. Early Hum Dev 1990;22:151–156.
52. Howe RS, Isaacson KJ, Albert JL, et al: Embryonic heart rate in human pregnancy. J Ultrasound Med 1991;10:367–371.
53. May DA, Sturtevant NV: Embryonal heart rate as a predictor of pregnancy outcome: A prospective analysis. J Ultrasound Med 1991;10:591–593.
54. Benacerraf BR: Ultrasound evaluation of the fetal face. In: Callen PW, ed: Ultrasound in Obstetrics and Gynecology, 3rd ed. WB Saunders, Philadelphia, 1993, pp 239–241.
55. Benirschke K: Incidence, etiology, and inheritance. In: Creasy RK, Resnik R, eds: Maternal-Fetal Medicine: Principles and Practice, 2nd ed. WB Saunders, Philadelphia, 1989, p 565.
56. Glass RH, Golbus MS: Habitual abortion. In: Creasy RK, Resnik R, eds: Maternal-Fetal Medicine: Principles and Practice, 2nd ed. WB Saunders, Philadelphia, 1989, p 437.
57. Hadlock FP, Deter RL, Harrist RB, et al: Fetal abdominal circumference as a predictor of menstrual age. AJR 1982;139:367–370.
58. Cleveland WS: The Elements of Graphing Data. Wadsworth Advanced Books and Software, Monterey, CA, 1985, pp 167–178.
59. Rossavik IK, Deter RL: Mathematical modeling of fetal growth: I. Basic principles. J Clin Ultrasound 1984;12:529–533.
60. Rossavik IK, Deter RL: Mathematical modeling of fetal growth: II. Head cube (A), abdominal cube (B) and their ratio (A/B). J Clin Ultrasound 1984;12: 535–545.
61. Rossavik IK, Hadlock FP: Variation in second trimester fetal growth and sonographic determination of gestational age (letter). J Ultrasound Med 1992;11:251–252.
62. Hadlock FP, Deter RL, Harrist RB, et al: Fetal head circumference: Relation to menstrual age. AJR 1992;138:649–653.
63. Jandel Scientific: Tablecurve v3.10. Jandel Scientific, 2591 Kerner Boulevard, San Rafael, CA 94901.
64. EXCEL, version 5.0; MicroSoft Corporation, PO Box 3021, Bothell, WA 98041-3021, 1993.
65. Rossavik IK, Fishburne JI: Conceptional age, menstrual age, and ultrasound age: A second-trimester comparison of pregnancies of known conception date with pregnancies dated from the last menstrual period. Obstet Gynecol 1989;73:243.
66. Bovicelli L, Orsins LF, Rizzo N, et al: Estimation of gestational age during the first trimester by real-time measurement of the fetal crown-rump length and biparietal diameter. J Clin Ultrasound 1981;9: 71–75.
67. Ott WJ: Accurate gestational dating. Obstet Gynecol 1985;66:311.
68. Nazari A, Check JH, Epstein RH, et al: Relationship of small-for-dates sac size to crown-rump length and spontaneous abortion in patients with a known date of ovulation. Obstet Gynecol 1991;78:369–373.
69. Filly RA: Ultrasound evaluation during the first trimester. In: Callen PW, ed: Ultrasound in Obstetrics and Gynecology, 3rd ed. WB Saunders, Philadelphia, 1993, pp 64–83.
70. Nyberg DA, Mack LA, Laing FC, et al: Distinguishing normal from abnormal gestation sac growth in early pregnancy. J Ultrasound Med 1987;6:23–27.
71. Nyberg DA, Filly RA, Filho DLD, et al: Abnormal pregnancy: Early diagnosis by ultrasound and serum chorionic gonadotropin levels. Radiology 1986;158:393–396.
72. Sabbagha RE, Cohen LS, Karins ML, et al: Early pregnancy evaluation. In: Sabbagha RE, ed: Diagnostic Ultrasound Applied to Obstetrics and Gynecology, 3rd ed. JB Lippincott, Philadelphia, 1994, p 596.
73. Filly RA: Ultrasound evaluation during the first trimester. In: Callen PW, ed: Ultrasound in Obstetrics and Gynecology, 3rd ed. WB Saunders, Philadelphia, 1993, p 89.
74. Nyberg DA, Hill LM: Normal early intrauterine pregnancy: Sonographic development and hCG correlation. In: Nyberg DA, Hill LM, Bohm-Velez M, et al, eds: Transvaginal Ultrasound. Mosby/Year Book, St Louis, 1992, pp 80–82.
75. Schats R: Transvaginal Sonography in Early Human

Pregnancy. Ter Verkriging van der Graad van Doctor, aan de Erasmus Universiteit Rotterdam, 1991, p 69.
76. Schats R, Jansen CAM, Wladimiroff JW: Embryonic heart activity: Appearance and development in early human pregnancy. Br J Obstet Gynaecol 1990;97:989–994.
77. Fine C, Cartier M, Doubilet P: Fetal heart rates: Values throughout gestation. Abstract 1569, Official Proceeding: 1988 World Federation for Ultrasound in Medicine and Biology. J Ultrasound Med 1988;7:S105–S106.
78. DuBose TJ, Dickey D, Butschek CM, et al: Letter to the editor. J Ultrasound Med 1988;7:237–238.
79. DuBose TJ, Porter L, Dickey D, et al: Fetal gestational days ± (fetal heart rate × 0.3) − 7. Official Proceedings, Society of Diagnostic Medical Sonographers, Boston, MA, 1989.
80. DuBose TJ, Porter L, Dickey D, et al: Sonographic correlation of fetal heart rate and gender. J Diagn Med Sonogr 1989;2:49–53.
81. DuBose TJ, Cunyus JA, Johnson L: Embryonic heart rate and age. J Diagn Med Sonogr 1990;6:151–157.
82. Kurtz AB, Wapner RJ, Kurtz RJ, et al: Analysis of biparietal diameter as an accurate indicator of gestational age. J Clin Ultrasound 1980;8:319–326.
83. Kurtz AB, Goldberg BB: Fetal head measurements. In: Kurtz AB, Goldberg BB, eds: Obstetrical Measurements in Ultrasound: A Reference Manual. Year Book Medical Publishers, Chicago, 1988, p 28.
84. DuBose TJ: Fetal biometry: Vertical calvarial diameter and calvarial volume. J Diagn Med Sonogr 1985;1:205–217.
85. DuBose TJ: 3D BPD correction. J Ultrasound Med 1988;7:S97.
86. Berman MC, ed: Winners of the 1986 Kenneth Gottesfeld Awards. J Diagn Med Sonogr 1986;2:182.
87. Goldberg BB, Kurtz AB: Atlas of Ultrasound Measurements. Year Book Medical Publishers, Chicago, 1990, p 278.
88. DuBose TJ: Assessment of fetal age and size: Techniques and criteria. In: Berman MC, ed: Obstetrics and Gynecology: Diagnostic Medical Sonography, A Guide to Clinical Practice, vol 1. JB Lippincott, Philadelphia, 1991, pp 279–289.
89. Goldstein RB, Filly RA, Simpson G: Pitfalls in femur length measurements. J Ultrasound Med 1987;6:203–207.
90. Winraub Z, Schneider D, Langer R, et al: Ultrasonographic measurement of fetal growth parameters for estimation of gestational age and fetal weight. Isr J Med Sci 1979;15:829–832.
91. Hoffbauer H, Pachaley J, Arabrin B, et al: Control of fetal development with multiple body measures. Contrib Gynecol Obstet 1979;6:147–156.
92. Kurtz AB, Goldberg BB: Fetal body measurements. In: Kurtz AB, Goldberg BB, eds: Obstetrical Measurements in Ultrasound: A Reference Manual. Year Book Medical Publishers, Chicago, 1988, pp 64–76.
93. Williamson MR, Williamson SL: Gamuts in Ultrasound. WB Saunders, Philadelphia, 1992, p 139.
94. Warsof SL, Gohari P, Berkowitz RL, et al: The estimation of fetal weight by computer-assisted analysis. Am J Obstet Gynecol 1977;128:881–892.
95. Shepard MJ, Richards VA, Berkowitz RL, et al: An evaluation of two equations for predicting fetal weight by ultrasound. Am J Obstet Gynecol 1982;147:47–54.
96. Li DFH, Woo JSK: Fractional spine length: A new parameter for assessing fetal growth. J Ultrasound Med 1986;5:379–383.
97. Sokal RR, Rohlf FJ: Biometry: The Principles and Practice of Statistics in Biological Research, 2nd ed. WH Freeman & Co, New York, 1981, pp 17–19.
98. Hair JF, Anderson RE, Tatham RL, et al: Multivariate Data Analysis with Readings, 3rd ed. Macmillan, New York, 1992, pp 2–16.
99. Kurtz AB, Goldberg BB: Combined fetal head and body measurements. In: Kurtz AB, Goldberg BB, eds: Obstetrical Measurements in Ultrasound: A Reference Manual. Year Book Medical Publishers, Chicago, 1988, p 146.
100. Erratum: Fetal weight error correction: Am J Obstet Gynecol 1982;143:485.
101. DuBose TJ: Fetal weight error perpetuated. Am J Obstet Gynecol 1990;162:876.
102. FrameWork IV integrated software, copyright 1991; Ashton-Tate Corporation, 6411 Guadalupe Mines Road, San Jose, CA 95120.
103. Hadlock FP, Harrist RB, Carpenter RJ, et al: Sonographic estimation of fetal weight. Radiology 1984;150:535–540.
104. Ferrero A, Maggi E, Giancotti A, et al: Regression formula for estimation of fetal weight with use of abdominal circumference and femur length: A prospective study. J Ultrasound Med 1994;13:823–833.
105. Fazekas I, Kosa F: Forensic fetal osteology. Heyden, Philadelphia, 1978, p 256.
106. Jordaan HVF: Estimation of fetal weight by ultrasound. J Clin Ultrasound 1983;11:59–66.
107. Hadlock FP, Harrist RB, Martinez-Poyer J: In utero analysis of fetal growth: A sonographic weight standard. Radiology 1991;181:129–133.
108. Render B, Stair RM: Quantitative Analysis for Management. Allyn & Bacon, Boston, 1994, pp 85–94.
109. Sokal RR, Rohlf FJ: Biometry: The Principles and Practice of Statistics in Biological Research, 2nd ed. WH Freeman & Co, New York, 1981, p 49.
110. Jeanty P, Rodesch F, Delbeke D, et al: Estimation of gestational age from measurements of fetal long bones. J Ultrasound Med 1984;3:75–79.
111. Sokal RR, Rohlf FJ: Biometry: The Principles and Practice of Statistics in Biological Research, 2nd ed. WH Freeman & Co, New York, 1981, p 583.
112. Lindgren BW: Statistical Theory, 3rd ed. Macmillan, New York, 1976, p 579.
113. Fay RA, Ellwood DA: Categories of intrauterine growth retardation. Fetal Maternal Med Rev 1993;5:203–212.
114. Fineberg HJ: Ultrasound evaluation in multiple gestation. In: Callen PW, ed: Ultrasound in Obstetrics and Gynecology, 3rd ed. WB Saunders, Philadelphia, 1993, pp 115–117.
115. Campbell S, Thomas A: Ultrasound measurement of the fetal head to abdomen circumference in assessment of growth retardation. Br J Obstet Gynaecol 1977;84:164–174.

CHAPTER 8

CRANIAL BIOMETRY

Terry J. DuBose

The fetal cranium is a three-dimensional (3-D) structure with an ellipsoidal (egg) shape.[1-5] The top of the cranium or calvarium normally has relatively smooth contours, whereas the base of the brain and calvarium lies in an irregular plane. These irregularities of the base are due to the four fossae—the frontal, occipital, and bilateral temporal—and their interposed divisions, which are formed by four bony structures, the bilateral anterior sphenoid wings and the posterior petrous ridges or pyramids (see Chapter 9, Fig. 9–6).

It has been acknowledged for more than 10 years that a transverse circumference of the fetal head is a more accurate sonographic measure of head and brain size than is a single diameter because of variations in shape and molding.[6] Figure 8–1 illustrates the sonographic acquisition of the standard transverse head circumference (THC) for a normally positioned fetus in a cephalic presentation.

Little attention has been given to the fact that the head can be molded in the vertical cranial diameter (VCD) as well as in the two diameters of the transverse plane, the biparietal diameter (BPD) and fronto-occipital diameter (FOD). Indeed, one of the primary purposes of the discussion in this chapter is to prove not only that the head molds in the vertical axis but that the VCD is the most dynamic diameter and the most sensitive to these changes in skull shape.

Figures 8–2 and 8–3 illustrate the 3-D nature of the human cranium. The first published description of the sonographic measurement of the VCD and the estimation of the growth of the 3-D volume of the fetal head was in 1985.[1] This research was recognized by the Society of Diagnostic Medical Sonographers, who honored it with the Gottesfeld Award in 1986.[2]

While I was preparing this manuscript, the artist pointed out that the VCD is not a new measurement but is only being revisited with sonographic methods. In actuality, Leonardo da Vinci described a similar dimension in 1489 (Fig. 8–2*A*).[7] On seeing this illustration, I asked the artist if she could draw a head in the da Vinci style but from a slightly different angle to show the sonographic measurements we were describing. She replied, "Knock off a da Vinci? Of course, everyone does it!" Figure 8–2*B* is the result. This drawing shows the basic measurements that are discussed in this chapter.

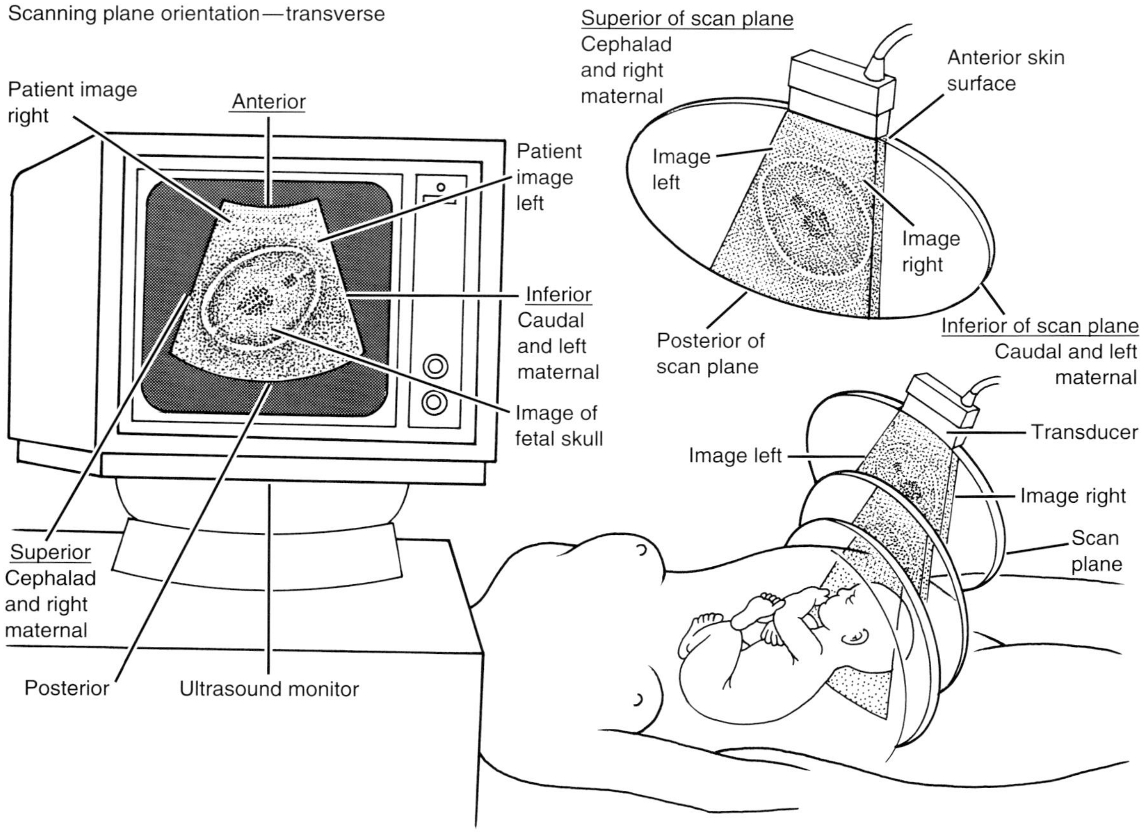

FIGURE 8–1.
Orientation of a normally positioned patient and sonographic monitor imaging the transverse head circumference. Note that the patient's right side is displayed on the left side of the monitor. Also, if the transducer were rotated 90 degrees to obtain the coronal head circumference, the woman's head would be toward the monitor's left and her feet would be toward the monitor's right.

Linear Geometry of the Fetal Cranium

LINEAR

Biparietal Diameter

Introduction to the Biparietal Diameter

The BPD is generally thought of as the shortest diameter of the ellipse of the THC[6,8–14]; however, this concept is very simplistic because it considers the BPD as if it only exists in flatland.[15] The BPD really resides in sphereland[16] or, more appropriately, in flat and curved space-time.[17] This latter way of looking at fetal morphology allows discussion of the fourth dimension of cranial solid geometry, the change in its measurements, shape, and volume across time.

The BPD of the fetal skull is a straight line that normally passes transversely through the middle of the thalamus, but it is much more than that. The BPD is the diameter of the fetal skull coronal circle. The BPD is equal to the average of the three diameters of the fetal calvaria. The BPD is the longest diameter that is perpendicular to the cerebral interhemispheric fissure. The BPD is also the widest dimension above the fetal ears. It is many things in the sonographic geometry of the fetal skull (see Figs. 8–2 and 8–3).

This chapter makes observations on the solid geometry of the fetal skull and its growth. The reader, whether novice or expert sonographer, should gain some degree of confidence about measurement of the BPD and other fetal head parameters.

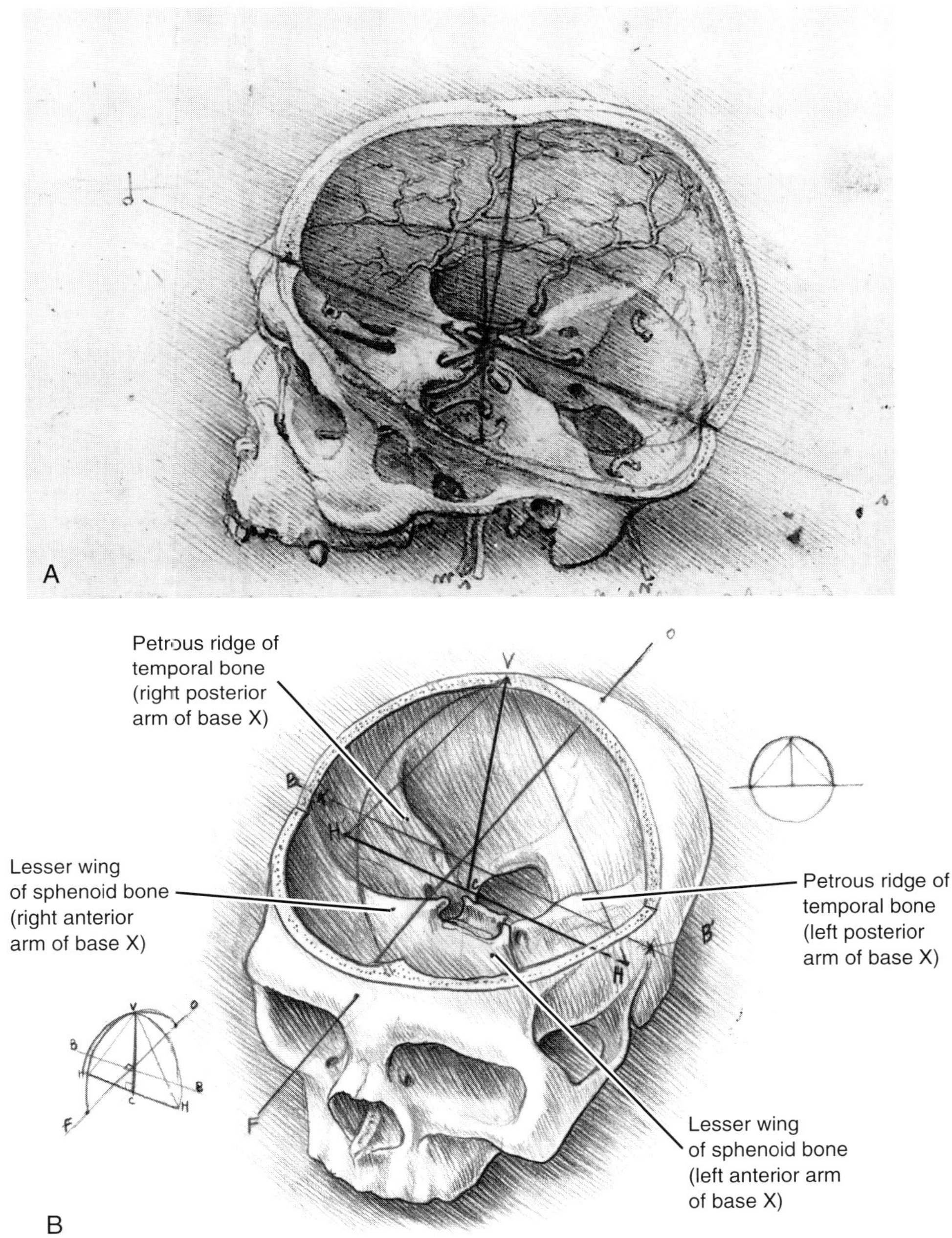

FIGURE 8–2.
Three-dimensional drawings of the interior of the human skull. *A*, This drawing by Leonardo da Vinci in 1489 demonstrates that there is nothing new under the sun. Leonardo had envisioned the vertical cranial diameter (VCD) well before it was illustrated sonographically in 1985. (From da Vinci L: The skull: Interior view. In: Leonardo da Vinci: The Anatomy of Man. Drawings from the Collection of Her Majesty Queen Elizabeth II, Windsor Castle, Royal Library; published by Museum of Fine Arts, Houston; Bullfinch Press of Little, Brown & Co, Boston, 1992, p 36.) *B*, Adaptation by Victoria Vescovo Alderman showing the relative locations of the various measurements discussed in this chapter. B–B′, biparietal diameter; F–O, fronto-occipital diameter; H–H, triangle base; H–V, two triangle sides; VC, vertical cranial diameter or height of triangle.

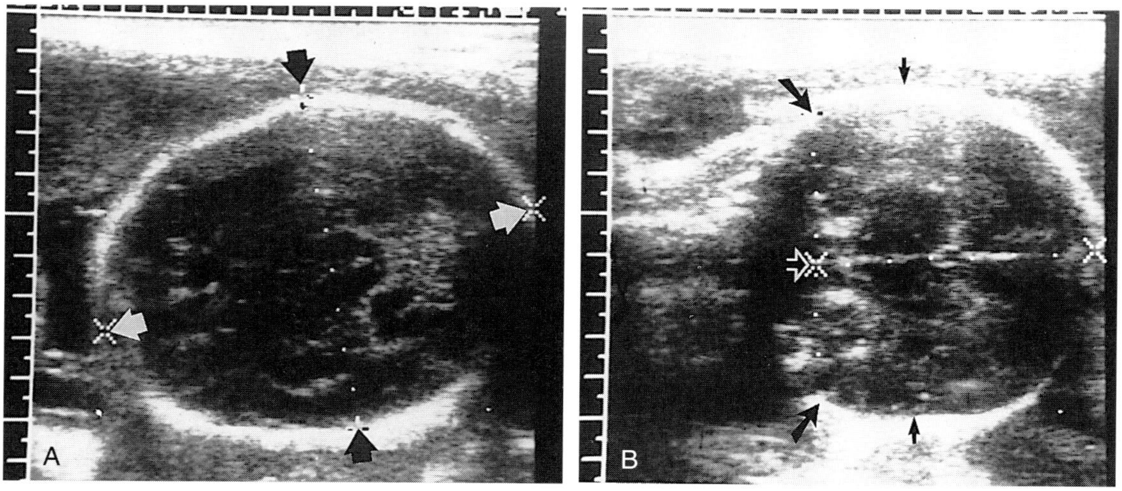

FIGURE 8–3.
Transverse and coronal head circumferences from the same normal fetus. *A*, This view of the fetal head is the most common. The thalamus is at the center of the head, with the dotted line of the biparietal diameter (BPD) (black arrows) passing through it. The BPD is measured leading edge to leading edge by the + cursors as 83 mm. The fronto-occipital diameter (white arrows) is measured midedge to midedge by the X cursors as 104 mm. The transverse cephalic index is normal at 0.80. *B*, The coronal view showing the coronal triangle measurement and the vertical cranial diameter (65 mm) between the X cursors (X at cranial vertex and X at center of the hippocampal base line [HBL], open arrow). The HBL (73 mm) is the dotted line between the diagonal black arrows and lies in the plane of the base X. The sides of the coronal triangle are between each end of the HBL and the vertex. A valid BPD can be measured between the small black arrows. Note the circular shape of the skull in this view. (LNMP = 31.7, AA = 32.5, multiple fetal parameter n = 8, range = 2.6 weeks, DKD)

Linear Geometry of the Transverse Fetal Skull

The first sonographic measurement of the fetal skull was the BPD.[8,18] The BPD is undoubtedly the most sonographically measured parameter of the human fetus, for good reasons. This measurement is shown as a line of dots between the two + cursors in Figure 8–3*A*. In this figure, it can be observed that the BPD is perpendicular to the interhemispheric fissure (midline), passes through the middle of the thalamus, and is the widest transverse diameter. It can also be observed that the BPD is usually not midway between the extents of the frontal and occipital bones. The BPD usually is slightly closer to the occipital bone at the posterior of the head because the human head is normally slightly wider toward the back.

The BPD is a highly accurate measurement to obtain. It has geometric features that make it easy to measure routinely. However, fetal skull molding causes variation in the length of the BPD. This variation in the BPD can be manifested as an increase in the length of the BPD (brachycephalic) or a decrease in length (dolichocephalic). This sounds contradictory, as many medical issues do. How can the BPD have high accuracy as a measurement and also exhibit large variation? Let us think about this dilemma.

First we address the measurement accuracy issue. If one takes several sonographic measurements of the same fetal BPD during the same examination or if different observers take measurements during the same examination, relatively consistent measurements are obtained.

Figure 8–3*A* shows the standard, or historically documented, head circumference. This is also the plane most commonly used to take BPD measurements. The head circumference is referred to as the THC throughout this text because the coronal head circumference (CHC), as well as a few other circumferences, is also discussed from time to time.

One reason for this interoperator accuracy is that the BPD is usually measured using axial resolution on the leading sides of the parietal bones (Fig. 8–4). This has been referred to as the leading-edge to leading-edge or outer-

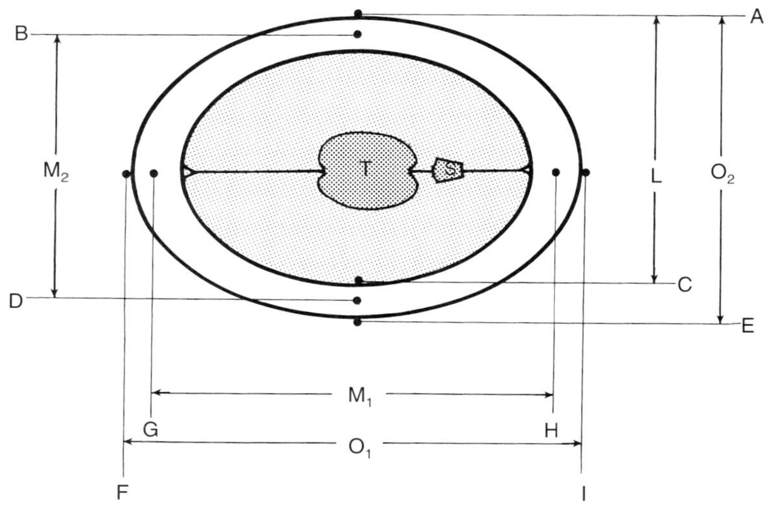

FIGURE 8–4.
Transverse head circumference. Various locations in which fetal skulls have been measured sonographically. O_1, outer-to-outer fronto-occipital diameter (FOD); M_1, mid-to-mid FOD; O_2 and M_2, outer-to-outer and mid-to-mid biparietal diameters (BPDs), respectively; L, leading-edge to leading-edge BPD; T, thalamus; S, cavum septi pellucidi. Algebraically, $O_2/O_1 = M_2/M_1$ and $L = M_2$; therefore, $O_2/O_1 = L/M_1$. Because the leading-edge to leading-edge BPD (L) is the most common and sonographically logical, it is recommended. Because the outer-to-outer FOD tends to be exaggerated owing to beam-width artifacts and because the mid-to-mid FOD (M_1) preserves the more normal BPD/FOD ratio, the M_1 measurement is recommended. If ellipse drawing tools are used, the ellipse AHCG or BHDG is recommended for the same reasons.

to-inner method.[19] The parietal bones are shallow cups or curved planes that form the sides of the fetal skull, with the concave sides of the cups facing each other. When the sonographic beam is relatively perpendicular to the parietal bones, these bones are strong reflectors of the sound waves. This strong reflection, along with the high resolution along the axial beam, results in the increased accuracy.

Another, less discussed, factor that affects the accuracy is the circular shape of the fetal skull in the midcoronal plane (see Figs. 8–2*B*, 8–3*B*, and 8–5). Because the normal fetal skull in this plane is usually a perfect circle, almost any diameter in the coronal plane is equal to the BPD. Figures 8–3*B* and 8–5 are coronal views of normal fetal skulls. Readers are cautioned not to confuse the sides of the triangle in Figures 8–2*B* and 8–5 with diameters. A diameter by definition must pass through the center of the circle. Observe how circular the perimeter of the skull is. The BPD was found to have a close correlation with the diameter of the circle that circumscribes the triangle, and no significant difference was found in the means at the 0.05 level (n = 300 random sample from 10,336, r = 0.993). In Figure 8–3*B*, the base of the triangle is the line between the + cursors and the height of the triangle is the midline between the X cursors (see also Fig. 8–5). How this coronal triangle is measured and how the diameter of the triangle circumference diameter (TriCD) is calculated are discussed later in the coronal plane section of this chapter.

Accepting for now that the coronal section of a normal skull is a circle, it can be easily observed in Figures 8–6 and 8–7 that the BPD lies in many potential planes. The BPD does not necessarily need to be perpendicular to the interhemispheric fissure (see Fig. 8–6). Figure 8–8*A* to *F* illustrates this fact. Because of the circular nature of the coronal view, it is possible to obtain very accurate BPD measurements from transverse head planes that are slightly oblique to the plane of the traditional THC. The only real requirements for an accurate BPD measurement are that it pass through the thalamus and be perpendicular to the long axis (FOD) of the skull, although it must be emphasized that planes that are perpendicular to the interhemispheric fissure make it easier to see the landmark anatomy

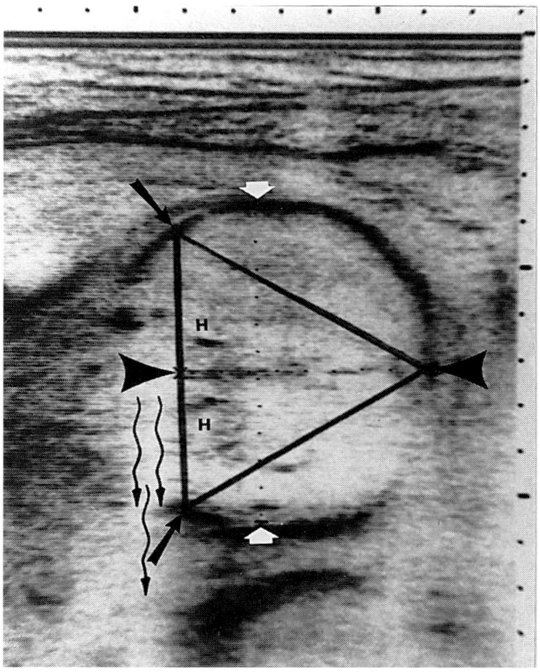

FIGURE 8–5.
Sonographic coronal view showing the circular nature of the coronal fetal skull. The vertical cranial diameter (between black arrowheads) is the height of the triangle. The base of the triangle (between diagonal black arrows), the hippocampal base line, is tangential to the bases of the bilateral circles of the hippocampal complexes (H) and the tops of the petrous ridges. The distal petrous ridge is obscured by the shadows (wavy arrows) from the proximal petrous ridge. A biparietal diameter (BPD) is measured between the white arrows. The circle that circumscribes the coronal triangle is equal to the BPD in normally shaped fetal heads. This is the image (black echoes on white background) on which the coronal triangle was first described in December 1983.

and help to ensure that the most accurate BPD measurement is being obtained. When the specular echoes from the midline fissure are seen, they help to confirm that the BPD is perpendicular to the FOD axis (see Figs. 8–3 and 8–8). The interhemispheric fissure is most easily seen with specular echoes. The strongest specular echoes are obtained from the fetal brain midline when the sonographic beam propagates perpendicularly or normal to the midline or midplane of the cerebral fissure.

Figure 8–8*A* to *F*, all from the same examination, show four different variations on the BPD measurement. The images demonstrate the fault-tolerant nature of the BPD. The mean of several BPD measurements in this case was 47.7 mm (measurement of record). In this case, all BPDs were less than 2% different from the BPD of record. The accepted tolerance for commercial sonographic machines using a large scale of view is an error of approximately 1.0% to 3.0%, or 1 to 3 mm per 100 mm.[20]

All of these reasons—the use of axial resolution, the strong specular reflections from the parietal bones, and the circular geometry of the coronal view—make the BPD a very accurate repeated measurement parameter during the same fetal examination.[21] However, what of the issue of BPD variability in a large population?

The BPD can be inaccurately exaggerated only if the measurement is taken obliquely to the FOD long axis, but the BPD can be inaccurately shortened in several ways. Erroneous shortening of the BPD is most often due to obtaining a plane of view that is not at the widest portion of the THC or coronal circle. This short BPD can be due to a plane of measurement that is too low in the cranium or, more often, too high (Fig. 8–9).

In Figure 8–9*A* and *B*, the transverse plane is too high in the fetal skull, and both a BPD and THC that are too small result. Also note that in both these images, the midline is almost continuous; in a THC through the thalamus, the midline is not continuous. In Figure 8–9*C* and *D*, the planes are too low in the skull. These images would also result in small BPDs and THCs. Note that in Figure 8–9*C*, a wing of the sphenoid bone (S) anteriorly and the top of the cerebellum (C) posteriorly can be seen. In Figure 8–9*D*, the plane is well into the cerebellum (C) and the pons of the brainstem (P) is seen.

It is common knowledge that the fetal skull does not normally complete its calcification until well after birth. The skull molds considerably during its passage through the birth canal. Indeed, a neonate's head has been called "plastic."[22,23] In general, the molding that normally takes place before passage through the birth canal is disregarded. Some research in the literature includes the sonographic study of fetal head molding, but not much.[3,6,23–25] One report that alludes to the possible effects of molding on the biometry of the fetal skull was by O'Keeffe and associates.[24] This research found that the head

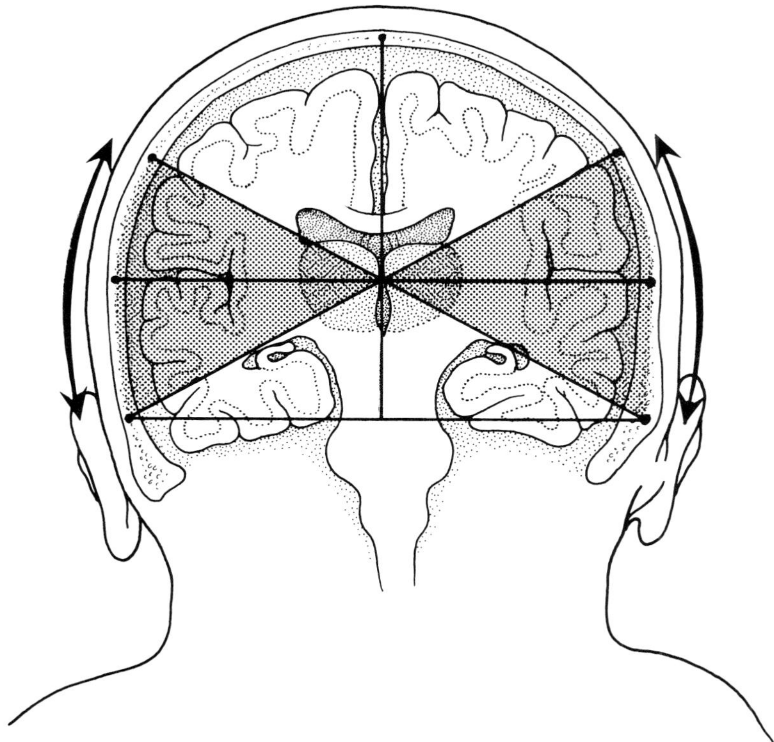

FIGURE 8–6.
This coronal drawing of a fetal head illustrates why the biparietal diameter (BPD) is such an accurate measurement. Any measurement that passes through the thalamus and lies between these two lines (planes on edge) is accurate. The circular nature of the coronal skull makes the BPD a fault-tolerant measurement.

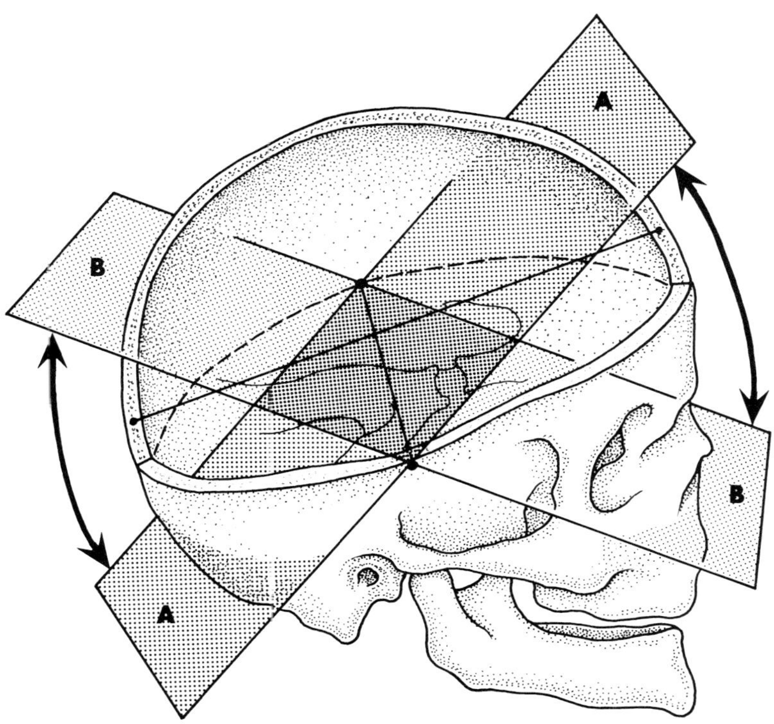

FIGURE 8–7.
A rendition of a fetal skull showing two possible planes from which a valid biparietal diameter (BPD) could be measured. An infinite number of planes from which a BPD can be measured exists between these planes. Plane A passes through the cerebellum and thalamus. Plane B passes through the orbits and thalamus. Not shown is the standard transverse plane of the head (THC), which would be approximately midway between planes A and B. The fronto-occipital diameter measurement is less fault tolerant than the BPD (see Figs. 8–8*A* to *F* and 8–10).

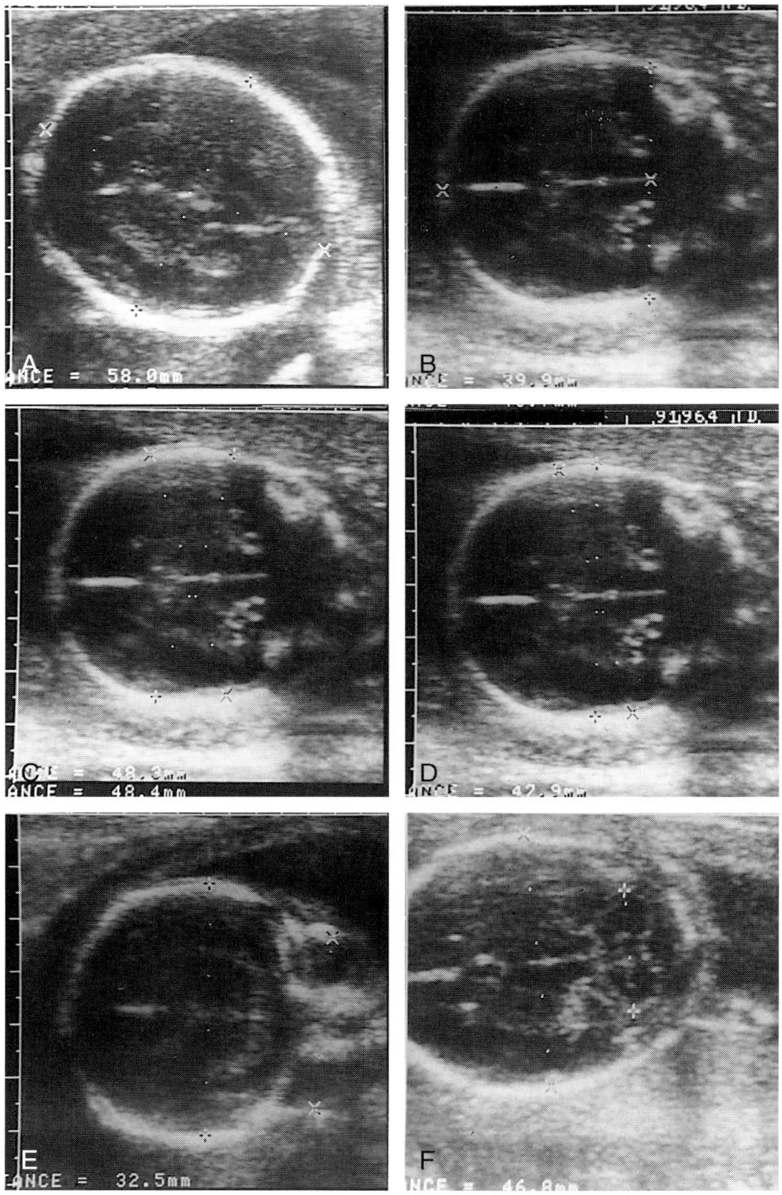

FIGURE 8–8.
These six sonograms all can yield biparietal diameter (BPD) measurements. The mean BPD measurement for the seven BPDs shown was 47.96 mm, with a range from 48.5 to 46.8, or 1.7 mm. The group average (BPD of record) had a mean of 47.7 mm. The BPD measurements in this case were within ±1.9% of the mean BPD of record, which is an acceptable tolerance. *A*, Standard transverse head circumference with fronto-occipital diameter (FOD) and BPD measurements (BPD = 48.5 mm). *B*, Coronal head circumference with vertical cranial diameter and hippocampal base line measurements. The same image is used in 8–8*C* and *D* for BPD measurements. *C*, Coronal head circumference with two diameter measurements that are approximately equal to the BPD (X = 48.3 mm, + = 48.4 mm). *D*, Same coronal view as in *B* and *C* . The true BPD (+ cursors) = 47.9 mm; the other coronal head diameter (X cursors = 47.9 mm) is exactly equal to the BPD. *E*, A view of the fetal head through the thalamus and orbits, demonstrating a BPD measurement (+ cursors = 47.9 mm). The outer binocular distance (X = 32.5 mm) is also measured. *F*, Another view through the lower thalamus and cerebellum. The BPD measurement here is the least (X cursor = 46.8 mm) because it is below the widest portion of the thalamus and skull and is not included in the averaging for the measurement of record. However, it is still less than 1 mm different (< 2%) from the BPD or record, which is acceptable according to most authors. The cerebellar width (+ cursors) is measured at 22.5 mm. (LNMP = 18.9 weeks, AA = 20.8 weeks, n = 9 parameters, range = 1.7 weeks, TD)

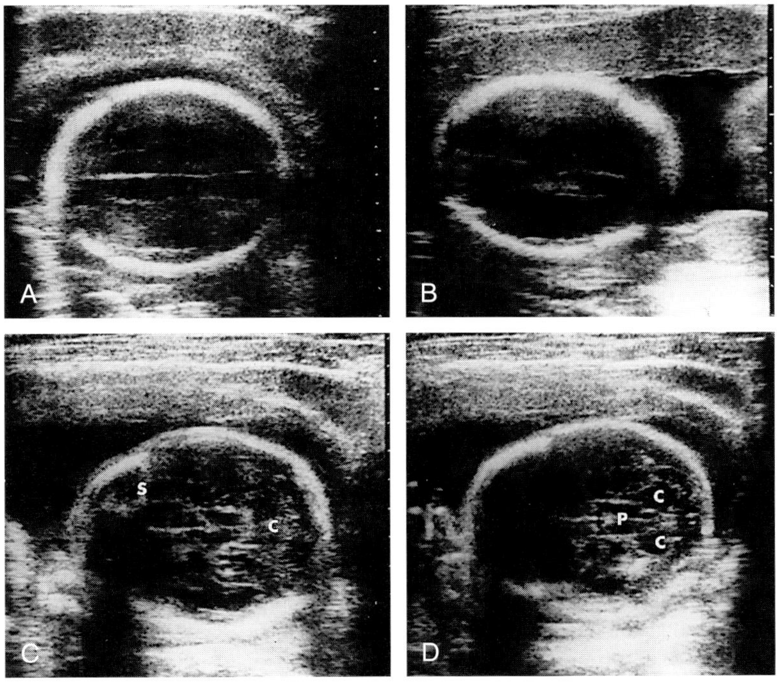

FIGURE 8–9.
These images demonstrate transverse planes that are too high or too low in the fetal cranium for valid biparietal diameter (BPD) measurements. *A*, This image is too high for an accurate BPD or fronto-occipital diameter (FOD) measurement; both would be underestimated. Note that the interhemispheric fissure is continuous from the front to the back of the skull. *B*, This transverse plane is also too high for accurate BPD and FOD measurements. Although it is lower than in *A*, it would also produce short measurements of the BPD and FOD. *C*, This transverse view is slightly too low for accurate BPD or FOD measurements. Note that the proximal sphenoid (S) is visible, as is the top of the cerebellum (C). *D*, This transverse plane is near the level of the base X of the sphenoid and petrous bones in the base of the skull. This plane is well into the cerebellar hemispheres (C) and below the thalamus. The tops of the petrous ridges can be seen as bright echoes on either side of the cerebellum. (LNMP = 24.9 weeks, AA = 25.9 weeks, n = 9, range = 2.7 weeks, TD)

molding resulting from oligohydramnios not only affected the accuracy of the BPD but also that in 55% of the cases the transverse cephalic index (TCI) was not able to predict head shape abnormalities. According to Goldberg and Kurtz, "It is possible that the fetal head had been misshapen by the oligohydramnios primarily in the craniocaudal dimension."[3]

This has been found to be true. If external bilateral pressure occurs along the axis of the BPD, the BPD is shortened. When this happens, another axis of the skull is exaggerated to compensate for the transverse compression. Most often, the axis that exaggeratedly compensates is the VCD rather than the FOD. The VCD has been found to be the most dynamic axis of the fetal skull (greatest variance). This skull molding and resulting effect on skull morphology are discussed in detail later in this chapter in the section on cranial volume.

Normal variation of the fetal skull shape and proportions must also be considered. Every person has, within limits, a unique appearance. Some have narrow, long heads; others have shorter, wider-shaped heads. Fetuses are no different. Some have dolichocephalic (long, narrow) head shapes, and others are brachycephalic (short, wide). These normal variations in head shape also increase the variation in the measurement of the BPD in a large population.

Because of small interoperator and intraoperator errors, the BPD is one of the easiest, best understood, and most accurate of fetal measurements that can be used if the head shape is normal. As pointed out earlier, however, the BPD has a relatively large variance in large populations. Hadlock has proved that the average age of multiple fetal parameter ages (MFP AA) is more accurate than any single fetal parameter used alone, especially the BPD, because of the shape/molding variation. This was confirmed in Chapter 7 when MFP ages were discussed.

Fronto-occipital Diameter

The long skull diameter, or front-to-back axis, is the least dynamic of the fetal cranial axes. This axis, the FOD, varies less than the BPD or the VCD (see the later section on 3-D cranial indexes for statistical analysis of these measurements).

The longest skull diameter (LSD)[14,26] has been referred to as the *occipitofrontal diameter*[11,27] and the FOD.[4,28,29] Although FOD has been used to refer to focus-object distance in radiological circles,[30-32] the acronym FOD seems to have more momentum and usage in the sonographic literature.

The FOD is best measured in the transverse head plane shown in Figures 8–3*A*, 8–4, and 8–8*A*. The FOD has been measured from both the mid-to-mid and outer-to-outer edges of the occipital and frontal bones. In an unpublished study of mid-to-mid and outer-to-outer measurements, the mid-to-mid measurements were found to be slightly more consistent (see Fig. 8–4). Hadlock hypothesized that the outer-to-outer measurements tended to add a bit of beam width.[6] This subject is discussed in more detail in the later section on the TCI. The FOD is most often measured in order to calculate the THC. I am not familiar with any fetal age tables or regressions calculated for the FOD alone.

The FOD can also be measured in the sagittal plane, but this plane is difficult to obtain in many cases, and the anatomical landmarks often are not well visualized (Fig. 8–10). For these reasons, it is recommended that the FOD measurement be taken from transverse planes in which the BPD may also be measured.

The FOD is the least dynamic of the fetal skull axes, but only slightly less. With fetal skull molding, it appears that most of the changes in morphology are in the coronal plane. The FOD is a relatively stable diameter, but its measurement is also affected by sonographic beam shape. The FOD is measured using lateral resolution in most cases. Because of beam width, lateral resolution produces more variation in measurements than axial resolution. The FOD is also more sensitive to slight variations in the plane of view or measurement. This is because the arcs of the frontal and occipital bones are smaller relative to the long axis of the measurement (see Fig. 8–10). It can be observed that relatively small changes in the plane along this axis can affect the FOD measurement.

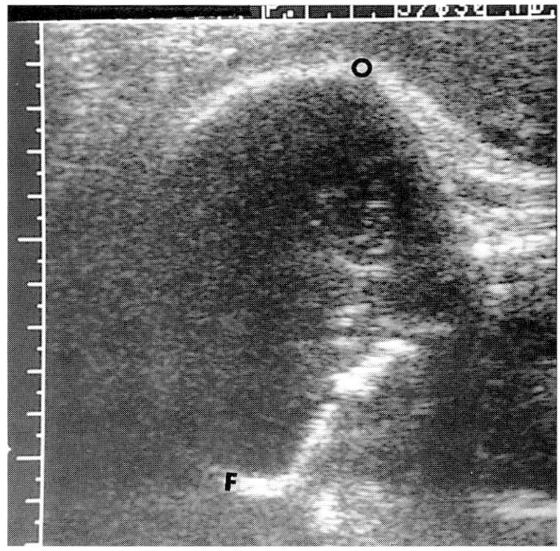

FIGURE 8–10.
Sagittal view of a fetal skull showing the location of the fronto-occipital (F-O) diameter (FOD). This plane is not used for making this measurement because the landmark anatomy is difficult to observe. It is presented here for demonstration purposes only. This shows that the FOD measurement is not as fault tolerant as the biparietal diameter. (LNMP = 32.0 weeks, AA =33.0, n = 9, range = 3.4 weeks, TD)

Coronal Fetal Head

The coronal view of the fetal skull has not been used as often for measurements[1,3,23,26,33,34]; however, I and others have found this view to be valuable for six different reasons:

1. The coronal view facilitates measurement of the VCD, which allows an estimation of the cranial volume and the 3-D BPD correction. Goldberg and Kurtz stated, "It is this measurement that makes the calculated head volumes theoretically more accurate."[3,4]
2. The coronal circumference of the fetal cranium is smaller than the THC; therefore, the coronal measurements can be obtained at term, when the FOD often

exceeds the field of view of many transducers.
3. The VCD is most sensitive to head molding. The use of the VCD in 3-D cranial ages provides more accurate dates for the pregnancy.
4. The coronal view provides anatomical images that include both the bodies and temporal horns of the lateral ventricles, thus allowing evaluation for hydrocephalus. Other cranial anatomy is also observable in this view (see Chapter 9).
5. The curve of the sagittal cranial calvaria gives the coronal measurements a fairly large tolerance of variation of the planes in which acceptable measurements can be obtained (Figs. 8–11 and 8–12).
6. Routine use of 3-D measurements ensures that the fetal cranium is studied more closely. Anomalies are less likely to be overlooked with this additional view.

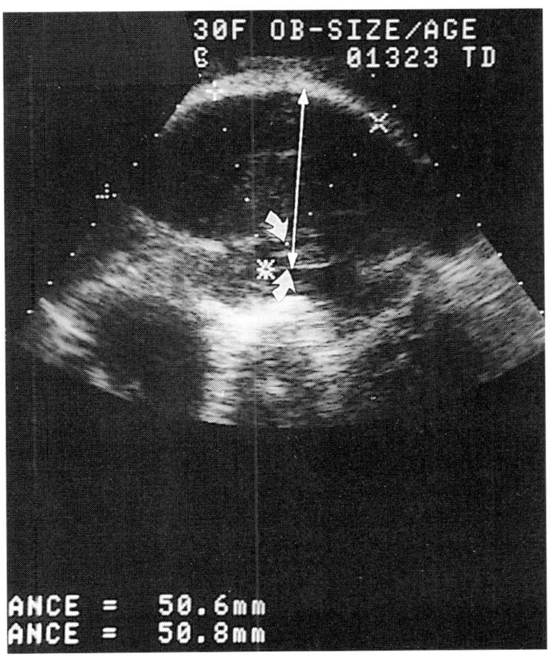

FIGURE 8–11.
Sagittal view showing the long axis of the hippocampal complex (between the curved arrows). The vertical cranial diameter is measured from the base of this structure to the vertex of the cranium (double arrow), which is approximately equal to the measurements by the cursors (X = 50.6 mm, + = 50.8 mm). This image demonstrates that the vertical cranial diameter is less fault tolerant than the biparietal diameter but more so than the fronto-occipital diameter. (LNMP = 32.6 weeks, AA = 31.5, n = 9, range = 2.5 weeks, TD)

This section discusses the geometry of the coronal view and how the measurements are taken. It also provides some statistical analysis of these measurements. The anatomy of the brain is discussed in Chapter 9, and the use of the coronal measurements used in combination with other measurements for cranial volume estimates is discussed later in this chapter. Figure 8–3*B* shows a coronal view of the fetal skull with the measurements that are discussed here. The BPD in this view was discussed earlier. This discussion begins with the coronal triangle and its various measurements.

Cranial Coronal Triangle

The coronal views of the fetal skull shown in Figures 8–3*B* and 8–5 are perpendicular to both the interhemispheric fissure and the plane of the base X of the fetal cranium (see Fig. 8–2). Because the common transverse view of the fetal cranium from which the BPD is usually measured is parallel to the base X, this midcoronal view is also perpendicular to the transverse view.

The appropriate coronal view is easily obtained from the base X view by turning the transducer 90 degrees and finding the thalamus, the interhemispheric fissure, and the bilateral hippocampal gyri (see Fig. 8–3*B*). The best view should include the thalamus, brainstem, both hippocampal gyri, and the bodies of the lateral ventricles. It may include either the anterior spine or esophagus. This at first feels awkward, but it is really no more difficult than obtaining an accurate FOD. When a fetus is facing straight forward or backward in a woman's uterus, the coronal view can be almost impossible to obtain. In a population of 2001 living fetal measurements made in 1992 by 12 sonographers, the VCD was measured in 90% of the fetuses in which a BPD was also measured. The FOD was measured 99% of the time.

From this coronal view, five different measurements can be taken: the BPD, the VCD, the hippocampal base line (HBL), and the two sides of the equilateral triangle (Figs. 8–13, 8–5, and 8–3*B*). These measurements, in conjunction with the FOD, can be used to calculate five fetal age estimates: the BPD, the cranial volume (CV), the triangle circumference diameter (TriCD), the CHC, and the 3-D aver-

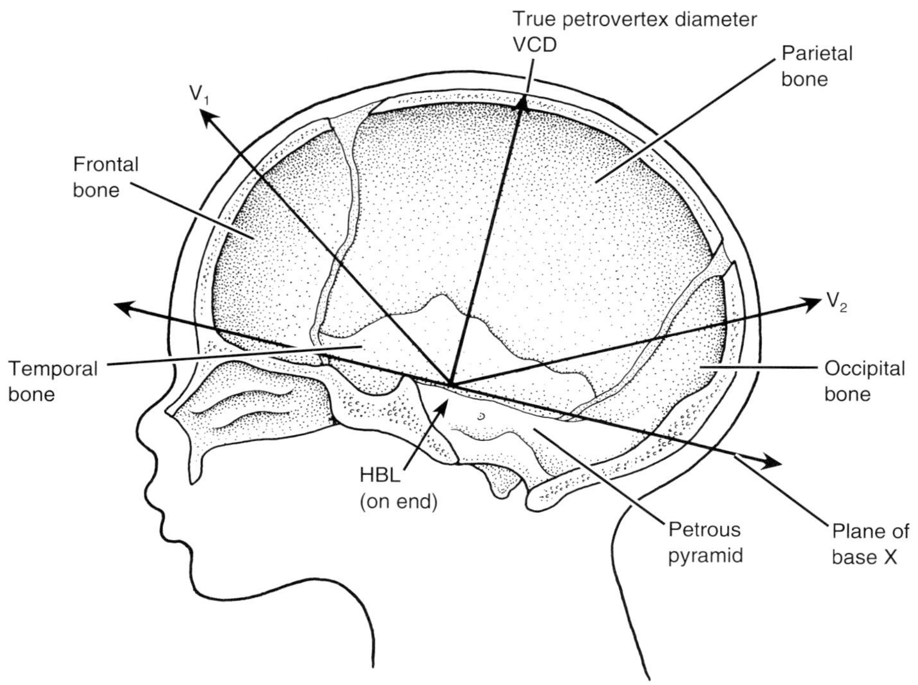

FIGURE 8–12.
An illustration of the sonogram in Figure 8–11. A fairly accurate vertical cranial diameter (VCD) measurement can theoretically be obtained from any coronal plane between V_1 and V_2 because of the arc of the sagittal calvarium. The hippocampal base line (HBL) is a point (line on end) represented by the intersection of all lines (planes on edge). The fronto-occipital diameter (not shown) would be the greatest measurement from the middle of the frontal to the middle of the occipital bones and parallel to the plane of the base X. Any petrovertex diameter measurement between the angle formed by V_1 and V_2 is acceptable.

age or 3-D BPD correction. It is interesting that the BPD, TriCD, and 3-D BPD all are equal in normally shaped heads (Fig. 8–14). These measurements and their statistical analysis follow shortly.

Many will question the need for taking so many measurements of the fetal skull. It is true that 3-D head measurements do not make a significant difference if the head is normally shaped. However, if the cephalic index (CI) is off the mean by very much, the 3-D measurements become more important. Routinely using the coronal measurements also encourages sonographers to observe the head in another way. I believe that this facilitates closer observation of the cranial anatomy and ensures that abnormal anatomy is not overlooked. It is also appropriate in a textbook documenting normal fetal development that this geometry be presented.

In Figures 8–3*B* and 8–5, it can be seen that the HBL is tangential to the inferior edges of the circles around the bilateral hippocampal complexes. The anatomy around the hippocampi is made up of several structures that form the appearance of circles in the true coronal view. The detail of this anatomy is discussed in Chapter 9. The HBL is also across or tangential to the tops of the petrous ridges and has been referred to as the *interpetrous base line*[1] or the *interpetrosal portion of the base of the skull*.[3,4] In this text, this line is simply referred to as the HBL.

The HBL is an imaginary line that forms the base of the coronal triangle and is the bitemporal squamosal diameter. The HBL is a transverse line in the plane of the base X. The sides of the triangle are from the vertex of the cranium to the bilateral HBL-temporal bone intersections.

Several different calculations of the cranial geometry, mentioned earlier, can be obtained from this triangle; some are used in conjunction with the BPD and FOD. The following discussion moves from the simple to the more complex volumetric calculations.

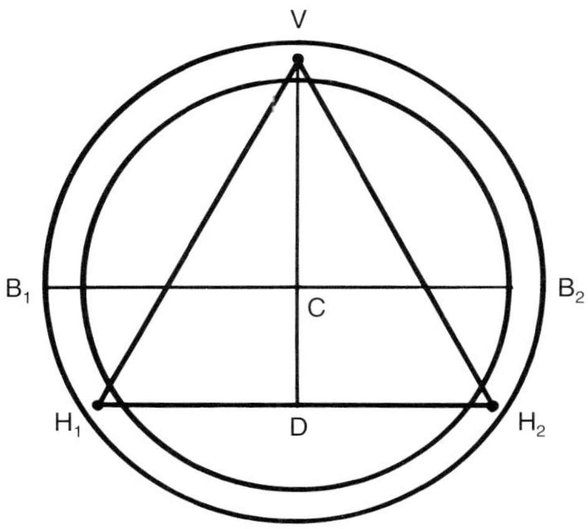

FIGURE 8–13.
Coronal triangle and measurements. All the measurements from the circle of the coronal head (see Fig. 8–2*B*). The biparietal diameter (BPD) is the leading-edge to leading-edge or outer-to-inner measurement between B_1 and B_2. The hippocampal base line (HBL) is between H_1 and H_2, the VCD is from the vertex (V) of the triangle to the middle (D) of the HBL, and the two sides of the triangle are between H_1 and H_2 and V. A complex mensuration formula calculates the circumference of the circle from the length of the HBL and the two sides. From this calculation, the coronal triangle circumference diameter (TriCD) can be derived. The TriCD is equal to the BPD in normally shaped heads. (r = 0.994, n = 1736). See text for the TriCD mensuration formula.

Vertical Cranial Diameter

The height of the triangle is from the apex to the middle of the HBL and is the VCD from the vertex of the skull to the midbase X of the skull (see Fig. 8–13). The VCD passes vertically through the central thalamus and third ventricle and is perpendicular to the BPD and FOD. It lies in both the plane of the interhemispheric fissure and the coronal plane (i.e., at their intersection).

As stated, the VCD is the height of the coronal triangle. It is coincidental that in a normally shaped fetal head, the VCD length is less than the BPD by approximately the difference of the FOD and BPD. That is to say,

$$\text{VCD} = \text{BPD} - (\text{FOD} - \text{BPD})$$

or

$$\text{BPD} = \text{VCD} + (\text{FOD} - \text{BPD})$$

In a sample of 234 living fetuses in which all three diameters were measured (from a random sample of 300 from a population of 3952 consecutive referrals), no statistically significant difference was found in the means or the variances for the foregoing relationships (Table 8–1).

This relationship means that the average of the three diameters (3-D) is also equal to the BPD. This 3-D calculation can be useful for estimating fetal age and weight when the fetal head is abnormally proportioned. This 3-D BPD correction is discussed in detail later in this chapter.

The VCD has been used in a formula that is similar to that used to calculate the more traditional THC. This calculation using the BPD and VCD to estimate the circumference of a circle was called the CHC because it uses the same formula as the THC and not because it is a true CHC. It is addressed later in the section on circumferences.

Triangle Circumference Diameter

The coronal triangle that is shown in Figures 8–5 and 8–13 can be used to calculate the circumference of the coronal view of the skull. The triangle measurements can be taken with two sets of cursors by anchoring and measuring the HBL with the first set. The second set of cursors, with one cursor anchored at the cranial vertex, is used to measure the triangle sides and height. It is shown that this circumference is usually a perfect circle in normally shaped heads. Because the transverse diameter of the coronal skull is the BPD, as shown earlier, it logically follows that the diameter of this circle is also equal to the BPD. The diameter of this circle that circumscribes the triangle has been called the TriCD.[23] The mensuration formula that describes the TriCD comes from the *CRC Standard Mathematical Tables*.[35,36]

$$\text{TriCD} = 2((\text{HBL} \times \text{TriS}_1 \times \text{TriS}_2)/(4 \times \sqrt{(s \times (s - \text{HBL}) \times (s - \text{TriS}_1) \times (s - \text{TriS}_2))}\,))$$

where

$$s = .5 \times (\text{HBL} + \text{ANGS}_1 + \text{ANGS}_2)$$

where TriS_1 and TriS_2 are the sides of the triangle and HBL is the base of the triangle.

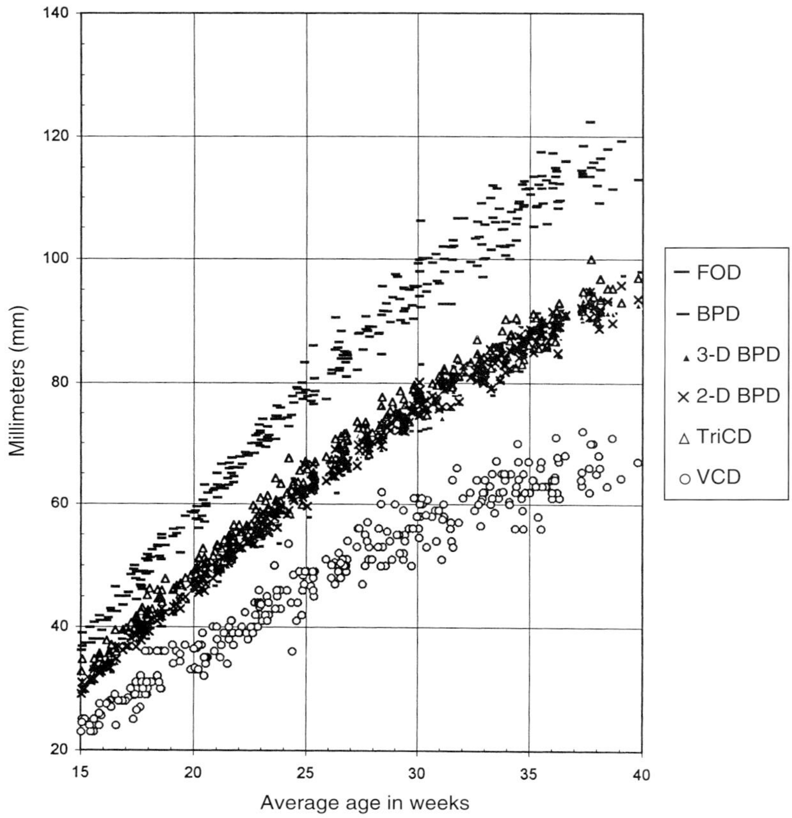

FIGURE 8–14. An XY scatter plot of the growth curves for six linear cranial parameters from 300 random fetuses older than 15 weeks. FOD, fronto-occipital diameters; BPD, biparietal diameter; 3-D BPD, three-dimensional BPD; 2-D BPD, two-dimensional BPD; TriCD, triangle circumference diameter; VCD, vertical cranial diameter. The BPD, 3-D and 2-D BPD, and TriCD are theoretically equal in normally shaped heads (analysis of variance, $P = 0.55$, $n = 300$, $r \geq 0.993$). In this graph, the BPD, 3-D and 2-D BPD, and TriCD all fall midway between the FOD and VCD and form a cloud of plots, making it difficult to distinguish one from the other. The VCD appears to have the greatest dispersion throughout pregnancy, and all plots appear to have slightly increased dispersion after 25 to 30 weeks.

In normally shaped heads, the most accurate construction of the TriCD is from a coronal triangle that is both an isosceles and equilateral triangle. However, the previous formula works for any triangle that is circumscribed by the coronal circumference of the head. If any side of the triangle approaches zero, then the standard error becomes greater because of small variations in cursor placement. The nearer the triangle is to equilateral (all three sides of the triangle being equal), the smaller the errors.

At this point, some definitions of head shapes seem useful. Most experienced sonographers are familiar with the terms *brachycephalic* and *dolichocephalic*. These terms have to do with the head shape as it relates to the comparison of the BPD and FOD. In general, *brachycephalic* implies that the head is relatively wide from side to side (BPD) and short from front to back (FOD). The head shown in Figure 8–15 is not truly brachycephalic (TCI = 0.83) but is slightly above the mean of 0.80. *Dolichocephalic* implies that the head is relatively long from front to back (FOD) and narrow from side to side (BPD), producing a THC less than 0.80. Figure 8–16 is an example of a true dolichocephalic with a THC of 0.69.

In this text, the terms describing head shapes are used relatively and not as absolutes, which is usually taken to indicate that the CI is outside ±2 SD. These terms are discussed in greater detail in the later section on CI. *Dolichocephalic* and *brachycephalic* do not describe changes in the vertical axis, the more dynamic VCD. Figure 8–14 is an XY scatter plot of the three diameters of fetal skull throughout pregnancy. This graph also includes the two-dimensional and 3-D BPD corrections and coronal TriCD. The significance of the equality of the BPD and 3-D average is discussed later. It can be observed in this graph that the BPD, TriCD, and two-dimensional and 3-D BPD correction lie midway between the FOD and VCD.

TABLE 8–1. TESTS OF MEANS AND VARIANCES: THREE-DIMENSIONAL CRANIAL EQUALITIES

FORMULAS	PAIRED TWO-SAMPLE STUDENT'S *t*-TEST FOR MEANS		RESIDUALS = Fn − MEASUREMENT		
	P	r	Sum (in mm)	Average (%)	Variance (%)
F1: 3PD = (FOD + BPD + VCD)/3 = 3-D BPD	0.849	0.993	−0.39	−0.6%	0.1%
F2: 3PD = (FOD + VCD)/2	0.774	0.983	−0.59	−0.8%	0.3%
F3: BPD = VCD + (FOD − BPD)	0.566	0.933	−1.18	−1.7%	1.0%
F4: FOD = BPD + (BPD − VCD)	0.659	0.962	1.18	1.7%	0.7%
F5: VCD = BPD − (FOD − BPD)	0.444	0.888	1.18	3.2%	1.9%

These five formulas are expressions of equalities in the fetal cranial geometry. Formula F1 is the three-dimensional biparietal diameter correction (3-D BPD). Formulas F2 to F5 are geometric relationships that exist in normally shaped heads. A two-sample Student's *t*-test for means was performed using 234 fetal examinations (from a random sample of 300 living fetuses) in which all three cranial parameters were measured. It is shown that there is no significant difference in these equalities ($P > 0.05$).

The r value is the correlation between the parameters and the equality formulas. It can be observed that the BPD = F1 (3-D BPD correction) has the highest correlation at 0.993 and the VCD = F5 has the least correlation with the transverse diameters (BPD and FOD), r = 0.888.

An analysis of variance (ANOVA) was performed on the residuals of each formula minus the respective parameter (i.e., F1 residual = F1 − BPD). It can be seen that the F1 residuals were always the smallest for the sum of the residuals, the average residuals as a percent of the parameter size, and the residuals' variance as a percent of the parameter size. Again, the F5 equality (VCD) is the largest in these categories.

It is notable that the residuals of F4 and F5 will always be equal and F3 will always have the same value with the opposite sign. This is because these residual formulas contain the same variables; in F3 the signs of the variables are reversed. Although this is interesting, I have found little clinical usefulness except for equality F1, which can be substituted for the BPD regardless of the fetal head shape or degree of molding.

From this analysis as well as from observation of thousands of 3-D cranial measurements, it was concluded that the VCD is the most variable of the fetal cranial diameters.

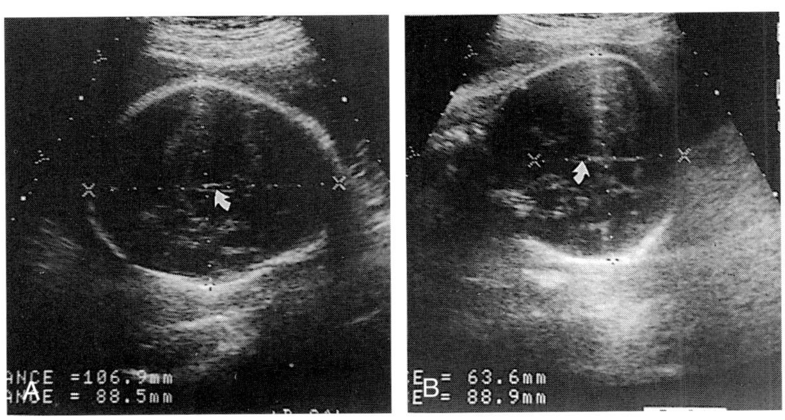

FIGURE 8–15. Platycephaly. This normal fetal head near term has a somewhat compressed vertical cranial diameter. *A*, The biparietal diameter (BPD) (+ = 88.5 mm) and the fronto-occipital diameter (X = 106.9 mm) are measured. The transverse cephalic index is 0.83, which is slightly greater than normal (normal = 0.8 ± 0.1) but still a relatively normal-shaped head. The curved arrow points to the third ventricle. *B*, In the coronal view, both BPDs can be seen to be bowing more than usual. This bowing causes the widest diameter actually to be above the third ventricle (curved arrow) and at the top of the thalamus. Note that at the widest, the BPD in this coronal view is 88.9 mm, or about 0.4 mm greater than in the standard transverse head circumference view. The point here is not that the difference in the two BPDs is great but that head shape does enter into their accuracy. (LNMP = 37.3 weeks, AA = 34.3, n = 9, range = 4.0 weeks, TD)

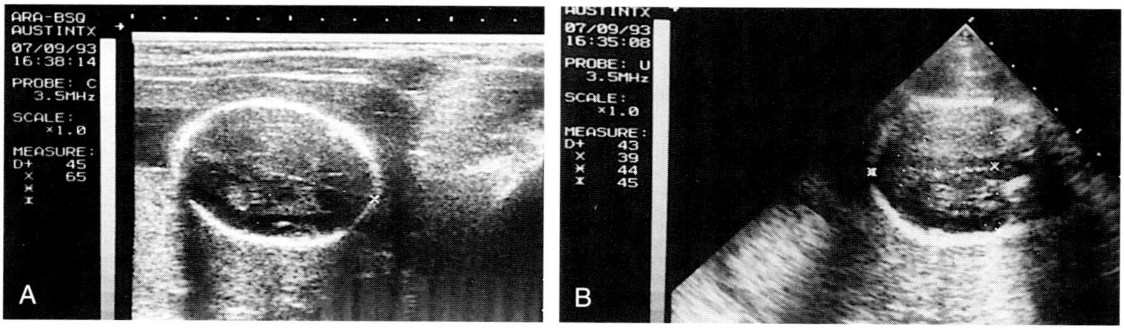

FIGURE 8–16.
Dolicho-oxycephaly. Breech fetus at midpregnancy. *A*, This transverse plane of a fetal head demonstrates a dolichocephalic fetal head with a transverse cephalic index of 0.69, which places it just outside −2 SD. The biparietal diameter (BPD) and fronto-occipital diameter (FOD) measured 45 mm and 65 mm, respectively. From this one view, one cannot make any judgment about the height of the vertical cranial diameter (VCD) or three-dimensional geometry. This fetus is breech, with its head squashed between the uterine wall anteriorly and the placenta posteriorly. The amniotic fluid was judged to be normal in other images. *B*, This coronal view of the same breech fetus shown in *A* demonstrates an exaggerated VCD (note that the coronal skull is not circular). Measurements (in millimeters) from this image were as follows: hippocampal base line = 43, VCD = 39, triangle side one ($TriS_1$) = 44, triangle side two ($TriS_2$) = 45. The five cranial parameters' calculated ages in LMP weeks were BPD = 19.4, transverse head circumference (THC) = 20.5, coronal head circumference = 20.2, triangle circumference diameter = 21.0, and cranial volume = 20.8. This is a range of 1.6 weeks, which is not extraordinary; this range is actually within ±2 SD by cranial age range analysis (see Chapter 7). However, consider the scenario in which another examination at 34 weeks shows the fetus in cephalic presentation, compressing the VCD and exaggerating the THC. If only the THC and abdominal circumference are compared on the two examinations, the fetus could appear to have progressive asymmetrical intrauterine growth retardation when actually only the head shape had changed as a result of molding. (LNMP = 20.3, AA = 20.7, n = 9, range = 1.3 weeks, LP)

If a fetus pushes its head against the uterine wall or the woman's pubic bone, the vertex of the head is somewhat compressed, shortening the VCD. This causes the top of the head to appear somewhat flat, or platycephalic. After about 32 weeks, the fetus may stretch, pressing the vertex of its head and causing a sort of self-induced platycephaly. The prefix *platy-* comes from the Greek *platys*, meaning "broad." The shape can also be thought of as a relatively flat top of the head, rather platelike. Vertical pressure on the skull causes the VCD to be compressed to some degree, and the BPD or FOD is exaggerated to compensate.[23] Figures 8–15 and 8–17 are examples of transverse and coronal views of a platycephalic fetus. Note that in the transverse view (Fig. 8–15*A*), the BPD measures 88.5 mm through the midthalamus and third ventricle; however, in the coronal view, it can be seen that the widest BPD is actually above the third ventricle and measures 88.9 mm. This is an example of the bending of the parietal bones, which is discussed in an excellent report on fetal head molding.[24] This article points out that "The preterm skull has weaker material properties and wider sutures. Thus, more molding at lower pressures is possible." This article went on to summarize earlier literature: "Further efforts to define the exact mechanism of molding led to the observation by Holland[37] in 1922 that the skull is a pliable shell composed of loosely joined plates attached to a rigid base. He speculated that the frontal and parietal bones actually bend under pressure." Although the example presented by Carlan and colleagues[25] is an extreme case of molding, lesser degrees of molding are common perinatal events that are measurable. It is also important to note that the TCI for the fetus shown in Figure 8–17 was relatively normal at 0.83, meaning that it is likely that both the BPD and FOD were compensatingly exaggerated by the compression of the VCD. Note that the coronal skull is not as perfect a circle in Figures 8–15 to 8–17 as it is in the earlier examples.

The inverse of the brachycephalic shape is one in which the VCD is exaggerated as a result of lateral skull pressure that compresses the BPD. The resulting head shape has a relatively high vertical axis and can be called *oxycephaly*. The Greek word *oxys* means "sharp" or "pointed." Therefore, oxycephaly indicates

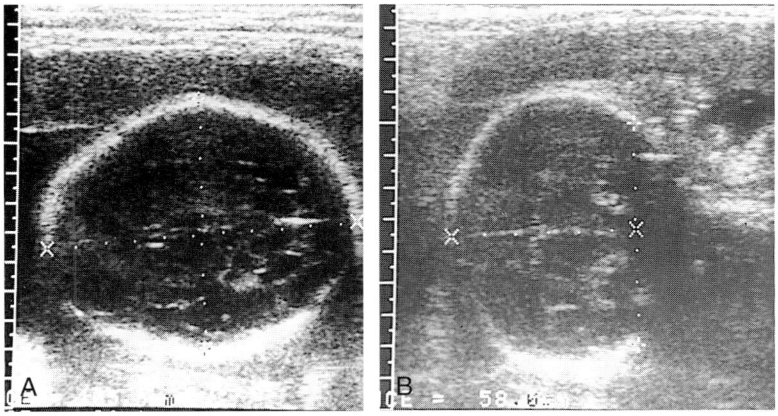

FIGURE 8–17.
Platycephaly. Transverse and coronal views of a fetal head in the third trimester. *A*, Normal-appearing transverse view of the head with a transverse cephalic index of 0.81, biparietal diameter (BPD) = 86.1 mm = 34.6 weeks, and fronto-occipital diameter = 105.5 mm = 34.3 weeks. *B*, In the coronal view, the skull does not appear circular but is flattened. In this case, the BPDs bow outwardly, but the widest BPD still passes through the midthalamus. Compare this molding with that in Figure 8–15*B*. They both result in a small degree of platycephaly, but the BPD molding is slightly different. (LNMP = 32.0, AA = 33.0, n = 9, range = 3.4 weeks, TD)

some degree of coneheadedness. Figures 8–16*A* and 8–16*B* are examples of transverse and coronal views of a relatively oxycephalic fetus. This fetus is breech and also exhibits slight dolichocephaly; therefore, it might be referred to as dolicho-oxycephalic.

The three diameters of the fetal skull achieve normal proportions before the end of the first trimester. These proportional relationships produce indexes that can be used to describe the head shape. The following is a discussion of these cephalic indexes.

THREE-DIMENSIONAL CRANIAL INDEXES

Transverse Cephalic Index

The ratio of the BPD to the FOD is commonly referred to as the CI.[6,38,39] The CI is the primary index of head shape that is used in sonographic literature. Because we are discussing the 3-D fetal skull, two more indexes or ratios are considered. For this reason, the CI, with which every experienced sonographer is familiar, is referred to as the TCI. The other two indexes are the coronal cephalic index (CCI) and the sagittal cephalic index (SCI).[1,23]

The TCI has been discussed extensively in the literature. Haas, using radiographs, found the TCI to be 81.7, with a range of 73.5 to 90.4, in 52 infants between the ages of 1 and 12 months.[38] Hadlock and colleagues reported that the TCI as measured by sonography was normally 78.3 ($\pm$2 SD = $\pm$9.4).[6] Jordaan measured the TCI directly in 50 neonates delivered by cesarean section and found the mean TCI to be 80.6.[39] Figure 8–18 is an XY plot of the TCI with a LOWESS (locally weighted smoothing) mean and $\pm$2 SD.

Hadlock and colleagues discussed these studies in detail.[6] They reported that Haas "noted that these values [Haas's] might be slightly higher than actual values because the distortion by projection of breadth was greater in his series than that of length." The Haas distortion is due to radiographic magnification. Of their own study, Hadlock and associates stated that "Our mean value of 78.3 is slightly lower than the values observed postnatally. This may be related in part to the greater distortion of the frontal and occipital bones resulting from the sonographic beam passing parallel to these structures rather than perpendicular." Hadlock was stating here that beam width can have an effect on the FOD measurement, and I concur in the opinion that measurement of the outer edges of the FOD tends to include some beam-width artifact in the measurement. The FOD measurements often have the additional difficulty of shadowing because the sound beam travels tangentially to the frontal and occipital

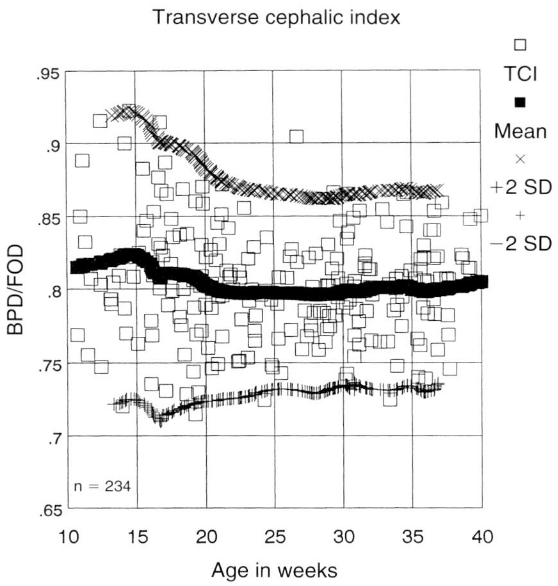

FIGURE 8–18.
An XY scatter plot (open squares) of the transverse cephalic indexes (TCI) for 234 fetuses in which head measurements were obtained in 300 randomly selected pregnancies. The solid black line is the LOWESS smoothed mean, the X plots are the LOWESS smoothed +2 SD, and the + plots are −2 SD. This x-axis is the average age in equivalent LMP weeks. Note that the TCI = biparietal diameter/fronto-occipital diameter is at or just above 0.80.

bones. Visualization can be particularly difficult with divergent fields of view from sector or curvilinear transducers. With these types of transducers, the true transverse view (the longest skull diameter) is placed in the shadow of the skull, which is more proximal to the transducer. In these shadowy conditions, an attempt to approximate the outer edges may often result in an overestimation of the FOD, whereas in the protocol of midedge FODs, slightly less variation is found. In a series of 167 obstetrical sonographic examinations, we (TJD, LP, DKD, LANB) measured every FOD using Hadlock's method of outer-to-outer edges of the frontal and occipital bones. We also measured these same FODs by placing the cursors at the estimated center of the frontal and occipital bone echoes (i.e., at the middle of the bone echoes). We found slightly less variation in the midfrontal to midoccipital bones than in the outer-to-outer measurements. We then established a protocol in which all FOD measurements are taken from the midfrontal to midoccipital bones and the BPD is leading edge to leading edge. We now have performed more than 10,000 fetal examinations using that protocol, with good results. The data presented here and in Chapter 7 were accumulated using this protocol.

The use of this BPD–leading edges and FOD-midedges protocol lends itself to a TCI that is in line with those published by Jordaan for the neonates born by cesarean section. This is because ratios for outer perimeter measurements are theoretically the same as the ratios produced by the protocol described here.[1] This is described in Figure 8–4. Algebraically, Figure 8–4 is interpreted as follows:

$$AE/FI = BD/GH \text{ and } AC = BD$$

therefore

$$AE/FI = AC/GH$$

Figure 8–18 is a time series XY plot of TCIs from a random population. In this graph, the TCI mean is the LOWESS smoothed mean. LOWESS smoothing is locally weighted smoothing; in financial circles, this is often called a *moving average* or *rolling average*. The mean standard deviation was determined by a similar LOWESS function for 2 SD.[40] It is easy to observe that Jordaan's consistency of the THC is confirmed. There is very little variation of this index from the mean of 0.80, and it is almost always less than 0.90 and more than 0.70.

This study of the three cephalic indexes of the fetal skull found the following relationships (see Table 8–2 for descriptive statistics):

Mean TCI = BPD/FOD = 0.81
($\pm$ 2 SD = $\pm$ 0.09 = 0.72 to 0.90)

Mean CCI = VCD/BPD = 0.74
($\pm$ 2 SD = $\pm$ 0.12 = 0.62 to 0.86)

Mean SCI = VCD/FOD = 0.59
($\pm$ 2 SD = $\pm$ 0.09 = 0.50 to 0.68)

The reader can observe that in this population from 300 random examinations, the CCI has the largest variation (2 SD = $\pm$ 0.12). We believe that this larger variation is due to head shapes and not to larger errors in meas-

TABLE 8–2. **DESCRIPTIVE STATISTICS FOR THREE-DIMENSIONAL CRANIAL INDEXES (RANDOM SELECTION)**

	TCI	CCI	SCI	FOD/3-D	BPD/3-D	VCD/3-D
Mean	0.81	0.74	0.59	1.25	1.01	0.74
Standard error	0.00297	0.00383	0.00286	0.00217	0.00220	0.00262
Median	0.80	0.73	0.59	1.26	1.01	0.74
Mode	0.81	0.70	0.58	1.28	1.02	0.73
Standard deviation	0.04661	0.05854	0.04377	0.03326	0.03372	0.04011
Variance	0.00217	0.00343	0.00192	0.00111	0.00114	0.00161
Kurtosis	16.12722	0.50876	0.34096	0.40242	0.43780	0.34311
Skewness	2.29508	0.14494	0.06274	−0.25585	0.03042	−0.12973
Range	0.47	0.31	0.30	0.23	0.19	0.22
Minimum	0.71	0.59	0.44	1.13	0.91	0.61
Maximum	1.18	0.90	0.74	1.36	1.10	0.83
Sum	198.94	172.15	137.99	293.53	235.58	172.89
Count	247	234	234	234	234	234
Confidence level (95%)	0.00581	0.00750	0.00561	0.00426	0.00432	0.00514

These statistics describe six indexes of the three-dimensional (3-D) cranial parameters: the transverse cephalic index (TCI = BPD/FOD), the coronal cephalic index (CCI = VCD/BPD), the sagittal cephalic index (SCI = VCD/FOD), and the 3-D indexes, shown as last three column headings. The TCI is shown graphically in Figure 8–18. The 3-D indexes are shown graphically in Figure 8–19*A* and *B*.

In the 3-D indexes, it can be observed that relative to the 3-D average, the FOD has the least standard error, standard deviation, and variance. The VCD has the greatest of these. This reiterates the fact that the VCD is the most variable of the three cranial diameters and the FOD is the least.

urements. Because of the malleable nature of the sutures and fontanelles and the recognized potential for skull molding as well as normal morphological variations, the VCD is thought to be the most dynamic axis of the fetal cranium. Analysis of variance (ANOVA) found a statistically significant difference in the mean CCIs between sonographers at the 0.05 level but not at the 0.01 level ($P = 0.029$, df = 226). No significant difference in the CCIs between laboratories was noted ($P = 0.847$, df = 226). This finding indicates that successful use of 3-D measurements depends on a sonographer's skill and experience.

Cephalic Indexes

The three independent CIs (TCI, CCI, and SCI) are sensitive to variations in the relationships of any two measurements, but it becomes an exercise in mental gymnastics to attempt to relate all three measurements, one to the other two, using this method. Also, because there is overlap of the variation in the three CIs discussed earlier, the XY plots of all three indexes are difficult to interpret. For this reason, it was decided to look at the ratios of the three axes to the average of the three measurements (3-D average).

Figure 8–19*A* shows the XY plot of the ratios of the FOD, BPD, and VCD to the 3-D average of these measurements. Shown in Figure 8–19*B* are the bar graph histograms for these indexes. This was done in order to observe the relative variation between the three measurements. Note that the BPD/3-D is approximately 1.002 (2 SD = 0.94 to 1.07). This means that the 3-D average is equal to the normal BPD and can be used to estimate the fetal age on a standard BPD table. The clinical importance of this fact and its use as a substitute for fetal age and weight estimates are discussed later in the section on the 3-D BPD correction. The following can be observed about these three measurements from Figures 8–19*A* and *B*. After about 15 menstrual weeks, all three measurements maintain a relatively constant proportion. Before 15 weeks, the tendency is toward relatively longer FODs and shorter VCDs; however, the transverse diameter, the BPD, appears to be more constant throughout gestation from as early as it can be measured sonographically.

The proportions of the fetal cranium are

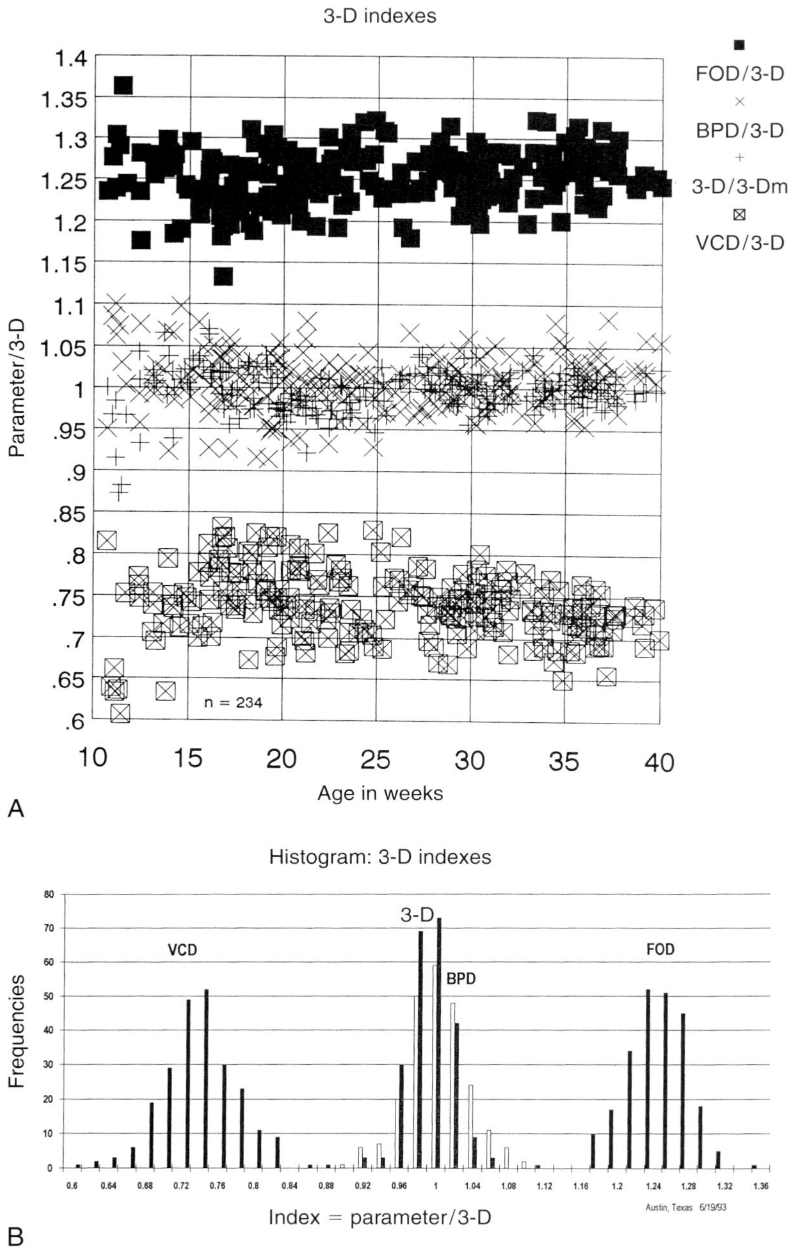

FIGURE 8–19. Three-dimensional (3-D) cephalic indexes and histograms. The 3-D indexes are a variation on the standard cephalic index. Each linear parameter (biparietal diameter [BPD], fronto-occipital diameter [FOD], and vertical cranial diameter [VCD], is divided by the average of the three (3-D). These are for 234 fetuses in which all three diameters were measured in 300 random cases. *A*, The XY time series plot of four ratios: the FOD/3-D index, the BPD/3-D index, the VCD/3-D index, and the 3-D index (3-DI = 3-D/3-Dm = 3D average/3-D LOWESS means). These indexes were devised because indexes such as the standard transverse cephalic index (TCI) compare only two parameters at a time. When dealing with more than two parameters, the use of simple ratios makes it more difficult to conceptualize the proportions, one to the others. The most important lesson from this time series scattergram is that the BPD/3-D is equal to 1, which means that the 3-D average of the BPD, FOD, and VCD can be substituted for the BPD for estimates of age or weight regressions regardless of head shape and molding. *B*, These bar graph histograms are for the 3-D indexes in *A*. They demonstrate the relative variation or dispersion for each index. The VCD, BPD, and FOD all are divided by the 3-D average. The 3-D is the 3-D/3-D LOWESS smoothed means because a simple 3-D/3-D would always produce a ratio of 1 (see LOWESS in Chapter 7). From this, it can be observed that the VCD has the greatest dispersion. It can also be observed that the BPD and 3-D ratio have the same mean of 1 and lie midway between the VCD and FOD.

about the only parameter relationships that remain relatively constant throughout gestation. All other ratios, such as the head to abdomen or extremities tend to vary through time. The ratios of the head are fairly simple to remember because, for example, the mean THC ratio is 0.80 (±0.1 = 2 SD) in most fetuses at any time during pregnancy. However, the THC/abdominal circumference ratio varies every week. Therefore, one must keep a chart or graph close at hand to determine normal values for these ratios. Even the humerus-to-femur ratio varies slightly. It is a perfect 1:1 ratio only at 16 weeks (more on this topic in Chapters 7 and 9).

Because the ratios of the fetal cranium measurements appear relatively consistent throughout gestation, several in addition to the THC can be rounded to provide numbers that are simple to describe and remember.

These are 3-D ratios that have not been previously published. The following are the rounded generalized ratios (see Table 8–2 for more precision):

$$\text{Mean BPD/3-D} = 1.00 \quad (\pm 2\text{ SD} = \pm 0.10 = 0.90 \text{ to } 1.10)$$

$$\text{Mean FOD/3-D} = 1.25 \quad (\pm 2\text{ SD} = \pm 0.10 = 1.35 \text{ to } 1.15)$$

$$\text{Mean VCD/3-D} = 0.75 \quad (\pm 2\text{ SD} = \pm 0.10 = 0.65 \text{ to } 0.85)$$

These ratios are good rules of thumb that allow for slightly more variation than our study population.

Circumference and Area Geometries of the Fetal Cranium

CIRCUMFERENCE AND AREA

The THC has been well studied.[14, 41–43] It is very accurate in terms of fetal age estimates if the VCD is normal. The THC is not, however, the ultimate in fetal biometry. Others have stated that "The BPD is very useful for dating pregnancy and evaluating growth of the fetus; however, it is subject to an artificial decrease or increase in size by normally occurring changes in head shape, such as dolichocephaly and brachycephaly; although these changes alter the BPD they do not change the HC measurement."[44] This statement completely ignores the 3-D nature of the head. The vertical axis is more dynamic and can increase or decrease as a result of the changes in head shape mentioned earlier, causing inverse and compensatory changes in the THC while often leaving the TCI normal (see Fig. 8–17).

The THC is calculated from the formula for an ellipse. The formula is actually a modified version of the circumference of a circle using two diameters rather than the one diameter of a circle. This is discussed in detail in the section on geometry in Chapter 5. The formula is

$$\text{THC} = 1.57\ (\text{FOD} + \text{BPD})$$

This formula yields the approximate circumference of an ellipse in the same units as the diameter measurements. The resulting circumference, the THC in this case, can then be used to estimate the age of a fetus or in a ratio with other parameters to estimate various proportions. It is probably the most commonly used fetal measurement to estimate fetal age since the mid-1980s. Most researchers report the THC to be accurate to within 1 to 2 weeks of age.

The dates of a pregnancy can be estimated by using the THC in a look-up table such as Table 7–1 or by using it in a regression formula. Hadlock and colleagues[14] developed the following formula using outer perimeter measurements:

$$\text{MA} = 8.8 + 0.55 \times \text{THC} + 2.8 \times 10^{-4}$$

$$(2\text{ SD} = \pm 1.8 \text{ weeks}, r^2 = 97.9\%)$$

where MA stands for menstrual age. Another regression that is slightly simpler and has similar accuracy has been developed. The following relationship is for leading-edge to leading-edge BPD and midedge-to-midedge FOD measurements.

$$\text{MA} = (2.815 + 0.01 \times \text{THC})^2$$

$$(2\text{ SD} = \pm 1.15 \text{ weeks}, r^2 = 94.5\%)$$

For raw BPD and FOD measurements, this becomes

$$\text{MA} = (2.815 + 0.01 \times (1.57 \times \text{FOD} + \text{BPD}))^2$$

The area of the fetal skull cross section has been less used. Goldberg and Kurtz found eight reports describing the transverse cross-sectional area of the fetal head in terms of age.[45] In their historical research of fetal head measurements, Goldberg and Kurtz stated that "The accuracy is not better than either the BPD or the [transverse] head circumference measurements and since the variation may be greater, it is felt that the head area is not a useful or proven method."[45]

I concur that the calculation of the cross-sectional area has no advantage over the THC and is less accurate than the 3-D measurements to be discussed shortly.

TWO-DIMENSIONAL BIPARIETAL DIAMETER

In 1984, a formula was published for correcting the effects of abnormal proportions of the standard transverse or transaxial head circumference on the BPD.[46] That is, if the TCI is abnormal, this formula adjusts or corrects the BPD based on the normal ratio of the FOD to the BPD.

$$\text{Corrected BPD} = \sqrt{((\text{BPD} \times \text{FOD})/1.265)}$$

The use of this formula on the two-dimensional measurements of the transverse fetal skull allows more accurate gestational age and weight estimations using formulas that require BPD measurements.

Although more accurate than the standard BPD, in some cases this method suffers from the same disadvantage as the standard BPD and THC, that being that it ignores the fact that the fetal cranium is a 3-D volume not a two-dimensional plane. For this reason, the 3-D BPD correction (discussed later) is recommended.

Volume of the Fetal Cranium

CALCULATION OF THE VOLUME

"The primacy of brain over somatic growth is a distinctive feature of normal fetal development that is preserved in asymmetric intrauterine growth retardation (IUGR)."[47] This is the concept of "head-sparing" IUGR. If uterine or placental perfusion is compromised, it is thought that the resulting reduction of fetal nutrition leads to slowed growth. It appears that in cases of asymmetrical or head-sparing IUGR, the natural priorities provide preferential perfusion to the brain over the body.

Little sonographic research has addressed the growth of the mass of the fetal brain or volume of the cranium. Goldberg and Kurtz[3] reported only four studies of the head volume. The first three of these derived a cubic function of the transverse diameters (FOD and BPD) of the fetal skull. Although the concepts of these three reports recognized that the fetal cranium is a 3-D volume, the use of only two diameters is not a valid way to estimate this volume. An additional way to estimate the growth of the cranial mass was proposed by Jordaan and colleagues.[47,48] Rather than estimate volume, these researchers estimated brain weight by using sonographic measurements on various regressions on the BPD, the largest THC, and the transverse neurocranial cross-sectional area.

All of these methods ignore the third dimension of the cranium, the VCD, except two. Jordaan and Dunn recognized "the ponderal size of the brain, which is a function of a three-dimensional or volumetric measurement." However, they went on to state that "no ultrasonic data on the vertical-auriculo-vertex diameter (VAV) are available in the literature."[49] Although this was true at the time of their publication, the VCD, which very nearly approximates the VAV that Jordaan and Dunn had envisioned, was published in 1985.[1] This VCD measurement was described earlier.

Head molding or normal variations in the calvarial proportions can result in changes in all three axes of the solid mass of the head. In fact, it appears that the VCD is the most dynamic of the three diameters of the fetal skull.[23]

If the membranes rupture prematurely, the resulting loss of fluid allows the uterine walls to collapse against the fetal skull. This can result, most often, in pressure along the transverse axis of the skull, the axis of the BPD measurements. This pressure causes shortening of the BPD. The VCD or the FOD is exaggerated to compensate, and some degree of dolichocephaly results. Although this hypothesis is difficult to prove, evidence of this effect is described in the literature.[3,24,25] Proof of this phenomenon is found later in the 3-D BPD correction section.

The original article on the CV used a nonstandard formula for an ellipsoidal volume. This nonstandard formula was naively derived using the average radii of the FOD, BPD, and VCD in the formula for a sphere[1]:

$$\text{CV} = 4.189[(\text{FOD} + \text{BPD} + \text{VCD})/6]^3$$

Although this formula yields accurate estimates for ellipsoidal shapes of the fetal skull that are compatible with life, it does not produce accurate estimates for more extreme ellipsoids with sausage or disk shapes. With this formula, the nearer the shape is to a true sphere, the more accurate is the estimate of the volume.

After considerable study, I realized the error and derived a formula that is based on the more common ellipsoidal formula[50]:

$$\text{Ellipsoid volume} = 1/6 \times \text{pi} \times A \times B \times C$$

where A, B, and C are the diameters of the ellipsoid. This is normally simplified to

$$0.52 \times A \times B \times C$$

or in the case of the fetal cranium,

$$CV = 0.52 \times FOD \times BPD \times VCD$$

This last formula produced a result that was slightly smaller than the first formula for the CV using the averaged diameters. Others have also found that the standard ellipsoid volume formula slightly underestimates biological volumes.[51] In order to make the more standard formula produce results that matched experiments on clay models in the approximate shapes of fetal calvaria, the formula was further modified:

$$\mathbf{CV = 0.555 \times FOD \times BPD \times VCD}$$

This last formula yields volumes that are cubes of the measurement units for the diameters—that is, millimeter measurements yield cubic millimeter volumes and centimeter measurements yield cubic centimeters (milliliters). In order to use millimeter measurements and to produce volumes in milliliters, use the following:

$$\mathbf{CV = 0.000555 \times FOD \times BPD \times VCD}$$

In this formula, the parameters are measured as described in the earlier section on linear cranial geometry. The last formula is used to estimate fetal age from Table 7–1.

It should be understood by readers that all the measurements, such as circumferences and volumes, that are calculated from linear measurements are actually estimates. For these calculations to yield accurate results, the parameter would have to be a perfect sphere, ellipse, or ellipsoidal shape. Few biological shapes exhibit perfectly smooth contours. The fetal brain is more or less flat on the bottom, with depressions into the surface where the petrous pyramids and sphenoid bones fit. Another factor is the four fossae between these bones, the frontal fossa, the occipital fossa, and the bilateral temporal fossae.

The fact that the organs are not perfect geometric shapes has little effect on the results of the formulas as long as the reader understands that these are consistent, reproducible functions of the actual geometry. This is to say, it really does not matter that we are not calculating the exact volume of the cranium as long as we use the same method for estimating the volume as was used by the original researcher when the chart or graph we are using was constructed. The measurement(s) must be taken in the same way as the researcher did, and the same formula(s) must be used to make estimates using the regression formula, chart, or graph. It is for this reason that if a sonographer does not know precisely how a researcher took the measurements to produce a nomogram, then the chart or graph is essentially useless. If the researcher used outer-to-outer BPD measurements for a chart and if the sonographer is using leading edge to leading edge, then the estimate will be in error.

Although the exponential increase in the CV produces accurate estimates of age, another 3-D function of the fetal cranium is both simple and useful. It is coincidental that the average of the three diameters—FOD, BPD, and VCD—are equal to the BPD in a normally shaped head. This has been called the *3-D BPD correction*.[26]

THREE-DIMENSIONAL BIPARIETAL DIAMETER

The three diameters and the 3-D average of the fetal head from a random sample of 234 from a large population are shown in Figure 8–14. It can be observed that the BPD and 3-D scatter plots reside midway between the FOD and VCD. However, the 3-D plot not only lies midway between the FOD and VCD but also exhibits slightly less dispersion than the BPD. From this observation, it was realized that the 3-D average can be used to estimate the fetal age from any standard BPD chart regardless of the head shape or molding. For this reason, it has been called the 3-D BPD correction.[26]

Several relationships can be derived from this phenomenon. Table 8–1 shows the algebraic expressions of these relationships. The statistical analysis of these relationships was performed using Excel for Windows.[52] The probability (P) of equivalence was tested using the t-test, assuming unequal variance ($n = 234$ random, $\alpha = 0.05$). The basic finding was that there is no statistical difference in the equalities (values across the equal signs) and the VCD has the lowest correlation and the greatest variance.

Although only the first of these equalities (3-D BPD correction, see Table 8–1) has much clinical usefulness, they are presented in order to document the various geometric relationships of the human fetal cranium. These relationships are constant throughout the fetal period in normally shaped heads. Of course, if the head is abnormally shaped, the first (the 3-D BPD correction) is most accurate.

The 3-D nature of the fetal cranium means that when one axis is compressed, one or both of the other two axes are exaggerated to compensate. Which of the axes compensate or what degree of compensation can be attributed to either of the other two axes appears to vary from case to case. This is discussed more in the next section.

THREE-DIMENSIONAL CRANIAL AGE ANALYSIS

Statistical gurus will probably consider the following discussion to be "voodoo statistics." Less fastidious sonographers may consider it hair splitting; after all, how much accuracy in fetal sonography is required . . . or possible? Most women do not remember the exact day or night when they conceived, and the duration of pregnancy can vary significantly. The term of a normal human pregnancy is generally considered to be between 38 and 42 weeks, with a mean of 40 weeks from the last normal menstrual period (LNMP).[53,54] This is a range of 4 weeks during which a pregnancy may be considered normal. So what's the difference of a few days or a week or two?

To respond to the latter issue, it is true that predicting the exact date of a normal labor and delivery is nearly impossible or at least is an educated gamble. However, the rate of increase in the size of a fetus is a reliable indicator of health. A diabetic woman's fetus may gain weight too fast and have difficulty in delivery as well as hydrops fetalis. In cases of IUGR or twins, one or both may increase in size too slowly and require close monitoring in order to determine the optimum time and method for delivery. For these last cases, all possible accuracy is advisable.

To test which of the various cranial parameters are most accurate for estimating fetal age, three different sets of fetal measurements and the average age of multiple fetal parameter ages (MFP AA) were compared with LNMPs as reported by the pregnant women. Each set contained 9 parameters and 22 resulting fetal ages estimated in different ways from these parameters (Tables 8–3 and 8–4). Figures 8–20*A* and *B* show four representative parameter measurements plotted against the LNMP and MFP AA in weeks from the 300 random set. Each fetus had attained an LMP age greater than 15 weeks and was included only once. The first group was a random sample of 300 examinations of 10,336 performed during the years 1984 to 1993, in which the three dimensions and a fetal heart rate were measured. The second group included only those fetuses of the 10,336 in which the three cranial dimensions were measured and a relatively dolichocephalic head shape was found with TCI of less than 0.74, resulting in a total of 357 living fetuses older than 15 weeks. The third group was similar to the second, except that it included only fetuses with relatively brachycephalic head shapes ($TCI > 0.86$, $n = 322$).

These sonographic examinations were performed by 12 registered sonographers (11 American Registry of Diagnostic Medical Sonographers, 1 eligible) in four laboratories using seven different sonographic machines from three different manufacturers. All measurements were entered into fetal size/age analysis software at the time of the examination. Preliminary analysis found no statisti-

TABLE 8–3*A*. FETAL PARAMETERS AND AGE DEFINITIONS

ABBREVIATION	AGE NAME
	Parameter Measurements for Correlation Matrices
BPD	Biparietal diameter (leading edge to leading edge)
CHC	Coronal head circumference = $(d_1 + d_2)1.57$
TriCD	Coronal triangle circumference diameter (see text)
CV	Cranial volume in ml = (FOD × BPD × VCD × 0.000555)
FemL	Femoral diaphysis length
THC	Transverse head circumference = $(d_1 + d_2)1.57$
2-D BPD	2-D BPD = $\sqrt{(\text{FOD} \times \text{BPD})/1.265}$
3-D BPD	3-D BPD correction = (FOD + BPD + VCD)/3

PARAMETER AGES FOR ANOVA		AGE DETERMINATION BY
AC wk	Abdominal circumference	See Table 7–1
Average body wk	Average age of AC wk, FEM wk, HUM wk, and CRL wk	Averaged
Average Cranial wk	Average age of CV wk, BPD wk, THC wk, CHC wk, and TriCD wk	Averaged
AA	Average age of MFPs from look-up table	Averaged
BiOD wk	Binocular diameter (outer to outer)	See Table 7–1
rBPD age	Biparietal diameter	Regression
BPD wk	Biparietal diameter	See Table 7–1
rCHC age	Coronal head circumference	Regression
CHC wk	Coronal head circumference	See Table 7–1
r2D BPD age	2-D BPD correction	Regression
rCV age	Cranial volume	Regression
CV wk	Cranial volume	See Table 7–1
Fem wk	Femoral length	See Table 7–1
Hum wk	Humeral length	See Table 7–1
LNMP	Last normal menstrual period (maternal history)	Maternal history
rTHC age	Transverse head circumference	Regression
THC wk	Transverse head circumference	See Table 7–1
rTHC Hadlock	Transverse head circumference regression (Hadlock)	Regression
rTriBPD age	Triangle circumference diameter	Regression
TriBPD wk	Triangle circumference diameter	See Table 7–1
r3D BPD age	3-D BPD correction	Regression_1
r3D BPD age_2	3-D BPD correction	Regression_2

These are the various parameters used in the analyses in Tables 8–4*A* to *F*. The abbreviations are used throughout the following tables. The *Age Name* column is the parameter or calculation used to estimate the fetal age, and the *Age Determination By* column tells if the parameter age was estimated from Table 7–1 or using a formula in a spreadsheet. Most abbreviations are preceded by *r* or followed by *wk*. The *r* indicates a formula (see Table 8–3*B*), and *wk* indicates Table 7–1. For the cranial ages, both r and wk age estimates are given. The wk age estimates for the fetal body parameters—Fem, Hum, and AC—are for comparison purposes. All look-up table estimates (wk) were by computer algorithm, which performs straight interpolation to 0.10 of a week.

cally significant differences between observers, laboratories, or machines.

A correlation matrix and an ANOVA were performed six times on the three different sets of data, twice on each set, once on all of each set of fetuses older than 15 weeks and once on only those fetuses that were older than 30 weeks. These three sets of data were tested in this way because most fetal head molding occurs late in pregnancy (after 30 to 34 weeks). Table 8–3*A* defines the parameter abbreviations, and Table 8–3*B* shows the regression formulas that were used to estimate parameter ages.

The correlation matrices were performed on the LNMP, AA, and the measurement data of nine parameters. Table 8–3 defines the parameters. The results of all six correlation ma-

TABLE 8–3*B*. **REGRESSION FORMULAS FOR FETAL CRANIAL AGES**

PARAMETER NAME	PARAMETER ACRONYM	REGRESSION FORMULAS FOR EQUIVALENT LMP AGE
Linear Measures		
Biparietal diameter	rBPD	$Age = 7.7 + 0.22 \times BPD + 0.0009 \times BPD^2$
3-D BPD correction (1st regression)	r3D BPD	$Age = 7.7 + 0.22 \times 3\text{-}D + 0.0009 \times 3\text{-}D^2$
3-D BPD correction (2nd regression)	r3D BPD_2	$Age = 5 + (0.0022 \times 3\text{-}D^2) + 1.46 \times \sqrt{(3\text{-}D)}$
Corrected BPD (2-D)	r2D BPD	$Age = 5 + (0.0022 \times 2\text{-}D^2) + 1.46 \times \sqrt{(2\text{-}D)}$
Triangle circumference diameter = BPD	rTriCD	$Age = 5 + (0.0022 \times TriCD^2) + 1.46 \times \sqrt{(Tri\ CD)}$
Circumferential Measures		
Transverse head circumference	rTHC	$Age = (2.815 + (0.01 \times THC))^2$
Coronal head circumference	rCHC	$Age = 4.2 + 0.000288 \times CHC^2 + 0.9633 \times \sqrt{(CHC)}$
Transverse head circumference (Hadlock et al)	rTHC Hadlock	$Age = 8.96 + 0.540(THC \times 0.1) + 0.0003(THC \times 0.1)^3$
Volumetric Measures		
Cranial volume	rCV	$Age = 9.5 + 1.4 \times \sqrt{(CV)}$

These are the regressions used to estimate various cranial ages. With the exception of the Hadlock et al regression (THC FPHrg), all other formulas were selected using curve-fitting software from more than 3300 linear and nonlinear equations. The equations used were selected using two criteria: a coefficient of determination greater than 0.99 (r^2) and an equation that was relatively simple. Note that the same type of equations is used for each type of measurement and calculation, linear and circumferential.

trices are shown at the top of Tables 8–4*A* to *F*.

The ANOVA was less straightforward because the parameters grow at different rates. Therefore, it is difficult to compare the variation in growth of a linear BPD measurement with that of the exponential cubic CV estimation. Thus, it was decided to compare the variation of the fourth dimension of the parameters rather than the actual measurements. To make this comparison, each parameter was converted to its equivalent size in time—that is, the fetal age in equivalent LMP weeks. It is at this point that many statisticians will think "voodoo statistics." However, this should not be a fatal flaw in the study because in a single fetus, the THC may measure to the equivalent age of 24 weeks and the abdominal circumference may measure 26 weeks of age. It is absurd to think that the fetal abdomen was conceived 2 weeks before the head. Thus, the parameter ages are not the true ages of those parameters but are the fourth dimension, the equivalent parameter size expressed as a function of time. This process is discussed in greater detail in Chapter 7 in the section on age range analysis.

Several steps or data treatments were necessary to arrive at values that could be compared using the ANOVA. Figures 8–20*A* and *B* show four representative parameters in XY scattergrams against the LNMP and the AA, respectively. Only four of the parameters were plotted for simplicity of observation and to demonstrate the differing rates of change in growth. It can be observed that the uncertainty of the LNMP adds to the variation in these growth curves. However, because the LNMP is the accepted standard (independent variable) for these kinds of studies, the correlation matrices were sorted in descending order of correlation with the LNMP.

Figure 8–21*A* shows the equivalent parameter ages for the femur and THC plotted against the AA in LMP weeks. This was done because we are attempting to view the relative parameter variation within individual fetuses without obscuration from the inherent

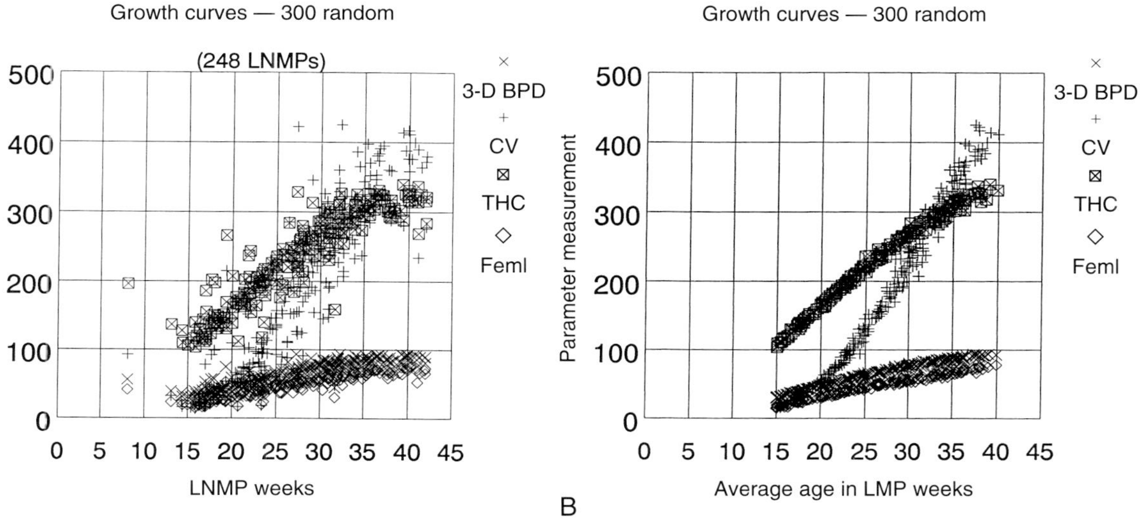

FIGURE 8–20.
Cranial three-dimensional (3-D) growth curves. Growth curves for 300 random fetuses of 10,336 fetuses measured between the start of 1984 and 1994. These curves are presented as examples of the larger number of parameters analyzed in Tables 8–4*A* through 8–4*F*. *A*, Four variables plotted against the reported last normal menstrual period (LNMP, maternal history). Plotted are the 3-D biparietal diameter (3-D BPD) (X = average of fronto-occipital diameter [FOD], BPD, and vertical cranial diameter [VCD]), the coronal volume (CV), the transverse head circumference (THC), and femur length (FemL). Note the wide variation in each parameter's curve; this primarily results from the wide variation in LNMPs. *B*, The same data as shown in *A* but plotted against the average age of multiple fetal parameters (n ≤ 9 parameters/case). Here each parameter's curve has much less variation.

variation of the LNMP. Again, these are only representative parameters. It can be observed that both parameters have a close correlation with the AA; however, the femoral age exhibits slightly greater variation around the trend line.

Once the equivalent ages were calculated for all parameters, the residuals were calculated by subtracting the MFP AA from each parameter age of each fetus. This process resulted in positive (+) residuals for parameters that were relatively larger (parameter age greater than the AA) and negative (−) parameters for those that were relatively smaller. The residuals for the femur length and THC are plotted in Figure 8–21*B*. It is easier to observe in Figure 8–21*B* that the femur length varies more than the THC throughout pregnancy. It can also be observed that the residuals increase as the AA increases—that is, the variation is a function of or is dependent on the time at which the parameter is measured. This was expected because it has been established that fetal parameters show more variation later in pregnancy.

The final treatment of the data was to express the parameter age residuals as a percentage of the AA. This was done to normalize the data and remove the dependency of the residuals on time. Figure 8–21*C* is an XY plot of the treatment. It is now easy to observe that the femur length has greater variation throughout pregnancy than does the THC. It can also be observed that the variation of both is a relatively constant percentage of the AA and that the femur length varies by less than about 9% to 10% and the THC varies by less than about 4% to 5% of the age. This fact is the basis of the age range analysis discussed in Chapter 7. After this final normalizing treatment of the data, the ANOVA was performed. The results were sorted in ascending values of variation. The ANOVA results are shown at the bottom of Tables 8–4*A* to *F*.

For some parameters, the fetal age was determined by computer software using an internal look-up table algorithm that interpolated each age to 0.1 week (0.1 week = approximately 17 hours).[55] Parameter ages determined from this computerized look-up table (see Table 7–1) have an abbreviation ending with *wk* (see Tables 8–3 and 8–4). Ad-

Text continued on page 196

TABLE 8–4A. **ANOVA AND CORRELATION: 300 RANDOM CASES OVER 15 WEEKS' AGE (OUT OF 10,336 CASES, 1984–1993)**

CORRELATION	LNMP	AA	FemL	2-D BPD	THC	3-D BPD	BPD	BiOD	CV	CHC	TriCD
LNMP	1.0000										
AA	0.9225	1.0000									
FemL	0.9167	0.9871	1.0000								
2-D BPD	0.9109	0.9933	0.9825	1.0000							
THC	0.9108	0.9929	0.9825	0.99995	1.0000						
3-D BPD	0.9083	0.9920	0.9813	0.9983	0.9985	1.000					
BPD	0.9081	0.9925	0.9787	0.9966	0.9957	0.9932	1.000				
BiOD	0.9072	0.9806	0.9699	0.9795	0.9791	0.9764	0.9778	1.000			
CV	0.90494	0.9853	0.9550	0.9716	0.9714	0.9728	0.9700	0.9448	1.000		
CHC	0.90490	0.9912	0.9782	0.9951	0.9949	0.9981	0.9939	0.9739	0.9730	1.000	
TriCD	0.9044	0.9898	0.9801	0.9938	0.9935	0.9952	0.9927	0.9760	0.9667	0.9957	1.00

ANOVA: SINGLE FACTOR SUMMARY

	(Parameter Age − AA)/AA			
Groups	*Count*	*Sum*	*Average*	*Variance*
Average cranial wk	300	−0.05	−0.0002	0.00026
rTHC age	300	0.23	0.0008	0.00040
r2D BPD age	300	−0.58	−0.0019	0.00040
r3D BPD age_2	300	0.52	0.0017	0.00041
THC wk	300	−0.95	−0.0032	0.00042
CV wk	300	−0.72	−0.0024	0.00043
rTHC Hadlock	300	−7.99	−0.0266	0.00045
CHC wk	300	−1.67	−0.0056	0.00058
rCV age	300	0.67	0.0022	0.00060

rCHC age	300	1.61	0.0054	0.00061
TriBPD wk	264	3.97	0.0150	0.00066
Average body wk	300	0.27	0.0009	0.00068
BPD wk	300	−0.84	−0.0028	0.00069
rBPD age_2	300	0.55	0.0018	0.00070
r3D BPD age	300	−4.20	−0.0140	0.00072
rBPD age	300	−4.34	−0.0145	0.00084
Fem wk	300	−0.40	−0.0013	0.00130
rTriBPD age	264	3.49	0.0132	0.00133
AC wk	300	1.38	0.0046	0.00135
Hum wk	300	0.48	0.0016	0.00155
BiOD wk	195	−0.75	−0.0038	0.00188
LNMP	248	1.69	0.0068	0.02502

ANOVA

Source of variation alpha = 0.001	SS	df	MS	F	*P* value	F crit
Between groups	0.48	21	0.0230	13.56	5.7E − 47	2.23
Within groups	10.77	6349	0.0017			
Total	11.25	6370				

Analysis of variance (ANOVA) and correlation matrices for the various parameters are shown. The correlations were performed twice on each in order to sort the correlation with the LNMP in descending order. The ANOVAs were sorted in ascending order. Three sets of data were used out of 10,336 consecutive referral cases examined from 1984 to the end of 1993 with fetal ages > 15 weeks (MSA: Austin, TX). A random set of 300, a set of 322/10,336 with TCI > 0.86, and a set of 357 with TCI < 0.74. The analysis was performed on each set and then a second time on a subset in which only the fetuses > 30 weeks were used. The correlations were performed on the LNMP, AA, and the measurement parameters shown. The ANOVAs were performed on the parameter age residuals as a percentage of the AA ({Parameter, age − AA}/AA). The analysis was done using Microsoft Excel 4.0 for Windows.

Correlation values are by definition between 1 and −1. The nearer to 0 the correlations are, the weaker the relationship. The nearer the correlation is to 1, then the stronger the correlation between X and Y (i.e., large values of Y will accompany large values for X). However, the nearer the correlation is to −1, the reverse is true: Larger values of Y will accompany smaller values for X. In fetal analysis, a negative correlation is impossible because it would mean that as one parameter grows larger the correlating parameter would grow smaller.

ANOVA, analysis of variance, is used to determine if the means of two or more samples are equal and to calculate sample variances. In these tests, the relative variances are the most important information. All ANOVAs found significant differences in the means, probably because of the large degrees of freedom (df) and the fact that some of the regressions are closely parallel but not precisely equal.

TABLE 8–4*B*. ANOVA AND CORRELATION: 105/300 RANDOM CASES OVER 30 WEEKS' AGE (OUT OF 10,336 CASES, 1984–1993)*

CORRELATION	LNMP	BiOD	FemL	AA	2-D BPD	THC	BPD	3-D BPD	CV	CHC	TriCD
LNMP	1.0000										
BiOD	0.7395	1.0000									
FemL	0.6132	0.7749	1.0000								
AA	0.5893	0.8916	0.8870	1.0000							
2-D BPD	0.5059	0.8131	0.7657	0.9489	1.0000						
THC	0.5033	0.8027	0.7623	0.9437	0.9991	1.000					
BPD	0.4897	0.8451	0.7439	0.9309	0.9462	0.9314	1.000				
3-D BPD	0.4866	0.7730	0.7546	0.9429	0.9720	0.9748	0.8931	1.000			
CV	0.4735	0.7695	0.7475	0.9379	0.9491	0.9510	0.8787	0.9942	1.000		
CHC	0.4670	0.7925	0.7381	0.9351	0.9195	0.9131	0.9142	0.9637	0.9763	1.000	
TriCD	0.4582	0.8325	0.7511	0.9257	0.8875	0.8809	0.8911	0.9079	0.9171	0.9292	1.00

ANOVA: SINGLE FACTOR SUMMARY

	(Parameter Age − AA)/AA			
Groups	*Count*	*Sum*	*Average*	*Variance*
Average cranial wk	105	0.35	0.0033	0.00035
r2D BPD age	105	0.44	0.0042	0.00052
r3D BPD age_2	105	0.39	0.0037	0.00058
rTHC age	105	−0.45	−0.0043	0.00059

CV wk	105	0.66	0.0063	0.00060
rTHC Hadlock	105	−1.97	−0.0188	0.00060
THC wk	105	0.29	0.0028	0.00065
rCHC age	105	0.44	0.0042	0.00067
r3D BPD age	105	−4.01	−0.0382	0.00067
rBPD age	105	−3.72	−0.0354	0.00069
rCV age	105	0.61	0.0058	0.00072
CHC wk	105	−0.11	−0.0010	0.00075
rTriBPD age	87	−2.12	−0.0244	0.00079
TriBPD wk	87	0.59	0.0068	0.00083
rBPD age_2	105	0.84	0.0080	0.00083
Average body wk	105	−0.35	−0.0033	0.00093
BPD wk	105	0.24	0.0023	0.00097
Fem wk	105	−1.28	−0.0122	0.00152
AC wk	105	0.70	0.0067	0.00158
BiOD wk	47	−0.52	−0.0111	0.00230
Hum wk	105	−0.39	−0.0037	0.00231
LNMP	91	1.81	0.0199	0.00824

ANOVA

Source of variation alpha = 0.001	SS	df	MS	F	*P* value	F crit
Between groups	0.44	21	0.0210	17.56	7.5E − 47	2.24
Within groups	2.60	2180	0.0012			
Total	3.04	2201				

*See footnote to Table 8–4*A*.

TABLE 8–4*C*. **ANOVA AND CORRELATION: MODERATE BRACHYCEPHALIC—ALL CASES OUT OF 10,336 WITH TCI > 0.86 AND FETAL AGE > 15 WEEKS (1984–1993)***

CORRELATION	LNMP	FemL	AA	3-D BPD	CHC	BPD	2-D BPD	THC	CV	TriCD	BiOD
LNMP	1.0000										
FemL	0.9667	1.0000									
AA	0.9662	0.9942	1.0000								
3-D BPD	0.9586	0.9911	0.9951	1.0000							
CHC	0.9582	0.9902	0.9941	0.9993	1.0000						
BPD	0.9582	0.9911	0.9951	0.9984	0.9968	1.000					
2-D BPD	0.9579	0.9910	0.9950	0.9989	0.9968	0.9996	1.000				
THC	0.9579	0.9909	0.9950	0.9989	0.9967	0.9995	0.999999	1.000			
CV	0.9548	0.9754	0.9898	0.9790	0.9790	0.9767	0.9771	0.9771	1.000		
TriCD	0.9523	0.9890	0.9934	0.9969	0.9965	0.9960	0.9960	0.9960	0.9751	1.000	
BiOD	0.9454	0.9877	0.9919	0.9903	0.9888	0.9914	0.9912	0.9912	0.9692	0.9890	1.00

ANOVA: SINGLE FACTOR SUMMARY

	(Parameter Age − AA)/AA			
Groups	*Count*	*Sum*	*Average*	*Variance*
Average cranial wk	322	1.28	0.0040	0.00018
CV wk	322	−5.48	−0.0170	0.00029
r3D BPD age_2	322	−4.73	−0.0147	0.00031
r2D BPD age	322	−4.83	−0.0150	0.00034

THC wk	322	−5.73	−0.0178	0.00038
rCV age	322	−5.13	−0.0159	0.00041
Average body wk	322	−1.19	−0.0037	0.00044
rTHC Hadlock	322	−11.59	−0.0360	0.00045
BPD wk	322	9.34	0.0290	0.00046
rBPD age_2	322	9.68	0.0301	0.00047
CHC wk	322	1.36	0.0042	0.00049
rTHC age	322	−4.76	−0.0148	0.00049
rCHC age	322	4.45	0.0138	0.00050
TriBPD wk	289	6.81	0.0236	0.00064
rBPD age	322	4.96	0.0154	0.00076
BiOD wk	215	−2.48	−0.0115	0.00095
Fem wk	322	−2.55	−0.0079	0.00103
Hum wk	321	−1.61	−0.0050	0.00106
r3D BPD age	322	−7.85	−0.0244	0.00112
AC wk	321	1.01	0.0031	0.00123
rTriBPD age	289	6.50	0.0225	0.00149
LNMP	271	3.71	0.0137	0.01013

ANOVA

Source of variation alpha = 0.001	SS	df	MS	F	*P* value	F crit
Between groups	2.22	21	0.1057	104.81	0.00E + 0	2.23
Within groups	6.89	6836	0.0010			
Total	9.11	6857				

*See footnote to Table 8–4*A*.

TABLE 8–4*D*. ANOVA AND CORRELATION: MODERATE BRACHYCEPHALIC—ALL CASES OUT OF 10,336 WITH TCI > 0.86 AND FETAL AGE > 30 WEEKS (1984–1993)*

CORRELATION	LNMP	FemL	AA	3-D BPD	CHC	BiOD	BPD	2-D BPD	THC	CV	TriCD
LNMP	1.0000										
FemL	0.7752	1.0000									
AA	0.7122	0.9091	1.0000								
3-D BPD	0.6344	0.8091	0.9611	1.0000							
CHC	0.6309	0.7866	0.9328	0.9810	1.0000						
BiOD	0.6241	0.7903	0.8894	0.7920	0.7595	1.000					
BPD	0.6202	0.8066	0.9507	0.9547	0.9013	0.8194	1.000				
2-D BPD	0.6150	0.8031	0.9516	0.9650	0.9013	0.8151	0.9917	1.000			
THC	0.6143	0.8025	0.9511	0.9651	0.9007	0.8144	0.9906	0.99997	1.000		
CV	0.6183	0.7891	0.9432	0.9918	0.9911	0.7681	0.9174	0.9289	0.9291	1.000	
TriCD	0.5591	0.7548	0.9105	0.9086	0.8935	0.7494	0.8777	0.8817	0.8814	0.8977	1.00

ANOVA: SINGLE FACTOR SUMMARY

	(Parameter Age − AA)/AA			
Groups	*Count*	*Sum*	*Average*	*Variance*
Average cranial wk	107	0.35	0.0033	0.00033
r3D BPD age_2	107	−2.55	−0.0238	0.00045
CV wk	107	−2.38	−0.0222	0.00046
rTHC Hadlock	107	−4.98	−0.0465	0.00050

r2D BPD age	107	−2.07	−0.0193	0.00053
THC wk	107	−2.83	−0.0264	0.00055
rTHC age	107	−3.42	−0.0320	0.00056
r3D BPD age	107	−6.87	−0.0642	0.00056
rBPD age_2	107	4.24	0.0396	0.00058
rCV age	107	−2.00	−0.0187	0.00061
rBPD age	107	−1.33	−0.0124	0.00061
BPD wk	107	4.18	0.0391	0.00066
Average body wk	107	−0.37	−0.0035	0.00075
rCHC age	107	1.25	0.0117	0.00079
CHC wk	107	1.08	0.0101	0.00079
rTriBPD age	101	−1.91	−0.0189	0.00094
TriBPD wk	101	1.77	0.0175	0.00109
Fem wk	107	−0.92	−0.0086	0.00136
Hum wk	106	−0.55	−0.0052	0.00150
AC wk	107	0.32	0.0030	0.00163
BiOD wk	56	−0.61	−0.0109	0.00174
LNMP	93	0.92	0.0099	0.00451

ANOVA

Source of variation alpha = 0.001	SS	df	MS	F	*P* value	F crit
Between groups	1.37	21	0.0650	69.41	9.6E − 47	2.24
Within groups	2.11	2254	0.0009			
Total	3.48	2275				

*See footnote to Table 8–4*A*.

TABLE 8–4*E*. ANOVA AND CORRELATION: MODERATE DOLICHOCEPHALIC—ALL CASES OUT OF 10,336 WITH TCI < 0.74 AND FETAL AGE > 15 WEEKS (1984–1993)*

CORRELATION	LNMP	AA	2-D BPD	BPD	THC	3-D BPD	CHC	FemL	CV	TriCD	BiOD
LNMP	1.0000										
AA	0.8939	1.0000									
2-D BPD	0.8885	0.9939	1.0000								
BPD	0.8883	0.9930	0.9988	1.0000							
THC	0.8883	0.9938	0.99996	0.9984	1.0000						
3-D BPD	0.8859	0.9935	0.9978	0.9957	0.9979	1.000					
CHC	0.8823	0.9908	0.9935	0.9926	0.9934	0.9984	1.000				
FemL	0.8817	0.9794	0.9742	0.9720	0.9743	0.9746	0.9715	1.000			
CV	0.8793	0.9859	0.9730	0.9717	0.9730	0.9741	0.9723	0.9463	1.000		
TriCD	0.8763	0.9908	0.9924	0.9913	0.9924	0.9958	0.9957	0.9688	0.9709	1.000	
BiOD	0.8583	0.9823	0.9798	0.9782	0.9797	0.9798	0.9767	0.9573	0.9488	0.9769	1.00

ANOVA: SINGLE FACTOR SUMMARY

	(Parameter Age − AA)/AA			
Groups	*Count*	*Sum*	*Average*	*Variance*
Average cranial wk	357	−2.83	−0.0079	0.00025
r3D BPD age_2	357	5.14	0.0144	0.00038
rTHC age	357	3.94	0.0110	0.00043
CV wk	357	3.91	0.0110	0.00044

BPD wk	357	−14.97	−0.0419	0.00044
r3D BPD age	357	1.26	0.0035	0.00048
rBPD age_2	357	−14.06	−0.0394	0.00048
THC wk	357	1.81	0.0051	0.00050
CHC wk	357	−6.76	−0.0189	0.00051
rCHC age	357	−2.20	−0.0062	0.00053
r2D BPD age	357	−0.04	−0.0001	0.00054
rCV age	357	4.47	0.0125	0.00055
Average body wk	357	4.70	0.0132	0.00057
rBPD age	357	−16.31	−0.0457	0.00058
rTHC Hadlock	357	−7.20	−0.0202	0.00059
TriBPD wk	291	2.79	0.0096	0.00062
rTriBPD age	291	3.88	0.0133	0.00106
AC wk	357	4.42	0.0124	0.00137
BiOD wk	231	−0.91	−0.0039	0.00143
Hum wk	355	5.06	0.0143	0.00147
Fem wk	357	5.07	0.0142	0.00153
LNMP	281	6.05	0.0215	0.01674

ANOVA

Source of variation alpha = 0.001	SS	df	MS	F	*P* value	F crit
Between groups	2.92	21	0.1389	107.99	0.00E + 0	2.23
Within groups	9.64	7496	0.0013			
Total	12.56	7517				

*See footnote to Table 8–4*A*.

TABLE 8–4*F*. **ANOVA AND CORRELATION: MODERATE DOLICHOCEPHALIC—ALL CASES OUT OF 10,336 WITH TCI < 0.74 AND FETAL AGE > 30 WEEKS (1984–1993)***

CORRELATION	LNMP	AA	3-D BPD	CV	THC	2-D BPD	BPD	CHC	TriCD	BiOD	FemL
LNMP	1.0000										
AA	0.4928	1.0000									
3-D BPD	0.4778	0.9598	1.0000								
CV	0.4717	0.9488	0.9911	1.0000							
THC	0.4715	0.9428	0.9606	0.9213	1.0000						
2-D BPD	0.4712	0.9446	0.9586	0.9197	0.9995	1.000					
BPD	0.4604	0.9362	0.9292	0.8933	0.9775	0.9837	1.000				
CHC	0.4524	0.9260	0.9678	0.9870	0.8696	0.8706	0.8601	1.000			
TriCD	0.3713	0.9255	0.9221	0.9190	0.8810	0.8819	0.8703	0.9102	1.000		
BiOD	0.3588	0.8798	0.8154	0.8193	0.7937	0.7988	0.8110	0.8075	0.7663	1.000	
FemL	0.3598	0.7202	0.6096	0.5951	0.6128	0.6121	0.5939	0.5673	0.5126	0.4334	1.00

ANOVA: SINGLE FACTOR SUMMARY

	(Parameter Age − AA)/AA			
Groups	*Count*	*Sum*	*Average*	*Variance*
Average cranial wk	86	−0.33	−0.0038	0.00028
r3D BPD age_2	86	2.04	0.0237	0.00037
r3D BPD age	86	−1.67	−0.0194	0.00045
rBPD age	86	−5.75	−0.0669	0.00049

CV wk	86	2.28	0.0265	0.00050
rTHC age	86	1.35	0.0157	0.00051
rCV age	86	1.77	0.0206	0.00053
r2D BPD age	86	1.41	0.0164	0.00054
rBPD age_2	86	−2.92	−0.0340	0.00055
rTriBPD age	69	−1.78	−0.0258	0.00057
BPD wk	86	−3.65	−0.0424	0.00059
TriBPD wk	69	−0.20	−0.0029	0.00063
rCHC age	86	−0.90	−0.0105	0.00064
rTHC Hadlock	86	0.06	0.0007	0.00064
THC wk	86	1.87	0.0217	0.00066
Average body wk	86	0.69	0.0080	0.00068
CHC wk	86	−1.68	−0.0195	0.00074
AC wk	86	1.60	0.0186	0.00119
Hum wk	85	0.26	0.0031	0.00150
BiOD wk	39	−0.71	−0.0182	0.00226
Fem wk	86	0.29	0.0034	0.00311
LNMP	71	2.41	0.0339	0.01024

ANOVA

Source of variation alpha = 0.001	SS	df	MS	F	P value	F crit
Between groups	1.12	21	0.0531	45.47	6.0E − 47	2.25
Within groups	2.07	1773	0.0012			
Total	3.19	1794				

*See footnote to Table 8–4*A*.

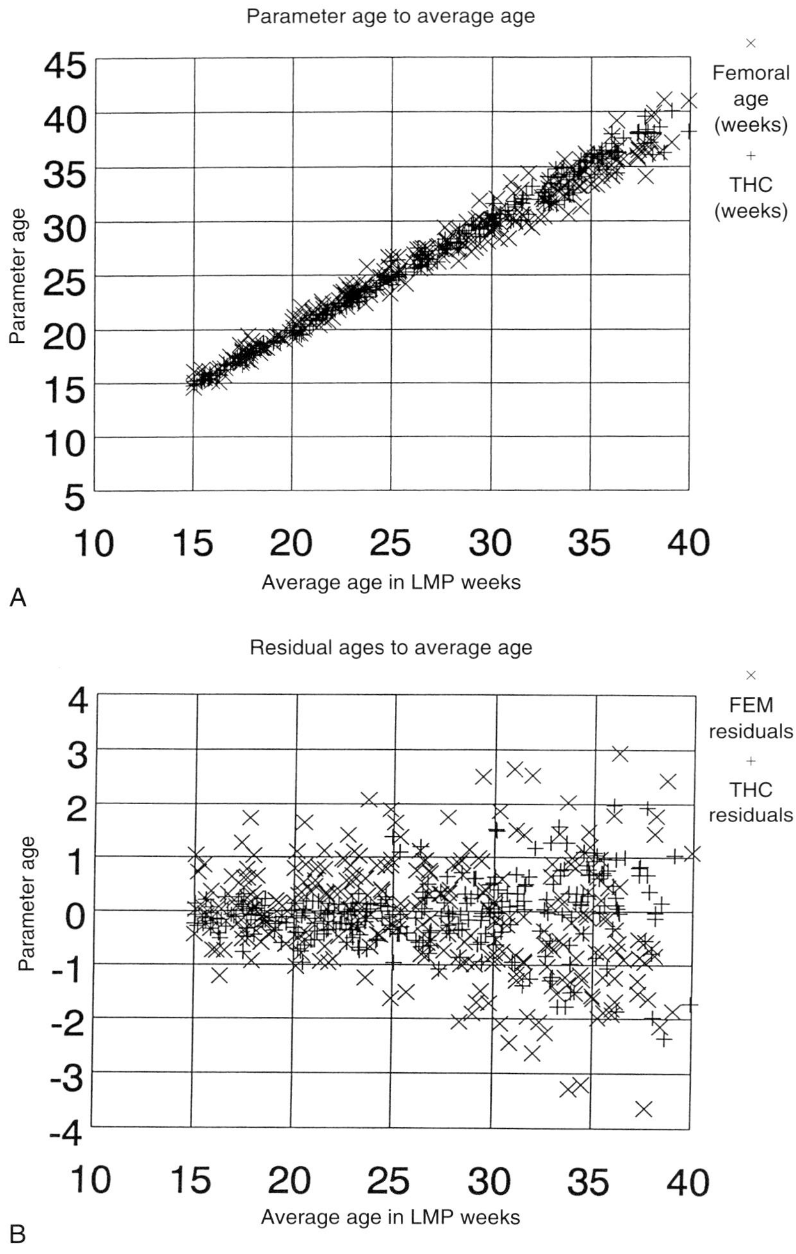

FIGURE 8–21.
Data treatments. Graphic representations of the data treatments used to arrive at the statistical analysis in Tables 8–4*A* through *F*. In these examples, only two parameters (femur length [FemL] and transverse head circumference [THC]) are shown because more parameters would produce graphs too confusing to discuss and because most sonographers are familiar with these. The same procedures were performed for each parameter in Table 8–3. *A*, Scattergram of the femoral and THC ages plotted against the multiple fetal parameter average age in equivalent LMP weeks. Each parameter age was determined by computer software from a look-up table; ages were interpolated to 0.1 week (17 hours). This view looks at parameter age as function of size in time, or a "size-age" or "sonographic age." Note that both the femoral age in weeks and THC in weeks correlate well with the average age. The femoral age can be observed to have greater variation because the X plots are always the most extreme above and below the trend. *B*, Residuals were calculated by subtracting the average age for a fetus from each parameter age for that same fetus. In this way, relatively large parameters yield residuals that are positive, and relatively small parameters yield negative parameters. Note that the residuals increase in dispersion (variation) with time.

ditional ages were estimated by regression formulas using a computer spreadsheet; these have abbreviations starting with *r* and ending with *age*. These regression formulas were derived using locally weighted smoothing functions (LOWESS)[40] to determine the mean age for each calculation. These LOWESS means were used in a computer program to perform multiple regressions on the data. The regressions finally used were chosen on the basis of two criteria, ease of use and a relatively high correlation coefficient. These regressions were then modified by trial and error using a spreadsheet to minimize the residuals' means and standard deviations. The resulting regression formulas are given in Table 8–3*B*. A regression formula for the age from the THC that was published by Hadlock and colleagues is included for comparison.[56]

The correlation matrices are sorted in de-

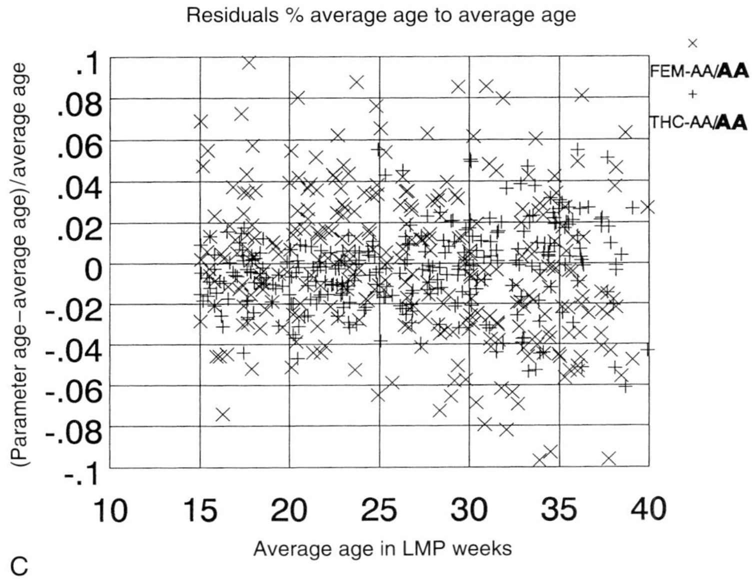

FIGURE 8–21. *Continued—C,* Normalized residuals. To remove the variations' dependence on time, each residual was divided by its average age to yield the residual as a percentage of that fetus's age. This makes the variation of the residuals relatively uniform throughout pregnancy. It is now easy to observe that the femur has a variation about twice that of the THC. The femur variation is less than ±10% of the age, and the variation of the THC is approximately less than ±5% of the age.

scending order of correlation with the LNMP ages—that is, the closest correlations are near the top. It is noted that in all sets, the AA and femur length ages correlate most closely with the LNMP except in the set of fetuses with a TCI less than 0.74 (relatively dolichocephalic). In one set, the femur dropped to the bottom of the correlation matrix and the 3-D BPD moved into the second highest correlation. The 3-D BPD also rated high in both sets (>15 and >30 weeks) with TCIs greater than 0.86 (relatively brachycephalic). It is also noted that in all cross-correlations, particularly the AA, the populations greater than 15 weeks of age have higher correlations than those greater than 30 weeks. This is because of molding and greater fetal individuation toward term.

The ANOVAs were sorted in descending order, with the smallest variations at the top and the greatest variations at the bottom of the column (variance). The ANOVA results for the random 300 data sets, which have a normal distribution of head shapes, reveal little pattern except that in general, head parameter ages have less variation than body parameters. In all sets, the body parameters (humerus length, femur length, and abdominal circumference) have variances that are twice as great as those of the cranial parameters. It is noted that the binocular distance always exhibits a relatively large variance toward the bottom with the body parameters. The LNMP, of course, always has the largest variation. In the fetuses with relatively brachycephalic and dolichocephalic heads, the 3-D parameters tend toward the smaller variances, particularly after 30 weeks, but this is not a hard-and-fast rule. The high *P* values in the ANOVAs mean that there is at least one parameter (group) for which the mean is statistically different from the other groups; however, this is also affected by the fact that the degrees of freedom are large.

Many will find this analysis tedious, confusing, and unnecessarily complex. Others may consider it simplistic and naive. It is presented here in the interest of documenting what has been learned about the solid geometry of the fetal cranium and its progressive growth. It is reiterated that in normally shaped heads, any cranial parameter is a reliable indicator of fetal age, as is the femur. The caveat is that if only one or two measurements are taken, then how is one to prove that the head is normally shaped? This becomes especially important when realizing that the fetal cranium can be compressed in the vertical axis, causing both the BPD and FOD to be slightly exaggerated and retaining a normal TCI (see Fig. 8–17). This latter situation is not uncommon after 30 weeks' gestation, and only 3-D measurements provide the most accurate size/age estimates. It is also possible for the reverse situation to occur when the BPD and FOD are compressed and the VCD exaggerated.

It can be seen from Table 8–4 that 3-D measurements in general have larger correlations and smaller variations as the fetal head becomes more abnormally shaped as a result of molding toward term, and that no one parameter is perfect in all situations. After 30 weeks, the 3-D BPD exhibits high correlation with the LNMP and AA while maintaining low variances. Of course, the MFP AA is always the best estimator of age, and the femur and humerus lengths are useful comparative parameters even though they exhibit the larger variations of the body.

These statistical analyses were performed using MicroSoft Excel 5.0 for Windows[52] on a 386sx personal computer. The fetal ages were determined using Basic Baby II[55] for the look-up table interpolation and FrameWork IV[57] for the spreadsheet LOWESS smoothing and regression formula modifications. The original regression formulas (except for Hadlock and colleagues, rTHC Hadlock) were derived using curve-fitting software called TableCurve.[58]

REFERENCES

1. DuBose TJ: Fetal biometry: Vertical calvarial diameter and calvarial volume. J Diagn Med Sonogr 1985; 1:205–217.
2. Berman MC, ed: Winners of the 1986 Kenneth Gottesfeld Awards. J Diagn Med Sonogr 1985;2:181–182.
3. Goldberg BB, Kurtz AB: Atlas of Ultrasound Measurements. Year Book Medical Publishers, Chicago, 1990, p 278.
4. Kurtz AB, Goldberg BB: Fetal head measurements. In: Kurtz AB, Goldberg BB, eds: Obstetrical Measurements in Ultrasound: A Reference Manual. Year Book Medical Publishers, Chicago, 1988, pp 22–35.
5. DuBose TJ: Assessment of fetal age and size: Techniques and criteria. In: Berman MC, ed: Obstetrics & Gynecology: Diagnostic Medical Sonography, A Guide to Clinical Practice, vol 1. JB Lippincott, Philadelphia, 1991, pp 279–289.
6. Hadlock FP, Deter RL, Carpenter RJ, et al: Estimating fetal age: Effect of head shape on BPD. AJR 1981;137:83–85.
7. Da Vinci L: The skull: Interior view. In: Leonardo da Vinci, The Anatomy of Man. Drawings from the Collection of Her Majesty Queen Elizabeth II, Windsor Castle, Royal Library; published by Museum of Fine Arts, Houston; Bullfinch Press of Little, Brown & Co, Boston, 1992, p 36.
8. Willocks J, Donald I, Duggan TC, et al: Foetal cephalometry by ultrasound. J Obstet Gynaecol Br Commonw 1964;71:11–20.
9. Campbell S: Ultrasonic fetal cephalometry during the second trimester of pregnancy. J Obstet Gynaecol Br Commonw 1970;77:1057–1063.
10. Davison JM, Lind T, Farr V, et al: The limitations of ultrasonic fetal cephalometry. J Obstet Gynaecol Br Commonw 1973;80:769–775.
11. Sabbagha RE, Barton FB, Barton BA: Sonar biparietal diameter: I. Analysis of percentile growth differences in two normal populations using same methodology. Am J Obstet Gynecol 1976;126:479.
12. Sabbagha RE, Barton FB, Barton BA, et al: Sonar biparietal diameter: II. Predictive of three fetal growth patterns leading to a closer assessment of gestational age and neonatal weight. Am J Obstet Gynecol 1976;126:485.
13. Kurtz AB, Wapner RJ, Kurtz RJ, et al: Analysis of biparietal diameter as an accurate indicator of gestational age. J Clin Ultrasound 1980;8:319–326.
14. Hadlock FP, Deter RL, Harrist RB, et al: Fetal head circumference: Relation to menstrual age. AJR 1982;138:649–653.
15. Abbott EA: Flatland, a Romance of Many Dimensions, by a Square, 6th ed. Dover, New York, 1952.
16. Burger D: Sphereland: A Fantasy About Curved Spaces and an Expanding Universe. Thomas Y. Crowell, New York, 1965.
17. Ellis GFR, Williams RM: Flat and Curved Space-Times. Oxford University Press, Oxford, 1988.
18. Kurtz AB, Wapner RJ, Kurtz RJ, et al: Analysis of biparietal diameter as an accurate indicator of gestational age. J Clin Ultrasound 1980;8:319–326.
19 Goldberg BB, Kurtz AB: Atlas of Ultrasound Measurements. Year Book Medical Publishers, Chicago, 1990, p 8.
20. McDicken WN: Diagnostic Ultrasonics: Principles and Use of Instruments. Churchill Livingstone, New York, 1991, p 150.
21. Goldberg BB, Kurtz AB: Atlas of Ultrasound Measurements. Year Book Medical Publishers, Chicago, 1990, pp 264–265.
22. Eastman NJ, Hellman LM: Williams' Obstetrics. Appleton-Century-Crofts, New York, 1961, pp 416–417.
23. DuBose TJ: Assessment of fetal age and size: Techniques and criteria. In: Berman MC, ed: Obstetrics & Gynecology: Diagnostic Medical Sonography, A Guide to Clinical Practice, vol 1. JB Lippincott, Philadelphia, 1991, p 287.
24. O'Keeffe DF, Garite TJ, Elliott JP, et al: The accuracy of estimated gestational age based on ultrasound measurement of biparietal diameter in preterm premature rupture of membranes. Am J Obstet Gynecol 1985;151:309–312.
25. Carlan SJ, Wyble L, Lense J, et al: Fetal head molding: Diagnosis by ultrasound and a review of the literature. J Perinatol 1991;11:105–111.
26. DuBose TJ: 3-D BPD correction. J Ultrasound Med 1988;7:S97.
27. Hansmann M, Hackeloer BJ, Staudach A: Normal fetal anatomy in the second and third trimester. In: Hansmann M, Hackeloer BJ, Staudach A, eds: Ultrasound Diagnosis in Obstetrics and Gynecology. Springer-Verlag, New York, 1985, pp 169–175.
28. Athey PA, Hadlock FP: Ultrasound in Obstetrics and Gynecology. CV Mosby, St Louis, 1981, pp 23–36.
29. Fiske CE, Filly RA: Ultrasound evaluation of the normal and abnormal fetal neural axis. In: Callen PW, ed: Ultrasonography in Obstetrics and Gynecology. WB Saunders, Philadelphia, 1983, p 100.
30. Selman J: The Fundamentals of X-Ray and Radium Physics, 4th ed. Charles C Thomas, Springfield, IL, 1965, pp 280–281, 295.
31. Selman J: The Fundamentals of X-Ray and Radium

Physics, 6th ed. Charles C Thomas, Springfield, IL, 1978, 6th ed., p 358.
32. Jenkins D: Radiographic Photography and Imaging Processes. University Park Press, Baltimore, 1980, p 143.
33. Goldkrand JW, Kuhlman T, Fox E, et al: Coronal biparietal diameter: A reliable alternative to the traditional transverse biparietal diameter. J Ultrasound Med 1990;9:555.
34. Weinraub Z, Herman A, Ron-El R, et al: Measuring coronal biparietal diameter. J Ultrasound Med 1991;10:486.
35. Hodgman CD, ed: CRC Standard Mathematical Tables, 12th ed. Chemical Rubber Publishing Co, Cleveland, 1959, p 397.
36. Beyer WH: CRC Standard Mathematical Tables, 28th ed. CRC Press, Boca Raton, FL, 1987, p 122.
37. Holland E: Cranial stress in the fetus during labor and the effects of external pressure on the intracranial contents, with an analysis of eighty-one cases of torn tentorium cerebelli and subdural cerebral hemorrhage. J Obstet Gynaecol Br Commonw 1922; 29:549.
38. Haas LL: Roentgenological skull measurements and their diagnostic applications. Am J Roentgenol 1952;67:197–209.
39. Jordaan HVF: The differential enlargement neurocranium in the fullterm fetus. S Afr Med J 1976; 50:1978–1981.
40. Cleveland WS: The Elements of Graphing Data. Wadsworth Advanced Books and Software, Monterey, CA, 1985, pp 169–179.
41. Law RJ, MacRae MA: Head circumference as an index of fetal age. J Ultrasound Med 1982;1:281–288.
42. Ott WJ: The use of ultrasonic fetal head circumference for calculating expected date of confinement. (abstract 507). AIUM Proceedings, New York, Oct. 18–21, 1983., p 246.
43. Goldberg BB, Kurtz AB: Atlas of Ultrasound Measurements. Year Book Medical Publishers, Chicago, 1990, pp 274–277.
44. DalCompo S, Sabbagha RE: Intrauterine growth retardation. In Berman MC, ed: Diagnostic Medical Sonography, vol 1. Obstetrics and Gynecology. JB Lippincott, Philadelphia, 1991, p 463.
45. Goldberg BB, Kurtz AB: Atlas of Ultrasound Measurements. Year Book Medical Publishers, Chicago, 1990, p 277.
46. Doubilet PM, Greens RA: Improved prediction of gestational age from fetal head measurements. AJR 1984;142:797–800.
47. Jordaan HV, Sattar FA, Shah P, et al: Simplified method of determining fetal brain weight in utero. Obstet Gynecol 1980;55:673–677.
48. Jordaan HVF, Clark BW: Prenatal determination of fetal brain and somatic weight by ultrasound. Am J Obstet Gynecol 1980;136:54–59.
49. Jordaan HVF, Dunn LJ: A new method of evaluating fetal growth. Obstet Gynecol 1977;51:659–665.
50. Beyer WH: CRC Standard Mathematical Tables, 28th ed. CRC Press, Boca Raton, FL, 1987, pp 130–131.
51. Hopman WPM, Rosenbusch G, Jansen JBMJ, et al: Gallbladder contraction: Effect of fatty meals and cholecystokinin. Radiology 1985;157:37–39.
52. Excel and Windows software. MicroSoft, P.O. Box 3011, Bothell, WA 98041-3011.
53. Resnik R: Post-term pregnancy. In: Creasy RK, Resnik R, eds: Maternal-Fetal Medicine: Principles & Practice. WB Saunders, Philadelphia, 1989, p 505.
54. Cunningham FG, MacDonald PC, Gant NF, eds: Williams Obstetrics, 18th ed. Appleton & Lange, Norwalk, CT, 1989, pp 2, 741–742.
55. Basic Baby II. Obstetrical Software, 811 West 31st Street, Austin, TX, 78705-2109.
56. Hadlock FP, Deter RL, Harrist RB, et al: Estimating fetal age: Computer assisted analysis of multiple fetal growth parameters. Radiology 1984;152:499.
57. FrameWork IV, Integrated Software. Ashton-Tate, 20101 Hamilton Avenue, Torrance, CA 90509-9972.
58. TableCurve. Jandel Scientific, 2591 Kerner Boulevard, San Rafael, CA 94901.

CHAPTER 9

FETAL HEAD AND SPINE

Terry J. DuBose
J. Neal Rutledge

Modern real-time sonographic equipment allows detailed study of the anatomy of the fetal head. Many early fetal cranial studies were concerned with the geometry, as described in Chapter 8. This chapter illustrates and discusses the anatomy of the normal fetal head and spine.

Although the stated purpose of this text is to describe the normal fetus sonographically, some relatively common and important abnormalities are discussed from time to time as appropriate. At these times, some of the techniques that researchers have developed to assist sonographers in distinguishing the subtle abnormalities from normal fetal anatomy are highlighted.

Embryonic

ORDER OF DEVELOPMENT

The embryonic head and brain tissue begin to differentiate by day 17 after conception or in the early fourth week after the last menstrual period (LMP).[1] This is about the time a woman usually begins to realize that she may be pregnant.

Sonographically, the embryonic disk or embryonic pole becomes visible during the fifth menstrual week (LMP). It is in the late fourth or early fifth week that the embryonic heartbeat may be first detected by transvaginal sonography. At 5 to 6 weeks of gestation, or 7 to 8 LMP weeks, the head becomes distinguishable from the embryonic body. The head at this early time is as large as the embryonic body.[2] When a transabdominal approach is used, identification of the beating heart may be the only way to determine which end is which.

By the end of the eighth LMP week, the head with its cystic rhombencephalon is easily distinguishable from the body and spine (Figs. 9–1*A* to 9–2*B*). The spine in the early embryonic stages is simply two rows of echoes (see Fig. 9–2*B*). The head may even be measured; however, the crown-rump length (CRL) remains the measurement of choice until the end of the first trimester because of its greater accuracy due to its relatively larger size. The head is still so small at this stage that any slight error in plane of view or cursor placement results in relatively larger errors in age estimates (see Chapter 8 for a discussion of head biometry; see Chapter 18 for week-by-week sonographic depiction of first-trimester development).

In the ninth LMP week, the head can be easily measured, even transabdominally (Fig. 9–3*A* and *B*). In these images, the head is measured in the transverse and coronal

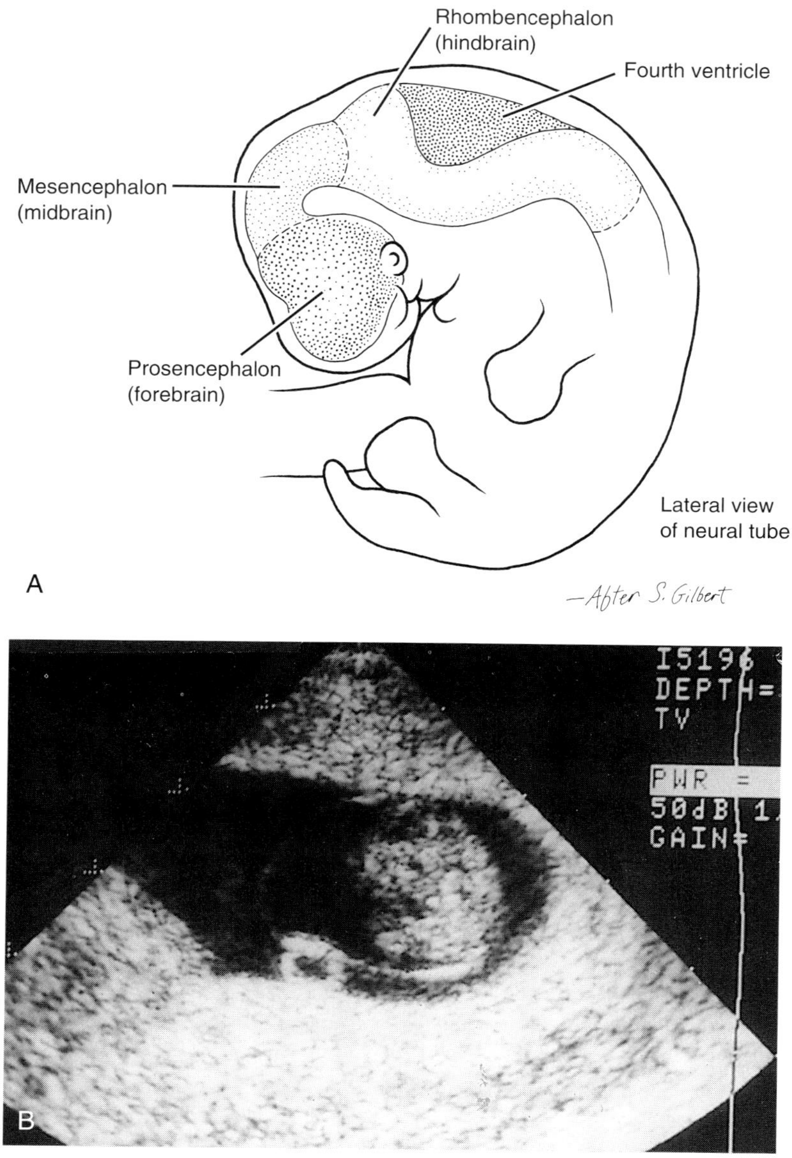

FIGURE 9–1.
Sagittal 8-LMP-week embryo. *A*, The major portions of the embryonic brain are seen at approximately 37 conceptual days (7–8.0 LMP weeks), Streeter's Carnegie stage 16–17. The prosencephalon or forebrain is divided into approximately two halves at the eye. The more anterior portion is the telencephalon, and the more posterior half is the diencephalon. (Adapted from Gilbert SG: Pictorial Human Embryology. University of Washington Press, Seattle, 1989, p 129.) *B*, Transvaginal sonogram of an embryo that correlates with the schematic in *A*. (AA = 7.7, n = 4, range = 0.7 weeks)

planes. Note that the interhemispheric fissure (midline) is obvious at this time. The echogenic areas at the bottom of the midline are the developing facial bones (see Fig. 9–3*A*). This is a normally proportioned embryo well within 1 SD of the mean for the range parameter ages (see Chapter 7 for more discussion of the age range analysis and size/age analysis).

The embryogenic period is completed by the end of the 10th LMP week. The fetus has human features, but the head is proportionately larger than the body and makes up almost half of the embryonic mass.[3] After the embryonic period, all the fetal tissues are present, and the primary change thereafter is in the size of the organs as growth proceeds rapidly.

RHOMBENCEPHALON

In the seventh and eighth LMP week, the most sonographically discernible component of the embryonic head is the rhombencephalon (see Figs. 9–1*A* and *B*).[4] The rhombencephalon, a cystic structure in the posterior

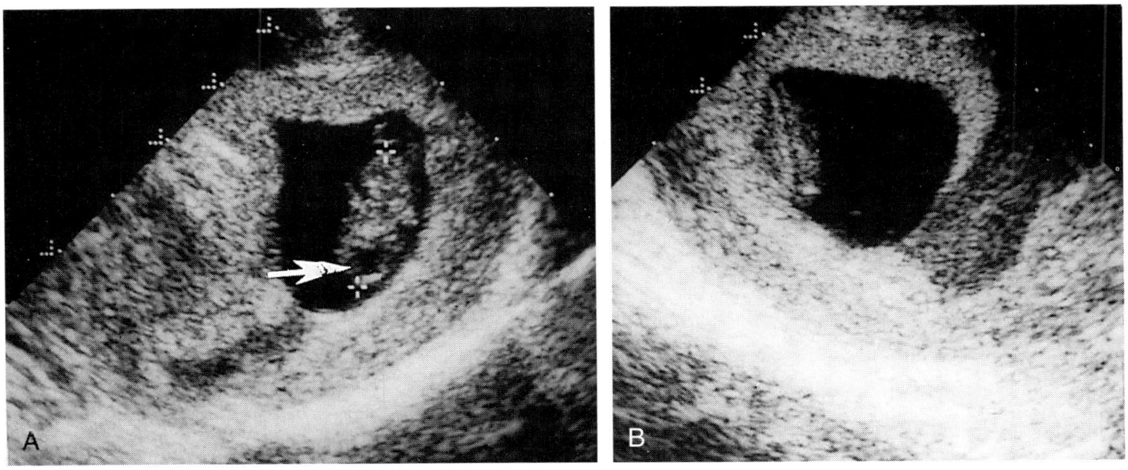

FIGURE 9–2.
Coronal 8-LMP-week embryo. *A*, This embryo with its head down is approximately the same age as the one in Figure 9–1. The crown-rump length measured 17.6 mm. The cystic formation (arrow) is the roof of the developing fourth ventricle and is posterior to the rhombencephalon, which comprises the metencephalon and myelencephalon. *B*, This image is more posterior in the embryo. Note that the spine appears as a double row of echoes. (AA = 8.3 LMP weeks, n = 5, range = 1.0 weeks, TD)

portion of the head, develops into the fourth ventricle and hindbrain, including the pons, cerebellum, and medulla oblongata.[5–7]

Sonographers must take care not to mistake the cystic yolk sac, which is in close proximity to the embryo, for the cystic rhombencephalon. This mistake could lead to erroneously long CRL measurements.

Second and Third Trimesters

SKULL

In fetal life, the skull is made up of several discrete bones and cartilaginous connective tissues. The primary areas are the two frontal eminences, the two parietal eminences, the occipital bone, and the chondrocranium or cartilaginous base of the skull[8] (Figs. 9–4 and 9–5).

The bones of the calvarium are separated by fibrous areas called *sutures*; the sutures intersect at the fontanelles. Figure 9–5 sonographically demonstrates the metopic suture above the nose. These fibrous connective tissues are hypoechoic and allow the skull to mold or change in response to external pressures. This molding is commonly recognized during passage through the birth canal. Molding has received less attention in the prenatal period because little was known about it until sonography allowed accurate measurements in utero.[9]

Frontal Bone

The fetal skull frontal bone is made up of two curved or cup-shaped plates, the frontal eminences, which cover the anterior aspect of the brain. Between these two plates is the frontal or metopic suture, which joins superiorly into the anterior fontanelle (see Figs. 9–4 and 9–5). On either side and posterior to the frontal eminences are the left and right coronal sutures, which also join the anterior fontanelle at the top of the head.[10, 11]

The area of the frontal bone is commonly known as the forehead. This is one of the terminal points of measurement for the fronto-occipital diameter (FOD)[12–15] of the skull and is the longitudinal skull diameter (LSD).[16–18] This diameter of the fetal skull is also sometimes known as the occipitofrontal diameter.[19, 20] Here we use the more common FOD.

Occipital Bone

The occiput or occipital bone encloses the posterior base of the brain (Figs. 9–4 and 9–6). The occipital bone forms the posterior portion of the foramen magnum around the

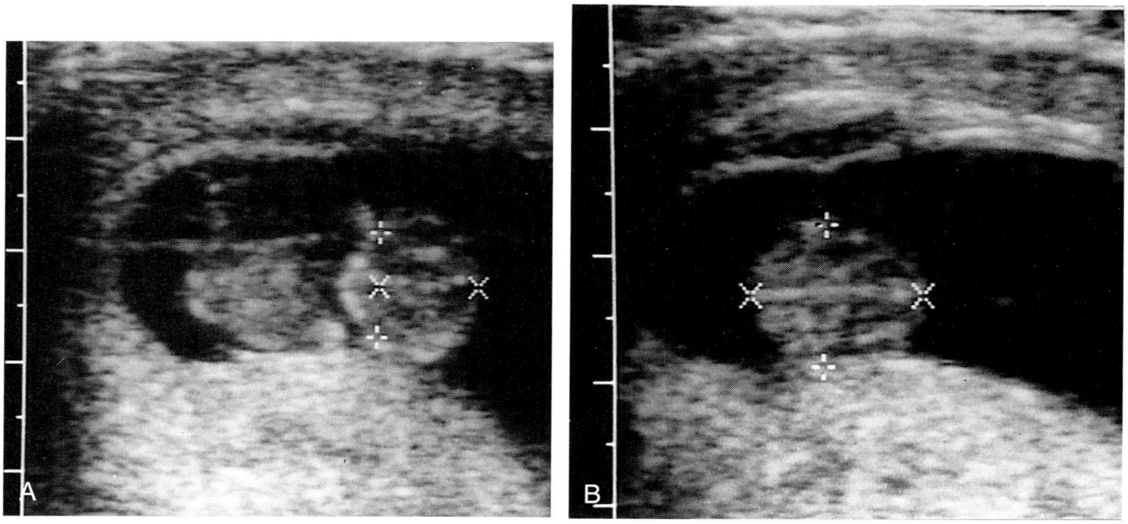

FIGURE 9–3.
Embryonic head in the ninth LMP week. *A*, In this coronal plane of the embryo, the head can be observed to be larger than the body. The interhemispheric fissure, midline, of the brain can be observed (ventrical cranial diameter [VCD] between X cursors = 9.6 mm). The + cursors are measuring the hippocampal base line (HBL = 9.6 mm) or the base of the coronal triangle. Note the very circular appearance of the cranium in this view. *B*, This is the transverse head circumference from the same embryo. The interhemispheric fissure is clear. The biparietal diameter (+ cursors) measured 11.4 mm, and the fronto-occipital diameter measured 14.2 mm. Using the VCD measurement from image *A* as the third dimension of the skull, the cranial volume was calculated to be 0.9 ml. (AA = 9.5 LMP weeks, n = 8, range = 1.2 weeks, TD)

spine. It is a curved, somewhat triangular bone that is bounded on the sides by the left and right lambdoid sutures. These sutures join at the top of the occipital bone with the sagittal suture to form the posterior fontanelle. The posterior is the smaller of the two fontanelles at the top of the head.

The occipital bone is the terminal point at the back of the head for the FOD of the skull.

Parietal Bones

Posterior to the frontal eminences and the coronal sutures are the two parietal eminences. The parietal bones are cup-shaped bones that form the sides and top of the head. These are the largest bony plates of the human skull. They come together bilaterally at the top of the head along the sagittal suture and extend caudally to the squamous suture, which extends between the parietal and temporal bones. At the anterior and posterior ends of the squamous suture are two more fontanelles. The left and right anterolateral fontanelles are somewhat elongated triangular shapes at the junction of the frontal, parietal, temporal, and sphenoid bones. The squamous suture extends posteriorly, between the parietal and temporal bones, to the posterolateral fontanelles. The posterolateral (mastoid) fontanelles are at the intersections of the sagittal suture and the bilateral lambdoid and temporo-occipital sutures (see Fig. 9–4).

The parietal bones are relatively flexible, and they bow when pressure is exerted against the vertex of the skull.[9] Toward term, a fetus becomes more crowded in the uterus and has a tendency to press the top of its head against the lower uterine walls and pelvic bones. This pressure can cause outward bowing of the parietal bones and resulting exaggeration of the biparietal diameter (BPD). These bones also tend to flatten slightly when pressure is exerted along the transverse axis, somewhat shortening the BPD. This flattening most often occurs when a fetus is in a breech position.

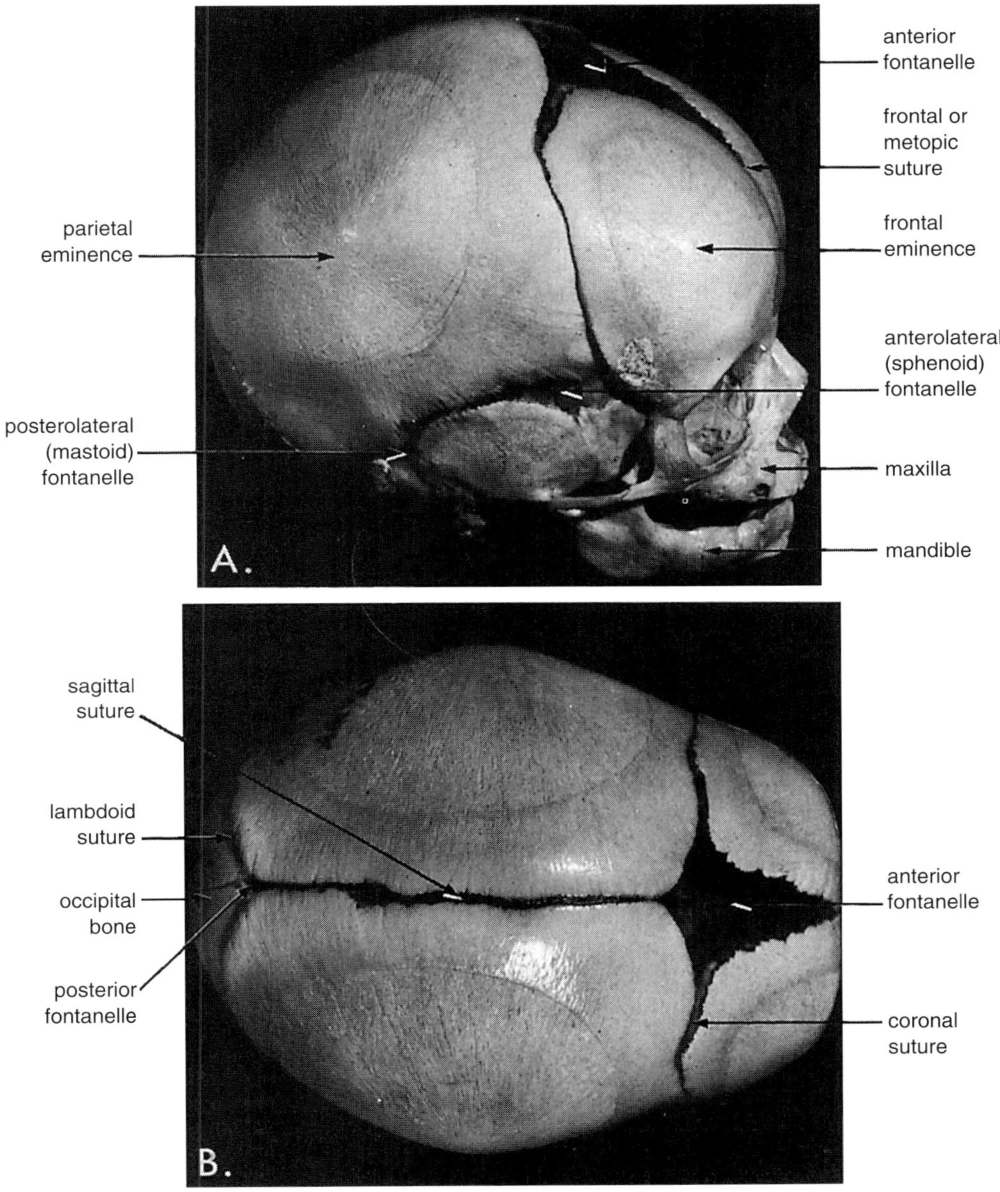

FIGURE 9–4.
Photographs of a fetal skull showing the sutures and fontanelles. *A*, Oblique lateral view. *B*, Superior view. The bony plates of the normal skull do not fuse until after birth, some not until adult life. These sutures are flexible and allow the skull to mold before and during birth. (From Moore KL, Persaud TVN: The Developing Human: Clinically Oriented Embryology, 5th ed. WB Saunders, Philadelphia, 1993, p 362.)

Sectional Anatomy of the Head

Base of the Skull

Base X. By the end of the first trimester, the various portions of the cartilaginous base of the skull have fused to form the chondrocranium.[8] The cartilaginous petrous portion of the temporal bone fuses with the occipital bone to form the ring of the foramen magnum, through which the spinal cord passes. The petrous pyramids contain sinuses, which can occasionally be observed sonographically as less echogenic than the more medial ossific portions (Figs. 9–6 and 9–7).

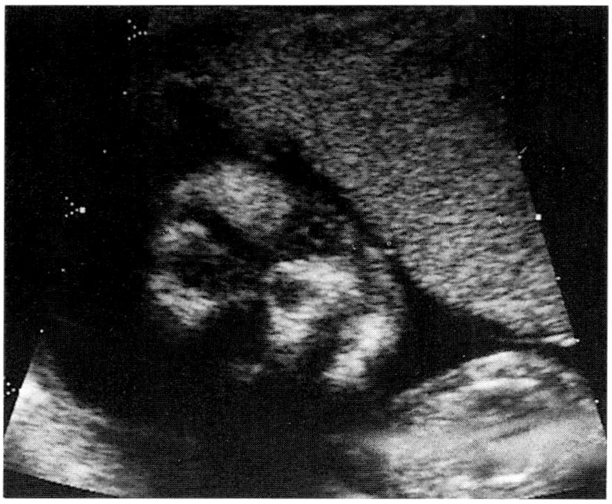

FIGURE 9–5.
The two frontal eminences are separated by the metopic suture. The maxilla and mandible form the lower face. Compare this image with Figure 9–4. The circle of echoes in the left orbit is around the lens of the eye. (AA = 18.5 LMP weeks, n = 10, range = 1.6 weeks, TD)

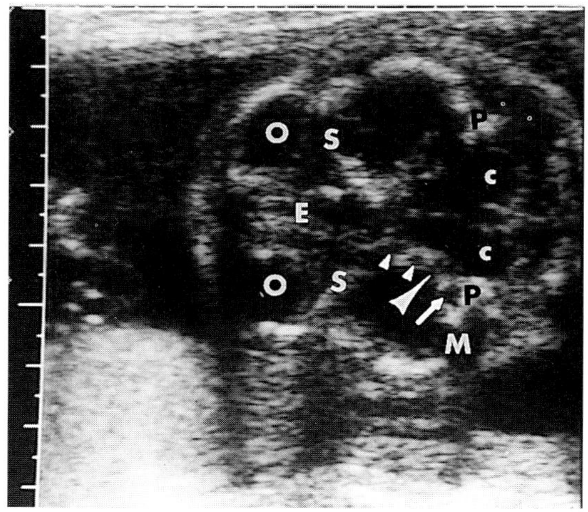

FIGURE 9–7.
Transverse sonogram of the fetal skull base X. Anteriorly, the plane of view is through the orbits (O), below the orbital plate of the frontal bone. The cerebellum (c) lies between the petrous ridges (P) in the posterior fossa. Ethmoid sinuses (E) lie posterior to the echoes of the crista galli and olfactory bulbs and anterior to the hypoechoic sphenoid sinuses. Small arrowheads, internal carotid artery siphon (petrous portion); large arrowhead, jugular bulb; arrow, sigmoid sinus; M, mastoid sinus. (AA = 23.5 LMP weeks, n = 9, range = 1.2 weeks, TD)

Various sonographic researchers have recognized the base X in the base of the fetal cranium as landmark anatomy for purposes of orientation of the scan planes.[21–24] The bilateral sphenoid and petrous pyramid bones in the base of the skull are echogenic structures that form the arms of the base X (Figs. 9–6 to 9–8).

The base X is important for orienting fetal cranial measurements. The plane in which the base X is visualized is parallel and caudate to the standard plane used to measure the transverse head circumference (THC). The plane of the base X is crossed transversely by the hippocampal base line (HBL), and the coronal triangle is perpendicular to the plane of the base X (see Chapter 8 for more on fetal cranial biometry).

Sphenoid Bones. The lesser wings of the sphenoid bones are above and posterior to the bilateral orbits of the eyes. The great wings of the sphenoid extend inferiorly, posterior to the orbits. The optic nerves emerge from the optic canal in the posteromedial portions of the lesser wings into the cranial cavity and optic chiasm. The lesser wings of the sphenoid bones form the anterior arms of the sonographic base X of the fetal skull (see Figs. 9–6 to 9–8).

Petrous Pyramids and Temporal Bones. The petrous pyramids of the temporal bones are the posterior arms of the base X. These pyramids are bony structures that house the inner ear and mastoid cells and have a linear axis that normally lies approximately 45 de-

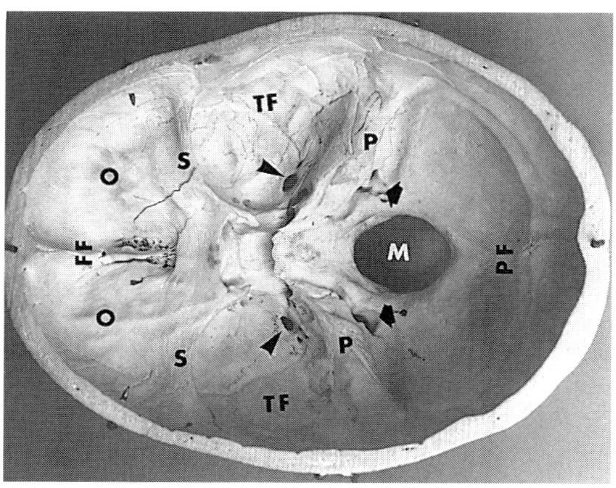

FIGURE 9–6.
Photograph of the interior of the base of an adult skull. The base X is made up of the bilateral sphenoid bones (S) anteriorly and the petrous ridges (P) posteriorly. The orbital plates of the frontal bone (O) cover the orbits and form the frontal fossa (FF). Arrowheads, foramen ovale; arrows, jugular foramen; M, foramen magnum; FF, anterior cranial or frontal fossa; TF, bilateral middle cranial or temporal fossae; PF, posterior cranial fossa.

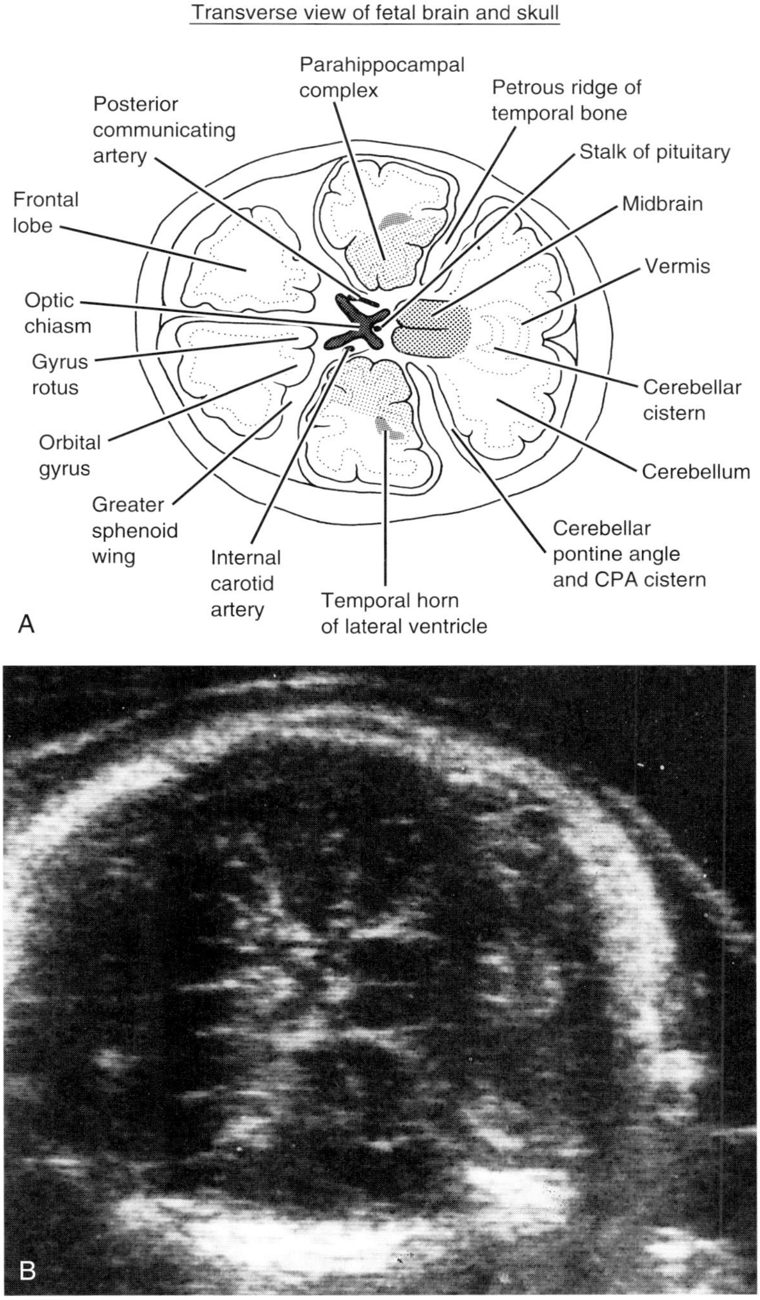

FIGURE 9–8.
Base X of fetal skull. *A,* This schematic was drawn from the sonogram in *B*. *B,* The base X of the fetal skull can be seen. The optic chiasm forms a small hypoechoic x at the center of the larger base X. The anterior portion of the plane is just superior to the orbital plates of the frontal bones and lobes of the cerebrum posteriorly (compare this with Figure 9–7, which passes below the orbital plates).

grees to the midline of the cranium. The HBL passes transversely across the anterior portion of the petrous pyramids. The foramen magnum, through which the spinal cord exits the skull, lies midway between the more posterior portions of the pyramids (see Figs. 9–6 to 9–8).

Transverse

Orbits. The orbits are the facial bones that contain the eyes. Each orbit is made up of parts of seven different bones: the frontal bone superiorly; the maxilla, palatine, ethmoid, and lacrimal inferiorly and medially;

the zygoma laterally; and the sphenoid posteriorly[25] (see Figs. 9–4 to 9–7).

Sonographic measurements have been published for the orbital diameters, the inner-to-inner distances between the orbits, and the outer-to-outer distances between the outer edges of the orbits. This last measurement has the greatest distance and therefore exhibits the least percentage of error because of slight variations in the plane of view and placement of the cursors (see Figs. 9–7 and 9–8).

Transverse Head Circumference. The most common sonographic measurement of the fetus is the BPD. The term BPD is sometimes used to describe the common view used to measure the THC, but this is not the best use of the term. The BPD measurement is a line that passes transversely through the brain, the thalamus, and the third ventricle and is perpendicular to the interhemispheric fissure. It is also the widest transverse distance across the skull above the ears (Figs. 9–9 and 9–10).

In the transverse view, the thalamus is a hypoechoic oval structure with a slitlike third ventricle at its center. Sonographers should become thoroughly familiar with the anatomy of this important sonographic plane of view (see Fig. 9–9). An accurate BPD measurement passes through the center of the thalamus.

Coronal

The coronal view of the fetal skull has received less attention than the transverse view. However, it is as important and may be more important in some cases than the transverse view. This is because the coronal view can be used to measure the BPD, but it can also be used to measure the very dynamic vertical cranial diameter (VCD).[17, 26–34] The VCD and coronal circumference are more dynamic owing to fetal skull molding than are the diameters of the THC (see Chapter 8 for discussion of the geometry of cranial molding and head shape).

It is possible to view important cranial anatomy in the coronal view (see Fig. 9–10). In this view, the thalamus is again observed along with the interhemispheric fissure. The bodies of the lateral cerebral ventricles are at the top of the thalamus, and the corpus callosum forms the roof of the ventricles. The temporal horn of the lateral ventricles forms the superolateral aspect of the bilateral circles of the hippocampal complexes. The cavum vergae may be observed in the midline at the top of the thalamus until approximately the 28th LMP week and occasionally until term. An accurate BPD can be measured through the midthalamus in this plane.

Sagittal

The sagittal view of the fetal cranium can be difficult to obtain because the top of the fetal head is most clearly approached only when a fetus is breech or transverse. Figure 9–11 includes some of the best sagittal images we have ever obtained, and they cannot be reproduced routinely. Although the sagittal plane can be interesting for the study of brain anatomy and is common in neonatal neurological studies, it is less useful in perinatal sonography because it is difficult to obtain. To date no fetal growth measurements have been published using this view of the fetal head.

BRAIN

Brain Growth

The fetal cerebral hemispheres are relatively smooth at first and develop sulci as gestation progresses (Fig. 9–12).[35] The lateral sulcus develops into the sylvian fissure toward term and can occasionally be observed in the transverse and coronal views (Fig. 9–13).

Midbrain

Where the spinal cord passes into the base of the skull, a bulbous area, the pons, is just anterior to the cerebellum (see Figs. 9–8 and 9–11). Sonographically, in the transverse view, the pons appears as two ovoid structures separated by a thin echogenic line (see Fig. 9–8). Just anterior to the pons is the optic chiasm, which forms an X at the center of this image. The chiasm is where the optic nerves from each eye join at the midbase of the brain.

Cerebellum

The cerebellum is located in the posterior or occipital fossa just behind the foramen

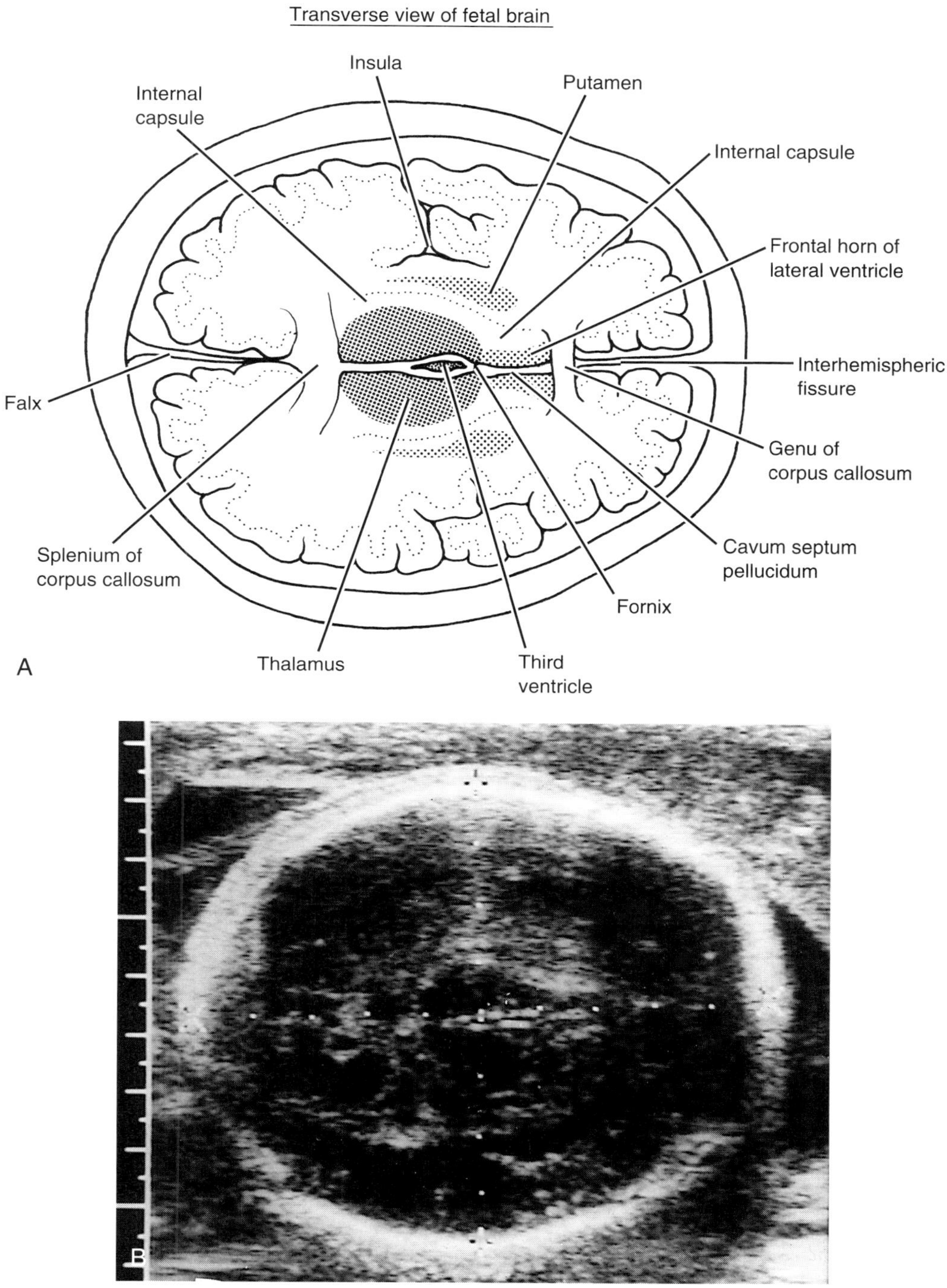

FIGURE 9–9.
Transverse head circumference. *A,* A schematic of the proper plane of view for measuring the transverse head circumference. This drawing corresponds to the sonogram in *B. B,* Transverse head circumference. + = BPD = 79 mm; X = FOD = 97 mm.

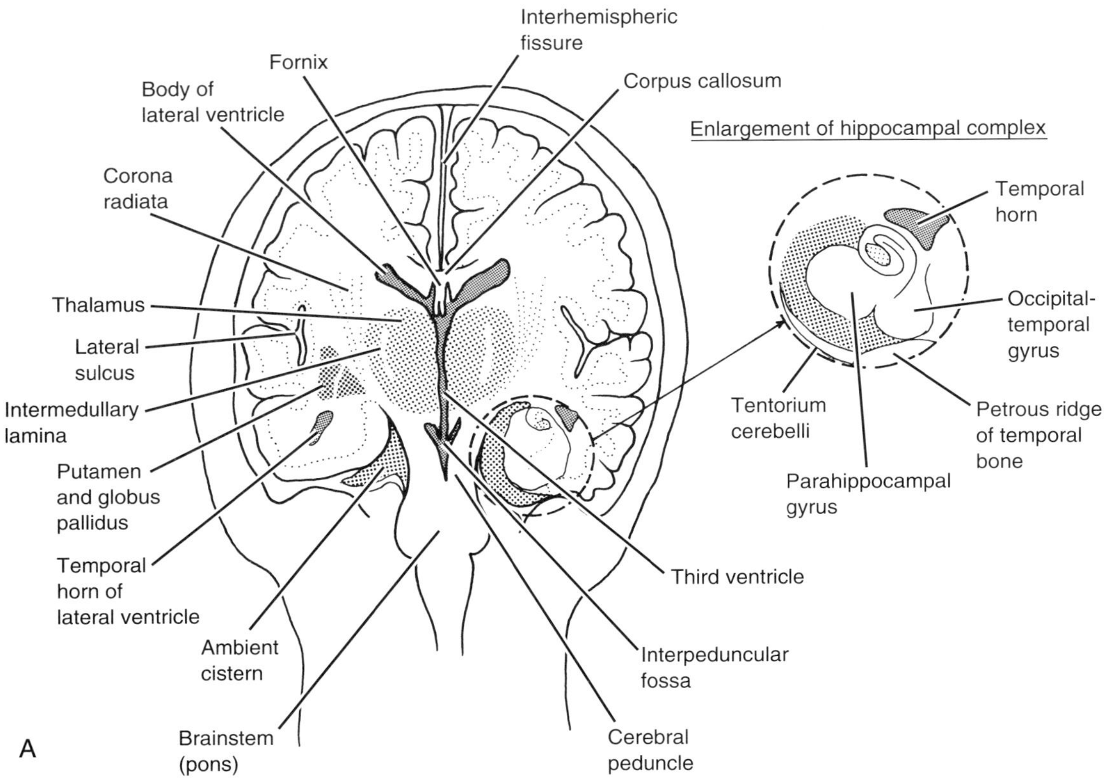

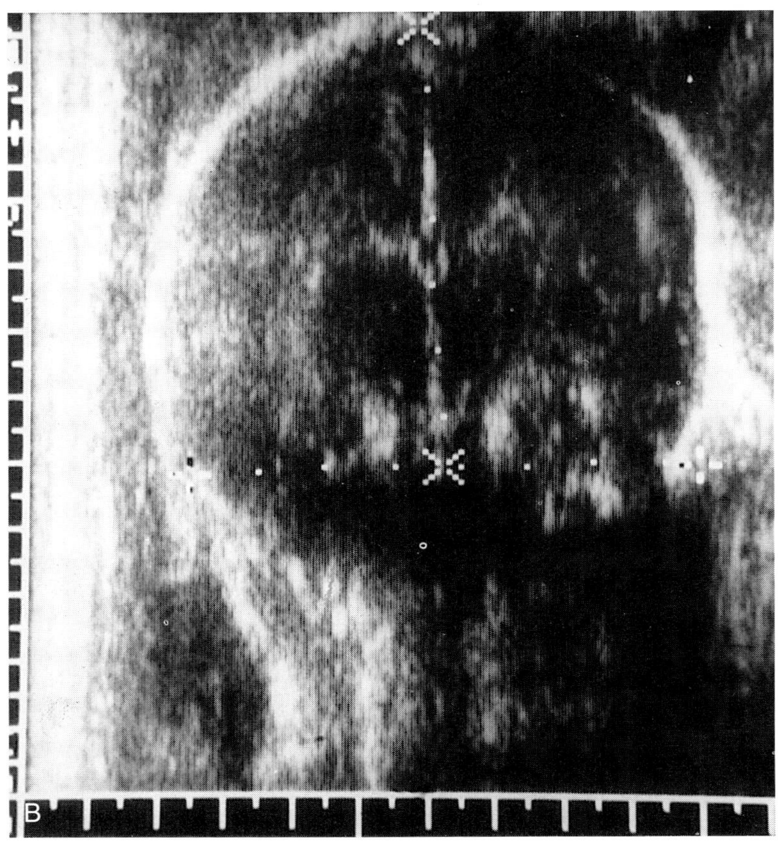

FIGURE 9–10.
Coronal head. *A,* This drawing of the sonogram in *B* shows the anatomy of the coronal view of the fetal skull, with detail of the hippocampal complex or formation. (Adapted from Mark LP, Daniels DL, Naidch TP, et al: Hippocampal anatomy and pathologic alterations on conventional MR images. AJNR 1993;14:1237–1240.) *B,* In this coronal sonogram, the two circles around the bilateral hippocampal complexes are obvious. The hippocampal base line (HBL, + cursors) passes tangential to the inferior edges of these circles and across the tops of the bilateral petrous pyramids. The third dimension of the fetal skull (vertical cranial diameter, VCD = 67 mm) is measured from the vertex of the skull to the center of this imaginary line. (AA = 33.8 LMP weeks, n = 8, range = 2.1 weeks, DKD)

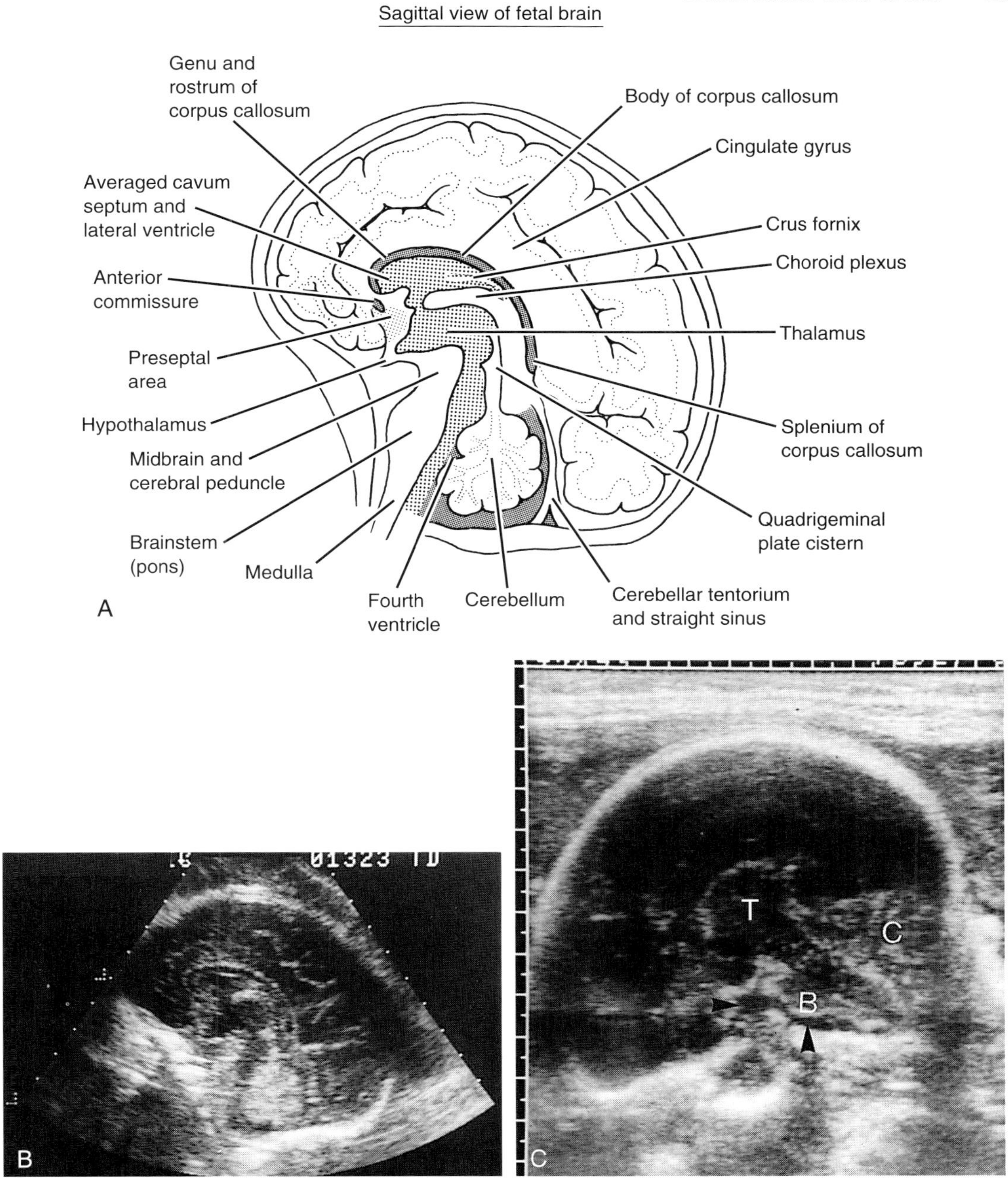

FIGURE 9–11.
The sagittal view of the fetal skull is often difficult to obtain and is not normally used for cranial measurements. *A*, This drawing correlates with *B*. *B*, Sonographic view through the anterior fontanelle and sagittal suture and slightly lateral to the midline. The lateral ventricle and the cavum septi pellucidi and cavum vergae are probably volume averaged by the beam width. *C*, This view is similar to *B* but is through the posterior fontanelle. T, thalamus; C, cerebellum; B, basilar pons; black arrowheads, prepontine cistern. Note that the echogenicity of the brain tissues may change with changes of view. This is because much of these tissues is fibrous and appears more echogenic when the fibers are perpendicular to the direction of sound beam travel. Reverberations also affect the appearance of the tissues.

magnum and brainstem. This is between the petrous pyramids at the back of the head. The cerebellum is made up of two hemispheres divided by the cerebellar vermis. Sonographically, the vermis appears more echogenic than do the cerebellar hemispheres on either side (Figs. 9–14 and 9–15). A view of the base X often provides a clear view of the cerebellum, other landmark anatomy, the orbits, the cisterna magna, and the bony structures (see

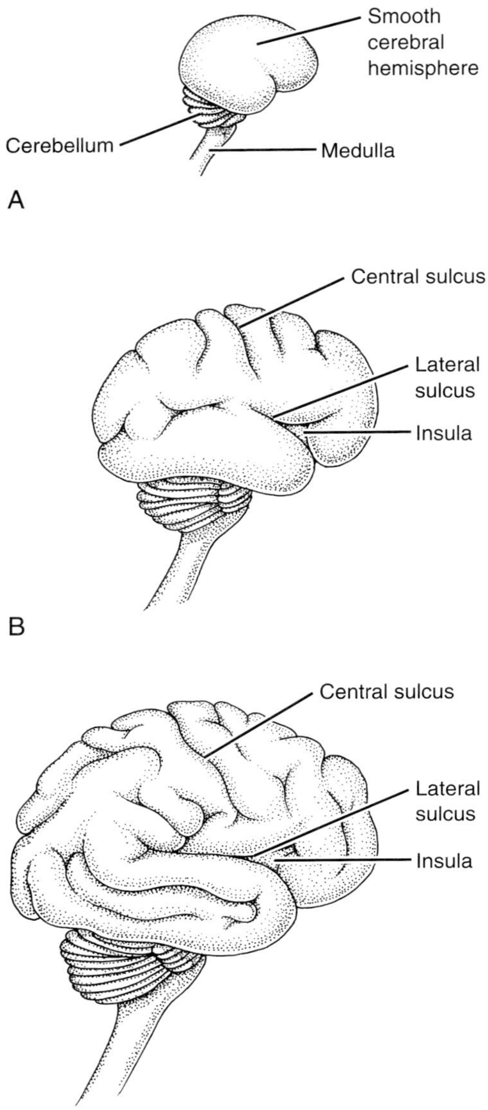

FIGURE 9–12.
Brain surface development. Successive stages of the development of the sulci or fissures. Lateral views of the right hemisphere. *A*, 15 LMP weeks. *B*, 28 LMP weeks. *C*, 37 LMP weeks. (Adapted from Moore KL, Persaud TVN: The Developing Human: Clinically Oriented Embryology, 5th ed. WB Saunders, Philadelphia, 1993, p 411.)

Figs. 9–6 to 9–8, 9–11, 9–12, 9–14, and 9–15).

Just inferior and posterior to the cerebellum is the cisterna magna, which is a fluid-filled space between the cerebellum and occipital bone (see Fig. 9–14). Observation of the cisterna is sonographically important because in cases of spinal cord defects, the cord may become tethered or anchored by the defect, and as a result, the brainstem and cerebellum can obliterate this fluid space as the body and spine grow. Faint septa can occasionally be observed sonographically within the cisterna magna, crossing from the vermis of the cerebellum to the internal occiput sulcus (see Fig. 9–14). One or more cisterna magna septa may be identified; they represent portions of the leptomeninges[36] or associated veins, not the straight sinus, and should not be confused with pathological entities. One study identified these septa in 94% of fetuses after 15 LMP weeks.[37] A Dandy-Walker malformation results from absence of the cerebellar vermis and is associated with various degrees of cerebellar hypoplasia. The result is an enlarged cisterna magna, which may communicate directly with the fourth ventricle.[38]

Measurements of the transverse cerebellar diameters throughout gestation have been published (see Table 7–1 for cerebellar diameter correlation to fetal age). Early in pregnancy (before 15 LMP weeks) and late (after 30 weeks, when the skull is becoming more calcified), the cerebellum may be difficult to measure. During midpregnancy (15 to 25 LMP weeks), the cerebellum in millimeters is approximately equal to the fetal age in weeks (± 2 SD = 2.8 weeks) (see Chapter 7).

Cerebrum

Ventricular System

Early Ventricles and Choroid Plexus. Early in the fetal period, which begins with the 11th LMP week,[39] the ventricles are almost completely filled by the choroid plexus. The echogenic choroid plexus is one of the major sonographic features of the fetal brain until about the 18th LMP week (Figs. 9–16 and 9–17 and the 15th week of Chapter 19).

Figures 9–18 and 9–19*A* are of a plastic cast of the adult cerebral ventricular system. The relative proportions of these casts are similar to those of the fetal ventricles in the last half of gestation. In Figures 9–17 and 9–19*B*, a lateral ventricle can be observed to contain the more echogenic choroid plexus. The posterior horn is filled with hypoechoic cerebrospinal fluid (CSF) which the choroid plexus secretes (see Fig. 9–19*B*).

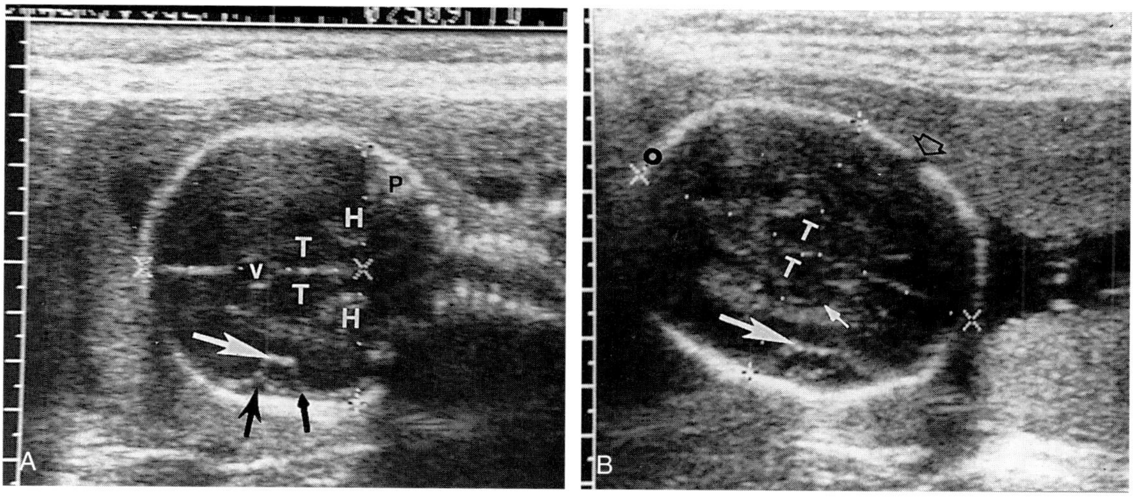

FIGURE 9–13.
A, Coronal sonogram demonstrating the lateral sylvian fissure (large black arrow) and sylvian cistern (large white arrow) during the 23rd LMP week. The sylvian or lateral fissure is a horizontal sulcus or crease in the anterolateral aspect of the brain. This sulcus extends deep to approximately midhemisphere, where it terminates at the insula or isle of Reil. Just inferior to the sylvian fissure is the superior temporal sulcus (small black arrow), which approximately parallels the sylvian. Other anatomy visible is the line of the interhemispheric fissure, which is interrupted by the cavum vergae (V), the petrous portion of the temporal bones (P), two lobes of the thalamus (T), and circles of the hippocampal complex (H). The petrosquamous sutures are under the + cursors. The anatomy of the near hemisphere is obscured by acoustic reverberation. Note slight compression and flattening of the parietal bones, with loss of the circular shape of the coronal skull; the vertical cranial diameter (VCD) (45.5 mm) is only slightly exaggerated. *B*, More standard transverse (transverse head circumference) view of the same fetal skull with biparietal diameter (BPD = 56.9 mm) and fronto-occipital (FOD = 75.1 mm) measurements. The slight compression of the BPD and exaggeration of the VCD (slight oxycephaly) result in a tendency toward dolichocephaly (transverse cephalic index = BPD/FOD = 0.76); this is common in a breech fetus. The sylvian cistern is a linear echogenic line (large white arrow) that approximately parallels the skull; the hypoechoic area medial to this cistern is the insula. In the near skull, the coronal suture (open arrow) is shown. Small white arrow, putamen; o, occipital bone. (AA = 23.6 LMP weeks, n = 9, range = 1.6 weeks, TD)

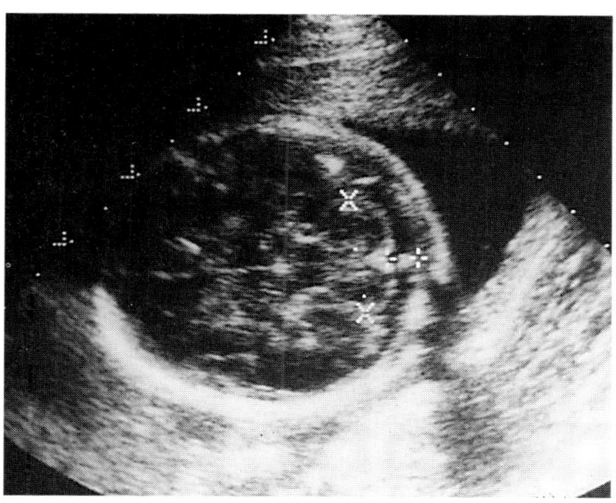

FIGURE 9–14.
Transverse cerebellum. This plane is below the standard transverse head circumference plane and demonstrates the correct measurement of the transverse cerebellar diameter (X = 23.8 mm). The fluid space of the cisterna magna (+ = 6.6) is observed posterior to the cerebellum. A septum or veins (leptomeninges) observed between the + cursors is normal. There may be none, one, or more of these septa. (AA = 24.0 LMP weeks, n = 9, range = 2.1 weeks, TD)

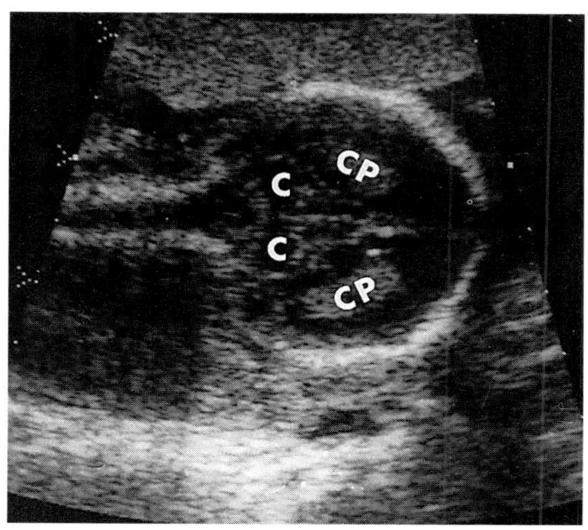

FIGURE 9–15.
Coronal cerebellum and ventricles. Here the two hemispheres of the cerebellum (C) can be seen posterior to and above the spine. Earlier in pregnancy, the choroid plexus (CP) fills the lateral ventricle antrum and bodies. (AA = 18.5 LMP weeks, n = 10, range = 1.6 weeks, TD)

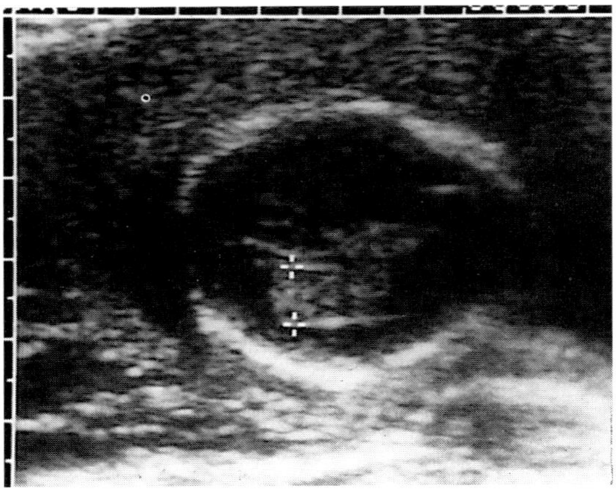

FIGURE 9–16.
Oblique, transverse view of the antrum of the lateral ventricle. Here (16 weeks) the antrum measures approximately 7 mm. This measurement should be less than 10 to 12 mm throughout gestation. The choroid plexus fills the body of the ventricle early in pregnancy. (AA = 16.1 LMP weeks, n = 10, range = 1.3 weeks, TD)

Lateral Ventricles

Anterior. The lateral cerebral ventricles are closest to each other at the anterior horns (see Fig. 9–18*A*). The anterior horns are separated by the septum pellucidum. The most anterior portion of the frontal horns flares out slightly.

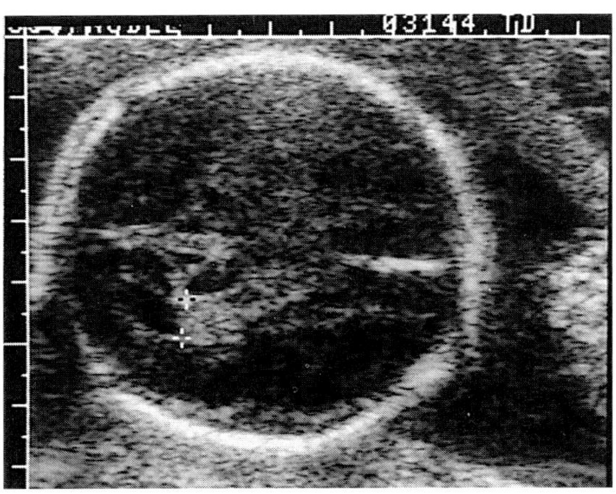

FIGURE 9–17.
This measurement of the lateral ventricle antrum is 6.1 mm in the 24th LMP week. In this image, the antrum is only 1 mm different from the one in Figure 9–16, yet it appears to be much smaller. This is because the ventricular antrum varies little in width while the skull and brain enlarge around it. Note that the echogenic choroid plexus (between + cursors) does not extend into the cerebrospinal fluid–filled posterior horn of the ventricle. (AA = 24.6 LMP weeks, n = 9, range = 1.3 weeks, TD)

The cavum septi pellucidi (CSP) and its related cavum vergae are discussed later.

Body. The bodies of the lateral cerebral ventricles are curvilinear slits in the anteroposterior (long) axis of the skull. The slitlike nature of the lateral ventricles can be appreciated in the coronal view of the fetal skull (see Fig. 9–10). Figures 9–18 and 9–19 also help in understanding the complex shape of the cerebral ventricular system. The cross-sectional axis of the body of the lateral ventricle in the coronal plane of view is approximately 45 degrees oblique to the midline structures at the top of the head.

The choroid plexus develops from an attachment that is approximately at the midpoint of the medial wall of the lateral ventricle near the ependymal roof of the third ventricle.[40] The point of choroid plexus attachment is also near the foramen of Monro.[41] From this midpoint, the choroid plexus extends posteriorly into the antrum of the lateral ventricles. The antrum is the area where the bodies and the temporal and posterior horns of the lateral ventricles communicate.

In cases of hydrocephalus or ventriculomegaly, the bodies of the ventricles balloon out to become more like curved, oval tubes than curved slits. As this enlargement of the ventricles increases, the tethered choroid plexus dangles by gravity into the fluid of the more dependent ventricle. This dangling choroid sign was first described by Filly and associates. The angle of the choroid is normally about 14 degrees from the midline and should not exceed 29 degrees.[42]

Antrum and Occipital Horn. The choroid plexus extends posteriorly into the antrum of the lateral ventricle but not into the occipital horn (see Fig. 9–19*B*). The posterior occipital horn contains only CSF. On examination and measurement, the normal ventricular system was defined as having an antral width of 10 mm or less.[43–46] Others have found that ventricle antrum measurements as much as 11 to 12 mm or even as much as 15 mm may be normal.[47,48] Monteagudo and colleagues[48] give nomograms for several different measurements of the lateral ventricles. The variation in the maximum acceptable measurement of the antrum (10 to 12 mm) may be due

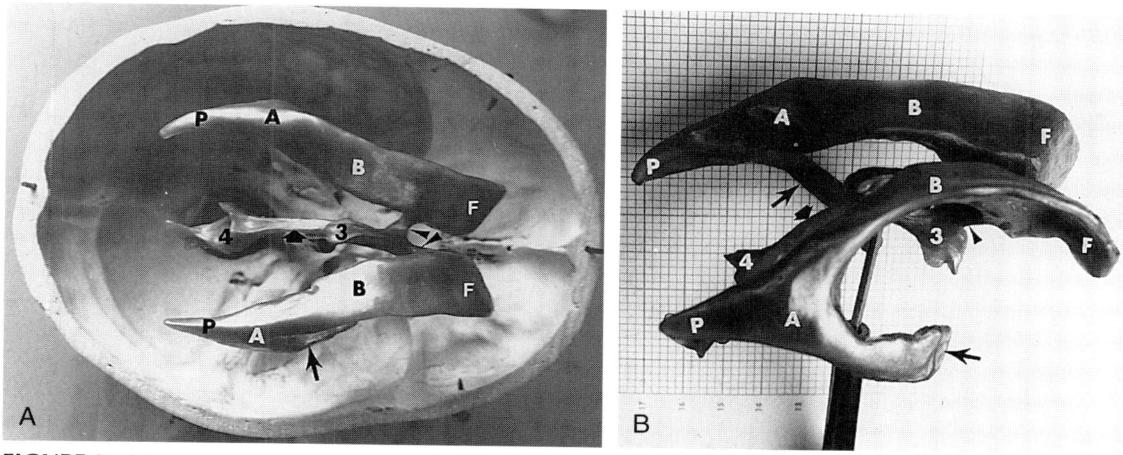

FIGURE 9–18.
A plastic cast from an adult ventricular system. Although the fetal head and brain are smaller than an adult's, the proportions are approximately the same, particularly late in gestation. (Cast provided by David Nichols, MD.) *A*, The cast is held in an approximately normal location within the skull cavity. Note the divergent angle of the lateral ventricles from front to posterior. The third ventricle is near the center, and the fourth ventricle is directly superior to the foramina magna. *B*, Oblique, lateral view of the ventricular system. The parts of the ventricles: F, frontal horns; B, bodies; P, posterior or occipital horns; long arrows, temporal (inferior) horns; A, antrum; 3, third ventricle; 4, fourth ventricle; wide arrow, cerebral aqueduct of Sylvius; small arrowheads, interventricular foramen of Monro.

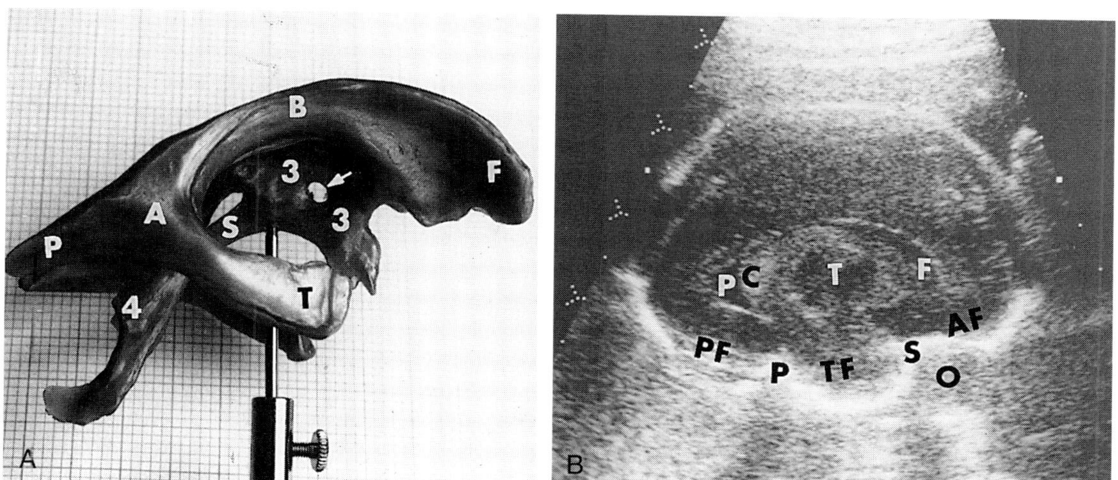

FIGURE 9–19.
Lateral view of the ventricular cast and corresponding sonogram of one lateral ventricle for comparison. F, frontal horn; B, body; P, occipital (posterior) horn; black T, temporal (inferior) horn; A, antrum; 3, third ventricle; 4, fourth ventricle; S, cerebral aqueduct of Sylvius; small arrow, massa intermedia; C, choroid plexus; white T, thalamus. *A*, Lateral photograph of the adult ventricular cast. *B*, Oblique sagittal sonogram showing a fetal lateral ventricle. The choroid plexus (C) does not extend into the posterior (occipital) horn (P). Note that the thalamus (white T) sits within the curve of the lateral ventricle bodies, antra (C), and temporal (inferior) horns. In this image, the temporal horn extends outside the plane of view. Observe that the base of the skull, anterior fossa (AF), temporal (middle) fossa (TF), and posterior fossa (PF) are separated from one another by the sphenoid (S) and the petrous pyramid bone (P). O, orbit. (AA = 26.3 LMP weeks, n = 9, range = 3.4 weeks, TD)

to the angle of the plane of view to the antrum. The antrum is not a perfect cylinder, and the degree of obliquity may affect the variability of the measurement (see Figs. 9–18 and 9–19).

Temporal/Inferior Horns. The temporal or inferior horns of the lateral ventricles extend inferiorly and anteriorly from the antrum of the ventricles (see Figs. 9–18 and 9–19). The more anterior portions of the temporal horn lie superolateral to the hippocampus.

Third and Fourth Ventricles

Third. Sonographically, the third ventricle is most commonly observed as a narrow slit at the center of the thalamus in the THC view of the fetal skull (see Figs. 9–10, 9–18, and 9–19).

Fourth. The fetal cerebral fourth ventricle is not normally observed sonographically. The area of the fourth ventricle may be observed in the sagittal plane of view (see Figs. 9–11, 9–18, and 9–19).

Choroid Plexus

Normal. The choroid plexus is tissue within the lateral ventricles. By sonography, it generally appears more echogenic than the surrounding tissues.

During the first half of pregnancy, the choroid plexus appears relatively large and fills the bodies of the lateral ventricles and most of the cranium (see Figs. 9–16 and 18–12*F*). As the fetal cranium and ventricles grow, the choroid plexus appears relatively smaller, although it does not actually shrink. Figures 9–16 and 9–17 show two fetal heads at 16.1 and 24.6 LMP weeks, respectively. The choroid plexus in each is well visualized. The lateral ventricle and choroid plexus occupy a larger percentage of the head in the earlier pregnancy. Comparison of the choroid plexus width with the scale at the edge of the images shows very little actual change in the size. The head simply enlarges around the choroid plexus.

As stated earlier in the section on the lateral ventricles, the long axis of the choroid plexus should be approximately 14 degrees (±4.3 degrees) from the midline. An angle greater than 29 degrees in the distal ventricle is indicative of ventriculomegaly.[45]

Cysts. Cysts of the choroid plexus are occasionally observed by sonography. Figure 9–20 shows bilateral choroid plexus cysts at 18.6 LMP weeks. These cysts are most often observed posteriorly in the antrum of the lateral ventricles. The cysts have been documented to resolve spontaneously and without consequence.[49]

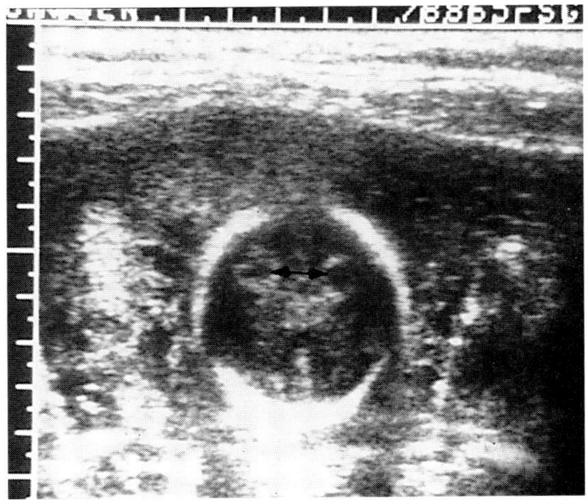

FIGURE 9–20.
This sonogram shows bilateral choroid plexus cysts (double arrow) in the area of the ventricular antra. These cysts may or may not be significant to the outcome of the pregnancy, but they have some association with certain genetic syndromes and warrant further study. These cysts have also been found to resolve by birth and to be asymptomatic. Care should be taken not to confuse the normal hippocampal complex and the abnormal choroid plexus cysts, which may have similar appearances. (AA = 18.6 LMP weeks, n = 9, range = 0.9 weeks, SG)

A case study of a fetus with a large, bilateral choroid plexus cyst at 16 weeks found the cyst to regress partly by the 19th week and to be gone completely by the 28th week. Another 16-week fetus was found to have small bilateral cysts that were completely resolved by the 21st week.[50]

In vitro sonographic studies of fetal specimens, followed by autopsy, have suggested an association between choroid plexus cysts and chromosomal abnormalities.[51] This study found cysts in 5 of 14 (35%) fetuses with trisomy 18. If only the trisomy-affected fetuses studied before 26 menstrual weeks are considered, then these five become 71.4% of that population (age < 26 weeks). The researchers concluded that "the finding of such cysts on a second-trimester ultrasound examination should suggest further evaluation, including chromosome analysis." Other investigators have supported this opinion.[52]

Another study of 234 second-trimester fetuses with sonographically identified choroid plexus cysts concluded, "the yield of abnormal karyotypes in fetuses with isolated CP [choroid plexus] cysts is low and may not justify the risk of amniocentesis."[53] Although these researchers found a lower association of abnormal karyotype, they did point out that when cysts were associated with genetic problems, the size of the cysts was not important.

One case study of cysts in the brain investigated postmortem diagnosis of neonatal isoimmune thrombocytopenia.[54] However, these cysts were found throughout the brain parenchyma and were not localized to the choroid plexus.

Cysts of the fetal choroid plexus have not been exclusively associated with genetic abnormalities, and controversy has been expressed about their significance.[55–57] It is safe to say that in the presence of these cysts, follow-up sonography and genetic analysis may be indicated.

Ventricular Enlargement: Hydrocephalus. When the ventricular system has an obstruction that prevents CSF from circulating out of the cerebrum, hydrocephalus results. Diagnostic medical sonography has provided a good way to study this condition.

The literature describes three basic approaches to sonographic evaluation of the fetal cerebral ventricles. One of these, the lateral ventricular width/hemispheric ratio, has been shown by the original researchers to be invalid. These three methods are briefly discussed here, and a fourth method is proposed.

Figure 9–21*A* and *B* shows images of a fetus with mild idiopathic ventriculomegaly at 29 menstrual weeks. The ventricular antrum measured 13.9 mm, and the angle between the interhemispheric fissure and the choroid plexus was approximately 45 degrees. Both criteria indicate enlargement of the ventricle. This condition has been associated with trisomies.[58] At this writing, this fetus has not yet been delivered, and no definitive diagnosis can be proposed; the fetus is sonographically normal, except for the cerebral ventriculomegaly.

Dangling Choroid Plexus. Cardoza and associates found that in cases of ventriculomegaly, the choroid plexus was free to move in the posterior aspect. The result of the movement was that the anterior attachment of the plexus remained in place near the midline while the posterior portion was free to respond to gravity. Therefore, the dependent choroid plexus dangled from the attachment as a result of gravity. They found that the long axis of the normal choroid plexus had an angle from the cerebral midline between 6 and 22 degrees. They also pointed out that an angle greater than 29 degrees was associated with ventriculomegaly.[59]

In Figure 9–21*A*, readers can use a protractor to measure the angle between the interhemispheric fissure (midline) and the long axis of the distal choroid plexus. This angle is found to be greater than 45 degrees and thus meets the criteria for ventriculomegaly.

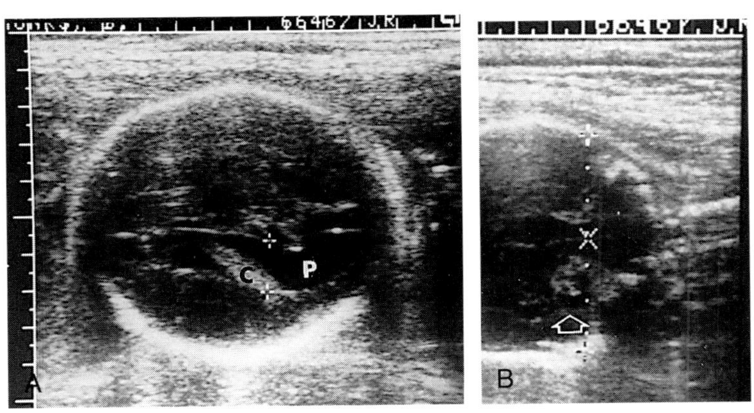

FIGURE 9–21.
Slight enlargement of the ventricular system. *A*, Transverse, oblique showing measurement of the ventricular antrum (13.9 mm). Use a protractor to measure the angle between the choroid plexus and the midline; this should not be more than 29 to 30 degrees. *B*, Coronal view of the same fetal head. Note the enlargement of the temporal horn (open arrow) at the lateral aspect of the hippocampal complex. (AA = 29.0, n = 8, range = 1.1 weeks, JR)

Measurement of the Antrum. Cardoza and associates also proposed measuring the width of the antrum of the lateral ventricle. They found that the antrum is less than 10 mm throughout pregnancy.[45] This is one of the easiest and most dependable empirical measurements of the ventricular system. The antrum is the area where the ventricular lateral body, temporal horn, and occipital (posterior) horn are joined (see Figs. 9–18 and 9–19).

The best image to measure the antrum is slightly cephalic to the plane used to measure the THC.[60] The ventricle on the side away from the transducer is usually easiest to see. The nearer ventricle can be very difficult to see or to measure, depending on a woman's body habitus, the transducer, the contrast resolution of the equipment, and of course the skill of the observer.

In Figure 9–21, the + cursors are measuring the antrum to be 13.9 mm in a 29-LMP-week fetus. This measurement meets the foregoing definition of ventriculomegaly.

Ventricular Width/Hemispheric Ratio. Jeanty and colleagues described the lateral ventricular wall/hemispheric width ratio in 1981.[61] In this report, they proposed a transverse view of the fetal head just above the plane used for the THC in which two lines can be seen (Fig. 9–22*D* and *E*). These lines are thought to be white matter tracts and not the walls of the lateral ventricles. They are in the area of the bilateral centrum semiovale and corona radiata.[62] In the textbook that Jeanty coauthored, this method of measuring ventriculomegaly was considered inaccurate.[63]

Coronal View. The transverse view of the fetal head showing the antrum of the lateral ventricles or the choroid plexus can occasionally be difficult or impossible to obtain because of fetal position. In this case, another method may be helpful. We propose viewing the ventricle bodies and temporal (inferior) horns of the lateral ventricles in the coronal view.[64]

Figure 9–21*A* and *B* shows transverse and coronal views of the same fetal head. In Figure 9–21*B*, the temporal horn of the lateral ventricle is an anechoic (without echoes) fluid-filled area that is just lateral to the circle about the hippocampal gyri. The temporal horn is also observed just cephalic to the HBL, which is demarcated by the dotted line between the + cursors.

If Figure 9–21*B* is compared with a normal coronal view of the fetal head such as Figures 9–10 and 9–13, the differences can be appreciated. The temporal horns form the superolateral portion of the circles around the hippocampal gyri in the normal fetus but cannot be seen as fluid structures.

If the coronal view of the fetal head (see Fig. 9–21*B*) reveals fluid in the temporal horns lateral to the hippocampal gyri, we suggest that every attempt should be made to obtain direct ventricular antrum measurements. If necessary, the examination can be repeated at a later time; it is hoped that the fetus will have changed position to permit better visualization.

Cavum Septi Pellucidi and Cavum Vergae

The CSP is a fluid-filled cavity that lies in the midline immediately anterior and superior to the thalamus (Figs. 9–22 and 9–23). The CSP should always be in the correct plane for measuring the THC (see Figs. 9–9, 9–18*A*, and 9–22*A*). Most discussion of the CSP in the sonographic literature relates to its use as a landmark for the THC.

The CSP does not normally exist after birth. "A cavum septi pellucidi, although beginning to involute just before term, is seen in about 80% of infants at term and persists in approximately 15% of adults."[65] In adults, the CSP is normally a very small space at the top of the septum just inferior to the corpus callosum.[66] The CSP has been called the fifth ventricle.[67] In some cases, the CSP may be dilated. This abnormal dilation "is thought to be a characteristic pathological change seen in boxers who have experienced a great number of blows to the head."[68] There appears to be some confusion about the nature of the cerebral "cava" in the fetus. In some literature, the fetal CSP is often illustrated as a cystic space or box.[69–72] In other publications, the CSP appears septated.[73–75] Still others have expressed the opinion that a "linear echo is often seen within cavum, parallel to the walls. This is most likely averaging of superior aspect of cavum septum pellucidum with inferior falx cerebri. . . . "[76]

The cavum vergae, or sixth ventricle, ex-

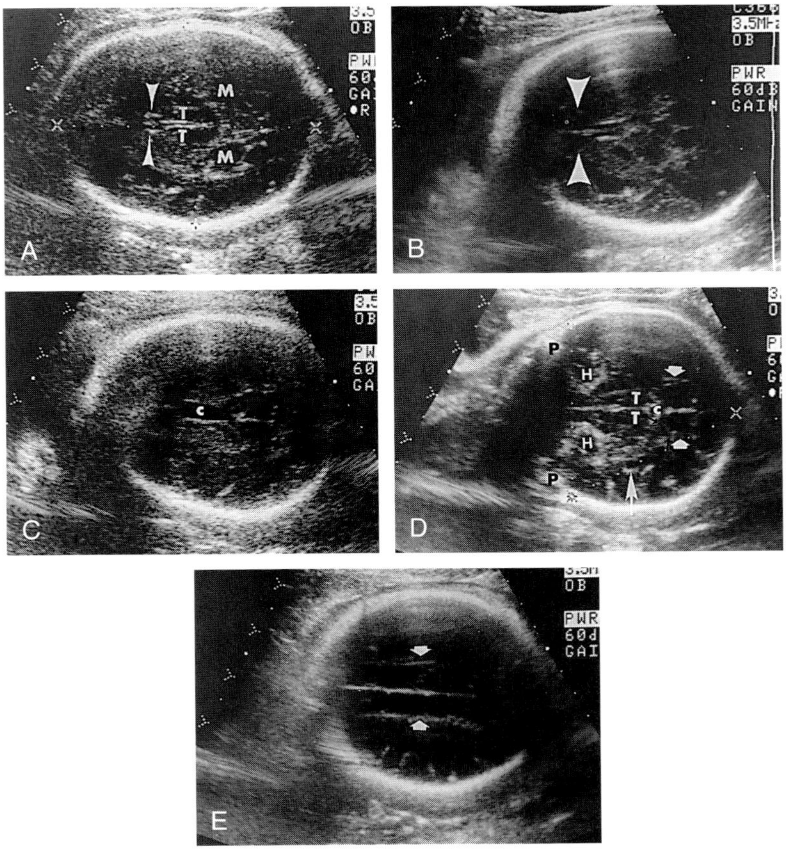

FIGURE 9–22.
Ventricles, cavum septi pellucidi, and cavum vergae. Five sonograms from the same examination. There appears to be some confusion in the literature about the sonographic appearance of the cavum septi pellucidi and the posterior portions of the anterior horns of the lateral ventricles, and scant attention has been paid to the cavum vergae. *A*, Standard view of the transverse view with biparietal diameter (+ = 77.2 mm) and fronto-occipital diameter (X = 96.1 mm) measurements. The third ventricle is the thin fluid space in the midline of the thalamus (T). Just anterior to the third ventricle are three short parallel lines (between arrowheads) that are thought to represent the walls of the posterior portions of the anterior horns of the lateral ventricles. The hypoechoic area posterior and lateral to the thalamus has been called the hippocampus minor (M); this should not be confused with the true hippocampal formation. *B*, A slight change in the plane from the previous image and image smoothing by frame averaging make the broad, superior portions of the anterior horns visible between the arrowheads and separated by the septum pellucidum (compare with Fig. 9–16*A* and *B*). *C*, This image is superior to and rotated higher in the posterior aspect above the thalamus, which cannot be seen. The linear fluid space (c) in the midline is the cavum septi pellucidi (more anterior portion) and the cavum vergae (more posterior portion). These cava begin contracting from the posterior at about 24 weeks. The cavum septi pellucidi begins to involute near term and is present in 80% of neonates. *D*, By rotating the plane of view 90 degrees from the transverse view above (*A*), the coronal view is obtained. In this view, the cavum vergae (c) may be seen atop the thalamus (T) as an apparent interruption of the interhemispheric fissure. The imaginary line of the hippocampal base line, tangential inferiorly to the circles of the hippocampal complex (H), is measured (+ = 66.8 mm) as well as one side (X = 69.3 mm) of the coronal triangle (near isosceles in normally shaped heads). Note that in this view the body of the lateral ventricle (between small black arrows) is a narrow slit that is approximately perpendicular and inside the apex of the triangle. Also, the sylvian fissure (long white arrow) is just outside the triangle. The two echogenic lines (wide white arrows) that extend superiorly from the lateral walls of the ventricle bodies are white matter tracts (see Fig. 9–19*E*). P, Petrous portions of temporal bones. *E*, High above the thalamus and ventricles in this transverse view, three parallel lines can be observed. The strong echoes from the falx cerebri are midline. On either side are parallel tracts of cortical white matter (arrows). These are the same lines as observed in the coronal view (*D*) and are not the walls of the lateral ventricles. These echoes are in the area of the medial portions of the bilateral centrum semiovale and corona radiata. (AA = 31.6 LMP weeks, n = 9, range = 2.5 weeks, TD)

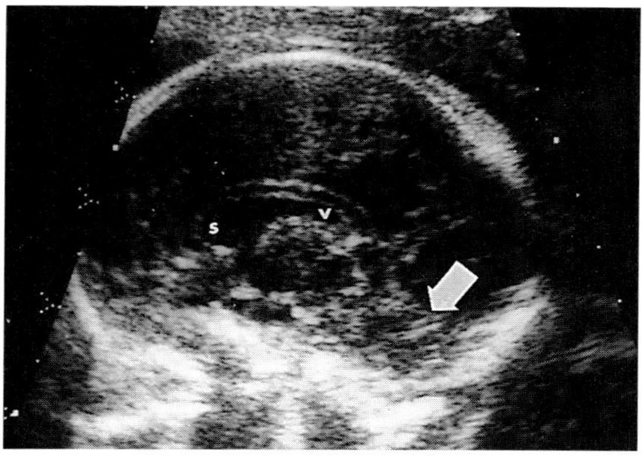

FIGURE 9–23.
Sagittal cavum septi pellucidi and vergae. This midline sagittal plane was obtained through the anterior fontanelle and sagittal suture. The hypoechoic fluid-filled cavum septi pellucidi (s) can be observed to be continuous in its extension into the cavum vergae (V) above the thalamus. These structures are beneath the well-demarcated corpus callosum, which appears as a thin anechoic line with bright edges. Although the corpus callosum appears sonographically similar to fluid, it is actually a very homogeneous tissue that has such a fine texture that there are no tissue interfaces to reflect the sound beam. The cerebellar vermis (arrow) appears relatively small in this midline projection. (AA = 26.2 LMP weeks, n = 9, range = 3.0 weeks, TD)

tends posteriorly from the CSP and above the thalamus. Figures 9–11, 9–22, and 9–23 show the cavum vergae and pellucidi. The view in Figure 9–22*C* of the CSP and cavum vergae in long axis is obtained by rotating the transducer from the previous, standard THC plane (see Fig. 9–22*A*). This rotation changes the plane so that the view is tangential to the top of the thalamus and the anterior CSP is in line with the more posterior cavum vergae.

The cavum vergae is not observed as often after approximately 31 weeks and may begin involuting in some fetuses after this time. The CSP and cavum vergae normally communicate[65]; however, there is some confusion about whether or not these cava communicate with the ventricular system. An older text states flatly, "It has no communication with the ventricular system and it has a different lining from the other ventricles."[67] A more modern publication states about the CSP and cavum vergae, "Most often they communicate with the ventricular system through the interventricular foramina."[77] An even more recent report states that "These cava are not considered part of the true ventricular system, since they are not lined with ependyma and rarely communicate with the lateral or third ventricles."[65,78]

We believe that the CSP and its related cavum vergae vary slightly in their presence and appearance, especially toward term.[65,79] Subtle changes in the angles of the transverse plane of view can cause the posterior portions of the anterior horns of the lateral ventricles and the midline septum pellucidum to be confused with a cavum septum or cavum vergae. In the long axis of the CSP and cavum vergae, their appearance is indistinguishable (see Fig. 9–22*C*). A fluid space, the cavum veli interpositi (CVI), is occasionally present above the third ventricle and cavum vergae and below the body and splenium of the corpus callosum. Antenatal sonographic observation of the CVI has been reported.[80] "The cavum veli interpositi is seen more often in infants and children and only occasionally in adults." Its presence may be associated with mental retardation.[81–83]

These midline structures clearly deserve further sonographic research into observation frequency and definition of their destiny in the developing human.

Thalamus

The thalamus is an important anatomical landmark in fetal sonography. It is at the center of the cranium and as such is always crossed transversely by an accurate BPD measurement (see Figs. 9–9, 9–22, and 9–24). A detailed discussion of the BPD and geometry of the fetal cranium is presented elsewhere (see Chapter 8).

The thalamus is made up of two ovoid gray nuclear masses that form the lateral walls of the third ventricle. Sonographically, the two halves of the thalamus appear hypoechoic relative to the cerebral cortex surrounding them (see Figs. 9–10*A* to 9–11*C* and 9–24). Functionally, most sensory stimuli are received by the thalamus, except for olfactory stimuli and some older diffuse pathways.[84,85]

In the transaxial view commonly used to measure the THC, the thalamus appears as relatively ovoid with a central line. In sonograms of particularly clear definition, the third ventricle may be seen as two parallel

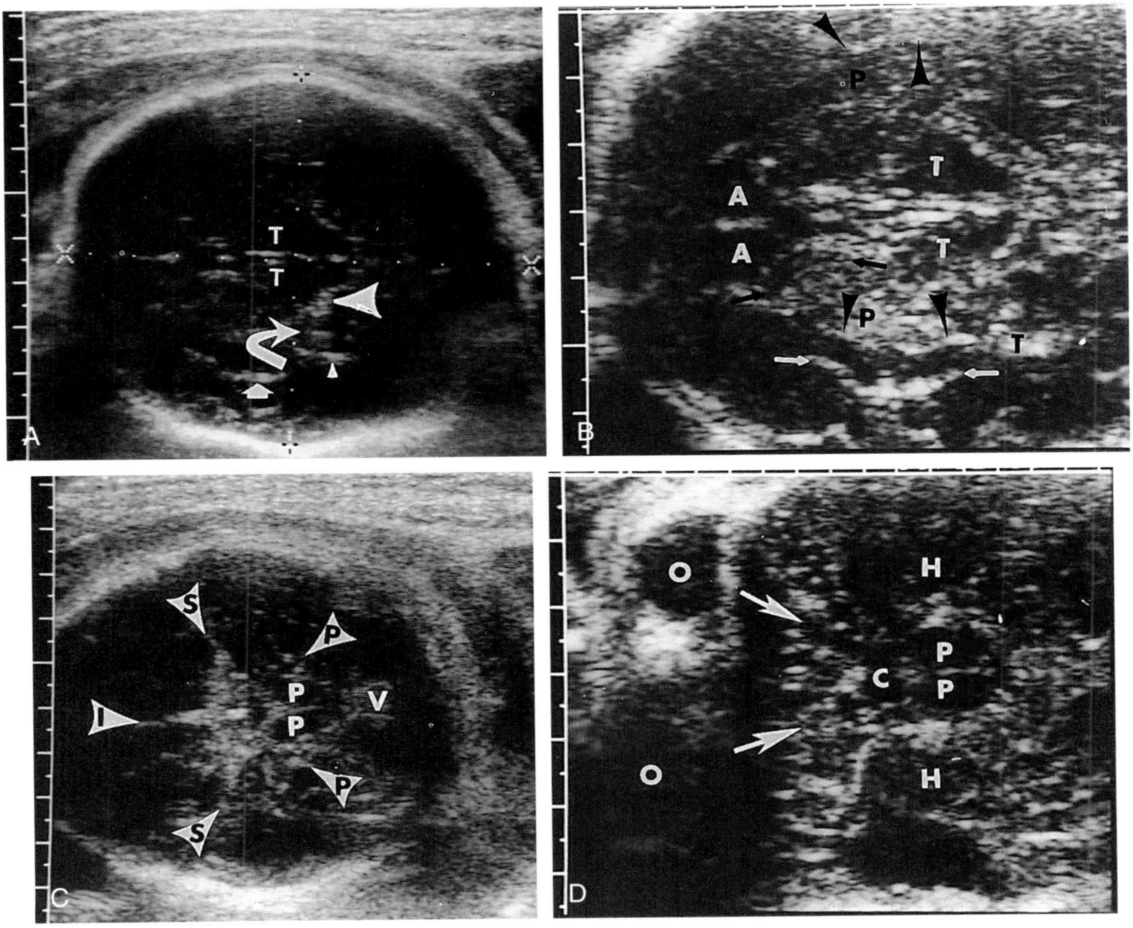

FIGURE 9–24.
Midbrain structures. Sonography of the very complex midbrain can be misleading for two reasons. Textures may vary depending on the directions of tissue fibers in relation to the sound beam, which may change the reflectiveness of the tissue (see Fig. 9–11*B* and *C*). In addition, the plane of view has beam width that may combine or average very small, close structures into a single image. *A*, Standard transverse head circumference with biparietal diameter (82.9 mm) and fronto-occipital diameter (105.6 mm) measurements. The cavum septi pellucidi is not seen, but the fornix and anterior horns of the ventricles are shown. The thalamus (white T) is hypoechoic, and the third ventricle appears as an anechoic slit between two bright echoes at the midthalamus. The sylvian sulcus (wide arrow) and temporal horn of the ventricles (small arrowhead) appear as echogenic lines. The hippocampus (curved arrow) can be seen between the temporal horn and the echogenic, fibrous geniculate nucleus (large white arrowhead). Heads of the caudate nuclei are not well visualized in this image (see *B*). *B*, This is an enlargement with increased gain from the same plane as image *A*. The distal head of the caudate nucleus (between small black arrows) is just posterolateral to the anterior horns of the ventricles (A). The anterior horns appear wider than they actually are, most likely because of beam-width averaging of the curved horns. Because the curving anterior horns are separated by the homogeneous tissue of the corpus callosum, which does not add echoes to the image, the horns appear much wider than they actually are. The hippocampus is again seen medial to the strong echoes from the temporal horn (black T). The sylvian fissure and insula (small white arrows) are particularly well demonstrated. P, putamen; black arrowheads, external capsule; T, thalamus. *C*, This image is slightly lower in the head than *A* and *B*. The third ventricle appears as the brightest echo at the center of the echogenic suprasellar cistern, anterior to the peduncles of the midbrain or brainstem (P). The interhemispheric fissure (I arrowhead) extends forward from the suprasellar cistern, and the sylvian fissure (S arrowheads) continues anterolaterally and inferiorly along the top of the lesser wings of the sphenoid bones. The lateral pontine cisterns (P arrowheads) extend posteriorly on either side of the peduncles. The echoes of the interhemispheric and the bilateral sylvian fissures and lateral pontine cisterns form a five-pointed star (arrowheads), six pointed if the echoes of the midbrain stem are included. The cerebellar vermis (V) is directly posterior to the brainstem. *D*, Image just inferior to *C*. Arrows point to the optic nerve tracts, which extend from the back of the orbits (O) to the optic chiasm (C). The more distal orbit is only faintly seen in the shadow of the nasal bones. P, peduncles of midbrain; H, hippocampus. (AA = 33.0 LMP weeks, n = 9, range = 1.4 weeks, TD)

lines with a thin layer of fluid between them (see Figs. 9–9 and 9–24).

In the coronal view, the two halves of the thalamus take on the shape of a stylized heart, as in a valentine, with the point (apex) of the heart representing the brain stem (see Figs. 9–10, 9–13*A*, and 9–22*D*).

In the less commonly obtained sagittal view of the fetal cranium, the thalamus is seen as a widening of the brainstem with a rounded top (see Fig. 9–11*C*).

The bodies of the lateral ventricles are above and lateral to the thalamus and can occasionally be visualized in the coronal view as fluid-filled slits with echogenic walls. In Figure 9–10, the ventricles are demonstrated in a coronal view. The roof of the bodies of the lateral ventricles is formed by the corpus callosum.

The thalamus is not usually measured but is used as an anatomical marker for planes that pass through the midbrain. However, in a very small, unpublished, informal survey of BPDs from 28 to 94 mm, we found the ratio of the thalamus width/BPD to decline slowly from a mean of 42% to a mean of 37% and to be between 30% and 50% at the 95% confidence levels ($n = 17$, $P > 0.05$). The population mean was 40%. This change of percentage in time is not significant.

Hippocampus

Description. The hippocampi are curvilinear structures that lie bilaterally in the temporal lobes. Each hippocampus is approximately 2.25 to 2.5 cm long in an adult. Anteriorly, a portion of the hippocampus is closely associated with the fimbria, dentate gyrus, cornu Ammonis, and subiculum. These form bilateral bulbous areas called the *hippocampal formations* or *complexes*, which are in the most anterior and medial portion of the inferior (temporal) horns of the lateral ventricles (see Figs. 9–10 and 9–24*D*).[86]

Each hippocampal complex has an echo density that is similar to the echo texture of the cerebral cortex. The structures surrounding the formation are hyperechoic. These structures appear as bilateral echogenic rings around the hippocampal complexes in the midcoronal view. These rings are made up of the temporal horn of the lateral ventricles laterally and superiorly and the tentorium medially and inferiorly. Identification of the rings of the coronal hippocampi may assist in evaluation of ventricular temporal horn dilation (see Fig. 9–21*B*). Other structures that lie within these echogenic rings are the ambient cistern, lateral geniculate nuclei, tails of the caudate nuclei, the bilateral parahippocampal gyri, and their associated collateral fissures.[87, 88]

Coronal Hippocampal Gyri. In the midcoronal view of the fetal cranium, the hippocampal gyri appear within two circles (see Fig. 9–10*A* and *B*). These landmark structures can be useful in identifying normal anatomy in the coronal view of the fetal skull. By drawing an imaginary line tangential to the inferior edges of these two circles, the VCD can be measured from the midpoint of this base line (HBL) to the vertex of the skull (see Chapter 8 for a discussion of the three-dimensional geometry of the fetal cranium).

Corpus Callosum

The corpus callosum appears hypoechoic sonographically because the tissue has a high density. It forms the roof of the lateral ventricles, CSP, and cavum vergae (see Figs. 9–9 to 9–11 and 9–23). It forms the major structure of communication between the two cerebral hemispheres.

Agenesis of the corpus callosum may be identified sonographically because the third ventricle tends to be enlarged and is high riding.[89] The lateral horns may also be enlarged and higher than usual in the head.

Cisterna Magna

Description

The cisterna magna is a fluid-filled space posterior to the cerebellum. It may or may not have one or more septa or veins that appear as linear echoes extending sagittally from the cerebellar vermis. Figures 9–7 and 9–14 show the transverse cerebellum and cisterna magna. Figure 9–15 shows the cerebellum in the coronal view. Figure 9–11 demonstrates the sagittal view of the cerebellum and cisterna magna.

Measurement and Size

The cisterna magna can be affected by spinal cord anomalies that are far distant from the cisterna itself. This is because a spinal cord defect can tether the cord. As a fetus grows, the cord is not allowed to move in the canal; therefore, it is fixed or tethered. This tethering causes a downward positioning of the cord and brainstem, which in turn results in a downward positioning of the cerebellum in the occipital fossa of the cranium. As a result, the cisterna magna is obliterated.[90]

In a well-documented study of 638 pregnancies, the cisterna magna was found to increase significantly with age in normal fetuses. The size at 14 weeks was 2 to 4 mm; between 17 and 19 weeks, the range was 2 to 10 mm; and by 21 weeks, the range was 4 to 7 mm. This same study found the cisterna magna measurement to be normal for 28 fetuses with abnormal karyotypes.[91]

Composite Analysis of Central Nervous System Development

Ventricular Antrum and Cisterna Magna

Filly and associates proposed a method of evaluating the development of the fetal central nervous system (CNS) that is relatively simple and quick. Using their method, they expressed confidence that 95% of CNS abnormalities could be ruled out.[46] This composite method requires measurement of the ventricular antrum (<10 to 12 mm) and the presence of the cisterna magna. If both these measurements are normal, 95% of CNS abnormalities can be ruled out, even if the lower spine cannot be adequately seen because of fetal position. Figure 9–21 demonstrates a slightly enlarged ventricular system.

Fruit Signs

Lemon

The so-called lemon sign is a slight depression of the bilateral temple region on a transverse head image. The lemon sign has been reported as being specific for myelomeningocele.[92]

Another study found that the lemon sign was not exclusively associated with myelomeningoceles.[93] This study found that out of 23 fetuses with lemon signs, 12 had myelomeningoceles, 6 had encephaloceles, and 5 had various structural anomalies not involving the neural tube. Some researchers have found that the lemon sign is most valid before 24 weeks.[94] It has been proposed that the lemon sign represents deformation of the frontotemporal calvarium from reduced pressure due to downward positioning on the brain by the tethered spine.[95] It was further suggested that the reduced pressure is increased by the obstructed CNS fluid buildup, hydrocephaly, causing the lemon sign to become more normal in appearance.

Although the actual cause of the lemon sign is unclear, there is no question that if a lemon sign is present, the fetus should receive close scrutiny.

Banana

When a spinal defect tethers the cord, the brainstem and cerebellum tend to remain fixed as the fetus grows. This low positioning causes the fluid in the cisterna magna to decrease and the cerebellum to conform to a shape that has been described as resembling a banana. This is better known as the Arnold-Chiari deformity or syndrome, which was described in the 1800s by two German pathologists, Julius Arnold and Hans Chiari.[96] More recently, this condition has been referred to as the *banana sign* in the sonographic literature. A London study found the banana sign in 72% of fetuses with spinal defects before 24 weeks. This same study found that after 24 weeks, in 81% of the fetuses with spinal defects, the cerebellum was sonographically absent.[95,97] This absence was described as downward pressure with "herniation of the brain through the cisterna magna."[95]

Vascular

Two-dimensional real-time color Doppler sonographic imaging has made study of the fetal cerebral vasculature possible. The circle of Willis can be easily demonstrated. Figure 9–25 is a black-and-white color Doppler image of the anterior circle of Willis. The bilateral middle cerebral and the anterior cerebral arteries are visualized. A small portion of the

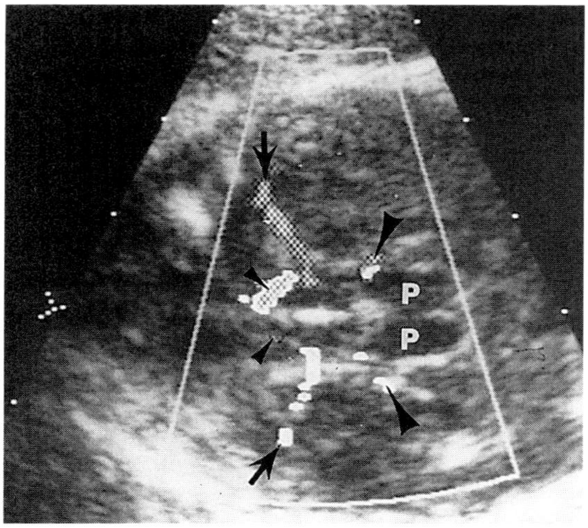

FIGURE 9–25.
Circle of Willis. Transverse plane near base X of the skull with color Doppler showing portions of the cerebral vascularity. P, peduncles of midbrain; arrows, middle cerebral arteries; small arrowheads, anterior cerebral arteries; large arrowheads, posterior cerebral arteries. (AA = 19.3 LMP weeks, n = 9, range = 0.9 weeks, TD)

posterior cerebral artery is also demonstrated. In this image, a velocity tag has been used to outline flow away from the transducer in contrasting white. The color Doppler shift is imaged as a checkered area. We are not aware of any reports of abnormal fetal cranial vasculature detected by sonography (see Chapter 13 for more on fetal Doppler sonography).

One study systematically evaluated the middle cerebral, vertebral, and intracerebellar arteries.[98] This study found similar (not significantly different) pulsatility indexes in the middle cerebral and vertebral arteries. However, the intracerebellar artery had consistently lower pulsatility indexes, indicating lower resistance to blood flow.

Other studies have found that in head-sparing or asymmetrical intrauterine growth retardation (IUGR), the body has a natural priority that causes the resistance to blood flow in the head to drop while the resistance to flow in the body tends to increase. The theory is that this favoring of the head allows the brain to continue to develop while the body is relatively starved in the presence of hypoxia and hypoglycemia due to the reduced perfusion.[99]

SPINE

Cervical

The cervical spine consists of seven vertebral bodies and intervening disk spaces. A slight flaring of the spine is seen at the top. This area at the base of the skull is a relatively common site for spinal defects. Figures 9–26 to 9–28 demonstrate normal fetal cervical spines.

Thoracic

Between the base of the neck and the small of the back, above the lumbar spine, are 12 thoracic vertebral bodies. All the thoracic vertebral bodies have rib articulations.

The thoracic spine normally exhibits some curve, depending on the fetal position. Because of this curvature, the entire thoracic spine may be difficult to observe in a single plane (see Figs. 9–26 to 9–28). The thorax is relatively uniform in appearance, vertebral body to vertebral body.

Because the vertebral bodies of the thorax and lumbar regions are similar in size, they may be used to estimate fetal growth and age.[100] This method measures seven complete thoracolumbar vertebral bodies and spaces (see Fig. 9–28). The thoracolumbar fractional

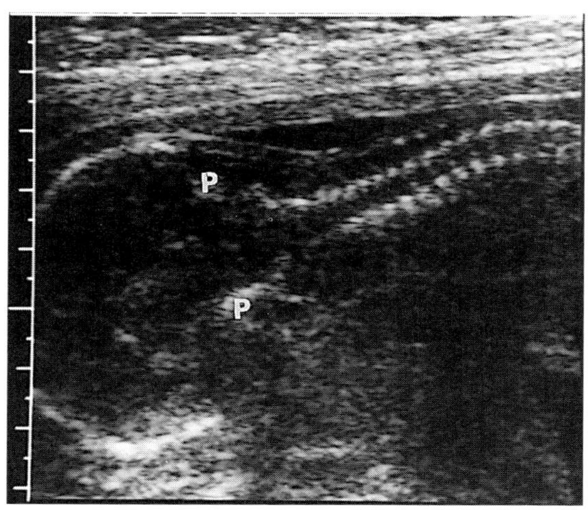

FIGURE 9–26.
Normal coronal view of a fetal cervical spine. Note that the spine widens into the posterior fossa of the cranium between the petrous pyramids (P). This is one of the more common locations of spinal defects. (AA = 22.5 LMP weeks, n = 9, range = 1.6 weeks, TD)

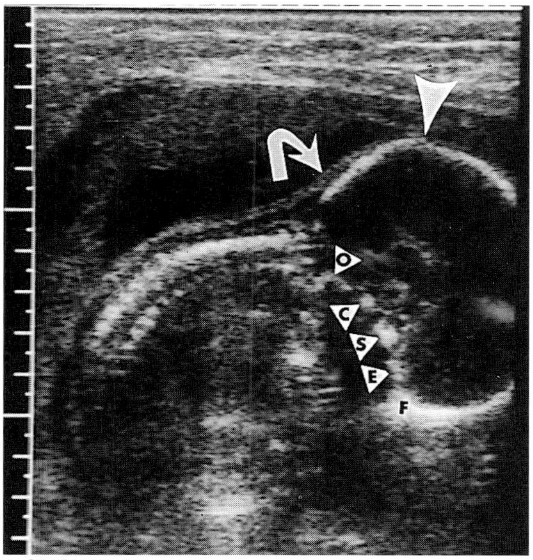

FIGURE 9–27.
Posterior sagittal view of the cervical spine and skull. The curved arrow points to the nuchal area over the base of the posterior occipital bone, where the skin may be thickened in some genetic syndromes. The large arrowhead points to the lambdoid suture/posterior fontanelle between the occipital and parietal bones. Triangles point to bones in the base of the skull. O, basilar portion of occipital bone; C, posterior clinoid; S, sphenoid bone; E, ethmoid or clinoid bone; F, frontal bone. The foramen magnum, through which the brainstem passes, is at the top of the cervical spine, just inferior to the 0 triangle (see Fig. 9–6). (AA = 22.5 LMP weeks, n = 9, range = 1.6 weeks, TD)

spine length (FSL) was suggested by Li and Woo because they found that this area could be observed in a single sonographic plane in 98.2% of the cases whereas longer or other spinal segments could less often be observed and measured in a single image.[101] These researchers found that the FSL correlated well with fetal age ($r^2 = 0.92$, $P < 0.0001$, n = 214). Their second-order regression follows:

$$FSL = -37.62 + 4.36 \times age - 0.04 \times age^2$$

where FSL = 7 vertebral bodies and spaces, and age = LMP weeks. A simplified version of this regression, which provides similar results, is

$$\mathbf{FSL = -40 + 4.4 \times age - 0.04 \times age^2}$$

Table 7–1 can be used to estimate fetal age from this FSL.

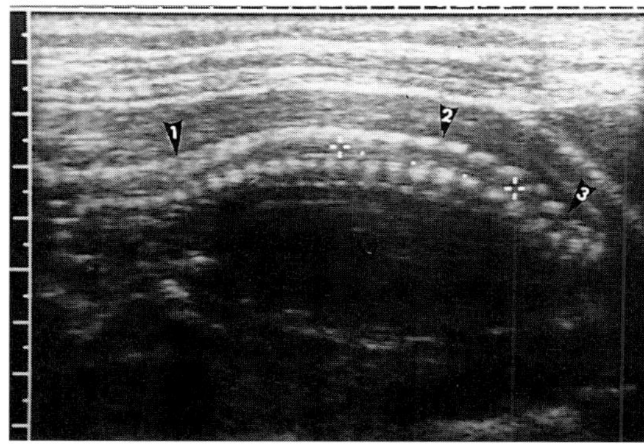

FIGURE 9–28.
Fetal spine and fractional spine length. Earlier in pregnancy, with transducers that provide large fields of view, the entire fetal spine can be observed in a single image, with appropriate fetal position. Here the entire spinal column is shown: Arrowhead 1 is between the cervical and thoracic portions, 2 is between the thoracic and lumbar portions, and 3 is between the lumbar and sacrum. The + cursors (34.5 mm) show the measurement of the fractional spine length, which should include seven thoracolumbar vertebral bodies and spaces. (AA = 20.8 LMP weeks, n = 9, range = 1.7 weeks, TD)

Li and Woo also found that the FSL/abdominal circumference (AC) ratio was relatively constant from the 19th to 42nd week of pregnancy.

$$FSL/AC \times 100 = 20.4 \pm 3.1 \ (\pm 2\ SD)$$

They found that the FSL was outside −2 SD for only 1 of 10 small-for-gestational-age (SGA) fetuses and was normal for both thanatophoric dwarfs in their study. This may mean that the FSL is less affected by variations in fetal size than are other parameters. In addition, Li and Woo pointed out, "The FSL may therefore be more useful in the assessment of fetal growth aberration starting from this early period. As it is possible that the length of the fetus which this parameter reflects is more closely related to the weight of the fetus than gestational maturity (similar to the AC)."[101] The FSL is demonstrated in Figure 9–28.

Lumbosacral

The lumbar spine contains five vertebral bodies; the sacrum is just inferior to the lumbar spine. The sacrum and coccyx taper to a point at the base of the spine (Figs. 9–28 and 9–29).

This region of the spine is a relatively common location of spinal defects. Figure 9–30 demonstrates a spinal defect that was diagnosed sonographically in one of two twins. Although this text is primarily concerned with normal fetuses, these images are included because spinal defects are among the most common of fetal anomalies and in the United States occur in 1.5 to 2.0 births per 1000.[102]

A complete study of the fetal spine should include transverse real-time study of the entire spine (Fig. 9–31). These views of the spine should demonstrate the three ossification centers of the vertebrae.

The fetal sacral length (SL) has also been measured and correlated with gestational age[103] (see Fig. 9–29). The sacrum is located between the iliac bones of the pelvis (Fig. 9–32). The wings of the iliac may cause shadowing and make the sacrum difficult to visualize. This measurement is also approximately one third shorter than the FSL, and any errors in cursor placement result in relatively larger percent errors.

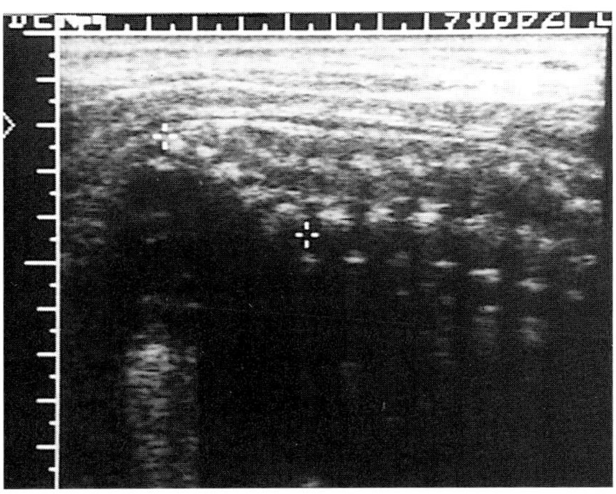

FIGURE 9–29.
Sacral length measurement between + cursors (37.9 mm). The sacral length includes the five sacral bodies from the anterosuperior margin of S1 (sacral promontory) to the inferior tip of S5. In this case, the fetus was diagnosed as being small for gestational age (SGA), based on two examinations approximately 30 weeks apart. Examination 1 was normal with a reported LNMP of 8.3 weeks, and the sonographic average age calculated to 8.2 LMP weeks. (AA = 8.2, n = 3, range = 0.9 weeks, RRG) At 38.1 LNMP weeks, a second examination was performed (this image), and the sonographic average age was calculated to be only 35.7 LMP weeks, a reduction in fetal growth of 2.4 weeks. This sacral length of 37.9 mm calculates to an LMP age of 37.0 (±0.7) weeks, very close to the LNMP age. This was considered SGA rather than intrauterine growth retardation because the abdominal circumference at 37.0 weeks was leading the cranial ages, which averaged to 35.0 LMP weeks. (AA = 35.7, n = 8, range = 4.1 weeks, LP)

Sherer and associates[103] reported the following simple linear regression equations for the SL and fetal age:

$$SL = -0.108 + 0.102 \times \text{age}$$

$$(r^2 = 0.959, P < 0.001, n = 506)$$

$$\text{Age} = 2.14 + 9.37 \times SL$$

where SL is in centimeters and age is LMP weeks. Sherer and colleagues' study[103] reported the standard deviations in only tabular and graphical forms. However, observation of the table for fetal age indicates the ±2 SD range to be approximately ±10% of the age. This is similar to the ranges found for most fetal parameters using age range analysis (see Chapter 7).

FACE

Lips and Palate

A complete sonographic study of the fetal head includes the face, particularly the lips and nose, to rule out clefts. This diagnosis is important because facial clefts are associated with other congenital abnormalities approximately 50% of the time.[104] The lips and nose are best imaged with real-time because they are not perfectly flat and slight cross-plane rocking can facilitate imaging the complete face. In Figure 9–33, approximately one half of the lips and one nostril are well visualized.

Approximately 50% of the time, a fetus is touching its face and head with its hands (see Chapter 15 for more discussion of fetal hand activities). These head and face hand activities may make evaluation of the face difficult because of shadowing from overlying extremity bones. The occasional sucking motion of the lips on the fingers or umbilical cord may, however, be a delight to the observing prospective parents. Sucking and swallowing motions have been reported as early as the

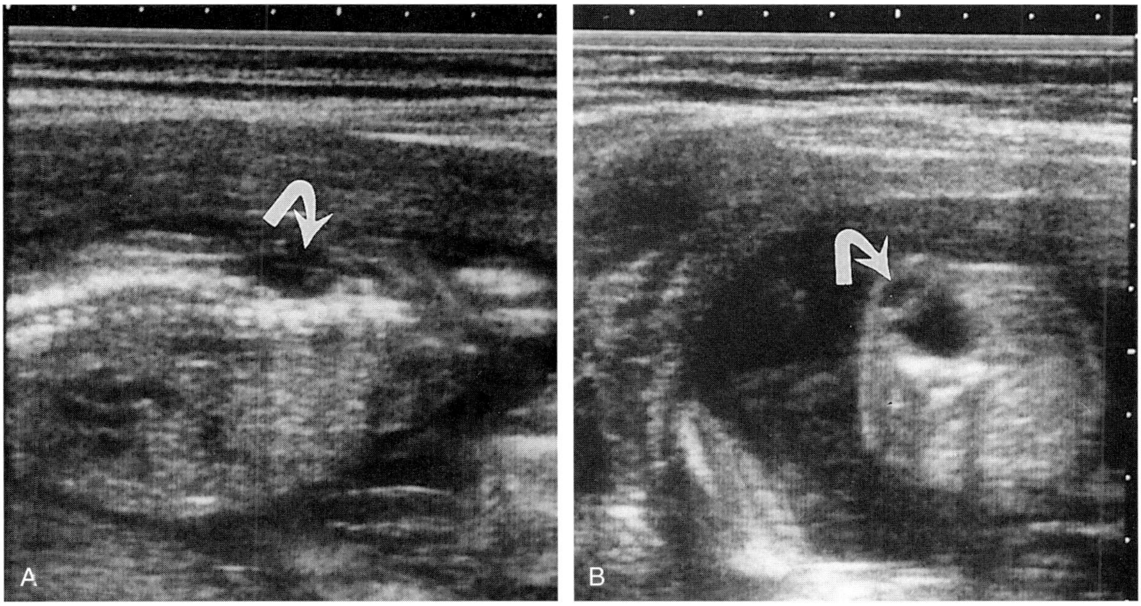

FIGURE 9–30.
Spinal defect. Although this text is concerned with normal fetuses, these images are included to give some idea of the appearance of a spinal defect. From these images, it is not possible to determine if this spina bifida (curved arrows) is a meningocele (protruding meninges with spinal fluid) or a meningomyelocele (protruding meninges with neural tissue). It was determined that the defect was closed (covered with skin), which means that results of the alpha-fetoprotein test might be normal. *A*, Posterior sagittal plane showing lumbosacral spinal defect (curved arrow) in the smaller of twins. *B*, Posterior transverse plane showing a lumbosacral spinal defect (curved arrow) in the same twin. (AA = 19.3 LMP weeks, n = 9, range = 2.5 weeks, JR)

12th LMP week. Other lip motions that may be observed are associated with jaw movements, yawning, and sticking the tongue out between the lips.[105]

The sagittal view of the face has also been shown to be important in the diagnosis of clefts in the hard palate because of an associated protrusion of the alveolus of the maxilla and the premaxilla tissue.[106] Figure 9–34 demonstrates a normal sagittal view of the fetal face.

One study measured the cheek-to-cheek distance (CCD), which correlated well with fetal age ($n = 234$, $r^2 = 0.806$).[107] This study found a linear relationship with age as follows:

$$\text{LMP age} = 9.77 + 4.16\ \text{CCD}$$

However, the study found the CCD $\pm$ 2 SD for the age throughout pregnancy to range from 50% of the age early in pregnancy to approximately 23% of age at term. This is a much larger variation than is shown by the skeletal structures, which usually exhibit a range of $\pm$10% of the age throughout pregnancy. The larger variation of the CCD may be an important indicator in variation in fetal fat and, therefore, weight. More study is needed.

Nose

The fetal nose can be observed with gentle cross-plane rocking of the field of view as the face and lips are studied (see Figs. 9–33 and 9–34). Clefts of the lip may extend up into either or both nostrils. The major difficulty in viewing the nose is a disadvantageous fetal position or a hand or arm overshadowing it.

Mandible

The mandible is best imaged in real-time. This allows gentle cross-plane rocking of the field of view to sweep across the front of the face for observation of the relative bone and tissue alignment and facial relationships (see

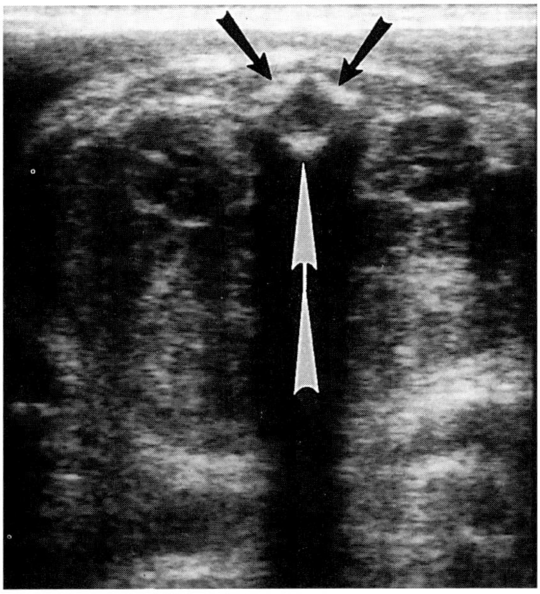

FIGURE 9–31.
Transverse fetal spine. The fetal spine should be observed in both the long and transverse views. The transverse view can rule out a lateral defect that a sagittal plane might not demonstrate. In the transverse view, the three ossification centers of the spine should form a triangular shape. The anterior center is the vertebral body (white arrow in acoustic shadow of spine). The two posterior echoes are the ossification centers of the lamina (black arrows). The skin covering the posterior spine should be smooth and uninterrupted. The spine should be observed from top to bottom in the transverse view using a cross-plane slide of the transducer. Note that the kidneys can be seen on either side of the spine. (AA = 39.0 LMP weeks, n = 8, range = 4.1 weeks, LP)

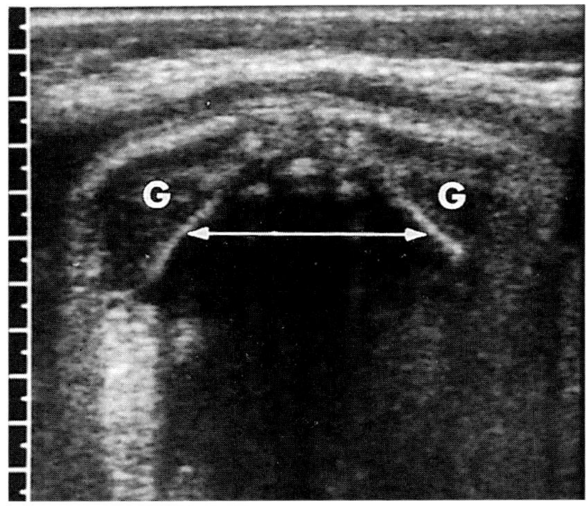

FIGURE 9–32.
Transverse sacrum and pelvis. The sacrum does not have the three ossification centers of the higher spine. This normal transverse sacrum shows both iliac bones of the pelvis (double arrow). The skin can be observed to have a smooth contour over the sacrum and gluteus maximus muscles (G). (AA = 36.7 LMP weeks, n = 8, range = 3.8 weeks, SG)

Fig. 9–33). The sagittal view is particularly useful for subjective comparison of the mandible and maxilla (see Fig. 9–34). A short mandible, micrognathia, is associated with many syndromes. This is also true of most congenital facial defects.

Tables for the measurement and correlation of the mandible have been developed for this evaluation (Table 9–1).[108] Another study reported results very similar to those in Table 9–1. The differences for the mean mandibular measurements between the two studies were usually less than ±2 mm for each week.[109] However, this latter study reported results only between 12 and 28 LMP weeks because "They [Otto and Platt[108]] commented that up until 30 weeks' gestation measurement is possible in most fetuses, but beyond this gestation they frequently encountered difficulties. Our experience would also suggest that accu-

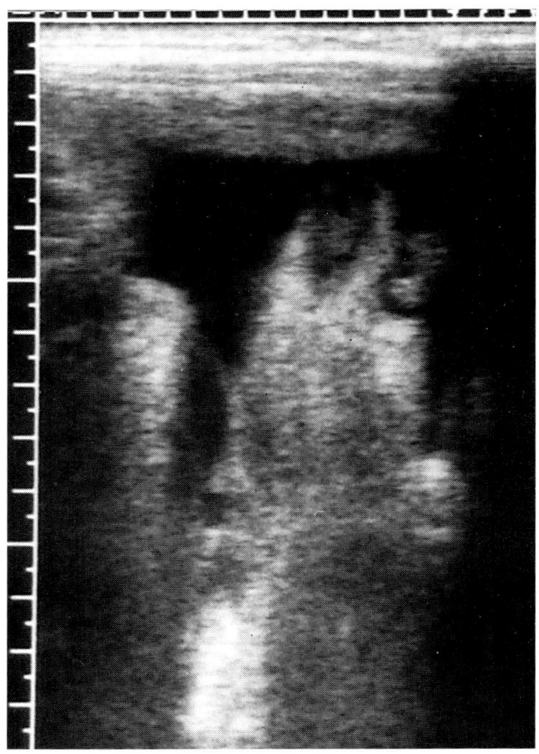

FIGURE 9–33.
Here half the lips and one nostril can be seen. The fetal face is best observed with real-time using a gentle cross-plane rocking in order to study the lips and nose. This cross-plane rocking allows complete study to rule out clefts. (AA = 39.0 LMP weeks, n = 8, range = 4.1 weeks, LP)

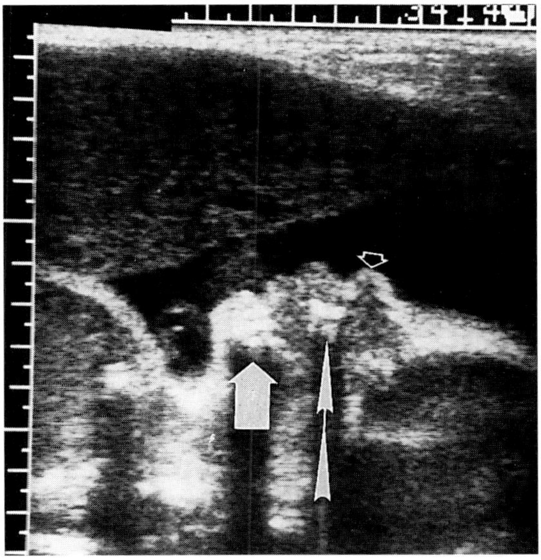

FIGURE 9–34.
Frontal sagittal image of fetal face profile. This image is from the larger of twins; the smaller twin is shown in Figure 9–10. Both were born normal males. This view is useful to observe the relationship of the facial bones. The mandible (wide arrow in mandibular acoustic shadow) should not be posterior to the maxilla (long arrow in maxillary acoustic shadow). A small mandible, micrognathia, is associated with certain genetic syndromes. A protruding maxilla and facial tags may be associated with facial clefts. The chin, lips, nose (open arrow), and forehead should exhibit a normal profile. (AA = 35.6 LMP weeks, n = 5, range = 1.4 weeks, DKD)

TABLE 9–1. FETAL MANDIBLE MEASUREMENT

GESTATIONAL AGE (WEEKS)	LOWER PL	MEAN	UPPER PL
14	0.8	1.2	1.6
15	1.0	1.4	1.8
16	1.2	1.6	2.0
17	1.5	1.9	2.3
18	1.7	2.1	2.5
19	1.9	2.3	2.7
20	2.1	2.5	2.9
21	2.2	2.6	3.1
22	2.4	2.8	3.2
23	2.6	3.0	3.4
24	2.8	3.2	3.6
25	2.9	3.3	3.8
26	3.1	3.5	3.9
27	3.2	3.7	4.1
28	3.4	3.8	4.2
29	3.5	4.0	4.4
30	3.7	4.1	4.5
31	3.8	4.2	4.6
32	3.9	4.4	4.8
33	4.1	4.5	4.9
34	4.2	4.6	5.0
35	4.3	4.7	5.1
36	4.4	4.8	5.2
37	4.5	4.9	5.3
38	4.6	5.0	5.4
39	4.7	5.1	5.5

This table can be used to evaluate the size of the mandible at various fetal ages in weeks. The mandibular sizes for approximately 95% of this population are expected to be between the lower and upper prediction limits (PL = 95% prediction limits). (From Otto C, Platt LD: The fetal mandible measurement: An objective determination of fetal jaw size. Ultrasound Obstet Gynecol 1991;1:12–17.)

rate measurement of the fetal mandible is not reliably obtained in the third trimester and it may be that a subjective assessment of jaw size at this stage of pregnancy is as reliable." Figure 9–35 shows a normal mandibular measurement. Table 9–1 can be used to compare mandibular size if micrognathia is suspected. Late in pregnancy, the subjective method described earlier may be useful (see Fig. 9–34). In Figure 9–34, it should be noted that the umbilical cord can be observed to be around the neck and under the chin of the fetus; however, there is no double loop and the skin line is not depressed, and this finding is probably not clinically significant unless it is found at the time of delivery (see Chapter 16 for more on nuchal umbilical cords).

Clefts

Clefts of the upper lip and palate have been diagnosed using sonography. In general, these diagnoses have been made from images that are tangential to the fetal face. In Figure 9–33, the lips and nose can be observed in a tangential view. The diagnosis of clefts should only be attempted using real-time sonography, usually with a transabdominal approach.

One study used transvaginal transducers to diagnose clefts.[110] The researchers proposed that the diagnosis could be made in sagittal planes by comparing the relative protrusion of the lower lip in relationship to the cleft of the upper lip, pseudoprognathism. If a fetus is in a suitable position for observation transvaginally, the diagnosis may be made as early as the 14th week with this method.

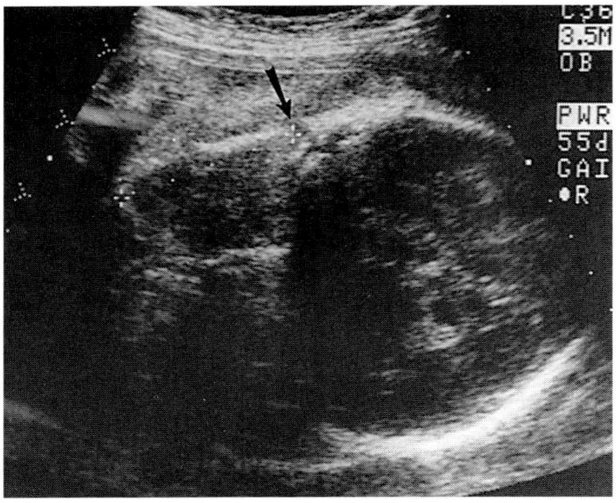

FIGURE 9–35.
Fetal mandibular measurement (+ cursors = 42.6 mm). This measurement is taken from the temporomandibular joint (arrow) to the anterior curve (symphysis) of the mandible. In this case, the 42.6-mm measurement is at or very slightly above the mean for age. Compare this measurement with Table 9–1. (AA = 31.2 LMP weeks, n = 9, range = 3.2 weeks, TD)

Eyes

The fetal eyes are obvious circular (spherical) structures at the front of the head and are useful for orientation. Their measurement can also be used to estimate age when other parameters are precluded by fetal position.[111, 112] The fetal eye measurement does, however, exhibit a relatively large variation. This is probably because of normal variation in hypertelorism and hypotelorism, as well as the less obvious reason of slight off-axis measurements (see Table 7–1 for outer binocular distance measurements and fetal age). The lens can often be observed, as well as the hyaloid artery (Fig. 9–36).

SCALP, EARS, AND HAIR

Scalp

Normal Scalp

The normal fetal scalp is less echogenic than the skull, and the skin over the calvarium usually is less than 4 or 5 mm. The skin thickness normally varies slightly, depending on the location, fetal body fat, and the time in gestation. Experience will give a sonographer a general feeling for the appearance of normal fetal skin (see Chapters 18 and 19 for representative normal fetal sonograms throughout pregnancy to use for comparison).

Some conditions can cause a generalized edema of the skin called *hydrops fetalis*. This may give the appearance of concentric layers or a halo. This condition can range from very subtle to quite severe and obvious.

Edematous Scalp

During the study of the cervical spine is a good time to observe the nuchal fold or nuchal occipital thickening.[113, 114] It was first reported in 1985 that nuchal skin thickening greater than 6 mm can be associated with certain syndromes such as Down's.[115, 116] The tissue thickness is measured over the inferior occipital bone, below the occipital protuberance (see Figs. 9–8, 9–14, and 9–27). It should be less than 6 mm.[116] The measure-

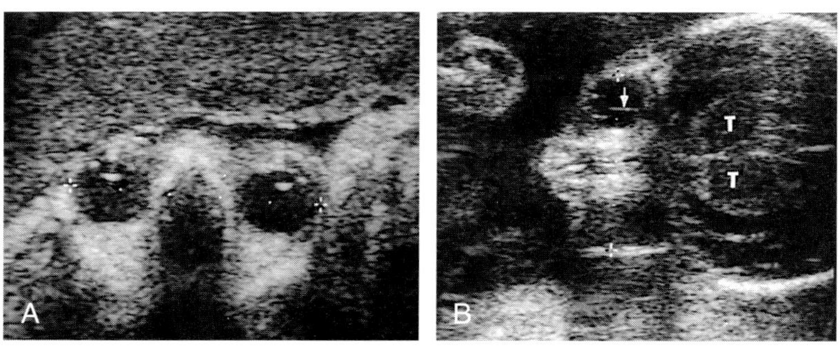

FIGURE 9–36.
Fetal eyes. The outer orbital distance (BiOD) can be useful if fetal position precludes easy measurement of other parameters. This measurement is taken to the inside of the zygomatic bones. (See Chapter 7 for fetal age tables.) *A*, Frontal view of the fetal eyes. The outer orbital distance is measured (+ cursors = 49.7) and evaluated to 30.5 LMP weeks. The bright echoes in the anterior part of the eye are from the posterior of the lens. (AA = 31.5 LMP weeks, n = 9, range = 2.5, TD) *B*, Transverse view of orbits with BiOD measurement (+ cursors = 40.9 mm = 24.8 weeks). Nasal bones tend to shadow the more distal orbit in this view. The thin line in the near orbit is the hyaloid artery (arrow), which supplies nutrition to the lens and is observed occasionally between the 15th and 29th LMP weeks. T, thalamus. (AA = 24.6 LMP weeks, n = 9, range = 1.3 weeks, TD)

ment is angle dependent and may result in false positives.[117]

Another major caution here is that a fat fetus with its neck extended may exhibit nuchal thickening. However, this in conjunction with other indicators such as short humeri and femurs could be an indication for further study. Measurement of long bones to predict Down's syndrome is controversial.[118]

Cystic hygroma of the nuchal area usually is cystic and septated and may be quite large. The fluid is a result of malformation of the lymph system.[121] Cystic hygroma is often associated with Turner's syndrome.[120] It has also been detected sonographically, only to resolve before birth. Echogenic fetal hair may also confound these observations late in pregnancy.[121]

During early pregnancy, the skin at the back of an embryo may appear cystic, or a fetus with its back to the amnion before fusion with the chorion may give the appearance of a cystic hygroma.

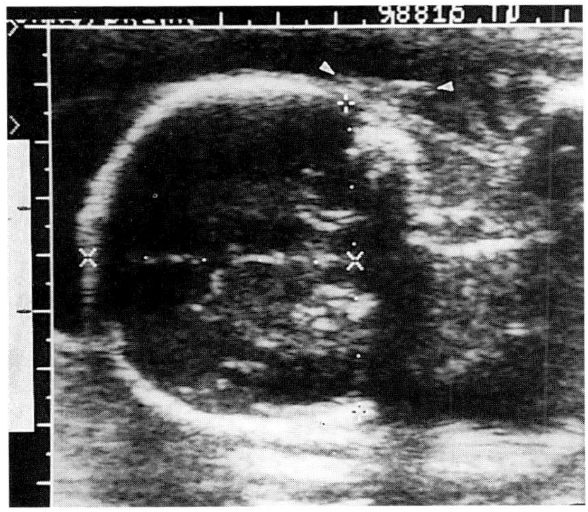

FIGURE 9–37.
The fetal ear (small arrowheads). The ear may be measured and compared with Table 9–2. In this image, using a paper straightedge to compare with the scale, the ear is approximately 18+ mm in length. This measurement would evaluate to approximately the 20th percentile or slightly above, which is normal for the fetal age. (AA = 24.0 LMP weeks, n = 9, range = 2.1 weeks, TD)

Ears

The ear has been measured and correlated with age and used in ratios of its width to length and to the BPD (Fig. 9–37). Table 9–2 gives the percentiles for the ear length (EL) to age. The ratio of the width to the length was found to be independent of age, between 82% and 49% in 95% of the population (±2 SD). After midpregnancy, the BPD/EL ratio for 95% of the population was between 245% and 360% (mean 303%). Ratio of BPD/EL declined very slowly from the 18th week to term, but not significantly.

The longest EL was found to increase linearly with menstrual age (LMP). Between the 14th and 25th LMP week, the normal EL can be approximated:

$$EL = (1.2 \times \text{age}) - 10$$

$$\text{10th to 90th percentiles} = \pm 15\%\ EL$$

where ear length is in millimeters and age is in LMP weeks.[122]

The ear is relatively small, however, and is more difficult to measure than the more accessible skeletal structures. It is therefore not recommended for fetal age determination. If ear abnormality is suspected, the foregoing comparative ratios appear more useful. An association of small ears has been found with second-trimester aneuploidy, an abnormal number of chromosomes.[123]

TABLE 9–2. **FETAL EAR LENGTH MEASUREMENT BY GESTATIONAL AGE**

GESTATIONAL AGE (WK)	EAR LENGTH (MM) PERCENTILE VALUES				
	10%	20%	50%	80%	90%
14	6	6	7	8	8
15	7	7	8	9	10
16	8	8	9	11	11
17	9	9	11	12	12
18	10	11	12	13	14
19	11	12	13	15	15
20	12	13	14	16	17
21	13	14	16	17	18
22	15	15	17	18	19
23	16	16	18	20	21
24	17	18	19	21	22
25	18	19	21	22	23

Ear lengths between the 14th and 25th LMP weeks with percentiles. The original report found that 10 of 14 fetuses with abnormal genes had ear lengths at or below the 10th percentile (total n = 424). (From Lettieri L, Rodis JF, Vintzileos AM, et al: Ear length in second-trimester aneuploid fetuses. Obstet Gynecol 1993;81:57–60.)

Hair

Fetal hair can often be observed sonographically late in pregnancy, particularly at the back of the head. Hair may not be observed on all fetuses, only those with a lot of hair or relatively coarse hair. The sonographic observation of hair has little diagnostic significance. The primary caution is that it not be mistaken for pathological processes such as the membranes of cystic hygroma.[121]

Future: Three-Dimensional Imaging

Already in existence are sonographic machines that can produce true three-dimensional images. The utility of these is yet to be proved, and they are not commercially available. One possible use of this technology would be to shorten the time to obtain all measurements from all planes of the fetal cranium from a single three-dimensional image made up of voxels (image volume of pixels). This would mean that once the three-dimensional data were acquired, the sonographer could use a track-ball device to select and fine-tune the proper planes for the THC, coronal head circumferences, binocular and cerebellar diameters, ventricular antrum width, and any other cranial parameters that might be desired—all from a single three-dimensional image. This would make cranial parameter measurement plane selection similar to the current cine-loop or video playback that is available on many modern real-time machines.

REFERENCES

1. Moore KL, Persaud TVN: The Developing Human. WB Saunders, Philadelphia, 1993, p 56.
2. Moore KL, Persaud TVN: The Developing Human. WB Saunders, Philadelphia, 1993, pp 89–91, 156.
3. Moore KL, Persaud TVN: The Developing Human. WB Saunders, Philadelphia, 1993, pp 87–91, 156.
4. Nyberg DA, Hill LM, Bohm-Velez M, et al: Transvaginal Ultrasound. Mosby/Year Book, St Louis, 1992, pp 134–137.
5. Goldstein SR, Woletz PS: Fertilization and embryology. In: Berman MC, ed: Diagnostic Medical Sonography: A Guide to Clinical Practice, vol I. JB Lippincott, Philadelphia, 1991, pp 202–203.
6. Moore KL, Persaud TVN: The Developing Human. WB Saunders, Philadelphia, 1993, p 208.
7. Thomas CL, ed: Taber's Cyclopedic Medical Dictionary, 16th ed. FA Davis, Philadelphia, 1989, p 1606.
8. Moore KL, Persaud TVN: The Developing Human. WB Saunders, Philadelphia, 1993, pp 360–363.
9. Carlan SJ, Wyble L, Lense J, et al: Fetal head molding: Diagnosis by ultrasound and a review of the literature. J Perinatol 1991;11:105–111.
10. Patel MD, Swinford AE, Filly RA: Anatomic and sonographic features of the fetal skull. J Ultrasound Med 1994;13:251–257.
11. Moore KL, Persaud TVN: The Developing Human. WB Saunders, Philadelphia, 1993, p 362.
12. Athey PA, Hadlock FP: Ultrasound in Obstetrics and Gynecology. CV Mosby, St Louis, 1981, pp 23–36.
13. Hadlock FP: Ultrasound determination of menstrual age. In: Callen PW, ed: Ultrasonography in Obstetrics and Gynecology, 3rd ed. WB Saunders, Philadelphia, 1993, p 93.
14. Hadlock FP, Deter RL, Harrist RB, et al: Fetal head circumference: Relation to menstrual age. AJR 1982;138:623–649.
15. Kurtz AB, Goldberg BB: Fetal head measurements. In: Kurtz AB, Goldberg BB, eds: Obstetrical Measurements in Ultrasound: A Reference Manual. Year Book Medical Publishers, Chicago, 1988, pp 22–35.
16. Hadlock FP, Deter RL, Carpenter RJ, et al: Estimating fetal age: Effect of head shape on BPD. AJR 1981;137:83–85.
17. DuBose TJ: Fetal biometry: Vertical calvarial diameter and calvarial volume. J Diagn Med Sonogr 1985;1:205–217.
18. DuBose TJ: 3D BPD correction. Proceedings of the WFUMB, AIUM, and SDMS (abstract 1506). J Ultrasound Med 1988;7:S97.
19. Hansmann M, Hackeloer BJ, Staudach A: Normal fetal anatomy in the second and third trimester. In: Hansmann M, Hackeloer BJ, Staudach A, eds: Ultrasound Diagnosis in Obstetrics and Gynecology. Springer-Verlag, Berlin, 1985, pp 169–175.
20. Sabbagha RE, Barton FB, Barton BA: Sonar biparietal diameter I: Analysis of percentile growth differences in two normal populations using the same methodology. Am J Obstet Gynecol 1976;126: 479–484.
21. Athey PA, Hadlock FP: Ultrasound in Obstetrics and Gynecology. CV Mosby, St Louis, 1981, pp 23–36.
22. Bowie JD: Real-time ultrasonography in the diagnosis of fetal anomalies. Clin Diagn Ultrasound 1982;10:228.
23. Fiske CE, Filly RA: Ultrasound evaluation of the normal and abnormal fetal neural axis. In: Callen PW, ed: Ultrasonography in Obstetrics and Gynecology. WB Saunders, Philadelphia, 1983, p 100.
24. DuBose TJ: Assessment of fetal age and size: Techniques and criteria. In Berman MC, ed: Obstetrics and Gynecology: Diagnostic Medical Sonography, A Guide to Clinical Practice, vol I. JB Lippincott, Philadelphia, 1991, pp 279–285.
25. Merrill V: Atlas of Roentgenographic Positions, 3rd ed. CV Mosby, St Louis, 1967, p 351.
26. Berman MC: Winners of the 1986 Kenneth Gottesfeld Awards for Outstanding Papers Published in the Journal of Diagnostic Medical Sonography. J Diagn Med Sonogr 1986;2:182.
27. DuBose TJ: 3D BPD correction (abstract 1506). J Ultrasound Med 1988;7:S97.
28. DuBose TJ: Fetal cranial plane and solid geometry (abstract 1505). J Ultrasound Med 1988;7:S205.
29. Kurtz AB, Goldberg BB: Atlas of Ultrasound Measurements. Year Book Medical Publishers, Chicago, 1988, p 35.

30. Goldberg BB, Kurtz AB: Atlas of Ultrasound Measurements. Year Book Medical Publishers, Chicago, 1990, p 278.
31. Goldkrand JW, Kuhlman T, Fox E, et al: Coronal biparietal diameter: A reliable alternative to the traditional transverse biparietal diameter. J Ultrasound Med 1990;9:555.
32 DuBose TJ: Assessment of fetal age and size: Techniques and criteria. In: Berman MC, ed: Obstetrics and Gynecology: Diagnostic Medical Sonography, A Guide to Clinical Practice, vol I. JB Lippincott, Philadelphia, 1991, p 286.
33. Weinraub Z, Herman A, Ron-El R, et al: Measuring coronal biparietal diameter. J Ultrasound Med 1991;10:486.
34. DuBose TJ: Coronal BPD revisited. J Ultrasound Med 1992;11:84.
35. Bowerman RA: Atlas of Normal Fetal Ultrasonographic Anatomy, 2nd ed. Mosby/Year Book, St Louis, 1992, p 75.
36. Bowerman RA: Atlas of Normal Fetal Ultrasonographic Anatomy, 2nd ed. Mosby/Year Book, St Louis, 1992, p 82.
37. Knutzon RK, McGahan JP, Salamat MS, et al: Cisterna magna septa: A normal anatomical finding (abstract 0999). J Ultrasound Med 1992;11:S13.
38. Sabbagha RE, ed: Diagnostic Ultrasound: Applied to Obstetrics and Gynecology, 3rd ed. JB Lippincott, Philadelphia, 1994, pp 422–423.
39. Moore KL, Persaud TVN: The Developing Human. WB Saunders, Philadelphia, 1993, pp 93–95.
40. Moore KL, Persaud TVN: The Developing Human. WB Saunders, Philadelphia, 1993, pp 407–409.
41. Filly RA: Ultrasound evaluation of the fetal neural axis. In: Callen PW, ed: Ultrasonography in Obstetrics and Gynecology, 3rd ed. WB Saunders, Philadelphia, 1993, p 213.
42. Cardoza J, Filly RA, Podrasky AE: The dangling choroid plexus: A sonographic observation of value in excluding ventriculomegaly. AJR 1988;15:167.
43. Chinn DH, Callen PW, Filly RA: The lateral cerebral ventricle in early second trimester. Radiology 1983;148:529–533.
44. Siedler DE, Filly RA: Relative growth of higher fetal brain structures. J Ultrasound Med 1987;6:573–576.
45. Cardoza JD, Goldstein RB, Filly RA: Exclusion of fetal ventriculomegaly with a single measurement: The width of the lateral ventricle antrum. Radiology 1988;169:711–714.
46. Filly RA, Cardoza JD, Goldstein RB, et al: Detection of fetal central nervous system anomalies: A practical level of effort for routine sonograms. Radiology 1989;172:403–408.
47. Pilu G: Opinion: Borderline fetal cerebral ventriculomegaly—the Twilight Zone. Ultrasound Obstet Gynecol 1993;3:85–86.
48. Monteagudo A, Timor-Tritsch IE, Moomjy M: Nomograms of the fetal lateral ventricles using transvaginal sonography. J Ultrasound Med 1993;5:265–269.
49. Chudleigh P, Pearce JM, Campbell S: The prenatal diagnosis of transient cysts of the fetal choroid plexus. Prenat Diagn 1984;4:135.
50. Benacerraf BR: Asymptomatic cysts of the fetal choroid plexus in the second trimester. J Ultrasound Med 1987;6:475–478.
51. Fitzsimmons J, Wilson D, Pascoe-Mason J, et al: Choroid plexus cysts in fetuses with trisomy 18. Obstet Gynecol 1989;73:257–260.
52. Klein VR, Chervenak FA: Fetal choroid plexus cysts (letters). Am J Obstet Gynecol 1993;168:277–278.
53. Nadel AS, Bromley BS, Frigoletto FD, et al: Isolated choroid plexus cysts in the second-trimester fetus: Is amniocentesis really indicated? Radiology 1992; 185:545–548.
54. Lester RB, Sty JR: Prenatal diagnosis of cystic CNS lesions in neonatal isoimmune thrombocytopenia. J Ultrasound Med 1987;6:479–481.
55. Perpignano MC, Cohen HL, Klein VR, et al: Fetal choroid plexus cysts: Beware the smaller cyst. Radiology 1992;182:715–717.
56. Porto M, Murata Y, Warneke LA, et al: Fetal choroid plexus cysts: An independent risk factor for chromosomal anomalies (abstract). Am J Obstet Gynecol 1992;166:356.
57. Platt LD, Carlson DE, Medearis AL, et al: Fetal choroid plexus cysts in the second trimester of pregnancy: A cause for concern. Am J Obstet Gynecol 1991;164:1652–1656.
58. Goldstein RB, Lapidus AS, Filly RA, et al: Mild lateral cerebral ventricular dilatation in utero: Clinical significance and prognosis. Radiology 1990;176:237.
59. Cardoza JD, Filly RA, Podrasky AE: The dangling choroid plexus: A sonographic observation of value in excluding ventriculomegaly. AJR 1988;151: 767–770.
60. Pilu G, Reece A, Goldstein I, et al: Sonographic evaluation of the normal developmental anatomy of the fetal cerebral ventricles: II. The atria. Obstet Gynecol 1989;73:250–255.
61. Jeanty P, Dramaiz-Wilmet M, Delbeke D, et al: Ultrasonic valuation of fetal ventricular growth. Neuroradiology 1981;21:127.
62. Schnitzlein HN, Murtagh FR: Imaging Anatomy of the Head and Spine, 2nd ed. Urban & Schwarzenburg, Baltimore, 1990, pp 11–17, 117.
63. Pilu G, Romero R, Rizzo N, et al: Prenatal diagnosis of cerebrospinal anomalies. In: Fleischer AC, Romero R, Manning FA, et al, eds: The Principles and Practice of Ultrasonography in Obstetrics and Gynecology. Appleton & Lange, Norwalk, CT, 1991, p 213.
64. DuBose TJ: Coronal BPD revisited. J Ultrasound Med 1992;11:84.
65. Williams AL, Haughton VM: Cranial Computed Tomography: A Comprehensive Text. CV Mosby, St Louis, 1985, p 317.
66. Schnitzlein HN, Murtagh FR: Imaging Anatomy of the Head and Spine, 2nd ed. Urban & Schwarzenburg, Baltimore, 1990, pp 27, 109.
67. Schaeffer JP, ed: Morris' Human Anatomy, 10th ed. Blakiston, Philadelphia, 1942, p 994.
68. Thomas CL, ed: Taber's Cyclopedic Medical Dictionary, 16th ed. FA Davis, Philadelphia, 1989, p 309.
69. Bowerman RA: Atlas of Normal Fetal Ultrasonographic Anatomy, 2nd ed. Mosby/Year Book, St Louis, 1992, pp 64–69.
70. Streltzoff J, Isaacson G, Chervenak FA: Normal anatomy of the fetal head, neck, and spine. In: Berman MC, ed: Obstetrics and Gynecology: Diagnostic Medical Sonography, A Guide to Clinical Practice, vol I. JB Lippincott, Philadelphia, 1991, p 222.
71. DuBose TJ: Assessment of fetal age and size. In: Berman MC, ed: Obstetrics and Gynecology: Diagnostic Medical Sonography, A Guide to Clinical Practice, vol I. JB Lippincott, Philadelphia, 1991, pp 284–286.
72. Kurtz AB, Goldberg BB: Fetal head measurements. In: Kurtz AB, Goldberg BB, eds: Obstetrical Measurements in Ultrasound: A Reference Manual. Year Book Medical Publishers, Chicago, 1988, p 44.

73. Hadlock FP, Deter RL, Harrist RB, et al: Fetal biparietal diameter: A critical re-evaluation of the relation to menstrual age by means of real-time ultrasound. J Ultrasound Med 1982;1:97–104.
74. Shepard M, Filly RA: A standardized plane for biparietal diameter measurement. J Ultrasound Med 1982;1:145–150.
75. McGahan JP, Phillips HE: Ultrasonic evaluation of the size of the trigone of the fetal ventricle. J Ultrasound Med 1983;2:315–319.
76. Bowerman RA: Atlas of Normal Fetal Ultrasonographic Anatomy, 2nd ed. Mosby/Year Book, St Louis, 1992, pp 69, 85.
77. Lee SH, Rao KCVG: Cranial Computed Tomography and MRI, 2nd ed. McGraw-Hill, New York, 1983, p 202.
78. Lowmann RM, Shapiro R, Collins LC: The significance of the widened septum pellucidum. AJR 1948;59:177–196.
79. Schnitzlein HN, Murtagh FR: Imaging Anatomy of the Head and Spine, 2nd ed. Urban & Schwarzenburg, Baltimore, 1990, p 187.
80. Hata K, Hata T, Ariyuki Y, et al: Ultrasonographic antenatal diagnosis of cavum veli interpositi. Int J Gynaecol Obstet 1991;36:141–148.
81. Epstein BS: Pneumoencephalography and Cerebral Angiography. Year Book Medical Publishers, Chicago, 1966, p 15.
82. Swischuk LE: Radiology of the Newborn and Young Infant. Williams & Wilkins, Baltimore, 1984, pp 822–825.
83. Taveras JM, Wood EH: Diagnostic Neuroradiology. Williams & Wilkins, Baltimore, 1976, pp 359–361.
84. Thomas CL, ed: Taber's Cyclopedic Medical Dictionary, 16th ed. FA Davis, Philadelphia, 1989, pp 1844–1845.
85. Matzke HA, Flotz FM: Synopsis of Neuroanatomy. Oxford University Press, London, 1972, p 6.
86. Schnitzlein HN, Murtagh FR: Imaging Anatomy of the Head and Spine, 2nd ed. Urban & Schwarzenburg, Baltimore, 1990, pp 31, 148–149, 160–161, 180–181.
87. Schnitzlein HN, Murtagh FR: Imaging Anatomy of the Head and Spine, 2nd ed. Urban & Schwarzenburg, Baltimore, 1990, pp 31, 117, 148–149, 160–161, 180–181.
88. Palacios E, Fine M, Haughton VM: Multiplanar Anatomy of the Head and Neck for Computed Tomography. John Wiley & Sons, New York, 1980, pp 16, 141–150, 179–183.
89. Filly RA: Ultrasound evaluation of the fetal neural axis. In: Callen PW, ed: Ultrasonography in Obstetrics and Gynecology, 3rd ed. WB Saunders, Philadelphia, 1993, pp 197–199.
90. Goldstein RB, Podrasky AE, Filly RA, et al: Effacement of the fetal cisterna magna in association with myelomeningocele. Radiology 1989;172:409–413.
91. Watson WJ, Katz VL, Chescheir NC, et al: The cisterna magna in second-trimester fetus with abnormal karyotypes. Obstet Gynecol 1992;79:723–725.
92. Nyberg DA, Mack LA, Hirsch J, et al: Abnormalities of fetal cranial contour in sonographic detection of spina bifida: Evaluation of the "lemon" sign. Radiology 1988;167:387–392.
93. Goldstein RB, Callen PW: The lemon sign: Not a specific indicator of meningomyeloceles (abstract 166). Am J Obstet Gynecol 1993; 346.
94. Nyberg D, Mack L, Hirsh J, et al: Abnormalities of fetal cranial contour in sonographic detection of spina bifida: Evaluation of the "lemon" sign. Radiology 1988;70:247–250.
95. Van den Hof MC, Nicolaides KH, Campbell J, et al: Evaluation of the lemon and banana signs in one hundred thirty fetuses with open spina bifida. Am J Obstet Gynecol 1990;162:322–327.
96. Thomas CL, ed: Taber's Cyclopedic Medical Dictionary, 16th ed. FA Davis, Philadelphia, 1989, p 138.
97. Nicolaides K, Campbell S, Gabbe S, et al: Ultrasound screening for spina bifida: Cranial and cerebellar signs. Lancet 1986;2:71–74.
98. Mari G: Regional cerebral flow velocity waveforms in the human fetus. J Ultrasound Med 1994;13: 343–346.
99. Fay RA, Ellwood DA: Categories of intrauterine growth retardation. Fetal Maternal Med Rev 1993; 5:203–212.
100. DuBose TJ: Assessment of fetal age and size: Techniques and criteria. In Berman MC, ed: Obstetrics and Gynecology: Diagnostic Medical Sonography, A Guide to Clinical Practice, vol I. JB Lippincott, Philadelphia, 1991, pp 280–281, 296.
101. Li DFH, Woo JSK: Fractional spine length: A new parameter for assessing fetal growth. J Ultrasound Med 1986;5:379–383.
102. Jones OW: Basic genetics and patterns of inheritance. In: Creasy RK, Resnik R, eds: Maternal-Fetal Medicine: Principles and Practice, 2nd ed. WB Saunders, Philadelphia, 1989, p 58.
103. Sherer DM, Abramowicz JS, Plessinger MA, et al: Fetal sacral length in the ultrasonographic assessment of gestational age. Am J Obstet Gynecol 1993;168:626–633.
104. Benacerraf BR: Ultrasound evaluation of the fetal face. In: Callen PW, ed: Ultrasonography in Obstetrics and Gynecology, 3rd ed. WB Saunders, Philadelphia, 1993, pp 239–242.
105. Walla CA, Platt LD: Observing fetal maturation through fetal movement and breathing. In: Berman MC, ed: Obstetrics and Gynecology: Diagnostic Medical Sonography, A Guide to Clinical Practice, vol I. JB Lippincott, Philadelphia, 1991, p 446.
106. Benacerraf BR: Ultrasound evaluation of the fetal face. In: Callen PW, ed: Ultrasonography in Obstetrics and Gynecology, 3rd ed. WB Saunders, Philadelphia, 1993, pp 238–242.
107. Abramowicz JS, Sherer DM, Bar-Tov E, et al: The cheek-to-cheek diameter in the ultrasonographic assessment of fetal growth. Am J Obstet Gynecol 1991;165:846–852.
108. Otto C, Platt LD: The fetal mandible measurement: An objective determination of fetal jaw size. Ultrasound Obstet Gynecol 1991;1:12–17.
109. Chitty LS, Campbell S, Altman DG: Measurement of the fetal mandible—feasibility and construction of a centile chart. Prenat Diagn 1993;13:749–756.
110. Bronshtein M, Mashia N, Blumenfeld I, et al: Pseudoprognathism—an auxiliary ultrasonic sign for transvaginal ultrasonographic diagnosis of cleft lip and palate in early second trimester. Am J Obstet Gynecol 1991;165:1314–1316.
111. Jeanty P, Cantraine F, Cousaert E, et al: The binocular distance: A new way to estimate fetal age. J Ultrasound Med 1984;3:241–243.
112. DuBose TJ: Assessment of fetal age and size: Techniques and criteria. In Berman MC, ed: Obstetrics and Gynecology: Diagnostic Medical Sonography, A Guide to Clinical Practice, vol I. JB Lippincott, Philadelphia, 1991, pp 279–285, 295–296.
113. Sabbagha RE, ed: Diagnostic Ultrasound: Applied to Obstetrics and Gynecology, 3rd ed. JB Lippincott, Philadelphia, 1994, pp 422–423.

114. Crane JP, Gray DL: Midtrimester sonographically measured nuchal skin fold thickness as a screening tool for Down syndrome. Obstet Gynecol 1991; 77:553.
115. Benacerraf BR, Barss VA, Laboda LA: A sonographic sign for the detection in the second trimester of the fetus with Down's syndrome. Am J Obstet Gynecol 1985;151:1078.
116. Benacerraf BR, Gelman R, Frigoletto FD: Sonographic identification of second-trimester fetuses with Down syndrome. N Engl J Med 1987;317:1371.
117. Manning FA: General principles and application of ultrasound. In: Creasy RK, Resnik R, eds: Maternal-Fetal Medicine: Principles and Practice, 2nd ed. WB Saunders, Philadelphia, 1989, p 218.
118. Winston YE: Down syndrome and femur length. Am J Obstet Gynecol 1988;163:1018.
119. Sabbagha RE, ed: Diagnostic Ultrasound: Applied to Obstetrics and Gynecology, 3rd ed. JB Lippincott, Philadelphia, 1994, p 435.
120. Holzgreve W: The fetus with nonimmune hydrops. In: Harrison MR, Golbus MS, Filly RA, eds: The Unborn Patient: Prenatal Diagnosis and Treatment. WB Saunders, Philadelphia, 1991, p 239.
121. Filly RA: Sonographic anatomy of the normal fetus. In: Harrison MR, Golbus MS, Filly RA, eds: The Unborn Patient: Prenatal Diagnosis and Treatment. WB Saunders, Philadelphia, 1991, p 96.
122. Shimizu T, Salvador L, Allanson J, et al: Ultrasonographic measurements of fetal ear. Obstet Gynecol 1992;80:381–384.
123. Lettieri L, Rodis JF, Vintzileos AM, et al: Ear length in second-trimester aneuploid fetuses. Obstet Gynecol 1993;81:57–60.

CHAPTER 10

FETAL THORAX AND NECK

Terry J. DuBose

The thorax includes all structures between the base of the neck and the diaphragm. The skeleton of the thorax includes the thoracic spine, ribs, scapula, and parts of the shoulder, clavicles, and sternum. The major thoracic soft tissues include the muscles, skin, connecting tissues, lungs, trachea and bronchial system, thymus, lymph glands, esophagus, and of course the heart and great vessels. The heart and vessels are detailed in Chapter 11.

Embryologic

During the first trimester, very little is observed in the thorax except the heartbeat. Even in the early second trimester, the lung echogenicity is similar to that of the liver, and these structures may be difficult to distinguish. The thorax and its contents are now starting to be studied during the early second trimester with transvaginal transducers.[1]

The embryonic heart rate is detailed in Chapter 12; however, the fact that the early heart rate accelerates rapidly and can be used to estimate embryonic age is emphasized here. From the start of the fifth week to the start of the ninth week, the heart rate accelerates at 3.3 beats per minute (B/M), a 10-beat increase in rate every 3 days or approximately 100 beats during the 30 days between 5.1 and 9.3 LMP weeks. The heartbeat begins at about 80 to 85 B/M when first detected at about 5.1 weeks by transvaginal sonography and accelerates linearly until the rate peaks between 9.0 and 9.5 weeks at about 165 to 195 B/M (Fig. 10–1).

Embryonic age can be estimated in LMP days by multiplying the heart rate by 0.3 and adding 6 days. To determine days from conception, subtract 8 days rather than adding 6. This age estimate is usually accurate within about ±8 days.

Skeletal

SPINE

The fetal spine is one part of the fetal anatomy that even a novice can usually identify. It often is the first structure that the parents can recognize. The spine is discussed in Chapter 9 as part of the neural axis, but some generalities are appropriate here.

The thoracic spine consists of 12 vertebrae

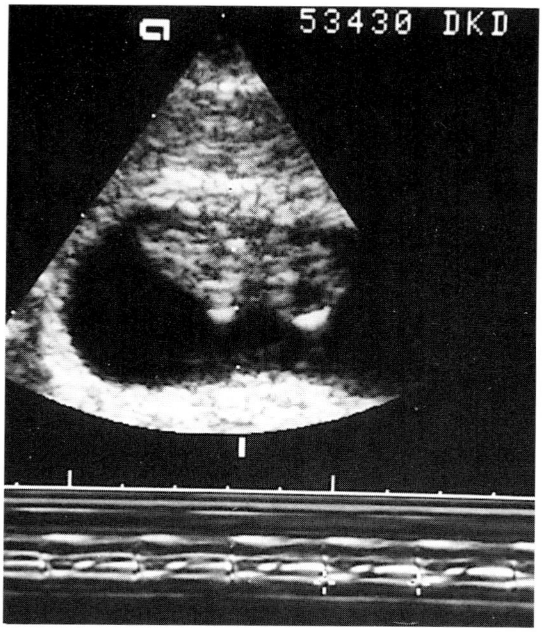

FIGURE 10–1.
Transvaginal sonogram of embryonic heart rate. Little can be defined of the thoracic contents, except that the heart rate is normal for age at 169 B/M, which evaluates to 8.0 (±1.2) LMP weeks. (LNMP = 9.0 weeks, CRL = 17 mm = 8.1 weeks, DKD)

and intervening spaces. In the thoracic area, the spine should be uniform in both its width and in the intervertebral spacing.

The fetal spine is best observed when a fetus is presenting its back to the transducer (Fig. 10–2). It can also be studied through the thorax and abdomen (Fig. 10–3).

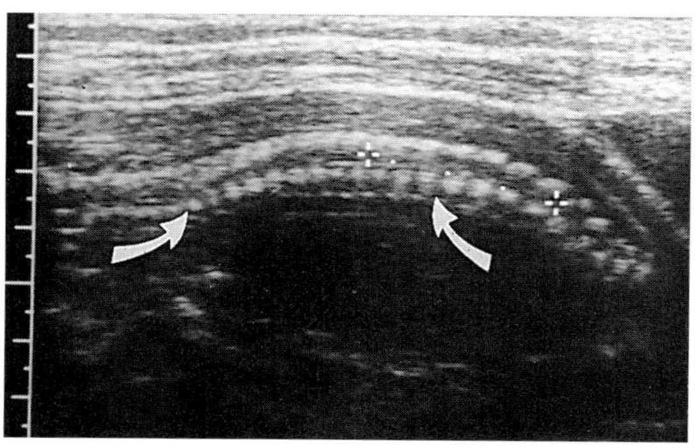

FIGURE 10–2.
The entire fetal spine from a posterior approach. The 12 vertebrae of the thoracic spine are between the arrows. The + cursors measure seven thoracolumbar vertebrae to be 34.5 mm, which equates to approximately 22.2 LMP weeks. (LNMP = 18.9 weeks, AA = 20.8 weeks, n = 9, range = 1.7 weeks, TD)

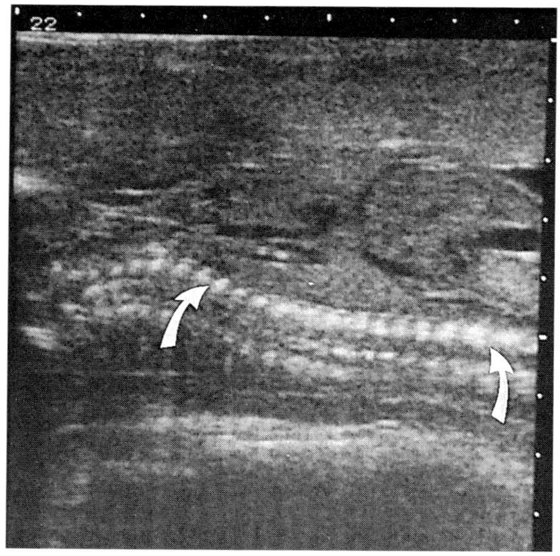

FIGURE 10–3.
Thoracic spine (between arrows) from the anterior view. The diaphragm can be seen as a curved hypoechoic line between the lung and liver. (LNMP = 24.0 weeks, AA = 21.0 weeks, n = 8, range = 1.6 weeks, TD)

The thoracic spine should be uniform from vertebra to vertebra in the cross-sectional view. Figures 10–4 and 10–5 show cross sections of normal vertebrae high in the thorax from the posterior view. The three ossification centers of each vertebra should form a trian-

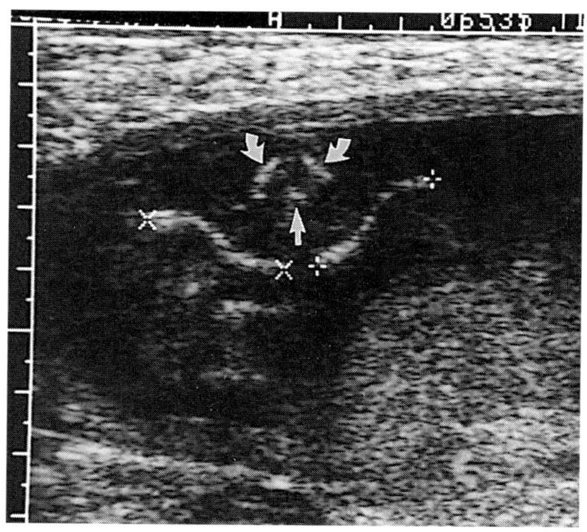

FIGURE 10–4.
Transverse of upper thorax. Arrows point to the three ossification centers of the spine, two posterior laminae (curved arrows) and a vertebral body (straight arrow). The clavicles are measured by the cursors (X = 24.1 mm, + = 23.8 mm). These measurements are above normal when compared with Table 10–3. (LNMP = ?, AA = 20.0 LMP weeks, n = 9, range = 1.8 weeks, TD)

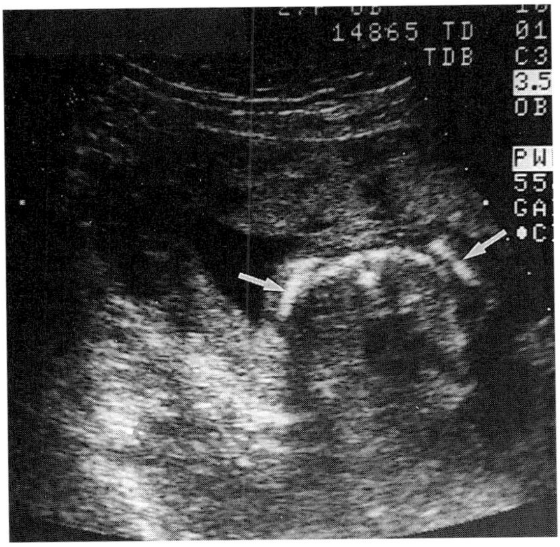

FIGURE 10–5.
Transverse thorax showing both scapulae (arrows) and three ossification centers of the transverse spine between. Ribs can be seen to curve under the scapulae. (LNMP = ?, AA = 20.3 LMP weeks, n = 9, range = 2.0 weeks, TDB/TD)

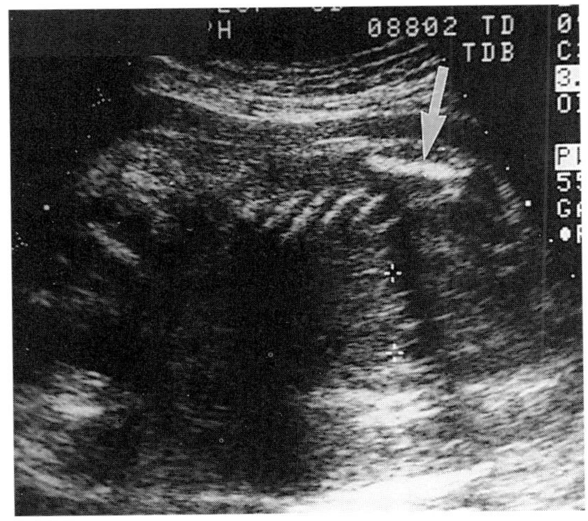

FIGURE 10–6.
The curved ribs can be seen emerging from beneath the scapula (arrow). The + cursors measure the coronal width of the thymus to be 19.1 mm. (LNMP = ?, AA = 28.1 LMP weeks, n = 9, range = 2.0 weeks, TDB/TD)

gle of three echoes. The two posterior echoes are the ossification centers of the lamina/pedicle junction, and the single anterior echo is the ossifying vertebral body or centrum.[2,3]

Spinal defects in the thoracic spine are not as common as they are in the cervical, lumbar, or sacral regions of the spine. A meningocele is a protrusion of the meninges through the spinal column. In a meningomyelocele, the protrusion also includes herniated neural tissue.[4] This congenital herniation of the spinal cord is also called spina bifida or myelomeningocele[5] (see Figs. 9–30*A* and *B*).

RIBS AND CHEST CIRCUMFERENCE

The fetal ribs usually are easy to identify sonographically. Figure 10–6 is a plane of view that is tangential to the lateral chest, showing ribs emerging from beneath the scapula. Fetal ribs should be smooth, curving lines of echoes when viewed in their length (see Fig. 10–6) and a row of echogenic dots when viewed in cross section (Fig. 10–7).

The rib cage should gradually enlarge toward the abdomen in a bell shape. The skin line of the chest and abdomen should be continuous and should have no abrupt angles or disruptions.

In some syndromes, the fetal chest is small relative to the abdomen. These cases have been described as having a champagne cork appearance because the thorax is narrow (bottom of the cork) and the abdomen suddenly bulges beneath the ribs (top of the cork).[6] These fetuses usually have other associated

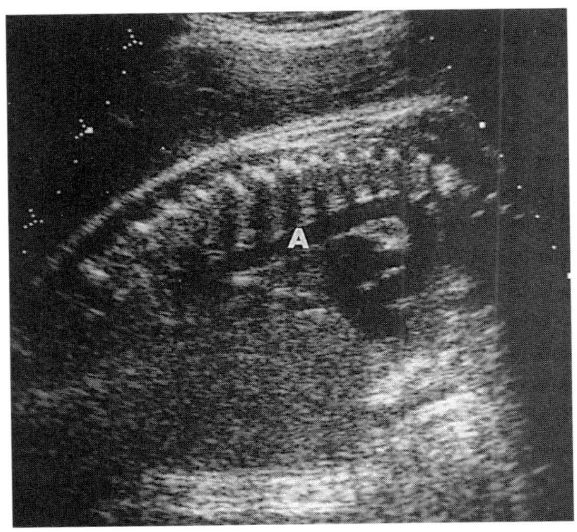

FIGURE 10–7.
Candy cane view of the descending aorta (A) and aortic arch from the left, posterior, parasagittal approach. This view is most easily obtained by lining up the plane of view with the posterior spine and then sliding slightly to the fetal left. The ribs in cross section are seen as bright echoes with intermittent acoustic shadows distally. (LNMP = 40.4 weeks, AA = 34.8 weeks, n = 9, range = 3.2 weeks, DG/TD)

forms of skeletal dysplasia such as short-limbed dwarfism and premature closure of the coronal and lambdoid sutures, which results in a cloverleaf skull. These thanatophoric (meaning "death producing," "death bearing," or "death seeking") dwarfs die of asphyxiating thoracic dystrophy and resulting compression of the lungs and heart.[7] Pena-Shokeir syndrome may also result in asphyxiation due to neuromuscular disorders, even though the chest circumference may be normal.[8] With osteogenesis imperfecta, the skeleton is poorly mineralized, and multiple fractures of the ribs as well as other bones can result.[9]

The chest circumference of fetuses has been measured, and the findings have been published (Table 10–1).[10] This measurement is made transversely at the level of the four-chamber heart view. One difficulty with this view is ascertaining that the plane is perpendicular to the long axis of the thorax. The thoracic measurement can be important in evaluating a fetus for syndromes that are associated with a hypoplastic chest. In these cases, a ratio of the chest circumference to the head or abdomen may be useful.

Chitkara and colleagues[10] determined these ratios from cross-sectional data in the same article as the original Table 10–1: the thoracic circumference (TC) to the transverse head circumference (THC) and the TC to abdominal circumference (AC). The TC/THC = 0.80 ± 0.12 (SD) and the TC/AC = 0.89 ± 0.06 (SD). They found that the TC/AC and the thoracic length/humerus length remained virtually constant from the 16th to the 40th week. The TC/THC ratio gradually increased from 0.72 to 0.89 from the 16th to the 40th week, respectively, but the change did not reach statistical significance (Table 10–2).

Another study using longitudinal data

TABLE 10–1. **FETAL THORACIC CIRCUMFERENCE MEASUREMENTS**

GESTATIONAL AGE (wk)	NO.	PREDICTIVE PERCENTILES								
		2.5	5	10	25	50	75	90	95	97.5
16	6	5.9	6.4	7.0	8.0	9.1	10.3	11.3	11.9	12.4
17	22	6.8	7.3	7.9	8.9	10.0	11.2	12.2	12.8	13.3
18	31	7.7	8.2	8.8	9.8	11.0	12.1	13.1	13.7	14.2
19	21	8.6	9.1	9.7	10.7	11.9	13.0	14.0	14.6	15.1
20	20	9.5	10.0	10.6	11.7	12.8	13.9	15.0	15.5	16.0
21	30	10.4	11.0	11.6	12.6	13.7	14.8	15.8	16.4	16.9
22	18	11.3	11.9	12.5	13.5	14.6	15.7	16.7	17.3	17.8
23	21	12.2	12.8	13.4	14.4	15.5	16.6	17.6	18.2	18.8
24	27	13.2	13.7	14.3	15.3	16.4	17.5	18.5	19.1	19.7
25	20	14.1	14.6	15.2	16.2	17.3	18.4	19.4	20.0	20.6
26	25	15.0	15.5	16.1	17.1	18.2	19.3	20.3	21.0	21.5
27	24	15.9	16.4	17.0	18.0	19.1	20.2	21.3	21.9	22.4
28	24	16.8	17.3	17.9	18.9	20.0	21.2	22.2	22.8	23.3
29	24	17.7	18.2	18.8	19.8	21.0	22.1	23.1	23.7	24.2
30	27	18.6	19.1	19.7	20.7	21.9	23.0	24.0	24.6	25.1
31	24	19.5	20.0	20.6	21.6	22.8	23.9	24.9	25.5	26.0
32	28	20.4	20.9	21.5	22.6	23.7	24.8	25.8	26.4	26.9
33	27	21.3	21.8	22.5	23.5	24.6	25.7	26.7	27.3	27.8
34	25	22.2	22.8	23.4	24.4	25.5	26.6	27.6	28.2	28.7
35	20	23.1	23.7	24.3	25.3	26.4	27.5	28.5	29.1	29.6
36	23	24.0	24.6	25.2	26.2	27.3	28.4	29.4	30.0	30.6
37	22	24.9	25.5	26.1	27.1	28.2	29.3	30.3	30.9	31.5
38	21	25.9	26.4	27.0	28.0	29.1	30.2	31.2	31.9	32.4
39	7	26.8	27.3	27.9	28.9	30.0	31.1	32.2	32.8	33.3
40	6	27.7	28.2	28.8	29.8	30.9	32.1	33.1	33.7	34.2

Use this table to determine if the thoracic circumference is normal for fetal age. Measurements in centimeters.

From Chitkara U, Rosenberg J, Chervenak FA, et al: Prenatal sonographic assessment of the fetal thorax: Normal values. Am J Obstet Gynecol 1987;156:1069–1074.

TABLE 10–2. VARIOUS THORACIC RATIOS*

RATIO	−2 SD	MEAN	+2 SD
TC/AC†	0.77	0.89	1.01
TC/THC†	0.56	0.80	1.04
TC/FemL	3.59	4.31	5.03
TC/HumL	3.37	4.03	4.69

*Means and ± 2 SD for thoracic ratios.

†Ratios did not vary significantly with gestational age.

TC, thoracic circumference at level of four-chamber heart view; AC, abdominal circumference at confluence of umbilical and portal veins (portal sinus); THC, standard transverse head circumference; FemL, femoral diaphysis length; HumL, humeral diaphysis length.

Adapted from Chitkara U, Rosenberg J, Chervenak FA, et al: Prenatal sonographic assessment of the fetal thorax: Normal values. Am J Obstet Gynecol 1987;156:1069–1074.

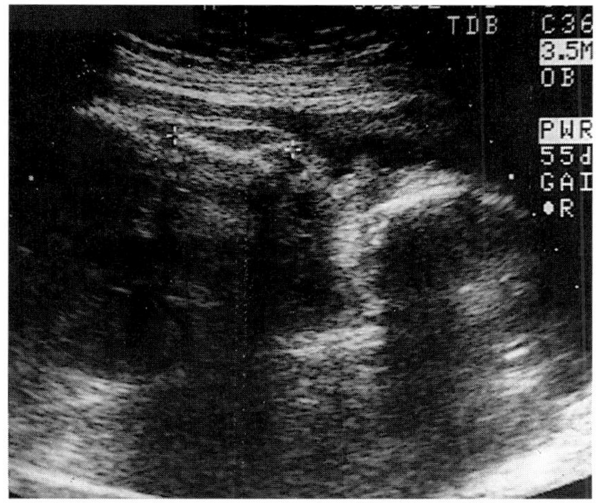

FIGURE 10–8.
Parasagittal view and measurement of the scapula. The + cursors measure from the inferior angle of the scapula to the tip of the acromion to be 27.6 mm. This is below the mean for age (mean = 29 mm) but within normal limits (5% = 24 mm) when compared with Table 10–4. (LNMP = ?, AA = 28.1 LMP weeks, n = 9, range = 2.0 weeks, TDB/TD)

from a smaller population found slightly smaller ratios for these same parameters.[11] This study found that the changes for the ratios were significantly different between the 20th and 40th weeks, although the researchers point out that the actual magnitude of the differences was small. The TC/THC ratio increased from a mean of 0.76 at 20 weeks to 0.82 at 40 weeks, and the TC/AC decreased from 0.87 to 0.80 during the same period.

A comfortable overlap of the ratios for the TC/THC was noted in the two studies, but less agreement was found in the TC/AC ratios. Therefore, the TC/THC is the safer ratio to use until a more definitive study is published.

SCAPULA

The scapulae, or shoulder blades, are prominent echogenic structures in a fetus. In Figure 10–6, the scapula can be seen as a bright line just proximal to the top of the ribs. The scapula may have a characteristic Y shape in a long-axis view (Fig. 10–8). This Y is a result of echoes from the body of the scapula forming the lower part of the Y, the acromion forming the fetal posterior portion, and the coracoid process forming the anterior portions of the top of the Y. The view to demonstrate this Y is not a true parasagittal plane but rather is slightly oblique, with the cephalic end of the plane farther from the spine than the inferior end. That is, the plane is from the bottom of the scapula out toward the shoulder.

Fetal scapular length has been measured, and the findings published.[12] Table 10–3 can be used to determine whether the scapular size is appropriate for age. This measurement may depend on the experience of the observer because of the shape of the scapula and the orientation of the plane of measurement. However, the investigators did not find a significant difference in the interobserver or intraobserver results. It is probable that the observers in this study were very experienced sonographers. Fetal age may be estimated using the following formula.

$$\text{LMP age} = 4.7702 + 0.9861 \times \text{scapular length in centimeters}$$

In this study, the ±2 SD was given as a constant ±8.4 weeks throughout pregnancy. This is a rather large variation. It is unlikely that the variation would be constant throughout pregnancy. Most parameters tend to become more variable as fetal age increases. The study used a fairly large population (515 fetuses across 27 weeks = approximately 19 measurements/week), which would indicate

TABLE 10–3. **SCAPULAR LENGTH PREDICTED BY GESTATIONAL AGE**

GESTATIONAL AGE (wk)	SCAPULAR LENGTH (cm)		
	−2 SD	Mean	+2 SD
14	0.6	1.0	1.4
15	0.7	1.1	1.5
16	0.8	1.2	1.6
17	0.9	1.3	1.7
18	1.0	1.4	1.8
19	1.1	1.5	1.9
20	1.2	1.6	2.0
21	1.3	1.7	2.1
22	1.4	1.8	2.2
23	1.5	1.9	2.3
24	1.6	2.0	2.4
25	1.6	2.1	2.5
26	1.7	2.2	2.6
27	1.8	2.3	2.7
28	1.9	2.4	2.8
29	2.0	2.4	2.9
30	2.1	2.5	3.0
31	2.2	2.6	3.1
32	2.3	2.7	3.1
33	2.4	2.8	3.2
34	2.5	2.9	3.3
35	2.6	3.0	3.4
36	2.7	3.1	3.5
37	2.8	3.2	3.6
38	2.9	3.3	3.7
39	3.0	3.4	3.8
40	3.1	3.5	3.9
41	3.2	3.6	4.0
42	3.3	3.7	4.1

Normal scapular lengths in centimeters by LMP age in weeks. Calculated by regression formula.

From Sherer DM, Plessinger MA, Allen TA: Fetal scapular length in the ultrasonographic assessment of gestational age. J Ultrasound Med 1994;13:523–528.

that the foregoing formula is relatively accurate; however, the statistics of variation may need refinement.

An apparent drawback to the scapular measurement is its relatively small dimensions. Because it is less than 4 cm at term, about half the size of the biparietal diameter (BPD) or femur, any error in the plane of measurement or placement of cursors results in relatively large percent errors. Figure 10–8 shows a measurement of the scapular length using the acromion as the upper endpoint of the measurement. The scapular length, which appears to be slightly longer than the age of this fetus would suggest, was underestimated using the published table. However, the scapula is often relatively easy to measure when a fetus is in a prone position; therefore, it may be useful for confirmation of ages when other parameters are abnormal or difficult to determine.

Anomalies of the scapula are associated with maternal exposure to retinoic acid, isolated and complete duplication, bilateral dysplasia, and Sprengel's deformity (the most common). The latter is an undescended scapula, usually unilateral and more common in women (3 : 1).[12]

CLAVICLES

The clavicles are slightly more straightforward for measurements than is the scapula. They have the drawback of being a relatively small parameter, reaching only about 4 cm at term. The clavicles are more often affected by various congenital anomalies than are scapulae. For this reason, the clavicular measurement may be more important in assessing these anomalies than for estimating age. Anomalies in which the clavicle may be affected are cleidocranial dysplasia, Holt-Oram syndrome, Goltz's syndrome, Melnick-Needles syndrome, and others.[13]

Figure 10–4 demonstrates the measurement of both clavicles. This image is from the posterior approach, with the cross section of the spine closer to the transducer. Note the characteristic curves of the clavicles.

Table 10–4 can be used to determine whether the clavicular measurements are appropriate for the age of a fetus.[13] However, it must be pointed out that this table, which spans 25 weeks, was constructed using only 85 fetuses. Therefore, only about three measurements per week were used to produce the table. This research needs to be replicated with a larger population to confirm its accuracy. In this study, the following formula for fetal age was given:

$$\text{LMP age} = 3.7177731 + 0.8272778 \times \text{clavicular length in millimeters}$$

The ±2 SD for age was given as a relatively constant ±8.9 weeks. Again, this is a rather large variation, which should normally in-

TABLE 10–4. **CLAVICULAR LENGTH PREDICTED BY GESTATIONAL AGE**

GESTATIONAL AGE (wk)	CLAVICLE LENGTH (mm) PERCENTILE 5th	50th	95th
15	11	16	21
16	12	17	22
17	13	18	23
18	14	19	24
19	15	20	25
20	16	21	26
21	17	22	27
22	18	23	28
23	19	24	29
24	20	25	30
25	21	26	31
26	22	27	32
27	23	28	33
28	24	29	34
29	25	30	35
30	26	31	36
31	27	32	37
32	28	33	38
33	29	34	39
34	30	35	40
35	31	36	41
36	32	37	42
37	33	38	43
38	34	39	44
39	35	40	45
40	36	41	46

Normal clavicle lengths in centimeters by LMP age in weeks.

From Yarkoni S, Schmidt W, Jeanty P, et al: Clavicular measurement: A new biometric parameter for fetal evaluation. J Ultrasound Med 1985;4:467–470.

crease with age. Because of the small population, discussed earlier, and the large constant variation, both the formula and variation are suspect.

STERNUM

The sternum, or breast bone, comprises the manubrium, at the top between the clavicles; the sternum, which extends inferiorly and connects with the ribs by way of the costal cartilage; and the xiphoid process, which protrudes from the bottom of the sternum. Not until adulthood do all parts of the sternum completely ossify. "The first ossification center appears in the fetal manubrium during the sixth fetal month [26–30 LMP weeks], and then three centers appear in the body of the sternum (mesosternum) at approximately 1-month intervals, progressing from above downward."[14] Therefore, through most of fetal life, the sternum is a hypoechoic line in the anterior chest.

The hypoechoic sternum is seen in the long axis in Figure 10–9*A* just anterior to the lung and beneath the skin. A transverse view of the chest also demonstrates the cartilaginous sternum (Fig. 10–9*B*). In this 27-LMP-week fetus, ossification centers are not demonstrated. The hypoechoic costal cartilage can be seen between the sternum and the rib. The ribs begin calcifying earlier, and they cast acoustic shadows.

Neck

The structures of the fetal neck can be studied using sonography. Figure 10–10 is a left parasagittal plane of a fetal head, neck, and chest at 18.4 LMP weeks. The clavicle can be seen in cross section, and the carotid artery is in long axis. The thyroid is also seen just inferior to the muscles associated with the tongue—the genioglossus, geniohyoid, and mylohyoid muscles. The left carotid artery passes posterior to the thyroid. A portion of the descending aorta is anterior to the spine and posterior to the heart.

Cross sections of the umbilical cord are seen under the fetal chin in Figure 10–10, as well as in front of the face. This appearance has been likened to the appearance of a fetus blowing bubbles.

Thymus

The thymus is proportionately larger in a fetus than in an adult. It is located in the anterior chest, just in front of the top of the heart and great vessels. It is sonographically homogeneous, with a texture similar to that of the lung. The thymus is shown in Figures 10–11*A* (longitudinal) and 10–11*B* (transverse). The thymus is currently of little interest in the

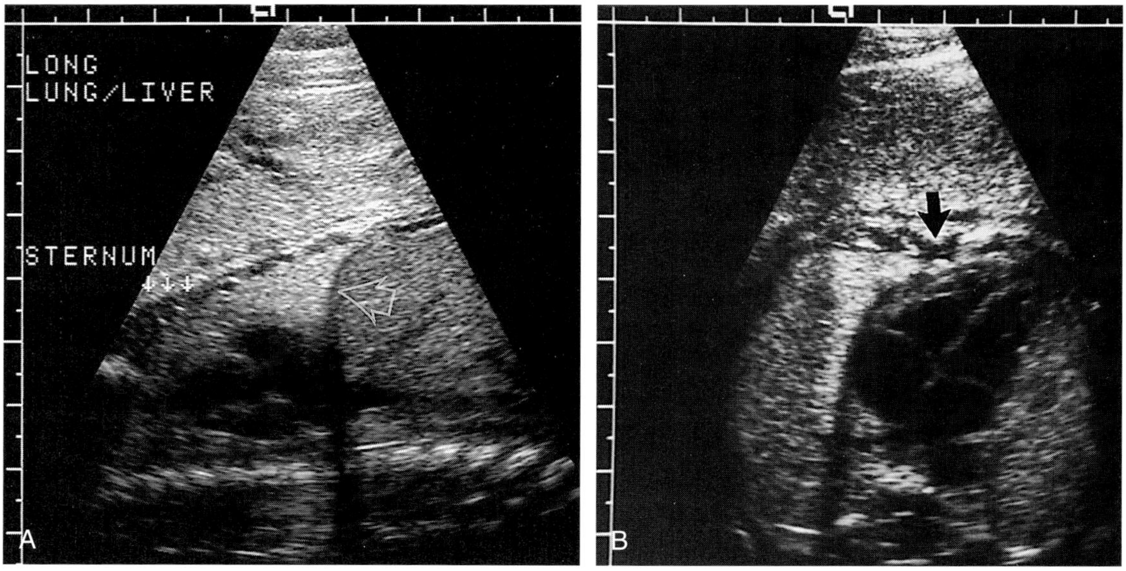

FIGURE 10–9.
Longitudinal and transverse images of the thorax and sternum in a 27-LMP-week fetus. *A*, the sternum is seen as a hypoechoic line (small arrows) of cartilaginous tissue between the skin and lung. The lung is more echogenic than the liver, with the diaphragm (open arrow) between. The inferior vena cava can be seen to penetrate the posterior diaphragm to enter the heart. *B*, Transverse thorax showing four-chamber heart and sternum (black arrow). The right ventricle is against the anterior chest just beneath the sternum; the left atrium is nearest the spine, at the lower portion of the image. (Images courtesy of ACUSON Corp., model XP10.)

field of sonography except to distinguish it from abnormal thoracic masses.

Heart

The fetal heart is an organ of major interest in the field of diagnostic medical sonography. Anomalies of the heart are relatively common and are associated with many syndromes, malformations, deformations, and sequelae. Almost 1% of all fetuses have heart defects, 1 in 100.[15] Because of the tendency for multiple anomalies to exist together, the observance of an anomaly anywhere in a fetus should give rise to a close study of its heart. Because of its importance, the normal fetal heart is discussed in detail elsewhere (see Chapter 11).

At present, the standard of care for sonography requires that a four-chamber view of the fetal heart be observed (Fig. 10–12*A* and *B*).[16] The four-chamber view can be obtained in most examinations after about 15 LMP weeks.[17] This view is obtained in a transverse view of the midthorax. The right ventricle is anterior, in the front of the chest. The left atrium is most posterior, nearest the spine. The right and left ventricles should be approximately equal in size, as should the two atria.[18] The interventricular septum should be free of defects, but the foramen ovale is seen between the atria. The valve of the foramen may be observed to flap into the left atrium with real-time. The short-axis view and outflow tract view are recommended for a complete study (see Chapter 11). The normal dimensions of the aortic and pulmonary outflow tract vessels have been published and are helpful for evaluation of abnormal conditions.[19, 20]

Real-time sonography can allow study of the moving heart even when the frozen image may be of lesser quality. Figures 10–12*A* and *B* are from two different fetuses of the same age. Using a scale size that enlarges the heart may help improve resolution. The cine-loop or video review function of modern sonographic machines is very helpful in the study of the heart, allowing an observer to step slowly through the frames.

The heart and vessels should be the only fluid-containing structures in the thorax on

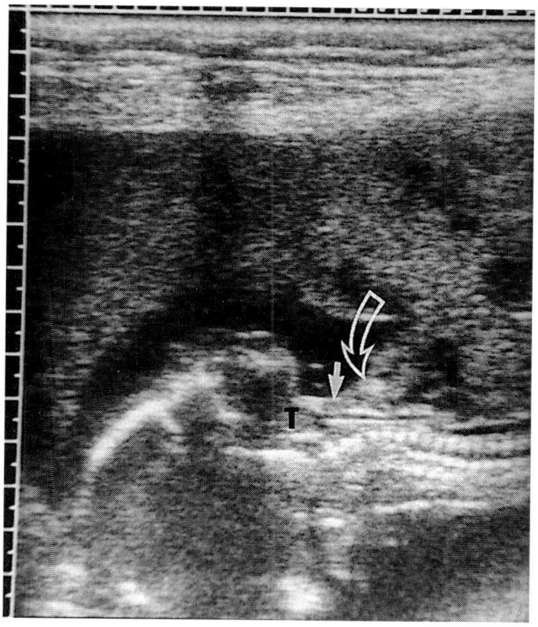

FIGURE 10–10.
Left parasagittal image of fetal neck. The genioglossus, geniohyoid, and mylohyoid muscles at the base of the tongue (T) are just cephalad to the thyroid (solid arrow). The linear left carotid can be seen passing posterior to the thyroid and clavicle in cross section (curved open arrow). The fluid tube just anterior to the spine is probably a portion of the aorta but may also be part of the fluid-filled esophagus. Loops of umbilical cord in cross section are anterior to the neck and face and appear as small circles or bubbles. (LNMP = 20.3 weeks, AA = 20.4, n = 8, range = 1.0 week, LG)

sonographic observation. If noticeable quantities of fluid are observed in the chest, an effort should be made to determine where the fluid is contained. Is it in the pericardium, the plural space, or the left or right chest, or are cystic-appearing structures seen? A diaphragmatic hernia with a portion or all of the stomach in the chest can resemble a cyst next to the left side of the heart (see the later diaphragm discussion).

Pericardial effusions are collections of fluid in the pericardial space or sac. Collections of this fluid up to 2 mm have been considered normal. One study found that collections as large as 7 mm may be normal if not associated with other abnormal conditions or anomalies.[21]

Pericardial effusions may develop with fetal hydrops. Figure 10–13 is an example of fetal hydrops with severe skin edema. This condition may result in fetal death due to congestive heart failure. It has been found that "umbilical venous pulsations are a generic sign of fetal congestive heart failure."[22, 23] The umbilical venous flow is usually at a constant amplitude. The researchers found that a pulsatile notch in the umbilical venous spectral Doppler flow predicted fetal mortality.[24]

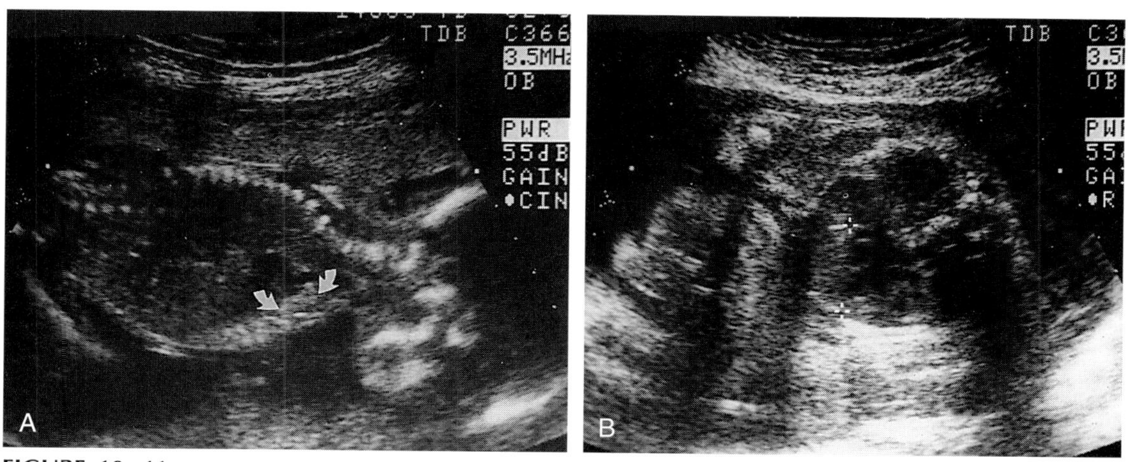

FIGURE 10–11.
The thymus is proportionally larger in a fetus than in an adult, but it can be difficult to image and recognize routinely. *A*, Posterior longitudinal view of the thorax and abdomen demonstrates the thymus (between arrows) in the anterior chest, just anterior to the top of the heart and great vessels. (LNMP = ?, AA = 20.3 weeks, n = 9, range = 2.0 weeks, TDB/TD) *B*, Transverse view of the thymus (+ cursors = 22.8 mm). This is the same fetus as in Figure 10–6 (which demonstrates the coronal view of the thymus). (Age via 15.0-week examination = 28.9 LMP weeks, AA = 28.1 weeks, n = 9, range = 2.0 weeks)

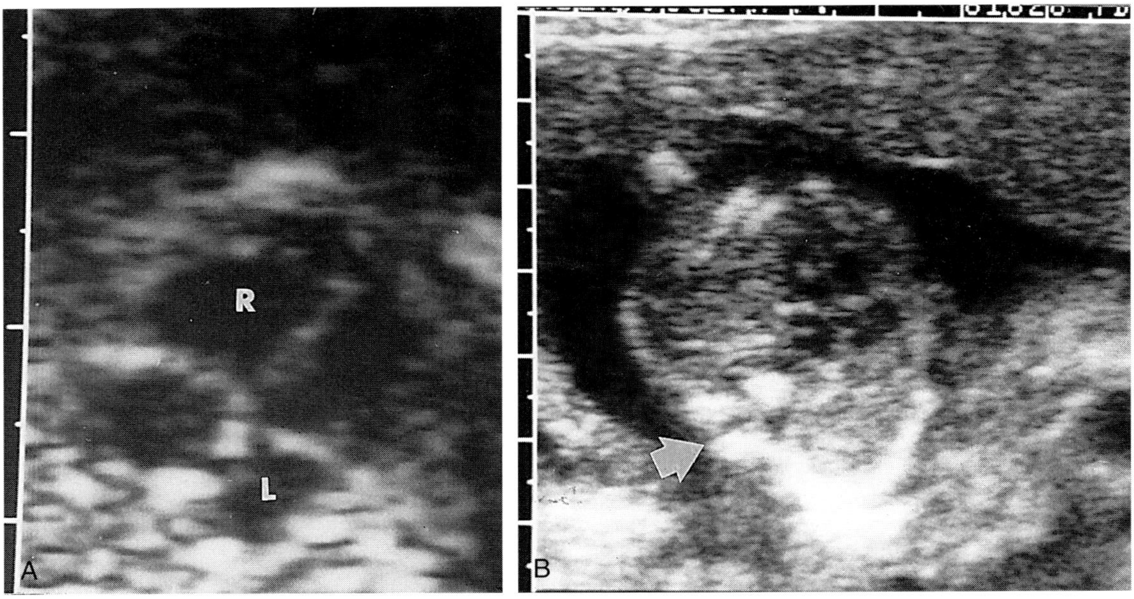

FIGURE 10–12.
Four-chamber views of the fetal heart in two fetuses of the same age. Real-time sonography is essential for evaluation of the fetal heart. Although static images can be obtained, they are often suboptimum. *A*, Four-chamber view of the heart, with presentation viewing the fetus from the feet toward the head. The right ventricle (R) is closest to the anterior chest wall and sternum. The left atrium (L) is nearest the spine, at the bottom of the image. The foramen ovale is seen as an opening in the septum between the left and right atria. (LNMP = 18.9 weeks, AA = 18.6, n = 10, range = 1.3 weeks, TD) *B*, This four-chamber heart is less clearly delineated than that in *A*, even though it is the same age. Real-time evaluation allowed confirmation that the heart was normal. This fetus was in cephalic presentation with the thorax viewed from the head toward the feet, the reverse of the previous image. The left atrium is still closest to the spine (arrow). (LNMP = 18.7 weeks, AA = 18.4, n = 9, range = 1.2 weeks, TD)

Vascular

AORTA

The ascending aorta carries blood from the left side of the heart, over the aortic arch, and into the descending aorta, which passes along the left anterior aspect of the spine. The descending aorta passes through the left posterior part of the diaphragm and into the abdomen (Fig. 10–14).

The thoracic portions of the aorta can usually be observed in a posterior, parasagittal plane along the left of the fetal spine. Figure 10–7 was produced in this manner. Acoustic shadows from the posterior ribs may cause intermittent obscuration of the aorta, but gentle rocking and sweeping of the plane of view should allow complete study.

From the anterior approach, the aorta may be seen in its entirety to the bifurcation into the iliac arteries. The aorta can be observed to pass anterior to the (left) spine in Figure 10–14. The umbilical vein in the abdomen is also shown.

Doppler study of the fetal aortic waveform can be compared with that of the head, neck, and umbilical cord to assess the preferential redistribution of blood flow to the brain in cases of intrauterine growth restriction (IUGR). As the resistance to flow in the umbilical cord increases, reducing placental perfusion and nutrients and oxygen to the fetus, a natural set of priorities is established, reducing the resistance to flow to the head in comparison with the aorta and body. This is discussed in more detail in Chapter 16, because these Doppler values are usually most beneficial when compared with those of the umbilical artery.

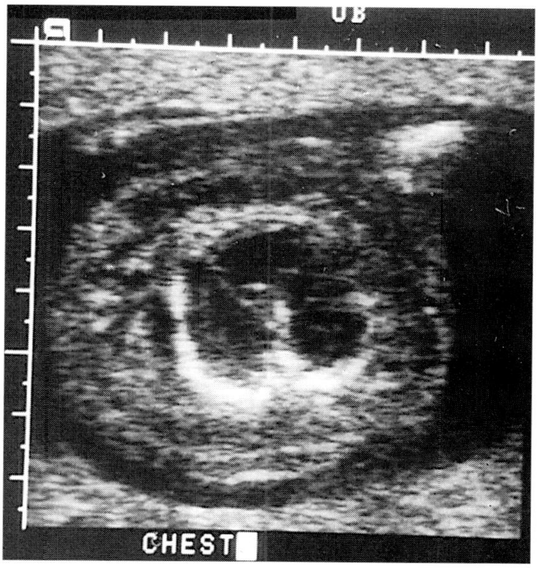

FIGURE 10–13.
Fetal hydrops with extreme edema. Note that the chest is the inner circle, with the very thick tissue concentrically around it. (Image courtesy of ACUSON Corp.)

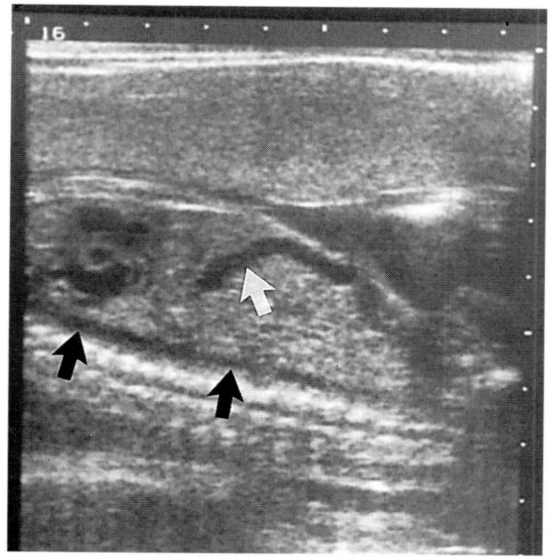

FIGURE 10–14.
The entire aorta (black arrows) can be seen from the arch to deep in the abdomen. The umbilical vein (white arrow) courses from the abdominal insertion into the liver. The aorta passes through the diaphragm approximately halfway between the black arrows. (LNMP = 24.0 weeks, AA = 21.0, n = 8, range = 1.6 weeks, SG)

VENOUS

The normal inferior vena cava (IVC) returns blood to the heart from the lower trunk. Below the diaphragm, the IVC courses anterior to the right side of the spine, parallel to the aorta. After the IVC passes through the diaphragm, it takes a more anterior tract toward the posterior heart to enter the right atrium (Fig. 10–15).

Pulmonary

DIAPHRAGM

The diaphragm forms the floor of the thorax and the top of the abdomen. The aorta, IVC, and esophagus are the only normal passages through the diaphragm. The aorta and esophagus are adjacent in the posterior left, and the IVC passes through the posterior right aspect of the diaphragm. All of these lie in close proximity to the spine.

The diaphragm can occasionally be clearly seen but at other times is difficult to observe. The maternal habitus, the position and age of the fetus, and the location of the placenta are factors in clarity. Figure 10–16 offers a good

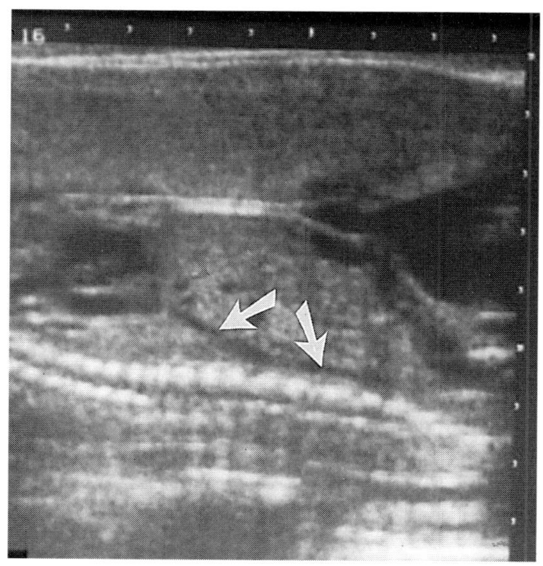

FIGURE 10–15.
The inferior vena cava (arrows) follows the left anterior spine until it approaches the diaphragm, where it courses anteriorly into the posterior of the right atrium of the heart. (LNMP = 24.0 weeks, AA = 21.0, n = 8, range = 1.6 weeks, SG)

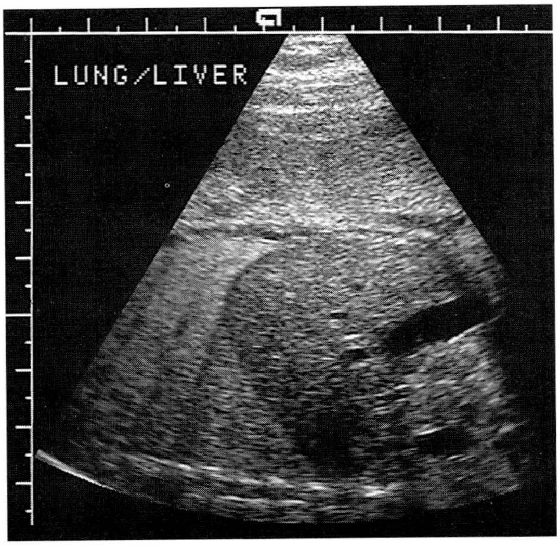

FIGURE 10–16.
The lung, diaphragm, and liver are clearly demonstrated. The lung has a typical homogeneous appearance that is more echogenic than the liver. This image demonstrates the clear resolution possible with modern sonographic equipment. (LMP = 27 weeks) (Image courtesy of ACUSON Corp., model XP10.)

look at the fetal diaphragm as well as the lung and liver. The diaphragm should be intact in its entirety, except for the passage of the three tubes mentioned earlier. The normal diaphragm appears as a hypoechoic line (Figs. 10–17 and 10–18). The IVC can be seen passing through the diaphragm in Figure 10–17, and in Figure 10–18, the diaphragm is a continuous line between the abdomen and thorax.

A fairly common fetal anomaly is the congenital diaphragmatic hernia (CDH), in which the opening around the esophagus is abnormal and the stomach and gastrointestinal tract can slide into the chest. Diaphragmatic hernias occur in 1:2000 to 1:5000 live births and are in the left diaphragm in 90% of cases. More severe cases can be fatal owing to compression and hypoplasia of the lungs. Less severe cases are surgically repairable at birth; however, if lung development has been impaired, the prognosis is not favorable. The mortality rate for CDH is between 30% and 50%.[25] At least one successful sonographic diagnosis and antenatal surgical repair has been reported.[26] With improved early transvaginal diagnosis, successful CDH repair will perhaps become more common.

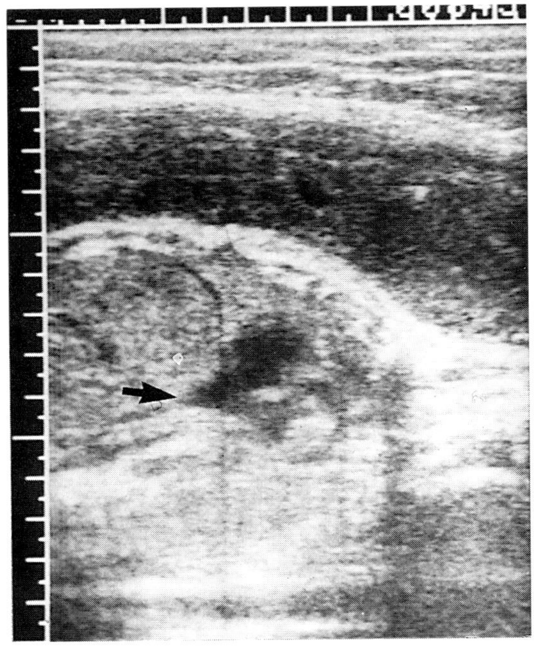

FIGURE 10–17.
Parasagittal plane showing the lung, liver, and diaphragm from the anterior approach. The diaphragm is the thin hypoechogenic line curving beneath the anterior chest wall toward the inferior vena cava (arrow), which can be seen to pass through the diaphragm. (LNMP = ?, AA = 35.3 weeks, n = 9, range = 2.5 weeks, LP)

Figure 10–19 is a schematic representation of a diaphragmatic hernia with the stomach in the chest. An innovative study of five fetuses observed on sonography to have CDH found that in only one could color

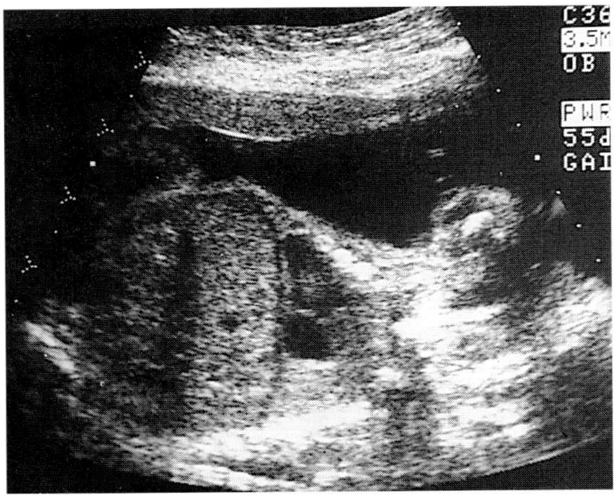

FIGURE 10–18.
Coronal view of the diaphragm, which is the dark, hypoechogenic line between the thorax (lung and heart) and the liver. (LNMP = 26.0 weeks, AA = 26.2, n = 9, range = 3.0 weeks, TD)

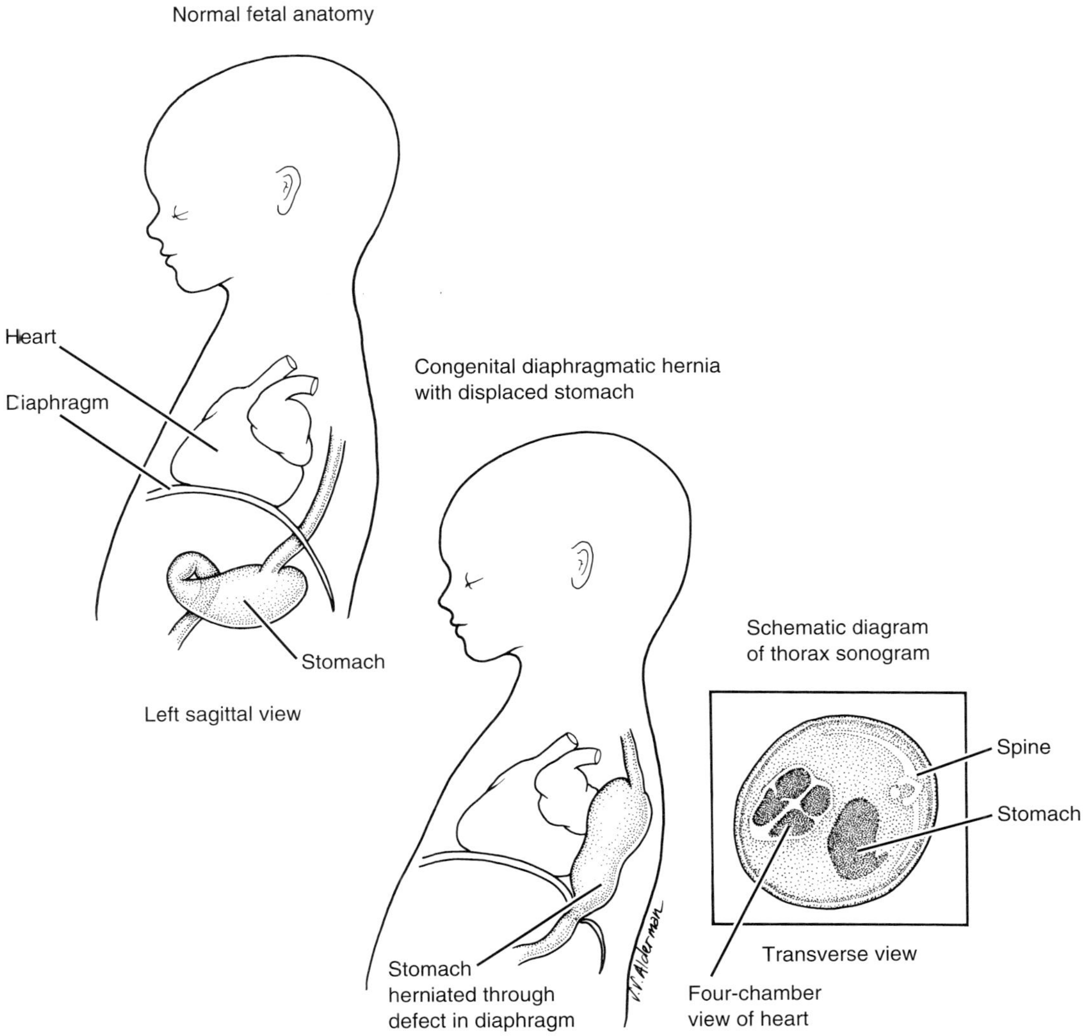

FIGURE 10–19.
Normal relationships of the heart, diaphragm, and stomach and the relationships that exist with congenital diaphragmatic hernia. In a cross section of the thorax, the stomach should not appear next to the heart.

Doppler not demonstrate amniotic fluid ebb and flow in the nasal and oropharyngeal area during fetal breathing motions. This one fetus died in the early neonatal period, but the other four survived this period. The researchers hypothesize that the absence of this amniotic color Doppler flow "is a useful marker for prenatal prediction of pulmonary hypoplasia"[27] (see Fig. 13–33 for images of this phenomenon).

A quick survey in the coronal view of the fetal body can demonstrate three fluid cavities: the heart, stomach, and bladder. Finding these cavities in normal relationships helps to rule out diaphragmatic hernia. The stomach should be approximately halfway between the heart and bladder and on the fetus's left side (Fig. 10–20). If the stomach or bladder is not visualized, waiting a few minutes, while continuing with other parts of the examination, should allow them to refill. If the stomach appears next to the heart, a hernia should be ruled out through closer examination (see Chapter 14 and Fig. 14–9*B*).

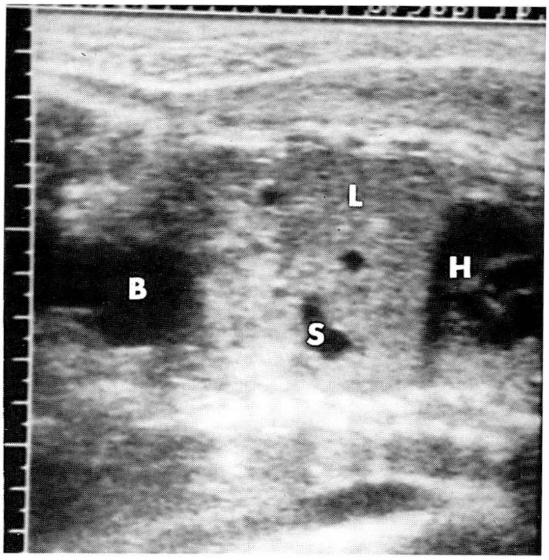

FIGURE 10–20.
Coronal view of a normal fetal trunk showing the three fluid cavities: urinary bladder (B), stomach (S), and heart (H). This view is used to rule out congenital diaphragmatic hernia by assessing the relationships of these fluid cavities. The liver (L) is seen to the right of the stomach. A short portion of the diaphragm can be seen between the liver and lung. (LNMP = 36.3 weeks, AA = 33.5, n = 9, range = 1.6 weeks, TD)

LUNGS

The lungs generally have a homogeneous texture and appear slightly more echogenic or isoechogenic to the liver. It has long been hoped that sonography would allow evaluation of fetal lung maturity.[28, 29] However, most positive results have been from indirect sonographic observations such as the rates of the fetal breathing motions, free vernix in the amniotic fluid, placenta grades, or possibly the BPD measurement.

The fetal lungs begin to produce surfactant by about the 23rd or 24th week. The surfactant is a complex substance of proteins, fatty acids, and lipids that reduces the surface tension in the maturing lungs. Absence or reduction of surfactant produces "Diminished aeration and high alveolar surface tension " . . . [which] . . ." leads to an increase in pulmonary vascular resistance."[30] This well-written report also states that with immature lungs, "The net effect is that a vicious circle is created leading to the development of the respiratory distress syndrome. This condition, which causes respiratory failure and is seen primarily in the preterm infant, has a high mortality rate if untreated and is the reason why obstetricians, in the past, delayed preterm delivery for as long as possible."[30]

When fetal breathing motions are observed, the thorax expands and contracts as if the fetus were breathing. This is a normal finding; indeed, it is abnormal for breathing motions not to occur for several seconds during a 30-minute period. The breath-to-breath intervals of the breathing motions become more regular after 34 to 36 weeks, and the intervals tend to be shortest in fetuses that eventually develop respiratory distress syndrome as neonates. This observation suggests that a mature pattern of regular, slower breathing motions is associated with mature fetal lungs. Peak fetal breathing motion occurs about 1 hour after maternal eating and correlates with high maternal blood glucose levels. Cigarette smoking reduces fetal breathing motions (for more discussion of normal breathing motions, see Chapter 17).

One study found an association with mature lecithin/sphingomyelin (L/S) ratios and therefore with lung maturity and a BPD measurement greater than 9.2 mm in nondiabetic pregnancies.[31] The assumed logic of this relationship is that the head size would be associated with fetal age and therefore lung maturity. However, McClure and Dornan stated that "this technique has generally not found favor, not least because the accuracy of measurement of the biparietal diameter is poor and the range of normality during the third trimester is extremely wide."[30] Slocum and colleagues, in the conclusion to their article, acknowledged occasional difficulties with the BPD and suggested that a study of the femur for this purpose might prove useful.[31] However, the femur also shows a large variation in comparison with the cranium. With more research, perhaps the use of three-dimensional BPD correction could improve on this technique (see Chapter 8). More likely, an integration of indicators of lung maturity such as fetal age by parameter size, breathing motions, placenta grade, and some sort of amniotic fluid vernix quotient similar to the biophysical profile will prove more successful. The issue of sonographic evaluation of fetal lung maturity is important and deserves more study.

Fetal pulmonary sequestration has been diagnosed by sonography. This is a relatively uncommon congenital abnormality in which an area of the lung is nonfunctioning and receives its blood supply from the systemic circulation. The sequestration presents as a hyperechoic mass in the chest. Doppler confirmation of systemic blood supply helps to confirm the diagnosis.[32] Other masses in the lung include teratoma, cystic adenomatoid malformation, bronchogenic cysts, bronchial atresia, rhabdomyoma, and enteric cysts, as well as diaphragmatic hernia, mentioned earlier.[33]

REFERENCES

1. Achiron R, Weissman A, Rotstein Z, et al: Transvaginal echocardiographic examination of the fetal heart between 13 and 15 weeks' gestation in a low-risk population. J Ultrasound Med 1994;13:783–789.
2. Bowerman RA: Atlas of Normal Fetal Ultrasonographic Anatomy, 2nd ed. Mosby/Year Book, St Louis, 1986, p 129.
3. Filly RA: Ultrasound evaluation of normal fetal anatomy. In: Callen PW, ed: Ultrasonography in Obstetrics and Gynecology, 3rd ed. WB Saunders, Philadelphia, 1993, p 165.
4. Streltzoff J, Isaacson G, Chervenak FA: Sonography of the abnormal fetal head, neck, and spine. In: Berman MC, ed: Diagnostic Medical Sonography, vol I: Obstetrics and Gynecology. JB Lippincott, Philadelphia, 1991, p 389.
5. Filly RA: Ultrasound evaluation of normal fetal anatomy. In: Callen PW, ed: Ultrasonography in Obstetrics and Gynecology, 3rd ed. WB Saunders, Philadelphia, 1993, pp 223–228.
6. Bader-Armstrong B: Normal and abnormal fetal limbs. In: Berman MC, ed: Diagnostic Medical Sonography, vol I: Obstetrics and Gynecology. JB Lippincott, Philadelphia, 1991, pp 437–438.
7. Williamson MR, Williamson SL: Gamuts in Ultrasound. WB Saunders, Philadelphia, 1992, p 119.
8. Goldstein RB: Ultrasound evaluation of the fetal thorax. In: Callen PW, ed: Ultrasonography in Obstetrics and Gynecology, 3rd ed. WB Saunders, Philadelphia, 1993, p 335.
9. Sabbagha RE, Toig RM, Sheikh Z: Skeletal abnormalities. In: Sabbagha RE, ed: Diagnostic Ultrasound Applied to Obstetrics and Gynecology, 3rd ed. JB Lippincott, Philadelphia, 1994, p 549.
10. Chitkara U, Rosenberg J, Chervenak FA, et al: Prenatal sonographic assessment of the fetal thorax: Normal values. Am J Obstet Gynecol 1987;156:1069.
11. Siddiqi TA, Beyer RA, Kofrhagen J, et al: A longitudinal study describing confidence limits of normal fetal cardiac, thoracic, and pulmonary dimensions from 20 to 40 weeks' gestation. J Ultrasound Med 1993;12: 731–736.
12. Sherer DM, Plessinger MA, Allen TA: Fetal scapular length in the ultrasonographic assessment of gestational age. J Ultrasound Med 1994;13:523–528.
13. Yarkoni S, Schmidt W, Jeanty P, et al: Clavicular measurement: A new biometric parameter for fetal evaluation. J Ultrasound Med 1985;4:467–470.
14. Silverman FN, ed: Caffey's Pediatric X-Ray Diagnosis: An Integrated Imaging Approach, 8th ed, vol 2. Year Book Medical Publishers, Chicago, 1985, p 1097.
15. Weaver DD: Classification of anomalies. In: Sabbagha RE, ed: Diagnostic Ultrasound Applied to Obstetrics & Gynecology. JB Lippincott, Philadelphia, 1994, p 325.
16. American Institute of Ultrasound in Medicine: Guidelines for Performance of the Antepartum Obstetrical Ultrasound Examination. AIUM Publications, 14750 Sweitzer Lane, Suite 100, Laurel, MD, 27070-5906, 1991.
17. Cyr DR, Guntheroth WG, Mack LA: Fetal echocardiography. In: Berman MC, ed: Diagnostic Medical Sonography, vol I: Obstetrics and Gynecology. JB Lippincott, Philadelphia, 1991, p 389.
18. Madden SJ, Peterson CL, Krew MA: Fetal echocardiography in conjunction with routine obstetric examinations. J Diagn Med Sonogr 1994;10:74–82.
19. Cartier MS, Davidoff A, Warnecke LA, et al: The normal diameter of the fetal aorta and pulmonary artery: Echocardiographic evaluation in utero. AJR 1987; 149:1003–1007.
20. Cartier MS, Doubilet PM: Fetal aortic and pulmonary artery diameters: Sonographic measurements in growth-retarded fetuses. AJR 1988;161:991–993.
21. Di Salvo DN, Brown DL, Doubilet PM, et al: Clinical significance of isolated fetal pericardial effusions. J Ultrasound Med 1994;13:291–293.
22. Reed KL: The role of venous Doppler in fetuses with non-immune hydrops: Opinion. Ultrasound Obstet Gynecol 1994;4:268–269.
23. Tulzer G, Gudmundsson S, Wood DC, et al: Doppler in non-immune fetal hydrops. Ultrasound Obstet Gynecol 1994;4:279–283.
24. Gudmundsson S, Huhta JC, Wood DC, et al: Venous Doppler ultrasonography in the fetus with non-immune hydrops. Am J Obstet Gynecol 1991;164: 33–37.
25. Wilcox DT, Karamanoukian HL, Glick PL: Care of the fetus/newborn with congenital diaphragmatic hernia. Fetal Maternal Med Rev 1994;6:81–94.
26. Harrison MR, Adzick NS, Lonaker MT, et al: Successful repair in utero of a fetal diaphragmatic hernia after removal of the herniated viscera from the left thorax. N Engl J Med 1990;322:1582–1584.
27. Fox HE, Badalan SS, Timor-Tritsch IE, et al: Fetal upper respiratory tract function in cases of antenatal diagnosed congenital diaphragmatic hernia: Preliminary observations. Ultrasound Obstet Gynecol 1993; 3:164–167.
28. Benson DM, Wladroup LD, Kurtz AB, et al: Ultrasonic tissue characterization of fetal lung, liver, and placenta for the purpose of assessing fetal maturity: AIUM/SDMS Official Proceedings. J Ultrasound Med 1983;2:97.
29. Cayea PD, Grant DC, Doubilet PM, et al: Inability of current clinical ultrasound to predict fetal lung maturity: AIUM/SDMS Official Proceedings. J Ultrasound Med 1984;3:99.
30. McClure BG, Dornan JC: Fetal lung maturation. Fetal Med Rev 1989;1:223–234.
31. Slocum WA, Martin JN, Martin RW, et al: Third-trimester biparietal diameter as a predictor of fetal lung maturity. Am J Perinatol 1987;4:266–270.
32. Sauerbrei E: Lung sequestration: Duplex Doppler diagnosis at 19 weeks gestation. J Ultrasound Med 1991;10:101–105.
33. Williamson MR, Williamson SL: Gamuts in Ultrasound. WB Saunders, Philadelphia, 1992, p 120.

CHAPTER 11

FETAL ECHOCARDIOGRAPHY

Julia A. Drose
Dale R. Cyr

Approximately 50% of childhood deaths due to a congenital abnormality are a result of congenital heart disease (CHD). Fetuses affected with CHD may be more numerous than published pediatric/newborn prevalence rates of 8 per 1000 live births and 27 per 1000 stillbirths.[1] These statistics illuminate the importance of fetal echocardiographic diagnoses.

In utero diagnosis of heart abnormalities, morphological or conductive, may alter the mode or site of delivery. In some cases, appropriate specialists also may be alerted for in utero therapy or immediate postpartum care. As with all sonography, the ability to recognize fetal heart anomalies results from experience and a thorough understanding of normal and abnormal anatomy, hemodynamics, and scanning techniques.

Embryology

The fetal cardiovascular system begins to form by the middle of the third embryonic week (5 weeks from the beginning of the last menstrual period) and is usually complete by week 8.[2] At this stage of development, a fetal crown-rump length of approximately 1.5 to 3 mm may be detected by endovaginal ultrasonography. A heartbeat may or may not be detected at this stage but should be consistently seen with an endovaginal transducer when the embryo achieves a crown-rump length of 5 mm, at approximately 6.5 weeks of gestational age.*[3]

Although some cardiac defects have been sonographically detected as early as 12 weeks' gestation, fetal heart size is usually not adequate for a thorough evaluation until 18 weeks' gestation. After 24 weeks' gestation, increased attenuation of the sound beam by the fetal spine, ribs, and limbs and the use of lower frequencies (e.g., 3 to 3.5 MHz) may make a fetal cardiac examination difficult.

Anatomy

Although anatomically similar to the pediatric and adult heart, the fetal heart offers significant differences. For instance, a fetal heart is

*Gestational age in this chapter is defined as menstrual age.

positioned within the chest more horizontally than an adult heart. Additionally, the fetal cardiovascular system contains three important shunts: (1) the ductus venosus, the (2) foramen ovale, and the (3) ductus arteriosus (Fig. 11–1). The ductus venosus lies between the umbilical vein and the inferior vena cava. It is responsible for carrying oxygenated blood from the placenta to the inferior vena cava, thereby allowing significant blood volume to bypass the fetal liver. The oxygenated blood within the inferior vena cava mixes with deoxygenated blood returning from the systemic circulation and enters the right atrium. From the right atrium, most of the blood (60%) is shunted into the left atrium via the foramen ovale. The remaining blood volume in the right atrium mixes with desaturated blood returning from the head and arms by way of the superior vena cava. The right atrial volume then traverses the tricuspid valve, during diastole, and enters the right ventricle. During systole, the right ventricular blood volume passes through the right ventricular outflow tract (RVOT) and into the main pulmonary artery. Because fetal lung metabolism is diminished throughout gestation, requiring less perfusion, the main pulmonary artery vascular resistance is increased, allowing a large portion of blood (90%) within the artery to be shunted through the ductus arteriosus into the descending aorta, largely bypassing the fetal lungs.

The oxygenated blood contained within the left atrium mixes with unsaturated blood from the fetal lungs, enters the left ventricle through the mitral valve during diastole, and is ejected through the left ventricular outflow tract (LVOT) into the ascending aorta.[4] Because of the foramen ovale and ductus arteriosus, blood within the fetal heart flows in a parallel fashion as opposed to the serial pattern of flow seen in the pediatric and adult heart.[5]

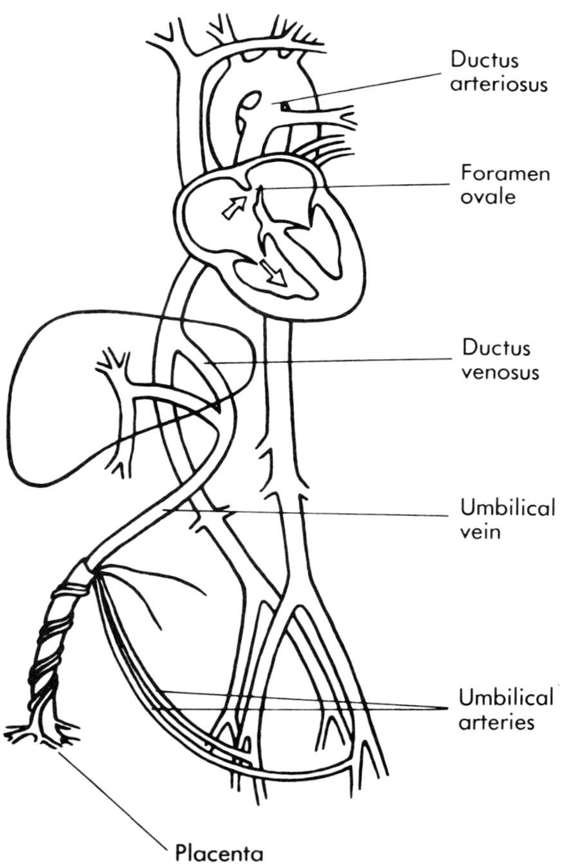

FIGURE 11–1.
Schematic demonstrating fetal intracardiac hemodynamics. (From Stamm ER, Drose JA, Thickman D: The fetal heart. In: Rumack CM, Wilson SR, Charboneau JW, eds: Diagnostic Ultrasound. Mosby/Year Book, St Louis, 1991, pp 800–827.)

Sonographic Technique

The spatial and contrast resolution necessary to evaluate the fetal heart requires state-of-the-art utlrasound equipment using the highest possible frequency. For fetal echocardiography, common frequencies typically are 5.0 or 3.5 MHz, depending on maternal body habitus, fetal and placental location, the amount of amniotic fluid present, and gestational age.

The first step in performing a fetal echocardiogram is to identify the position of the fetus within the uterus. Once fetal position is determined, the fetal heart should be seen within the left side of the chest with the apex of the heart pointing left, termed *levocardia*. A heart located more midline with the apex pointing anteriorly is defined as *mesocardia*. In *dextrocardia*, the heart is located in the right side of the chest and the apex points to the right. This should not be confused with *dextroposition*, in which the heart is usually displaced to the right by an external mass, which may be stomach or bowel, as in the case of diaphragmatic hernia or cystic adenomatoid malformation. It is important to note in dextrocardia that the apex of the heart remains pointing toward the left. It has been reported that abnormal position of the heart is associated with an 81% mortality, and abnormal axis of the cardiac apex carries a 50% mortality.[6]

FOUR-CHAMBER VIEW

The four-chamber view is both the primary and most significant view obtained when performing fetal echocardiography. The four-chamber view is acquired by scanning transversely through the fetal chest. Depending on the position of the transducer in relation to the fetus, the anatomy of the four-chamber view may be seen apically or from a subcostal scanning plane. The apical four-chamber view is visualized when the sound beam is directed parallel to the interventricular and interatrial septa (Fig. 11–2). This view allows identification and evaluation of both atria and the two ventricles, as well as the mitral and tricuspid valves. Doppler interrogation of the atrioventricular valves is optimal in this projection because the Doppler cursor is parallel to blood flow. It is important to image the atrial and ventricular septa as perpendicular to the insonation beam as possible, allowing septal defects to be better imaged. This is accomplished by imaging the fetus in a transverse plane and angling the transducer cephalically, under the ribs, from the superior aspect of the fetal liver, known as the *subcostal view*. Artifactual dropout of echoes may be seen in the apical four-chamber view, giving false appearances of septal defects, most commonly seen at the levels of the atrial septum secundum and the membranous portion of the interventricular septum. Color Doppler may also be used in this projection to evaluate the septa for any defects, keeping in mind that small septal defects may be beyond the resolution of either gray-scale imaging or color Doppler.

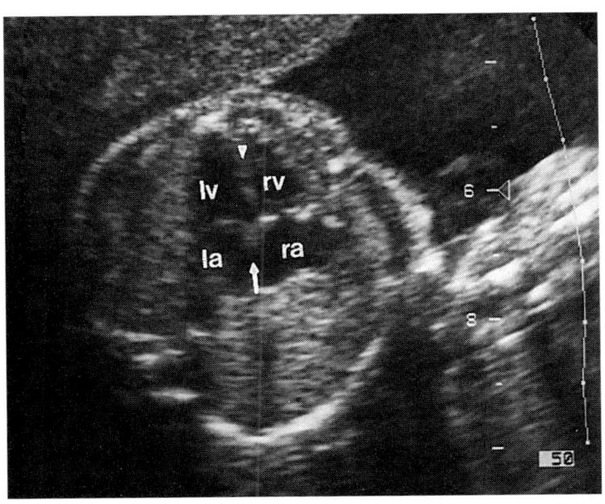

FIGURE 11–2.
Apical four-chamber view. la, Left atrium; ra, right atrium; lv; left ventricle; rv, right ventricle; arrowhead, moderator band; arrow, foramen ovale.

Four-chamber views are useful in providing additional anatomical information. The foramen ovale can be routinely seen as an echogenic flap within the left atrium, determining the morphological left side of the fetal heart. Doppler can be performed to identify the presence or absence of flow across the atrioventricular valves or to document normal right-to-left flow through the foramen ovale. The pulmonary veins may be seen connecting to the left atrium. Location of the moderator band, which is within the apex of the right ventricle, allows the observer to determine the fetal cardiac right side. Determining moderator band location is useful in questions about ventricular inversion.

In demonstrating the relationship of the aorta and main pulmonary artery, the diagnosis of CHD is improved. To achieve limited visualization of the aorta and main pulmonary artery from the four-chamber view, simply rotate or angle the transducer anteriorly, within the fetal heart, from the four-chamber view. Assuming that the sonographer is correctly oriented, specifically, to fetal cardiac anatomy (left and right sides, medial and lateral aspects), the first great vessel imaged is the aorta, arising from the left ventricle (Fig. 11–3*A*). This demonstrates continuity of the ascending aorta to the LVOT and left ventricle. The aortic valve is usually seen in this plane and offers promising angles for Doppler interrogation. Continued anterior angulation of the transducer from the aortic LVOT plane allows the main pulmonary artery and RVOT to be seen, arising from the right ventricle (Fig. 11–3*B*). Doppler interrogation of the main pulmonary artery (MPA) may be more difficult secondary to insonation angles approaching 90 degrees. A sweeping motion from the four-chamber view to the aorta/LVOT continuing anteriorly to the pulmonary artery/RVOT, allows the sonogra-

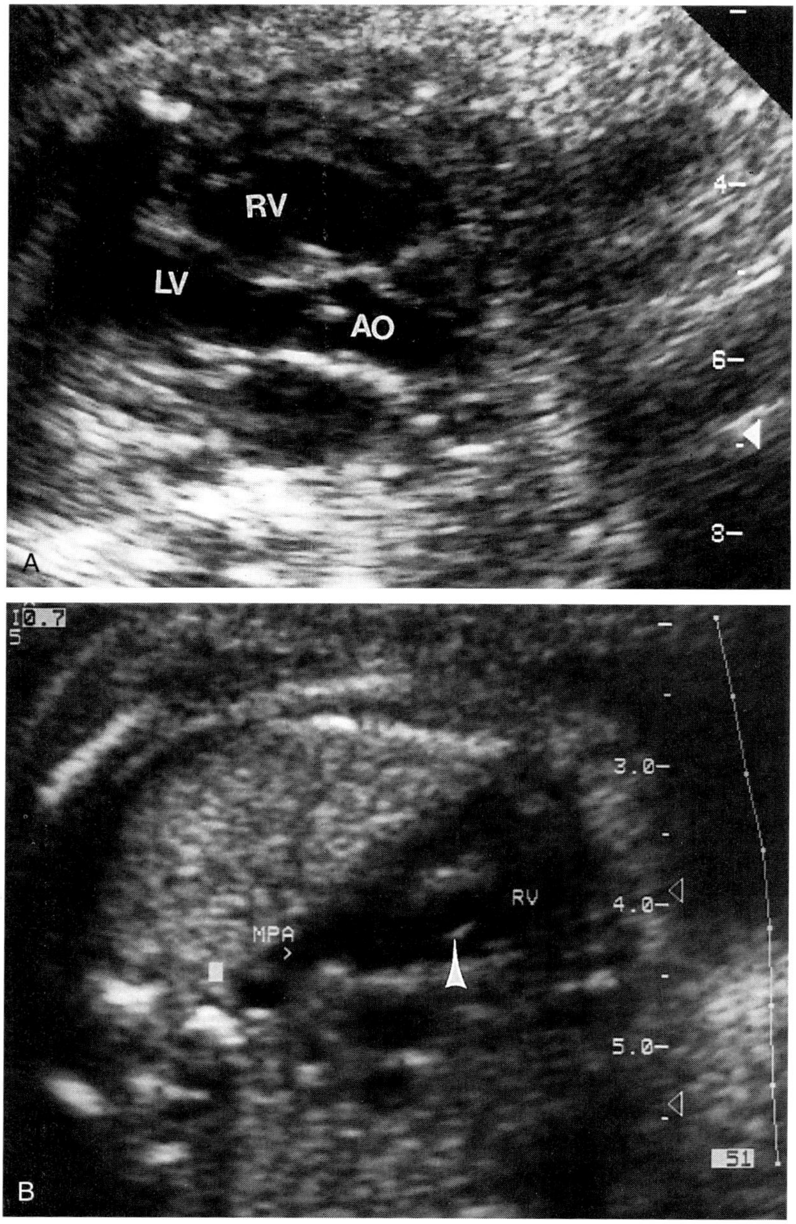

FIGURE 11–3.
A, Sonogram demonstrating aortic/left ventricular outflow view from an apical four-chamber view. RV, Right ventricle; AO, aorta; LV, left ventricle. *B*, Sonogram demonstrating pulmonary artery/right ventricular outflow tract, which is obtained by further anterior angulation from the aortic/left ventricular outflow tract. RV, Right ventricle; MPA, main pulmonary artery; arrowhead, pulmonary valve.

pher to view important anatomy to improve the diagnostic yield of CHD (see Fig. 11–3*B*).

LONG-AXIS VIEW OF THE FETAL HEART

From the subcostal four-chamber view, the transducer can be rotated 90 degrees or angled toward the fetal right shoulder to evaluate the fetal heart in a long-axis view. In this view, continuity between the anterior wall of the ascending aorta and the interventricular septum, as well as continuity of the posterior wall of the ascending aorta and the anterior leaflet of the mitral valve, can be evaluated. Doppler of the aortic valve may also be performed in this projection. The aorta should follow an anterior, leftward course. Continuing the transducer rotation toward the fetal right shoulder allows visualization of the pulmonary artery and right ventricular outflow tract. The pulmonary artery should course posteriorly and to the right of the aorta. Doppler study of the pulmonary artery can be obtained in this view.

SHORT-AXIS VIEW

Continuing a rightward transducer rotation results in a sagittal axis of the fetus. In this plane, a short-axis view of the fetal heart is imaged. In the short-axis view, multiple sections of the fetal heart should be obtained. The ventricles can be evaluated for size, and color Doppler may be used to evaluate the interventricular septum for defects. With the transducer in the same sagittal plane and sliding to the medial aspect of the fetus, or the fetal left, a short-axis view through the great vessels results (Fig. 11–4). This important view allows the great vessels to be seen in the anterior and posterior relationships to one another. The aortic valve should be seen in transverse axis, with the pulmonary artery draping anteriorly, demonstrating normal anatomical relationships. Failure to visualize this relationship of the great vessels may be indicative of an anomaly such as transposition of the great vessels. The short-axis view of the great vessels is also ideal for using Doppler to interrogate pulmonary artery flow.

The final structures to be evaluated during the course of a fetal echocardiogram are the aortic arch and the arch of the ductus arteriosus (ductal arch). These are usually seen by moving the transducer into a longitudinal, coronal view of the fetus. The aortic arch can be differentiated from the flatter, more caudally located ductal arch (Fig. 11–5) by identifying the three cephalic vessels arising from the transverse aortic arch. These vessels are the innominate (or brachiocephalic), left carotid, and left subclavian arteries. The aortic arch should be interrogated with Doppler from the aortic valve to the distal descending aorta, looking for increases in velocity that may be indicative of coarctation of the aorta. Coarctation, or narrowing, of the aorta may occur anywhere along the aortic arch. Some coarctations of the aorta are thought to be related to ductal closure; therefore, they may not occur until after birth. The purpose of visualizing the ductal arch is to confirm that it is patent; therefore, Doppler is also an important part of the evaluation. Ductal constriction may be related to a structural anomaly or associated with use of particular drugs such as indomethacin or analgesics.

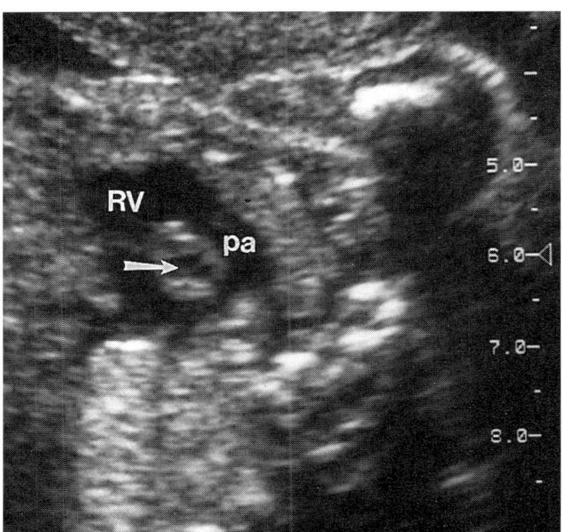

FIGURE 11–4.
Short-axis view of fetal heart at the level of the great vessels. RV, Right ventricle; pa, pulmonary artery; arrow, aorta.

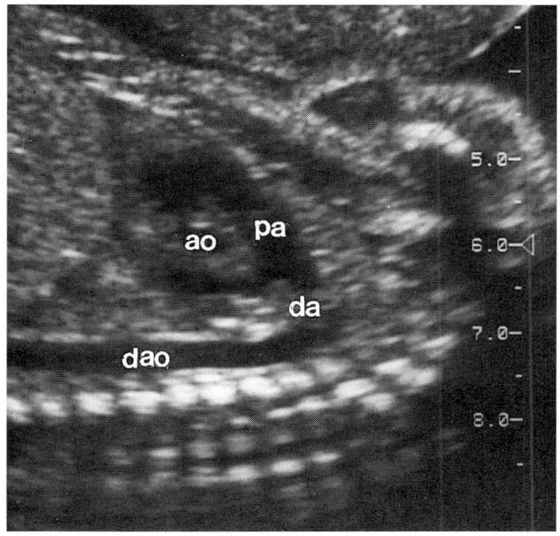

FIGURE 11–5.
Sagittal sonogram demonstrating the ductal arch. Ao, Aorta; pa, pulmonary artery; da, ductal arch; dao, descending aorta. Note that no cephalic vessels can be identified, distinguishing ductal arch from aortic arch.

Doppler Interrogation of the Fetal Heart

Pulsed Doppler is a useful adjunct to grayscale imaging when evaluating a fetal heart. All four valves in the heart should be evaluated proximal to the valve when looking for valvular insufficiency, and distal to the valve when concerned with valvular stenosis. Reversal of Doppler flow, which occurs during closure of a particular valve (during systole for the mitral and tricuspid valves and during diastole for the aortic and pulmonary valves) represents valvular insufficiency. The best view to evaluate Doppler flow in the atrioventricular valves typically is the apical four-chamber view. In this projection, the sample volume can be placed close to 0 degrees on either side of these valves. This four-chamber view also often allows an adequate angle to evaluate the aortic valve. If the ascending aorta cannot be visualized in this projection, a long-axis view of the aorta may provide the best angle for Doppler interrogation. The pulmonic valve is best evaluated in a short-axis view. A long-axis view of the pulmonary artery may also be useful, but the short-axis view usually provides the best Doppler angle for interrogation. Doppler should also be used to evaluate flow across the foramen ovale, normal flow should be seen as biphasic, occurring at a rate double that of the fetal heart.

Pulsed Doppler may also be valuable in assessing the interventricular septum for defects. Color Doppler of the interventricular septum in a subcostal four-chamber view usually is the best tool to look for septal defects. If a defect is present, color Doppler may be seen crossing the septum. Limitations in color Doppler spatial resolution may inhibit visualization of small septal defects. Most septal defects in a fetus, no matter how large they are, may cause only small bidirectional shunts.[7] This is because the pressures in both ventricles are similar in fetal life, secondary to the normal shunts present. The most common area for a ventricular septal defect to be located is in the membranous portion of the septum.[8] If a septal defect is detected by color Doppler, the pulsed Doppler sample volume can then be placed in the area of interest to confirm the presence of blood flow. Again, keep in mind that small septal defects in a fetal heart may be beyond the resolution capabilities of gray-scale, pulsed Doppler, or color Doppler.

Pulsed Doppler of both the aortic arch, looking for a coarctation, and the ductal arch to rule out constriction is also an important component of a complete fetal echocardiogram. See Chapters 13 and 16 for more on Doppler.

M-Mode

Although not routine in the evaluation of most fetal hearts, real-time directed M-mode echocardiography is a useful adjunct in some cases. In a fetus, subjective assessment with real-time gray-scale imaging by an experienced sonographer or sonologist may be the best method for evaluating chamber dimension, valve excursion, and wall motion. M-mode, however, allows a method of quantifying these parameters. Various nomograms that plot atrial and ventricular size, as well as septal and posterior heart wall thickness, against gestational age, femur length, or biparietal diameter do exist (Fig. 11–6).

M-mode is particularly useful in evaluating most fetal arrhythmias. M-mode is an effective method of measuring fetal heart rate and allows simultaneous display of atrial and ventricular wall movement. The semilunar and atrioventricular valves can also be evaluated, thereby allowing specific types of arrhythmias to be diagnosed. The best views for using M-mode to evaluate an arrhythmia are a short-axis view of the great vessels or a long-axis view of the LVOT. In both views, the M-mode cursor should be placed through the aortic valve and the left atrial heart wall. This allows the observer to see the motion of the atria via the left atrial wall and to see the motion of the ventricle, which would be reflected in the movement of the aortic root and valve. An atrial beat should normally be seen, followed immediately by a ventricular beat. If an arrhythmia is occurring, M-mode allows measurement of fetal heart rates and identification of the source of the arrhythmia (i.e., ventricular or atrial).

Heart Rate

Embryonic heart rate appears to increase rapidly to a mean peak of approximately 175 beats/minute during the first 47 to 52 days of life.[9] After this time, the cardiac acceleration in rate appears to reverse abruptly. By 20

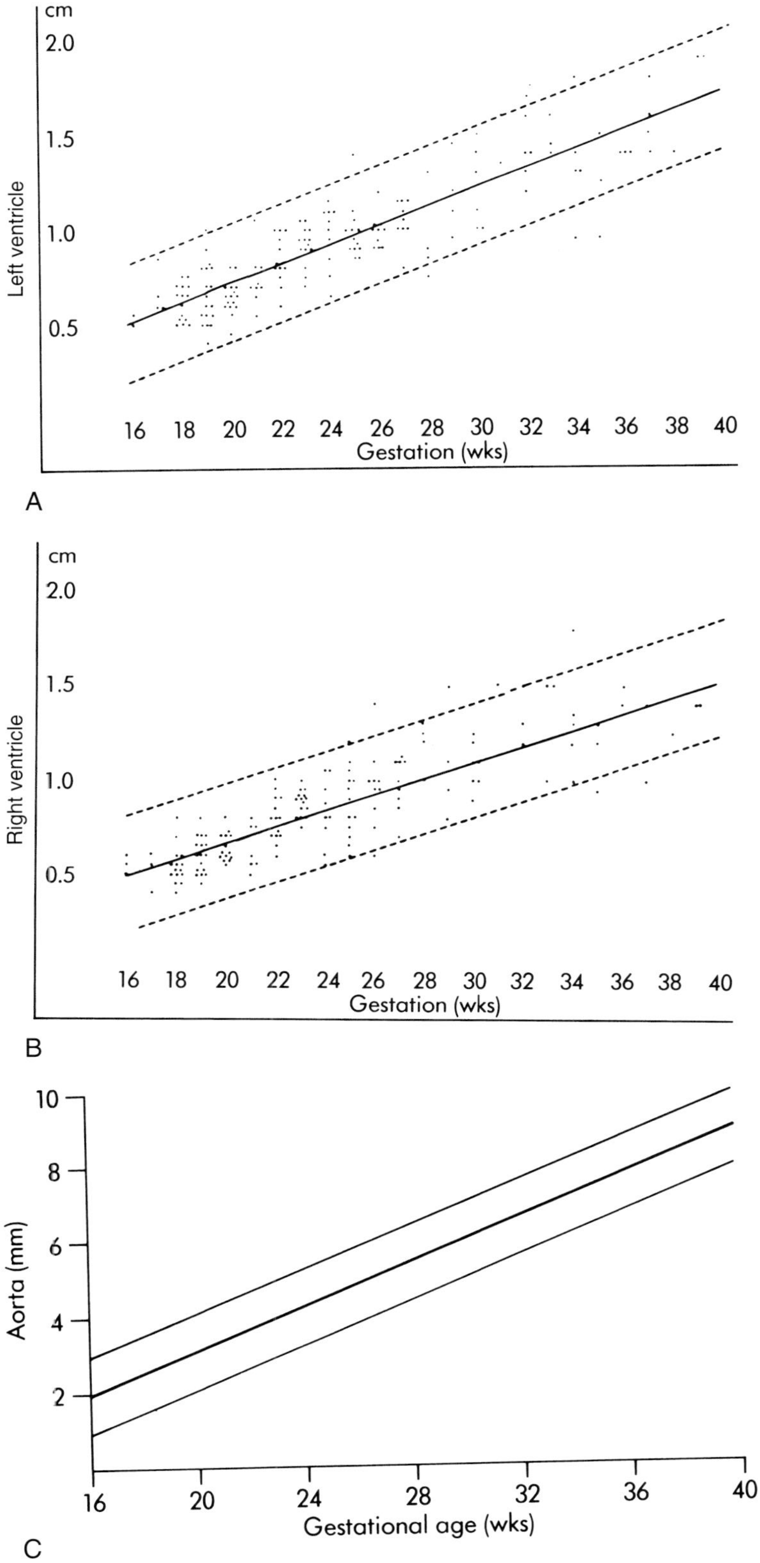

FIGURE 11–6.
A, Nomogram demonstrating left ventricular size in relation to gestational age. *B,* Nomogram demonstrating right ventricular size in relation to gestational age. *C,* Nomogram demonstrating fetal aortic size in relation to gestational age.

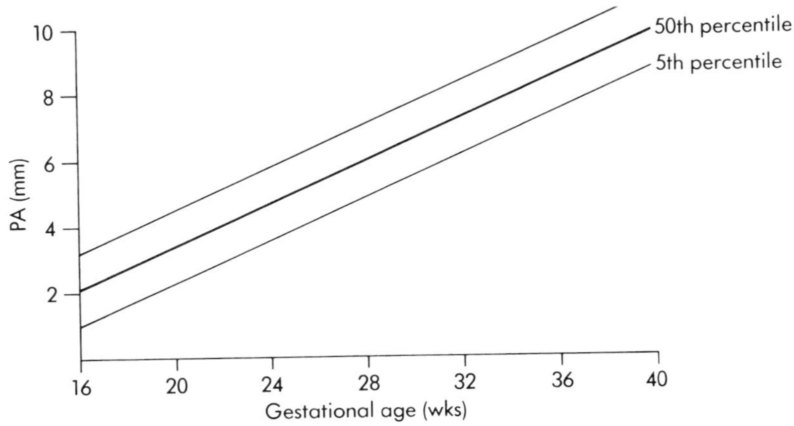

D

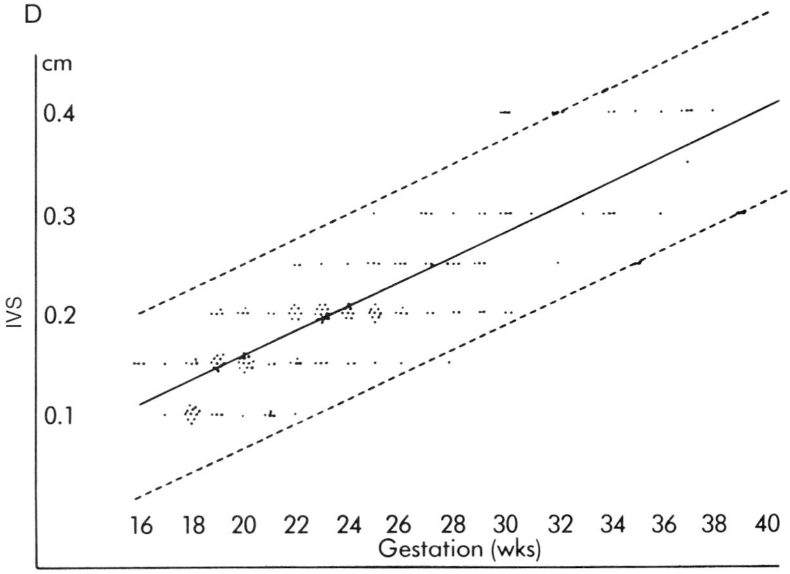

E

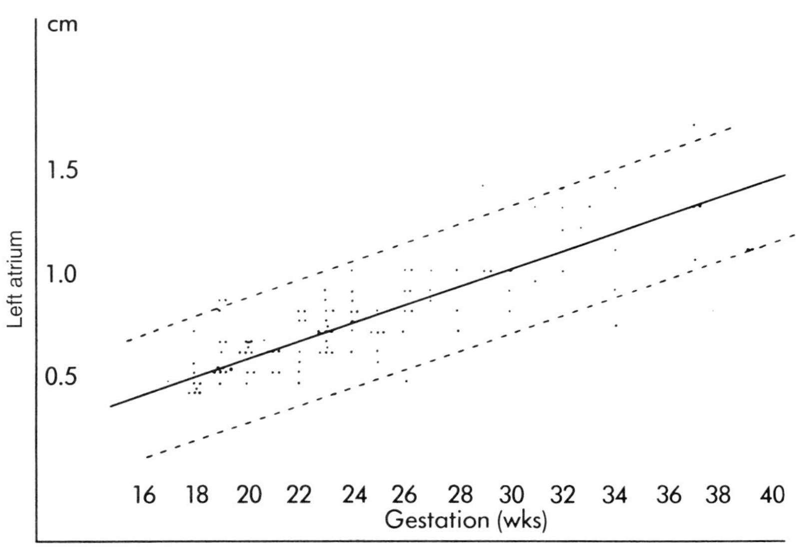

F

FIGURE 11–6 *Continued*
D, Nomogram demonstrating pulmonary artery (PA) size in relation to gestational age. *E,* Nomogram demonstrating interventricular septum (IVS) thickness in relation to gestational age. *F,* Nomogram demonstrating left atrial size in relation to gestational age. (With permission from Allan LD, Joseph MC, Boyd EGCA, Campbell S: M-mode echocardiography in the developing human fetus. Br Heart J 1982; 47:573–583.)

weeks' gestation, a normal fetal heart rate is 140 (±20) beats/minute and falls to approximately 130 (±20) beats/minute at term.[10] Tachycardia in a fetus is considered to be a heart rate greater than 180 beats/minute. Most fetal tachycardias are supraventricular and are categorized as paroxysmal supraventricular tachycardia (180 to 300 beats/minute), atrial flutter (300 to 400 beats/minute), or atrial fibrillation (400+ beats/minute).[11] Fetal bradycardia is defined as a heart rate of less than 100 beats/minute. The most common type of bradycardia noted in a fetus is transient bradycardia. This is usually caused by manual compression of the fetus with the transducer, causing a vasovagal response.[12] Reducing transducer pressure also alleviates bradycardia. Sustained bradycardia is usually a result of heart block in a fetus and presents a more dismal prognosis. Fifty percent of cases of complete heart block are associated with a structural abnormality of the heart.[13] Complete heart block is also more common in fetuses of mothers with collagen vascular disease, most commonly lupus.[14]

Occurrence Rate

Congenital heart malformations usually have a multifactorial etiology. Genetic predisposition in conjunction with environmental factors, such as maternal disease, antenatal infection, or maternal drug or alcohol use, account for 85% of cases. The remaining 15% are thought to be associated with chromosomal or monogenetic defects.[15] Recurrence risk for siblings of an affected infant are 2% to 3%. If two siblings are affected, the risk may be as high as 10% to 12%.[15,16] A fetus whose mother has a CHD has an occurrence rate of around 19% for CHD.

Approximately 25% of live-born infants with CHD have extracardiac anomalies.[17] Therefore, it is important that a complete obstetrical ultrasound examination be performed whenever a cardiac defect is suspected.

REFERENCES

1. Hoffman JIE, Christianson MA: Congenital heart disease in a cohort of 19,502 births with long-term follow-up. Am J Cardiol 1978;42:641–647.
2. Colvin EV: Cardiac embryology. In: Garson A, Bricker JT, McNamara DG, eds: The Science and Practice of Pediatric Cardiology. Lea & Febiger, Philadelphia, 1990, pp 71–108.
3. Levi CS, Lyons EA, Zheng XH, et al: Endovaginal US: Demonstration of cardiac activity in embryos of less than 5.0 mm in crown-rump length. Radiology 1990;176:71.
4. Sadler TW: Langman's Medical Embryology, 6th ed. Williams & Wilkins, Baltimore, 1990, p 223.
5. Reed KL: Fetal and neonatal cardiac assessment with Doppler. Semin Perinatol 1987;4:347–356.
6. Comstock CH: Normal fetal heart axis and position. Obstet Gynecol 1987;70:255–259.
7. Romero R, Pilu G, Jeanty P, et al (Eds): The heart. In: Prenatal Diagnosis of Congenital Anomalies. Appleton & Lange, Norwalk, CT, 1988, p 142.
8. Soto B, Becker AE, Moulaert AJ, et al: Classification of ventricular septal defects. Br Heart J 1980;43:332–336.
9. DuBose TJ, Cunyus JA, Johnson LF: Embryonic heart rate and age. J Diagn Med Ultrasound 1990;6:151–157.
10. Southall DP, Richards J, Hardwick RA, et al: Prospective study of fetal heart rate and rhythm patterns. Arch Dis Child 1980;55:506–510.
11. Shenker L: Fetal cardiac arrhythmias. Obstet Gynecol Surv 1979;34:561–563.
12. Mendoza GJ, Orlandino A, Steinfeld L: Intermittent fetal bradycardia induced by mid pregnancy fetal ultrasonographic study. Am J Obstet Gynecol 1989;160:1038–1040.
13. Crawford DC, Chapman MC, Allan LD: The evaluation of persistent bradycardia in prenatal life. Br J Obstet Gynecol 1985;92:941–944.
14. McCue CM, Mantakas ME, Tinglestad JB, et al: Congenital heart block in newborns of mothers with connective tissue disease. Circulation 1977;56:82–89.
15. Nora JJ, Nora AH: Maternal transmission of congenital heart disease, new recurrence risk figures and the question of cytoplasmic inheritance and vulnerability to teratogens. Am J Cardiol 1987;59:459–463.
16. Nora JJ, Nora AH: Update on counseling the family with a first degree relative with a congenital heart defect. Am J Med Genet 1988;29:137–1452.
17. Greenwood RD, Rosenthal A, Parisi L, et al: Extracardiac abnormalities in infants with congenital heart disease. Pediatrics 1975;55:485–492.

CHAPTER 12

HEART RATE

Terry J. DuBose

History of Sonographic Heart Rate

One of the earliest sonographic studies of the embryonic heart rate (EHR) was by Robinson and Shaw-Dunn.[1] This study, which was published in 1973, is still one of the best despite the fact that it used early M-mode on articulated arm, bistable (black and white, no shades of gray) machines. For this reason, the researchers were not able to document the heart rate before about 6.5 menstrual weeks. They were working at the limits of resolution for these early machines.

Robinson and Shaw-Dunn showed the EHR to accelerate from the middle of the sixth week to a peak at the start of the ninth postmenstrual week, with a mean of approximately 175 beats/minute (B/M), followed by a slow decline to the 15th week (Fig. 12–1). Their study was limited by the use of the LNMP for establishing the age of the embryo and the difficulty of documenting accurate crown-rump lengths (CRL) with the old static B-scanners. The data thus had a larger variation than is normal and caused the researchers to overlook the importance of the shape of the curve. The peak heart rate distribution (±2 SD) was between a high of about 200 and a low of about 150 B/M. This was remarkably accurate, given the early sonographic equipment with which Robinson and Shaw-Dunn were working.

Several studies have used M-mode with real-time instruments.[1–10] The results of these studies have been adapted in Figure 12–1 by entering their tables into a spreadsheet for plotting. It is easy to see the similarity of most of the graphs.

Other researchers have published EHR data without using M-mode to document the rates.[9–11] Most of these attempted to count the heart rate by watching the sonographic monitor. One even counted the EHR for three 15-second intervals and multiplied the average by 4 to estimate heart rates (see Fig. 12–1.)[9] However, it is almost impossible to accurately count a heart rate that can normally approach 190 B/M by simultaneously watching a video monitor and a stopwatch while holding a transducer steady on the faint heartbeat of an embryo. Nearly all of the researchers who tried visual counts of the EHR missed the high peak at 9 weeks and the gradual decline after 9 weeks.[9] The studies of visually counted heart rates tended to report that the EHR plateaued at about 140 to 160 B/M despite what some stated in subsequent publications.[12, 13]

An old myth is that the gender of a fetus can be predicted by its heart rate. While

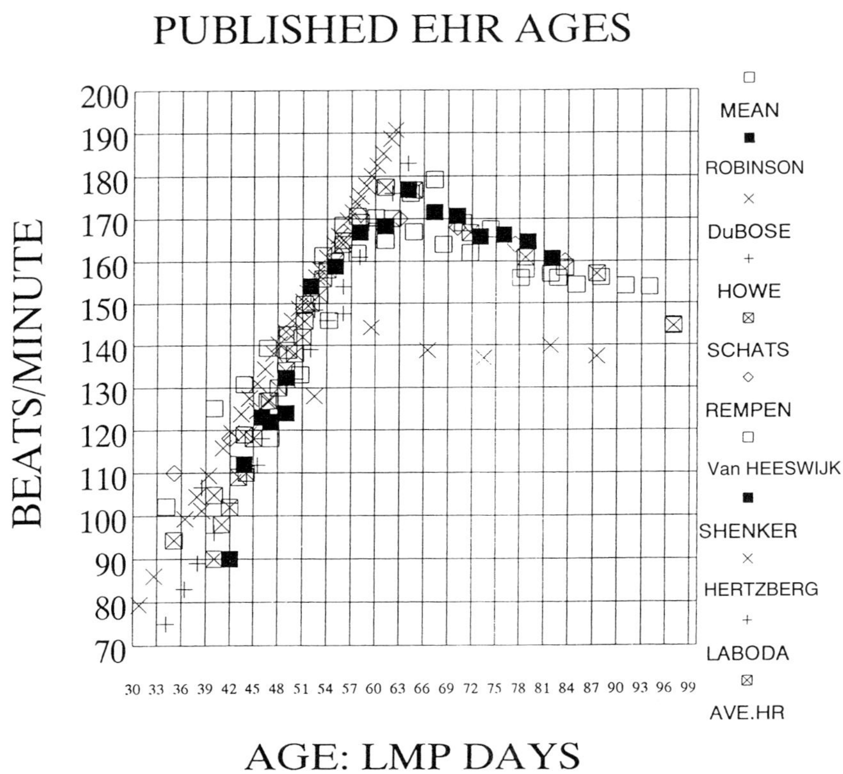

FIGURE 12–1.
This XY plot shows the similarity of several published tables of mean heart rates by embryofetal ages. The software allowed only six different symbols; therefore, the last five symbols are repeated. Most sets of data are so similar that it does not matter that the symbols are duplicated, except for the data of Hertzberg and colleagues[9] (X), which plateau below 150 M/B because they did not use M-mode to measure the heart rate. The other X symbol is the DuBose linear regression. The top open box (Mean) is a LOWESS smoothed mean of all tables. The average heart rate (boxed X) is the LOWESS means for the heart rate, which is unpublished and is presented for comparison (see Chapter 7 for a description of LOWESS smoothing).

attempting to determine our accuracy in fetal dating and weight estimates, our laboratory gave out 925 stamped self-addressed postcard questionnaires between 1984 and 1986 to sonographic obstetrical patients requesting birthing information. Fifty-one percent (474) of these cards were returned. One of the first and easiest questions answered was, Did the M-mode heart rate correlate with the resulting sex of the neonate? The heart rate data were divided into three groups—females, males, and those for whom no feedback card was received (no sex indicated). The study found no significant difference in female and male heart rates at any time during pregnancy. This research was rejected for publication in 1987 but was accepted as a letter to the editor in 1988.[14] This study offered one of the first suggestions that the heart rate might correlate with age. The full research was published by another journal the following year.[3] Analysis of variance of these data found no significant difference in the mean heart rates for all three groups (P = 0.48, n = 875). The mean rate for females was 149.26, males was 149.38, and unidentified sex was 150.5 B/M. The variance for females (variance = 190.5 B/M, n = 242) was greater than for males (variance = 170.9 B/M, n = 232). The no-sex-indicated group had a variance of 199.0 B/M, n = 401. The medians were females 150, males 149, and no sex 151 B/M; ±2 SD was ±26.2, ±27.6, and ±28.2 B/M, respectively. All three groups had a mode of 145 B/M.

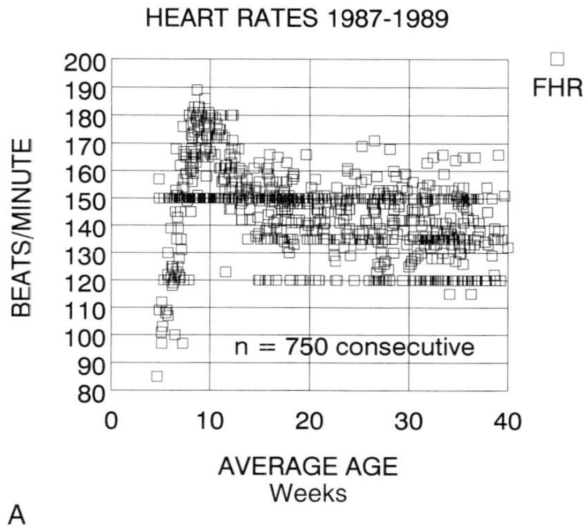

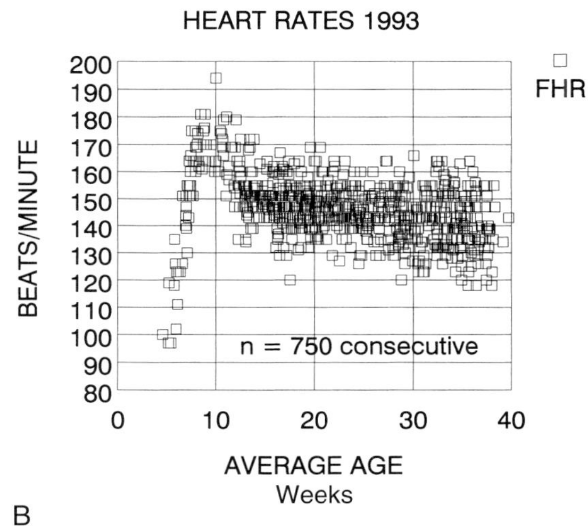

FIGURE 12–2.
A, HEART RATES TO AGE, 1987–1989. This plot of 750 consecutive examinations (from years 1987–1989) against fetal age throughout pregnancy demonstrates the need for accuracy. The accurate M-mode heart rates can be observed despite the horizontal lines of plots, all of which are from the same machine. This is similar to the errors achieved by counting the heart rate for 15 seconds and multiplying by 4 to arrive at beats per minute. This method always produces heart rates that are integers divisible by the multiplier. It is unclear what algorithm is used by the machine that produced the errors, but the manufacturer provided new software that corrected the problem in 1989. These data are similar to those in *B,* which contains data from another year and does not contain any erroneous M-mode heart rates. *B.* HEART RATES TO AGE, 1993. This plot is of 750 consecutive heart rates plotted against the average age of multiple fetal parameters. These are cross-sectional data (one measurement per patient) that were measured with M-mode by more than 12 sonographers using 10 different machines in 4 different diagnostic imaging laboratories. Note the very linear embryonic acceleration phase of the curve before 9 LMP weeks. Variation of the rates increases with time after the embryonic period.

Embryofetal Heart Rate

Figure 12–2 shows XY scattergrams from two different groups of 750 consecutive sonographic fetal examinations. Figure 12–2*A* is from examinations between 1987 and 1989, and Figure 12–2*B* is from 750 examinations in 1993. The two are shown together to make two points.

The first point is about accuracy of measurements. Figure 12–2*A* shows some distinct horizontal lines of plots at 150, 135, and 120 B/M. All of the heart rates in these lines were measured by M-mode on the same sonographic machine. In the fall of 1989, the manufacturer provided a software upgrade that corrected the problem. In these cases, the machine had an estimating algorithm that was similar to counting heart rates for 15 seconds and then multiplying by 4 to arrive at the beats per minute. This method always produces heart rates that are integers divisible by the multiplier. The need for accuracy whether using M-mode or trying to count the rates visually should be obvious.

The most accurate M-mode heart rate measurements are obtained by placing the M-mode vector across a rapidly moving echo such as one arising from a valve. Using the fastest M-mode tracing stretches out the heartbeats or in effect magnifies their length and reduces the percent error, which may result in variation in placement of the cursors. More accuracy can be achieved by measuring the M-mode tracing for larger numbers of heartbeats. Most sonographic machines do not give the user a choice in the number of beats measured, defaulting to only one or two beats; however, some machines allow the user to measure up to seven beats, which is much more accurate.

The second point is to show the similarity of the accurate heart rates in the two groups. Notice the narrow distribution of the EHRs before 9 weeks. For cross-sectional data that were gathered by more than 12 different sonographers in four different laboratories using 10 different machines, this appears to be a very linear increase.

Embryonic Heart Rate

EARLY

Embryologists identify the start of the embryonic heartbeat at 21 to 22 days after conception.[15] The heart rate is often the first firm sonographic evidence of an embryonic pole. Schats stated that "The most striking evidence of the presence of a [sic] embryonic pole is the appearance of cardiac activity."[16] Using the normal date for a 14-day ovulation for conception would establish the EHR as starting on the 35th day, or approximately the fifth week after the LMP. Schats, in a study of in vitro fertilization pregnancies, noted a 5-day window in which the EHR might be detected in pregnancies that appeared normal after the 11th week. This 5-day window was from the 25th to the 30th day after follicle aspiration. In addition, he found that the later in this window of time that the EHR was detected, the higher the chances of miscarriage in the first trimester. Schats reported that the time difference in the appearance of the EHR in continuing pregnancies and those that miscarried in the first trimester was significantly different within this 5-day variation ($P = 0.0028$).[5,17] Because the "difference in appearance of embryonic cardiac activity was associated with a difference in crown-rump length whilst the subsequent growth curve was normal, we ascribe these findings to different duration of the implantation stage."[5] A similar variation in implantation times was also noted by van Heeswijk.[6]

Another study by Goldstein found that the EHR was always detected by the time the embryonic pole, or CRL, measured 4 mm or greater.[18] The earliest cardiac activity this study found was in an embryonic pole of 2 mm. This would indicate that the EHR was found as early as 5.7 menstrual weeks and always by 6.1 menstrual weeks. These ages were estimated by correlating the CRL with age using Hadlock's 1992 table [19] (also see Table 7–1). Goldstein found one case in the literature (Brown and colleagues[20]) in which "a 4-mm embryo lacking cardiac activity then ultimately proved normal." For this reason, Goldstein suggested a threshold of 5 mm for absence of cardiac activity as a diagnosis of nonviable pregnancy.[15] Using Hadlock's CRL table (also see Table 7–1) would place this threshold at approximately 6.2 menstrual weeks (±2 SD = ± 0.8% = ± 3.5 days).[19] (For a more detailed discussion of the variation of fetal age as a percentage of that age, see Chapter 7, Age Range Analysis.)

This sonographically determined age for the start of cardiac activity in a developing human is approximately 1 week later than what embryologists judge to occur 21 days after conception, which is the equivalent of 35 days after menses. It is uncertain whether this difference occurred because most embryogenesis research used rhesus monkeys, before the advent of sonography. The findings are thought to be similar to those in humans but may vary slightly.[17,21] It may also be possible that sonography simply cannot detect the heartbeat until some time after the heart begins beating. What is clear is that the EHR may be as closely related to the stage of development of the embryo as is the CRL.

The EHR, when first detected sonographically, is close to the mother's heart rate, around 80 to 85 B/M between the early fifth and early sixth menstrual weeks. Because these very early EHRs are mere flickers of varying brightness at the edge of the yolk sac, it may be difficult to determine if one is observing an EHR or fluctuations in the maternal vessels. If this dilemma exists, it can often be resolved by taking M-mode tracings of both the EHR and maternal heart rates. Figure 12–3 is an example of this process during the fifth LMP week (CRL = 3.8 mm). In Figure 12–3*A*, the EHR is faintly observed and measured at 92 B/M between the + cursors on the M-mode tracing. In Figure 12–3*B*, the maternal heart rate is observed at 67 B/M as a "tissue thump" from the adnexal vessels. Both the maternal and embryonic heart rates may not be observable in the same image, but the maternal rate is readily ascertainable in the pelvic adnexa, which is an abundantly vascular region. Sonographic M-mode should always be used to measure both the embryonic and maternal heart rates because it is more accurate than counting while watching a clock, as explained earlier.

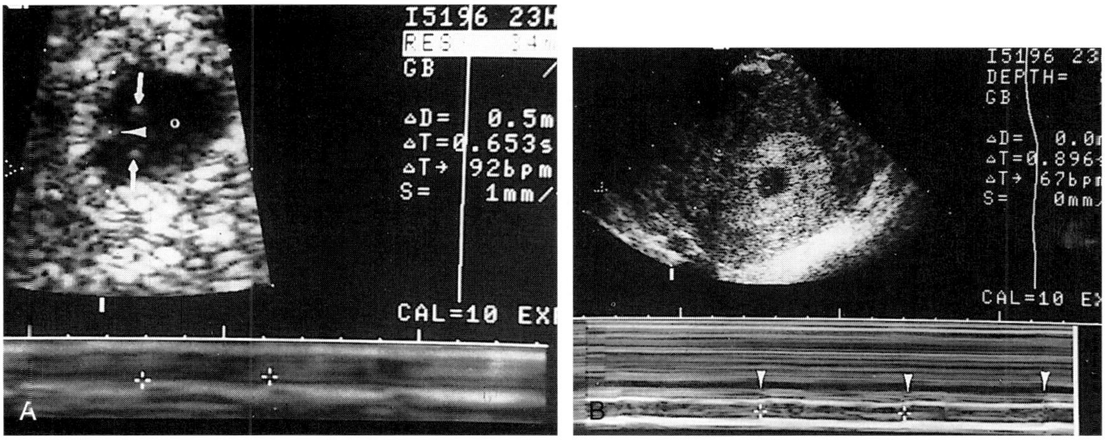

FIGURE 12–3.
A, This M-mode embryonic heart rate (EHR) was easily measured at 92 B/M. One beat is measured between the + cursors. This EHR was obtained for the embryonic disk at the edge of the faint yolk sac (arrowhead in the center of the yolk sac). Two specular echos (arrows) are observed at the yolk sac's anterior and posterior surfaces. The LNMP was reported to be 6.0 weeks prior, and the crown-rump length (CRL = 2.6 mm) age was 5.5 weeks. The 92 B/M EHR calculated to an equivalent 4.9 LMP weeks, or just 4.2 days (0.6 week) different from the CRL age, well within the 66 day (0.86 week) 95th percentile. This EHR age was calculated by the EHR linear regression: Age in LMP weeks = ((EHR × 0.3)+6)/7 (see Table 12–2). *B*, Here the maternal heart rate is measured by transvaginal M-mode at 67 B/M. The arrowheads mark the same points on three consecutive maternal heartbeats, which are registered from vessel/tissue thump in the right adnexa. This measurement was taken to confirm that the EHR (*A*) was different from the woman's heart rate.

After the EHR is first sonographically detected to be around 85 B/M early in the fifth LMP week, it usually accelerates rapidly and therefore normally is more rapid than the maternal heart rate. The only examinations in which I have observed maternal heart rates that exceeded that of their embryos' were in the fifth week in women who smoked cigarettes and smelled as if they had crushed out a cigarette just before entering the examination room.

The embryofetal heart rate in the first trimester is quite remarkable. Starting out at less than 90 B/M during the fifth menstrual week (LMP), it accelerates rapidly in a linear fashion until the early ninth LMP week. This acceleration appears to be constant in a large cross-sectional population (see Figs. 12–2 and 12–4A). In this population, the mean acceleration is 3.3 B/M per day, or approximately a 10 B/M increase every 3 days until the start of the ninth LMP week. A close correlation is noted between the EHR, CRL, and time in this acceleration phase of the cardiac development. Figure 12–4*A* shows the raw data for the embryofetal heart rate plotted against the CRL, with no data manipulation, to confirm the shape of this early acceleration phase. This graph has a slight curve in the acceleration phase due to the change in the CRL growth rate in time. The EHR appears to be more linear in acceleration when plotted against time (see Figs. 12–1 and 12–2). Figure 12–4*B* is a residual plot of these data. All EHRs that dropped 24 B/M or more below the regression line (mean) before the CRL reached 25 mm ended in embryonic demise (one case was unavailable for follow-up). The heart rates above the upper 95% confidence limits all were later found to be continuing as normal pregnancies or at delivery.

The EHR also appears to correlate with the maternal serum level of human chorionic gonadotropin. Figure 12–5 shows a similar acceleration and peak during the same time frame.[22, 23] No research has yet addressed the relationship of these two curves (EHR and human chorionic gonadotropin), but the similarity of the timing and shape is remarkable.

END OF EMBRYONIC PHASE

The peak EHR appears to occur when an embryo is between 22 and 25 mm, or

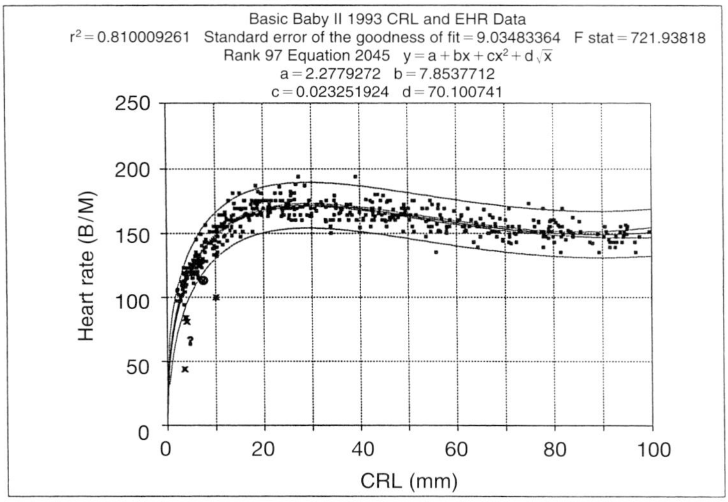

A

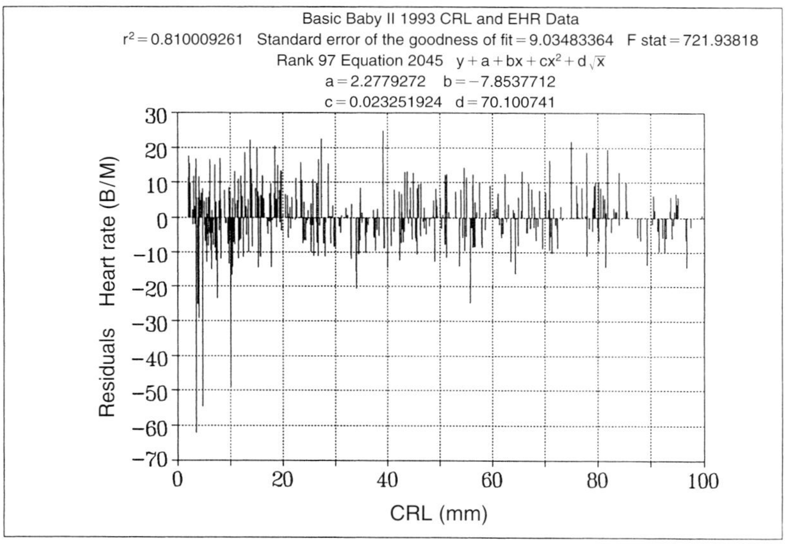

B

FIGURE 12–4.
A, Crown-rump length (CRL) and embryofetal heart rates (EHR). This XY plot and polynomial regression with 95th percentile confidence limits is shown to confirm the shape of the EHR curve. This figure is based on raw CRL and EHR data for all examinations during 1993 in embryos and fetuses with a beating heart and CRL <100 mm. Note the rapid acceleration phase before the CRL reaches 25 mm. This regression, as well as other estimates of the heart rate from embryofetal ages, is shown in Table 12–1. Follow-up on the six outliers below the lower 95% confidence limit found four embryonic demises (x). One was sonographically normal at 36 LMP weeks (O), and one was unavailable for follow-up (?). This graph and statistical analysis was produced using TableCurve, Jandel Scientific, San Rafael, CA 94901; (415) 453–6700. *B*, CRL and EHR RESIDUALS. These are residuals of the heart rates minus the regression line shown in *A*. These reveal a relatively constant variability throughout at approximately ±20 B/M. This regression appears to underestimate the EHR when the CRL is between about 18 and 23 mm, the period when the EHR peaks. This underestimation results in positive residuals at that time. In this population, five EHRs were more than 24 B/M below the mean before the CRL reached 20 mm; four ended in embryonic demise (one unavailable for follow-up).

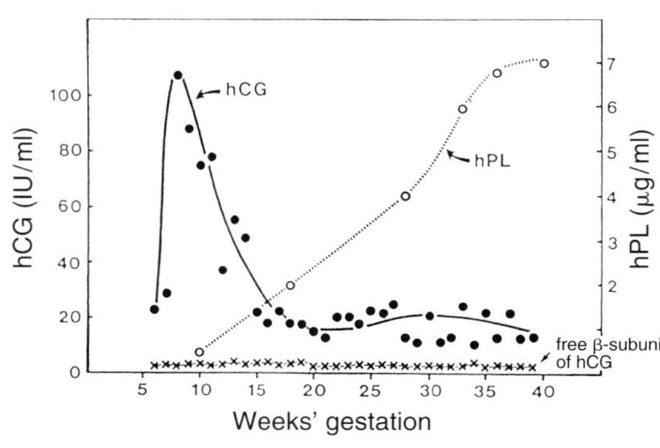

FIGURE 12–5.
This graph shows the mean concentration of human chorionic gonadotropin (hCG) and placental lactogen (hPL) throughout normal pregnancy. Note the peak in hCG at approximately 9 weeks. This is exactly the time of the peak in the embryonic heart rate (EHR). Although no study has attempted to correlate the EHR and hCG, the similarity in the early acceleration, peak, and slower decline in both is intriguing. Compare this curve with Figures 12–2*B* and 12–6. (From Selenkow HA, et al: Patterns of serum immunoreactive human placental lactogen [IR=HPL] and chorionic gonadotropin [IR-HCG] in diabetic pregnancy. Diabetes 1971;20(10):696. Reprinted with permission from *Diabetes*. Copyright © 1971 by American Diabetes Association, Inc.

between 8.9 and 9.2 LMP weeks (using Hadlock's 1992 CRL table), reaching a mean peak of 175 B/M (±2 SD = 20 B/M, $P < 0.001$). From this we can state that the EHR should never be less than 155 B/M when an embryo is between 22 and 25 mm in CRL (equivalent to 62 and 65 LMP days by Hadlock and colleagues). This rule of thumb does not apply to a woman's reported LNMP dates because the start of the LNMP is not as reliable a date, and this is a very narrow 3-day window of observation.

After the peak heart rate is reached at the start of the ninth LMP week, it starts a slow deceleration until term, at which time it normally is about 144 B/M, ±25 B/M (±2 SD, $P < 0.05$).[3] The shape of the embryofetal heart rate curve in time has the shape of a classical damping-feedback curve. This curve shape occurs in many control systems, from nuclear reactor temperature control to frog muscle response to electrical stimulation. These feedback or response curves are known in the engineering field as control systems.[24] To my knowledge, the recognition of the EHR as having the shape of a damping-feedback curve was first made independently by Dr. George Ellis, Professor of Cosmic Physics, SISSA, Trieste, Italy, and by Mark Maldenka, Petroleum Engineer of Midland, Texas.[4] The shape of this curve suggests the existence of variables that control the rates of acceleration and deceleration and the point at which the peak EHR occurs. This very interesting phenomenon deserves more study. It is possible that individual heart rate curve variations may be predictive of certain types of cardiac developmental problems.

A survey of embryology textbooks reveals that the period when the heart is highly susceptible to major malformations ends precisely at the time the EHR peaks and begins its deceleration phase (see Fig. 18–1),[25, 26] at the end of the eighth LMP week. This is also shortly after the closure of the interventricular foramen, completing the ventricular septum. Discussion of the mechanisms that might control the shape of the EHR curve has led to some speculation. Hill hypothesized a neural connection, which would mean that the peak in the EHR would correspond with some completion of a part of the cardiac neural pathways such as the bundle of His.[27] Nichols favored a hydraulic explanation in which the peak would come at the time the ventricular septum closes. In reality, it may be that feedback between neural, hydraulic, and perhaps hormonal influences controls the shape of the EHR curve. Only one case in our study population had a confirmed ventricular septal defect; in this case, the heart rate was found to remain high after the peak period (170 B/M at 14 weeks). This fetus also had other anomalies, including fetal ascites and cleft lip with a tag of tissue.

In the late embryonic period, after the start of the ninth LMP week, the heart rate begins its descent to term. The descent is relatively rapid until about 15 to 18 weeks, when deceleration slows or the curve flattens until term.

The variability of the EHR is low and may be due to errors in estimating the length of the heartbeats on the M-mode tracing as much as actual beat-to-beat variability. A small unpublished study of EHR variability using at least two M-mode measurements per examination found that the mean difference of the heart rate was 1.3 B/M (SD = 3.3, range 0 to 9, median = 0 B/M, n = 39), with observation intervals ranging from 10 seconds to 30 minutes (mean = 10 minutes). These results are of a similar magnitude to those of Schats and colleagues' study of in vitro fertilizations, in which the mean difference was 2.9 B/M in observation times of 15 to 60 minutes (SD = 1.7, range 0 to 4, median = 2, n = 47).[5, 16]

The statistics from this small study excluded one interesting embryo that exhibited high beat-to-beat variability. The reported LNMP was 10.1 weeks earlier, whereas the sonographic age was 5.4 LMP weeks by gestational sac diameter (14-mm chorionic cavity) and 5.6 LMP weeks by CRL (3 mm). The EHR by M-mode was first recorded at 88 B/M; 5 minutes later it had increased to 113 B/M, and after 2 more minutes it had dropped to 87 B/M. The pregnancy ended in embryonic demise before the eighth LMP week. The total range of heart rates for this case was 26 B/M in 7 minutes. Although one case does not constitute a study, the low variability in the two studies and the wild variation of this case does indicate that this is a fertile field for research on the embryonic heart.

REGRESSIONS

As stated earlier, several researchers have described the early acceleration of the EHR; however, few have performed regression analysis on the heart rate. Table 12–1 contains the regressions found by various investigators for predicting the EHRs (Fig. 12–6).

The first regression formula based on the EHR was presented by Fine and colleagues at the 1988 World Federation of Ultrasound in Medicine meeting in Washington, D.C. This formula was published in the proceedings' abstracts[28]; the research was never published in its entirety. This third-degree polynomial curve can be used to confirm appropriate heart rates from as early as the EHR can be observed until the 15th menstrual week. This estimation of the appropriate heart rate is accurate in 95% of the population to within ±22 B/M. Other higher-order regressions can be used to estimate the heart rate throughout pregnancy. After about 15 to 18 weeks and until term, the significance of the heart rate regressions is very low because the curve is almost flat, and short-term variability is normal.

The second publication of regressions on the heart rate was in 1990.[4] This article contained two linear regressions on the embryonic acceleration phase of the heart rate. One linear regression was for estimating the EHR from embryonic age (see Fig. 12–6), and the other was for estimating the appropriate age from the EHR (Fig. 12–7). Since that publication, other higher-order regressions that have been developed may be more accurate before the middle of the seventh LMP week. More research is needed in the very early embryonic period. Table 12–2 shows the regressions for estimating age from the EHR.

Second and Third Trimesters

DECELERATION

The heart rate in the early fetal period seems to have had the least study, certainly less than during the embryonic phase, at term, or in labor. The heart rate declines from a high of 160 to 190 B/M at the end of the embryonic period (ninth LMP week) until

TABLE 12–1. **REGRESSIONS: HEART RATE FROM AGE OR CROWN-RUMP LENGTH**

FIG. 12–6	REGRESSION FORMULA	± 2 SD	WHEN USED (VALID)	r^2
Fine et al[28]	$HR = -285.0316 + 117.4581 \times MA - 9.8594 \times MA^2 + 0.2642 \times MA^3$	±22 B/M	Before 15th LMP week	0.69
DuBose et al[4]	$EHR = ((MA \times 7) - 8.18)/0.285$	±26 B/M	Before 9th LMP week	0.78
DuBose *	$HR = 170 - 0.07 \times MA - 1700/MA^2 + 3.5 \times EXP(-LN(MA/8)^2/0.2) \times MA$	±22 B/M	Throughout pregnancy	0.36
DuBose and Meiss†	$HR = 140 + (20 \times (MA - 7)) \times MA^{(-.011 \times (MA - 7))}$	±21 B/M	Throughout pregnancy	0.44
CRL = HR	$HR = 6 - 7.6 \times CRL + 0.0225 \times CRL^2 + 68 \times \sqrt{CRL}$	±16 B/M	While CRL < 100 mm	0.82

These regressions are used to estimate the appropriate heart rate (see Fig. 12–6).

The regression formulas use the following variables: HR, embryofetal heart rate, EHR, embryonic heart rate; MA, LMP weeks; EXP, exponent; LN, natural logarithm; CRL, crown-rump length. Note that the CRL estimate of the heart rate (CRL-HR) is a rounded version of the equation plotted in Figure 12–4 and has an accuracy of ± 16 B/M for 2 SD.

*Unpublished regression. World Congress on Vaginosonography in Gynecology, June 14–17, 1990, San Antonio, TX; sponsored by the American Association of Gynecologic Laparoscopists.

†Unpublished regression in collaboration with James Meiss, Ph.D., Applied Mathematics, University of Colorado,

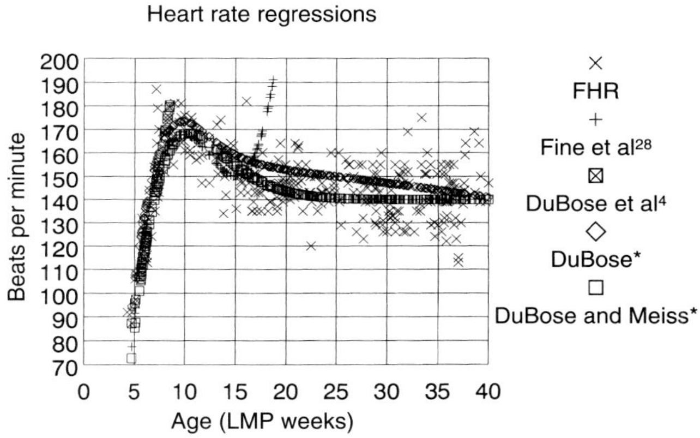

FIGURE 12–6.
Regressions for estimating the embryofetal heart rate from the age. The x-axis (independent variable) is the average age of multiple fetal parameters in equivalent LMP weeks. The estimated heart rates (dependent variables) are plotted on the y-axis. The + plots are the measured heart rates (FHR). The + plots are the Fine, Cartier, and Doubilet[28] (FCD) third-degree polynomial, which is valid to 15 LMP weeks. The boxed X plots are the linear regression, which is valid before 9 LMP weeks. The diamond and open-square plots are two polynomials that estimate the appropriate heart rate throughout pregnancy with various degrees of accuracy. All of these regressions are given in Table 12–1. Note the close agreement of all regressions before 9 LMP weeks, even though the FCD regression is from research in Boston and the others are from Austin (Unpublished regression. World Congress on Vaginosonography in Gynecology, June 14–17 1990, San Antonio, TX; Sponsored by the American Association of Gynecologic Laparoscopists.)

midpregnancy, when at 20 weeks it most often is between 120 and 170 B/M. The variability increases throughout the fetal period (see Figs. 12–2*A* and *B*, 12–4, and 12–6).

LATE PREGNANCY AND LABOR

Late Pregnancy

During the last half of pregnancy, the mean long-term heart rate does not vary much. In the late third trimester, it has a mean of approximately 144 B/M. However, the beat-to-beat variability during shorter periods varies more than it does during the early part of pregnancy.

This late pregnancy beat-to-beat variability is in response to external stimuli, maternal diet and hormones, and fetal motion. Variation at this time in pregnancy is expected, and its absence is considered abnormal. The causes and interpretations of these variations or the lack thereof are complex. Absence of variability in late pregnancy can signal fetal stress.

Changes of the fetal heart rate (FHR) of at least 15 B/M every 30 minutes are expected with an active fetus. The biophysical profile nonstress test requires two such changes for reactivity (see Chapter 17).

The antepartum fetal nonstress test includes three criteria for interpretation of the

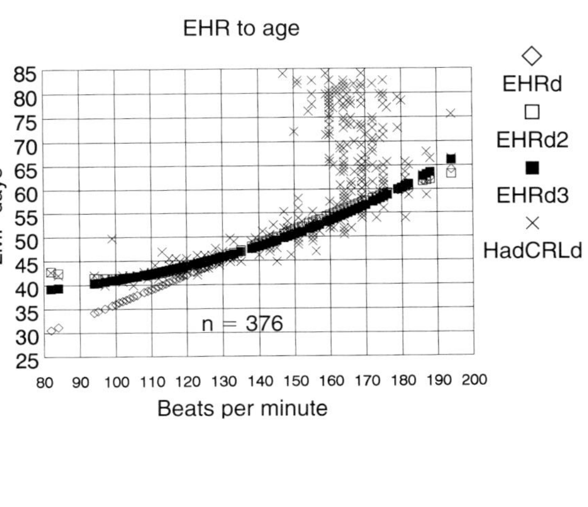

FIGURE 12–7.
Regressions: age from heart rate. Here the dependent and independent variables are reversed from those in Figure 12–6 in order to estimate the equivalent LMP age in days. The x-axis represents beats per minute. The first variable, EHRd (diamonds), is a linear regression. The second and third, EHRd2 and EHRd3, are polynomials and have an accuracy of ±4.7 and ±4.9 days (2 SD), respectively. For comparison, the X plots are the LMP ages in equivalent days as calculated using Hadlock and colleagues' 1992 CRL function (HadCRLd). All of these regression formulas are given in Table 12–2.

TABLE 12–2. REGRESSIONS: AGE FROM HEART RATE

FIG. 12–7	RESULTS	REGRESSION FORMULA	±2 SD	WHEN USED	r^2
EHRd	LMP days (MA)	$MA = EHR \times 0.3 + 6$	±6 days	Before 63 LMP days	0.84
EHRd	LMP days (MA)	$MA = EHR \times 0.285 + 8.18$	±6 days	Before 63 LMP days	0.84
EHRd	Conception days (CA)	$CA = EHR \times 0.3 - 8$	±6 days	Before 50 CA days	0.84
EHRd	Conception days (CA)	$CA = EHR \times 0.285 - 5.82$	±6 days	Before 50 CA days	0.84
EHRd2	LMP days (MA)	$MA = 7 \times (1.726 - 0.2745 \times EHR + 0.00205 \times EHR^2 - 0.0000044 \times EHR^3)$	±4.7 days	Before 63 LMP days	0.87
EHRd3	LMP days (MA)	$MA = 37 + 0.000004 \times MA^3$	±4.9 days	Before 63 LMP days	0.86

These regression formulas are used to estimate the embryonic age before the ninth LMP week. The first column lists are acronyms used in the graph in Figure 12–7. All formulas evaluate to the equivalent ages in days; weeks can be calculated by dividing the results by 7. The first four formulas are virtually the same linear regression and produce almost identical results for either LMP days (MA) or days from conception (CA) ($R = 0.99999$, at 0.01 significance level). Note that the embryonic heart rate (EHR) has a close relationship to age in the embryonic period. All regressions have ±2 SD of between 4.7 and 6 days. This means the normal EHR can estimate the dates of the pregnancy almost as closely as the normal crown-rump length.

results. In a reactive result, two fetal movements are followed by accelerations of the FHR by at least 15 B/M and a normal base line rate. Uncertain reactivity is a FHR with fewer than two movements and associated accelerations in rate; the base line rate may be normal or abnormal. A nonreactive result is lack of fetal motion or of variation in heart rate and an abnormal base line rate. A nonreactive test result is associated with poor fetal outcome.[29]

Labor

During labor, the heart rate should change with uterine contractions. Four basic FHR patterns are associated with uterine contractions[30]:

- Early decelerations start and end at the same time as a uterine contraction. As the uterus increases the pressure, the FHR decreases and vice versa. Early decelerations are not associated with fetal compromise.
- Late decelerations are similar to early decelerations but follow the uterine contractions by 10 to 30 seconds. This pattern is associated with decreased uterine blood flow. A more extreme late deceleration is nonreflex late deceleration, in which the variability of the FHR is absent. This indicates inadequate cerebral and myocardial oxygenation.
- Variable decelerations follow the rule of 60s, in which the FHR is 60 B/M below the normal base line and decelerations are below 60 B/M or longer than 60 seconds. These variable decelerations represent insufficient umbilical blood flow.
- Accelerations with contractions generally indicate a healthy, reactive fetus. These are thought to be similar to normal accelerations associated with fetal motions of the nonstress test.

This is a brief and simplistic presentation of a complex subject. A more complete discussion of the FHR during labor can be found in *Maternal-Fetal Medicine*.[30]

REFERENCES

1. Robinson HP, Shaw-Dunn J: Fetal heart rates as determined by sonar in early pregnancy. J Obstet Gynaecol Br Commonw 1973;80:805–809.
2. Shenker L, Astle C, Reed K, et al: Embryonic heart rates before the seventh week of pregnancy. J Reprod Med 1986;31:333–335.
3. DuBose TJ, Porter L, Dickey D, et al: Sonographic correlation of fetal heart rate and gender. J Diagn Med Sonogr 1989;2:49–53.
4. DuBose TJ, Cunyus JA, Johnson L: Embryonic heart rate and age. J Diagn Med Sonogr 1990;6:151–157.
5. Schats R, Jansen CAM, Waldimiroff JW: Embryonic heart activity: Appearance and development in early human pregnancy. Br J Obstet Gynaecol 1990;97: 989–994.
6. van Heeswijk M: Fetal heart rate in early pregnancy: Early pregnancy. Hum Dev 1990;22:151–156.
7. Rempen A: Diagnosis of viability in early pregnancy with vaginal sonography. J Ultrasound Med 1990; 9: 711–716.
8. Howe RS, Isaacson KJ, Albert JL, et al: Embryonic and human pregnancy. J Ultrasound Med 1991;10: 367–371.
9. Hertzberg BS, Mahony B, Bowie J: First trimester fetal cardiac activity. J Ultrasound Med 1988;7:573–575.
10. Laboda LA, Estroff JA, Benacerraf BR: First trimester bradycardia: A sign of impending fetal loss. J Ultrasound Med 1989;8:561–563.
11. May DA, Sturtevant NV: Embryonal heart rate as a predictor of pregnancy outcome: A prospective analysis. J Ultrasound Med 1991;10:591–593.
12. Hertzberg BS, Mahony BS, Bowie JD: Fetal heart rates. J Ultrasound Med 1989;8:407–408.
13. DuBose TJ, Butschek CM, Hill LW, et al: Fetal heart rates. J Ultrasound Med 1989;8:407.
14. DuBose TJ, Dickey D, Butschek CM, et al: Embryonic heart rate and gender (letter to the editor). J Ultrasound Med 1988;7:237–238.
15. Moore KL, Persaud TVN: The Developing Human: Clinically Oriented Embryology. WB Saunders, Philadelphia, 1993, p 310.
16. Schats R: Transvaginal Sonography in Early Human Pregnancy (Doctoral Dissertation). Universiteit Rotterdam, Jan 30, 1991, p 46.
17. Schats R: Transvaginal Sonography in Early Human Pregnancy (Doctoral Dissertation). Universiteit Rotterdam, Jan 30, 1991, pp 106–107.
18. Goldstein SR: Significance of cardiac activity on endovaginal ultrasound in very early embryos. Obstet Gynecol 1992;80:670–672.
19. Hadlock FP, Shah YP, Kannon DJ, et al: Fetal crown-rump length: Reevaluation of relation to menstrual age (5–18 weeks) with high-resolution real-time US. Radiology 1992;182:501–505.
20. Brown DL, Emerson DS, Felker RE, et al: Diagnosis of early embryonic demise by endovaginal sonography. J Ultrasound Med 1990;9:631–636.
21. Benirschke K: Principles and Management of Human Reproduction. WB Saunders, Philadelphia, 1972, pp 179–196.
22. Selenkow HA, et al: Patterns of serum immunoreactive human placental lactogen (IR-HPL) and chorionic gonadotropin (IR-HCG) in diabetic pregnancy. Diabetes 1971;10:696.
23. Yen SSC: Endocrinology of pregnancy. In: Creasy RK, Resnik R, eds: Maternal-Fetal Medicine: Principles and Practice, 2nd ed. WB Saunders, Philadelphia, 1989, p 386.
24. Voland G: Control Systems Modeling and Analysis. Prentice-Hall, Englewood Cliffs, NJ, 1986, pp XI, 135–160.
25. Sadler TW: Langman's Medical Embryology, 5th ed. Williams & Wilkins, Baltimore, 1985.
26. Moore KL, Persaud TVN: The Developing Human:

Clinically Oriented Embryology. WB Saunders, Philadelphia, 1993, p 156.
27. Hopper AF, Hart NH: Foundations of Animal Development. Oxford University Press, New York, 1980, p 425.
28. Fine C, Cartier M, Doubilet P: Fetal heart rates: Value throughout gestation. J Ultrasound Med (Abstract 1569) 1988;7:S105.
29. Parer JT: Fetal heart rate. In: Creasy RK, Resnik R, eds: Maternal-Fetal Medicine: Principles and Practice, 2nd ed. WB Saunders, Philadelphia, 1989, p 339.
30. Parer JT: Fetal heart rate. In: Creasy RK, Resnik R, eds: Maternal-Fetal Medicine: Principles and Practice, 2nd ed. WB Saunders, Philadelphia, 1989, pp 324–327.

CHAPTER 13

FETAL DOPPLER

Mark S. Cartier, RDMS

The applications of Doppler sonography in obstetrics are increasing. The primary indication for obstetrical Doppler ultrasound is the detection or confirmation of intrauterine growth retardation (IUGR), which is recognizable because of associated characteristic blood flow abnormalities. A subject of debate in the medical literature is whether Doppler sonography should be used only in those pregnancies in which this condition is already suspected (by history, laboratory data, or ultrasound findings) or whether it should be incorporated as a component of routine fetal imaging.[1,2] Whether as a screening test or as a directed investigation, the use of Doppler sonography to predict fetal distress and IUGR has been shown to be most effective when both the fetal and the maternoplacental circulations are studied.[3-6] The fetal vessels most commonly studied for IUGR and its complications are the umbilical arteries (of the umbilical cord), the descending aorta, and the middle cerebral artery (MCA), and the maternal vessels most commonly studied are the uterine arteries. Umbilical venous flow has also been measured to study IUGR, although not usually for clinical purposes. Research is being directed toward identification and characterization of blood flow in other fetal vessels, such as the renal arteries, which may provide further diagnostic clues in the diagnosis of IUGR.[7]

Doppler sonography has also become an indispensable tool in the prenatal diagnosis of cardiac abnormalities.[8] In particular, color Doppler sonography directly reveals cardiac chamber inflow and outflow currents, and pulsed Doppler quantifies peak systolic velocity and other parameters of this flow. A growing literature very clearly documents the diagnostic utility of this technique for a wide range of fetal cardiac lesions.

Doppler sonography is increasingly used in problem solving for fetal structural abnormalities found during conventional ultrasonography. Color and pulsed Doppler may be used to identify and trace aberrant blood vessels, to characterize the vascular supply of masses, or to reveal vascular compromise in a particular organ.[9] Finally, color Doppler flow maps have demonstrated fetal vessels not previously identified by pulsed or continuous wave Doppler, such as pulmonary artery branches, pulmonary veins, and the superior mesenteric artery (SMA), although the benefit of identifying these vessels has not yet been determined and requires further investigation.

The use of color and pulsed Doppler in obstetrical ultrasonography requires a foundation of knowledge of fetal vascular anatomy and an understanding of pulsed Doppler spectral waveforms, as well as technical competence in the use of Doppler controls and power levels. This chapter first reviews the essential technical factors for Doppler sonography and then presents the normal fetal circulation as revealed by color and pulsed Doppler sonography.

Safety

Of all the numerous uses for diagnostic sonography, only fetal examination has generated significant interest and concern about the extent of energy exposure. This concern derives from laboratory studies that have documented abnormal changes in cells exposed to elevated doses of ultrasound. However, diagnostic ultrasonography produces significantly lower doses than used in these laboratory studies. In numerous clinical studies, researchers have identified no abnormal effects on the fetus from diagnostic obstetrical ultrasonography.[10] Nevertheless, there remains particular concern about the use of fetal *Doppler* sonography because of the higher doses used with this technology than with conventional real-time sonographic imaging.[10] In response to these safety concerns, the United States Food and Drug Administration (FDA) has established upper limits for the insonating power used in obstetrical ultrasonographic examinations. Acceptable ultrasound power is maintained at a spatial peak temporal average (SPTA) intensity of less than 100 mW/cm^2.[11–14] Manufacturers may market ultrasound equipment with power levels exceeding these guidelines, but they are required also to provide settings for lower power levels more appropriate to fetal examination. In the absence of any more rigorously derived recommendations, the FDA guidelines have been widely accepted by the ultrasound community.

It seems prudent to maintain fetal exposure to Doppler ultrasound at a minimum. In addition to setting power controls to the lowest levels that can yield acceptable diagnostic information, responsible sonographers can reduce fetal exposure even further by limiting exposure time. Exposure time can be limited through a number of strategies. First and foremost among these strategies is thorough familiarity with the ultrasound equipment. A sonographer who fumbles through a Doppler sonographic examination, groping for knobs to turn and guessing at which parameters to adjust, surely increases fetal exposure by prolonging the examination. Next, a sonographer should possess a plan of action; an idea of what the Doppler examination might reveal and how best to confirm or preclude diagnostic hypotheses both reduces examination time and increases diagnostic yield. This assumes that the sonographer maintains a reasonable working knowledge of fetal vascular anatomy and circulatory physiology. Furthermore, use of color Doppler flow maps to guide pulsed Doppler interrogation shortens examination time by quickly identifying vascular foci.[13, 15] A large field of view color flow map, however, should be avoided because it both increases fetal exposure and degrades the color Doppler data.[15] Use of a small color box indicates that the sonographer is looking for specific information and is not making a haphazard search. The color Doppler examination can be shortened even more if it is recorded on videotape, because this allows reanalysis of the data after completion of the examination. See also Chapter 3.

A final word about safety. Most tests and procedures performed in medicine represent tradeoffs between their potential to cause harm and to yield useful information. Similarly, when performing fetal Doppler sonography, one must always consider the balance between potential harm and a possibly clearer understanding of the fetal status. One important implication of this concept is that when fetal Doppler is performed, the results should be analyzed and then relayed to the responsible physician or health provider. Otherwise, the Doppler examination yields only risk (albeit small) and no benefit.

Technical Factors

Sonographers' discussions about the quality of Doppler ultrasound often center on which manufacturer provides more sensitive equipment. The choice of equipment, although important, is not as critical to diagnostic yield as is the choice of correct settings. The quality and content of an obstetrical Doppler sonographic study are dependent on understanding the following technical factors, which are briefly elaborated on in this section:

1. Doppler sonographic technique
   a. Doppler gain
   b. Doppler angle: conventional sonographic imaging versus Doppler sensitivity and accuracy
   c. Low-velocity sensitivity versus high-velocity aliasing
   d. Frame rate versus depth and sample size
   e. Filters, motion artifact, and low-flow sensitivity
2. Data analysis
   a. Spectral gray scale
   b. Indexes of resistance
   c. Volume flow calculations
   d. Color flow map

DOPPLER GAIN

The lowest gain (or amplification) setting that displays adequate signals should be used. Gain set too high results in excessive background noise, making it difficult to identify and analyze the Doppler data. With pulsed Doppler, the spectral time–velocity tracing fills up with artifactual flow information that both distorts and obscures the vascular waveforms (Fig. 13–1*A*). With color Doppler, gain set too high causes artifactual flow information to be mapped outside of vascular structures and the depiction of actual flow to be distorted (Fig. 13–1*B* and *C*). On the other hand, gain set too low may reveal no or inadequate Doppler signal. The blood flow waveforms on a pulsed Doppler spectral tracing may not be seen at all, or if seen, so much data may be missing that analysis of the waveform yields incorrect blood flow measurements. Furthermore, a low-gain setting in color Doppler results in a deficient color flow map in which vascular flow is not detected. Unfortunately, proper gain setting is somewhat of a subjective decision. However, at least with pulsed Doppler, the audio output of the ultrasound system can assist the operator in arriving at a proper gain. Increase or decrease in Doppler gain changes the character of the audio output. When gain is set too high, the resulting distortion of the flow data can be recognized by the ear. When gain is set too low, the audio signal cannot be clearly heard.

Finally, proper gain setting for conventional gray-scale sonography in conjunction with color Doppler imaging is also crucial. Excessive gain on the two-dimensional image may actually obscure flow information on the color map.[15–17]

DOPPLER ANGLE: CONVENTIONAL SONOGRAPHIC IMAGING VERSUS DOPPLER SENSITIVITY AND ACCURACY

There is an inherent conflict between scanning strategies used in conventional gray-scale sonography and Doppler sonography. The transducer is often placed perpendicular to structures to be imaged with sonography because axial resolution is superior to lateral resolution and because ultrasound reflection is more effective at 90 degrees than at other angles. In contrast, the Doppler signal is greatest when the transducer is oriented 0 degrees relative to the direction of blood flow (parallel or "down the barrel"). At a 90-degree orientation of transducer and blood flow, the Doppler signal falls to almost nothing. Thus, a conflict in scanning strategies occurs because Doppler studies are guided by conventional sonographic imaging: Both the pulsed Doppler range gate and the color Doppler flow map are superimposed on the gray-scale image. Ultimately, however, gray-scale imaging is subordinate to Doppler interrogation during the Doppler portion of the sonographic examination, and the transducer should be oriented as close to 0 degrees with the blood flow as possible.

In addition to simply determining the strength of the Doppler signal, the orientation between transducer and blood flow is *the major factor* in the accuracy of the Doppler data. Ultrasound equipment reading out the results of pulsed Doppler in velocity (rather than just

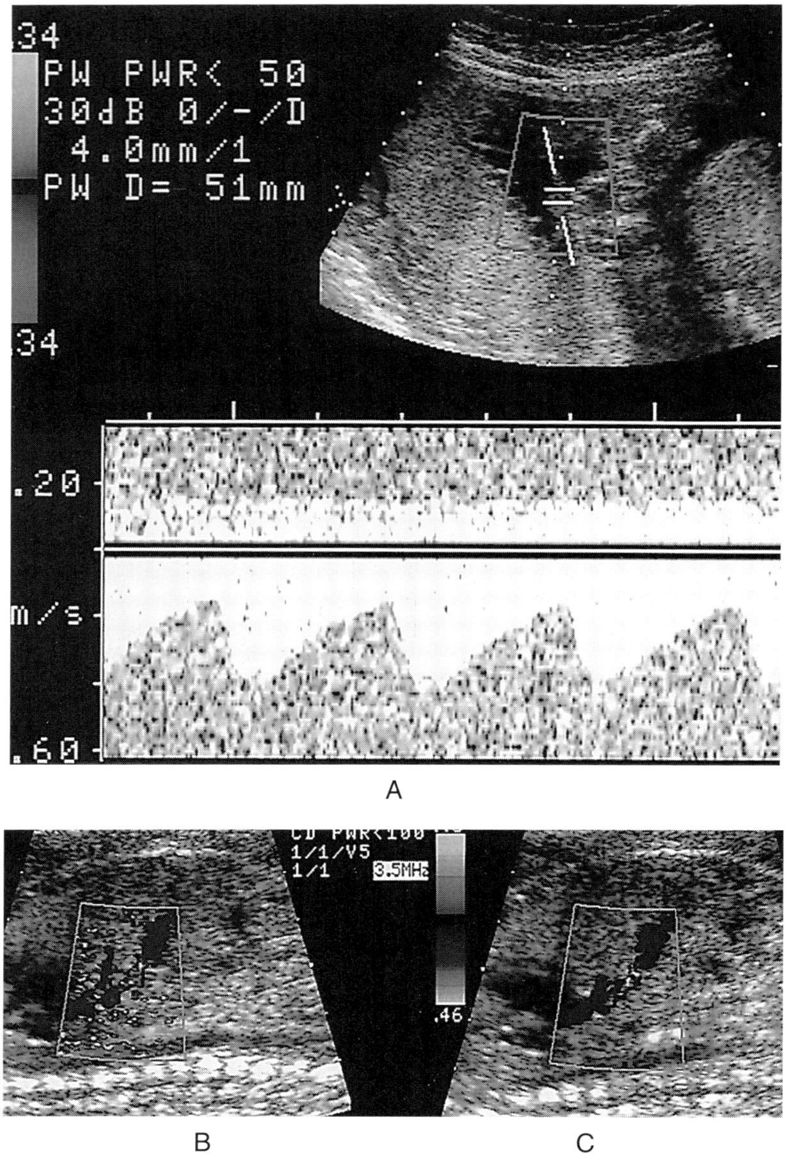

FIGURE 13–1.
A, Pulsed Doppler waveform of the umbilical artery with gain set excessively high. Notice the snowy appearance of the background as well as the filled-in arterial spectrum. *B* (see Color Figure 13–1*B*), Sagittal color Doppler image of umbilical vein and ductus venosus in a 20-week fetus. The inappropriately high gain setting exaggerates flow and vessel boundaries. *C* (see Color Figure 13–1*C*), Appropriate color gain setting in the same fetus provides more accurate flow data and depiction of vascular anatomy. With the proper gain setting, it is now possible to recognize the aliasing occurring in the ductus venosus as a result of normal high-velocity flow.

in Doppler shift frequency) requires the user to adjust an on-screen Doppler angle line in parallel with the blood flow (Fig. 13–2). It would seem, therefore, that any angle between the transducer and the direction of blood flow would be acceptable and equally accurate as long as one carefully sets the Doppler angle line. Unfortunately, that is not the case. As the angle between the transducer and axis of blood flow grows from 0 to 90 degrees, the error of the velocity measurement rapidly increases. For example, a 2% error is inherent in the velocity data at a Doppler angle between 5 and 10 degrees; the error rises to 45% at a Doppler angle of 65 to 75 degrees.[16] Thus, the Doppler angle must be minimized (and always less than 60 degrees) if velocity measurements are to be at all meaningful and clinically useful.

SENSITIVITY TO LOW VELOCITIES VERSUS ALIASING OF HIGH VELOCITIES

The pulse repetition frequency (PRF) is the *rate* at which an ultrasound transducer transmits the ultrasound pulses necessary for Doppler interrogation of blood flow. The PRF

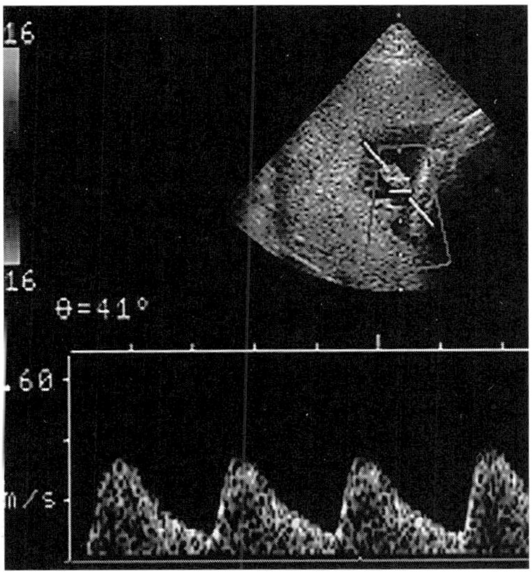

FIGURE 13–2.
(See Color Figure 13–2.) View of the umbilical artery with optimal gate and angle placement for proper pulsed Doppler interrogation. Demonstration of flow on the color Doppler flow map allows for more precise Doppler angle setting.

determines the highest-velocity flows that may be recorded without the occurrence of a particular type of signal distortion called *aliasing*. Using a higher PRF enables a higher velocity to be recorded without aliasing. As the distance between the transducer and the target blood vessel increases, however, the PRF must fall.[16,17] Thus, in obstetrical sonography, when a fetus is not close to the transducer, the peak velocity that can be accurately recorded may be limited. Use of a lower-frequency transducer may solve this problem because it has the effect of tolerating higher velocities without aliasing. The base line on the pulsed Doppler spectral waveform may be raised or lowered as yet another solution to the problem of aliasing[15] (Fig. 13–3). Why then would anyone need to use a low PRF setting? A low PRF is used because it increases the sensitivity for low-velocity blood flow and readjusts the optimal velocity scale for adequate graphic representation of such flow.[9,15,18]

PRF, transducer frequency, sample depth, and base line setting affect aliasing in high-velocity flow and sensitivity to low-velocity flow in both pulsed and color Doppler sonography. The manifestations of this aliasing are somewhat different, however, with one occurring on the spectral flow velocity tracing and the other on the color representation of the color flow map. Nevertheless, such aliasing in both pulsed and color Doppler has the potential for misinterpretation. Readjusting the ve-

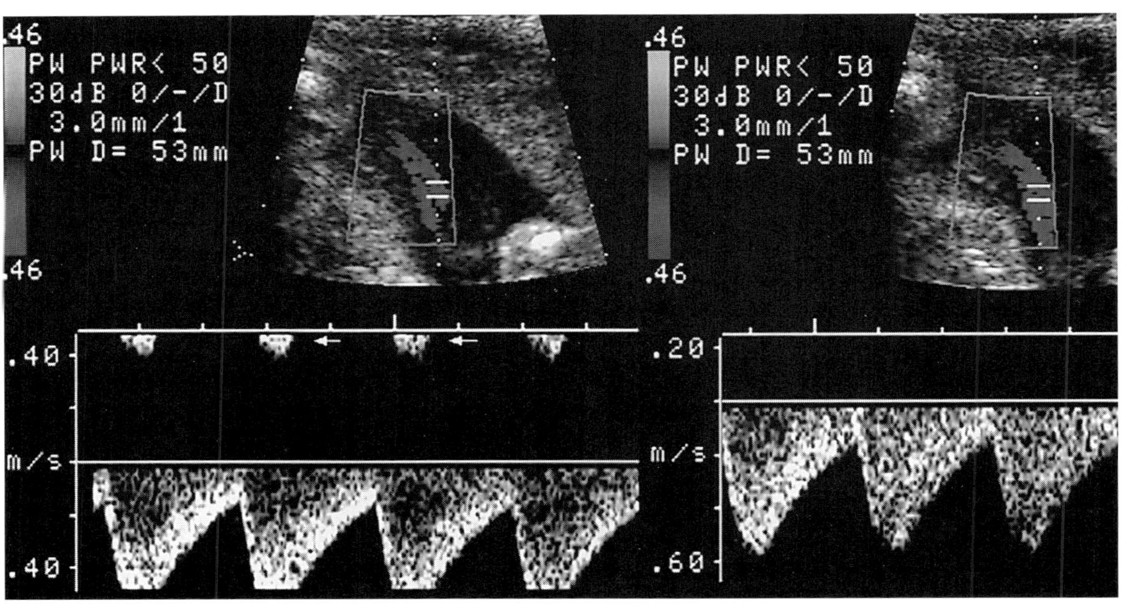

FIGURE 13–3.
Color and pulsed Doppler sonogram of the umbilical artery. The wraparound effect in the image on the left results when the scale of the spectrum is not adjusted properly, causing aliasing. The image on the right shows that adjustment of the base line can correct the aliasing without changing the overall scale.

locity scale of the pulsed Doppler spectral tracing and of the color Doppler flow map automatically readjusts the PRF.

FRAME RATE VERSUS DEPTH AND SAMPLE SIZE

Color Doppler frame rates affect how close to real-time the changes in flow are depicted on the ultrasound screen. It is worthwhile to try to use high frame rates in fetal color Doppler sonography because the fetal heart rate is approximately 2.5 times that of an adult. The greater the distance between the transducer and the target vessel, however, the lower is the resulting Doppler frame rate (because the PRF is diminished). On the other hand, the frame rate can be optimized by choosing a smaller color box (in axial dimensions).

FILTERS, MOTION ARTIFACT, AND LOW-FLOW SENSITIVITY

The high-pass filter establishes the threshold for the lowest frequencies or velocities (which tend to be artifactual) to be discarded from the display, on both the spectral tracing and the color flow map.[9,15,17] A high-pass filter set for a higher-frequency cutoff should be used near the fetal heart, where cardiac motion can cause artifactual distortion of the Doppler signal (Fig. 13–4). On the other hand, a lower-frequency cutoff setting should be used when there is little problem with motion artifact and the velocity of flow is low, such as in the fetal ductus venosus (Fig. 13–5). A problem occurs when one attempts to study low-flow blood vessels with Doppler close to a structure that causes motion artifact. Use of a higher cutoff frequency might not only reduce the motion artifact but could also eliminate the true low-flow signal. New, more sophisticated filtering techniques in color Doppler, based on real-time analysis of the returning signals, can eliminate motion artifact while preserving true low-flow information.

PULSED DOPPLER SPECTRAL GRAY SCALE

Pulsed Doppler provides usable vascular information in the form of the spectral time–velocity tracing. The velocity of red blood cells is sampled at regular intervals (determined by the PRF). This red blood cell velocity is plotted against time on the time–velocity tracing, yielding a waveform that is characteristic of flow within that vessel (Fig. 13–6). Because blood is a liquid, it does not move as one solid unit but rather as a

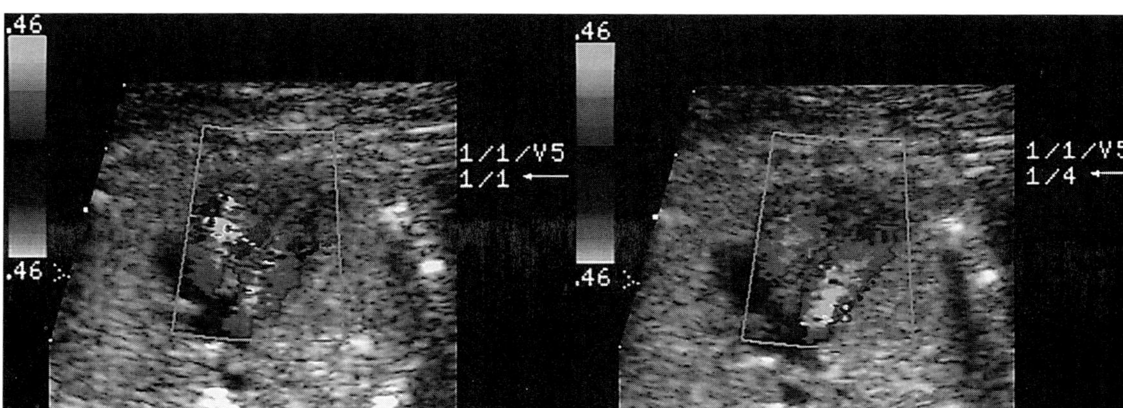

FIGURE 13–4.
(See Color Figure 13–4.) Color Doppler images of a fetal heart (apical four-chamber view) demonstrating use of the high-pass filter. The image on the left was obtained with the filter set for a low-frequency cutoff, resulting in distortion of flow information. The image on the right is the same view but with the filter set for a higher-frequency cutoff. The color flow information is well defined and interpretable.

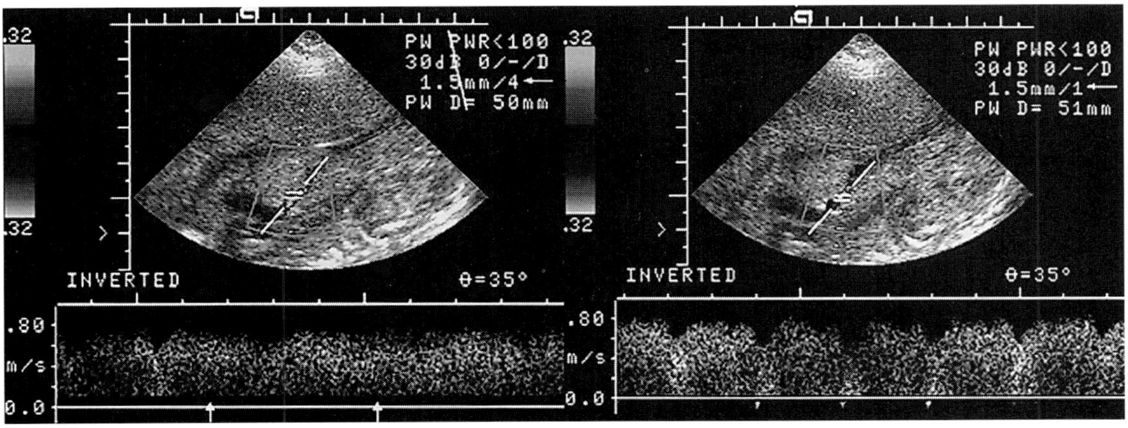

FIGURE 13–5.
Sagittal black and white, color, and pulsed Doppler ultrasonography of the ductus venosus. *Left*, An inappropriately high cutoff frequency (set at 4) is used for the pulsed Doppler high-pass filter, resulting in failure to depict the lowest red blood cell velocities at the bottom of the spectral tracing (small arrows). *Right*, Resetting the high-pass filter using a lower cutoff frequency results in display of the lower-velocity currents that were eliminated previously.

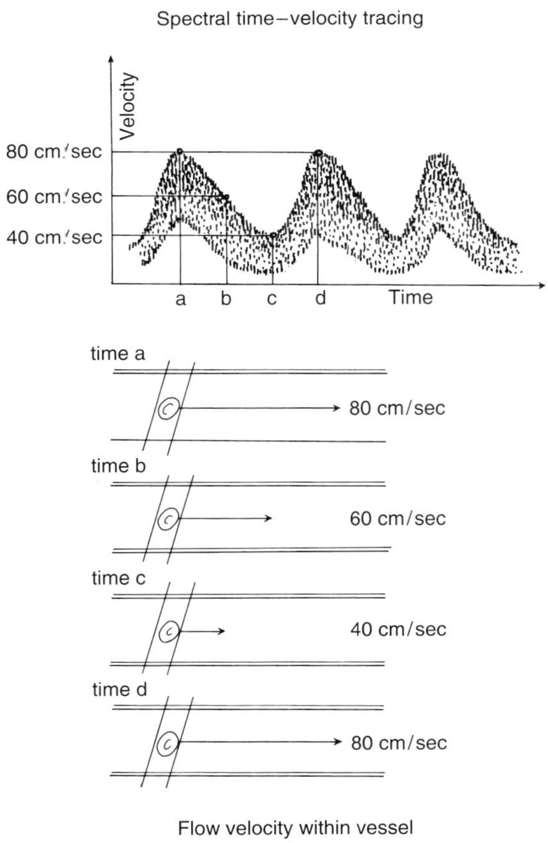

FIGURE 13–6.
Blood is moving at 80 cm/sec at time a, at 60 cm/sec at time b, at 40 cm/sec at time c, and at 80 cm/sec at time d. These points (plus many more in between) are plotted on the time–velocity Doppler tracing to yield a recognizable waveform.

composite of multiple individual components, with individual red blood cells representing the essential components for pulsed Doppler. Not all the blood cells travel at the same velocity; those in the center of the current move the fastest, and those near the vessel wall travel the slowest, with a spectrum of velocities between these two extremes. The pulsed Doppler tracing records this spectrum of velocities (hence the term *spectral tracing*) (Fig. 13–7).

The spectral time–velocity tracing records not only the different velocities of the blood cells at each moment in time but also the proportion of blood cells traveling at each particular velocity. This is accomplished through the use of a gray scale. Each dot on the spectral tracing represents a specific recorded velocity at a specific moment in time. If few blood cells are traveling at this particular velocity, the dot is lightly rendered. If many blood cells are traveling at this particular velocity, the dot is drawn in heavier.[16] Thus, on a white-on-black display, a dot representing very few cells is dark gray and a dot representing many cells is bright white (Fig. 13–8). The gray scale may be rendered in pseudocolor to improve visual recognition of waveform patterns (see Figs. 13–8, 13–29, and 13–30).

The particular time–velocity waveform

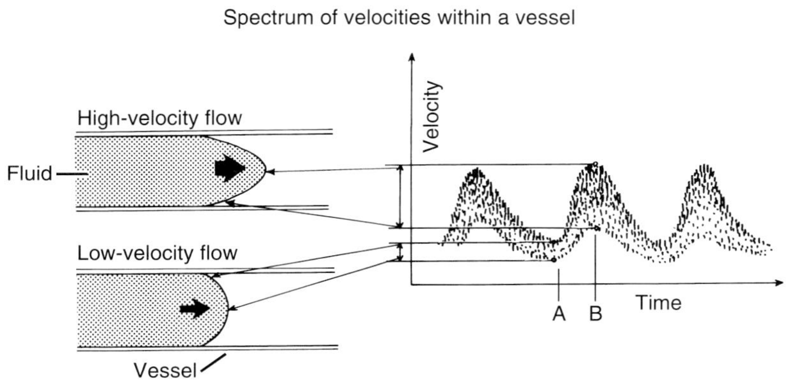

FIGURE 13–7.
At time A, during late diastole, blood flow is slower and there is less differential between the central faster current of blood and the peripheral slower current. That translates into a narrower plot on the time–velocity waveform. At time B, in early diastole, the overall blood velocity is higher and there is a greater differential between the central higher-velocity current and the peripheral slower current. This translates into a wider range of velocities on the plot of flow at time b.

rendered on the spectral tracing informs us of a number of factors influencing blood flow within an interrogated vessel: the nature of the vessel (artery versus vein), the vessel caliber, the degree of downstream resistance, and the heart rate and contractility. (Additional information is provided by the time–velocity waveforms from pulsed Doppler of the heart and great vessels: chamber compliance, valvular regurgitation, valvular stenosis, and the nature of arrhythmias.) A large fetal artery, such as the aorta, produces a time–velocity waveform that is rendered as a linear plot (see Fig. 13–27). The large caliber of the aorta is responsible for the very similar velocities of the bulk of the blood cells (with only a small difference between the faster central current and the peripheral slower current), thereby producing this "envelope" type of waveform. Narrower vessels produce a greater range in blood cell velocity, thereby producing a thicker waveform (called *spectral broadening*) (Fig. 13–9). The thickest waveforms, filled in from the top of the curve down to the base line, are produced by flow within very narrow vessels such as the fetal renal artery (see Fig. 13–19). The thickness of the waveform indicates that a wide range of blood cell velocities is occurring at any moment within this vessel. A filled-in waveform thus is not a sign of pathology in a small-caliber vessel, of which a fetus has many. It may denote abnormal turbulent flow, however, when found in a large-caliber vessel, such as in the fetal ascending aorta in the case of aortic valvular stenosis.

A number of technical matters should be kept in mind when using the pulsed Doppler spectral tracing. The pulsed Doppler range gate (the length of the Doppler sample) should extend over the entire width of the vessel to be sampled. If the range gate samples only a portion of the vessel diameter, the information within the spectral trace will be flawed. A narrow range gate centered over the periphery of a vessel detects only the slower-velocity peripheral blood cells, which vary less over time. A waveform with spuriously lower peak systolic velocity and overall pulsatility is thus produced, possibly leading to incorrect clinical impressions. Also, as described earlier, an improper gain setting can distort the gray-scale spectral tracing, thereby confusing the data.

INDEXES OF RESISTANCE

Flow data contained within the pulsed Doppler spectral tracing can be analyzed in a number of ways. The most obvious approach is to use the waveform to calculate volume flow within a vessel. This information would indicate something about the extent of blood flow to a particular organ, such as the placenta, and could be correlated with clinical status. However, a number of problems are associated with determination of volume flow, including measurement errors and the length of time required to perform the study.

Waveform analysis by calculation of an index of resistance represents an attractive al-

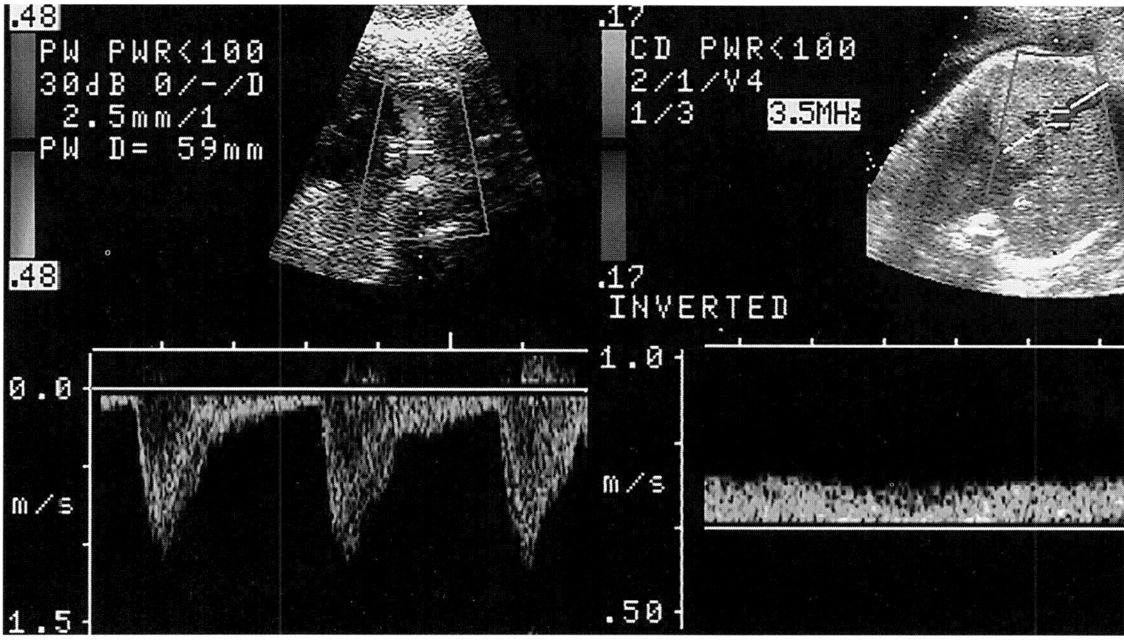

FIGURE 13–8.
(See Color Figure 13–8.) *Left,* Sagittal image of the ductus arteriosus revealing a spectrum of velocities on the time–velocity waveform. The brighter regions of the waveform are at the higher velocities and indicate that more of the blood is traveling at these velocities. *Right,* Axial image of the umbilical vein with color and pulsed Doppler. The homogeneous brightness of the waveform indicates that no one velocity predominates (i.e., equivalent numbers of blood cells are traveling at each of the represented velocities).

ternative to direct flow calculation and has become the standard in obstetrical Doppler for a number of reasons. The required measurement time is considerably less for indexes of resistance than for volume flow calculation. Furthermore, calculation error is reduced for the index of resistance because, unlike the volume flow measurement, vessel diameter is not a factor, the Doppler angle can be disregarded, and velocities need not be calculated from the raw Doppler shift data. (For similar reasons, indexes of resistance are well suited for continuous wave Doppler interrogation.) Finally, the index of resistance yields clinically useful vascular information related to volume flow. The index of resistance yields an

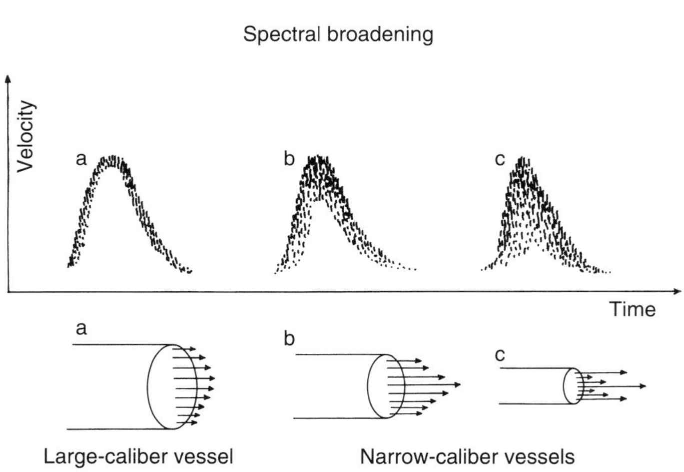

FIGURE 13–9.
Blood tends to move at a narrow range of velocities in larger vessels (a). The waveform appears as a relatively thin plot. In smaller vessels (b), there are greater differences in velocity between the central current and more peripheral currents. This is responsible for the thicker appearance of the waveform. In very small vessels (c), there is a very wide range of velocities, producing a "filled-in" waveform. This type of waveform is also seen in larger vessels when turbulence is present.

indication of downstream resistance to flow; that is, resistance to flow is measured in a blood vessel, but this resistance results from the anatomical and physiological status of the vascular bed located distal to this vessel. This downstream resistance is a major factor in the extent of blood flow supplying a vascular bed or organ. Thus, calculation of an index of resistance as a measure of downstream resistance yields some indication of extent of blood flow to that organ or vascular bed.

The theoretical basis for the use of indexes of resistance lies in the change in diastolic flow velocity as downstream resistance changes. As downstream resistance increases, diastolic velocity tends to fall. Systolic peak velocity may, in fact, also fall somewhat, but this is typically a smaller effect than in diastole. As resistance rises, diastolic velocity (measured at end-diastole) falls not only toward base line (velocity = 0 cm/sec) but may also cross the base line as a result of diastolic retrograde flow. Conversely, as resistance falls, diastolic velocity rises until, in vessels with extremely low downstream resistance, diastolic flow velocity nearly approaches systolic velocity. Thus, the heart of the analysis is the difference between systolic velocity and diastolic velocity or, in other words, the pulsatility of the arterial waveform. Furthermore, although each calculation is somewhat different, all of the three indexes of resistance are similar in that a higher number indicates elevated downstream resistance and a lower number indicates diminished resistance. The indexes are sensitive to fetal respirations and should be obtained during fetal apnea.

The systolic-to-diastolic ratio (S/D ratio, A/B ratio) is the easiest index of resistance to measure. One simply measures the peak systolic velocity (or kHz shift) and the highest end-diastolic velocity (or kHz shift) on the spectral tracing and divides the former by the latter (Fig. 13–10). This calculation is useful only in situations with forward diastolic flow. When diastolic flow velocity falls to zero, the S/D ratio climbs to infinity.[16,17] The resistive index (RI) provides similar information with nearly similar ease as the S/D ratio while correcting the limitations of the S/D ratio. Thus, the RI ((systolic peak velocity − end-diastolic velocity)/systolic peak velocity) also measures the difference between systolic and diastolic velocities but provides meaningful data when there is zero or retrograde diastolic

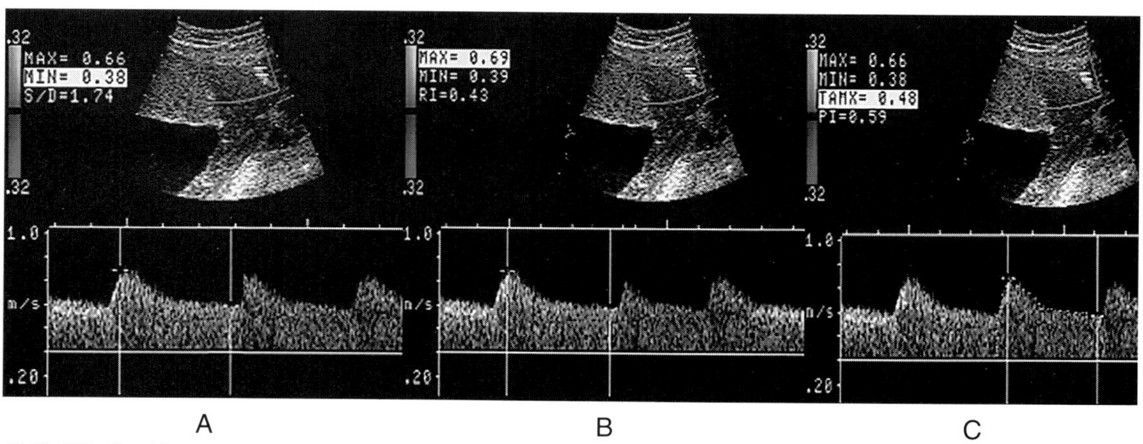

FIGURE 13–10.
Indexes of resistance of subplacental arterial flow. *A*, S/D ratio is calculated by measuring the maximal systolic velocity and the lowest peak diastolic velocity (usually found at end-diastole). *B*, Resistive index (RI) calculation is based on a different equation but the same measurements as the S/D ratio. *C*, The pulsatility index (PI) is based on maximum and minimum velocity measurements and the time-averaged maximum velocity. This average velocity is obtained by tracing the top velocities of the entire waveform throughout the cardiac cycle (dotted line) and averaging all the values of that curve.

flow (see Fig. 13–10). The highest measure of resistance in this calculation is 1.

The pulsatility index (PI) similarly measures the difference between systolic and diastolic velocities and provides meaningful data when diastolic flow falls to zero or below. The PI ((S−D)/mean velocity), however, adds another component to the calculation of downstream resistance, the overall time-averaged maximum velocity.[16,17] (see Fig. 13–10). The time-averaged maximum velocity is an average of the maximum velocities across the entire waveform. The operator simply traces the outline (or envelope) of the waveform, and the ultrasound machine's computer calculates the average velocity. The time-averaged maximum velocity contains information about downstream resistance in addition to that contained in the difference between systolic and diastolic velocities. A fall in resistance may cause a rise in this average, whereas an increase in resistance may produce a fall in this average.

The PI should theoretically provide the best information about downstream resistance. Nevertheless, the S/D ratio is the most widely used index of resistance in obstetrical Doppler because it is so easy to obtain. The RI is the next most popular index because it is only slightly more difficult to calculate, yet it is more versatile in abnormal flow conditions. The PI has been increasing in popularity as ultrasound equipment has become more advanced and capable of rapidly performing complex calculations.

VOLUME FLOW CALCULATIONS

Despite the greater time and expertise required and the inherent error associated with it, calculation of volume flow remains of interest in obstetrical Doppler, at least in the sphere of research. Volume flow of a vessel is determined by multiplying the cross-sectional area of that vessel by the mean velocity.[16] The diameter of the vessel is measured with two-dimensional sonography, and the cross-sectional area is calculated (area = $\Pi(\text{radius})^2$). Pulsed Doppler interrogation at the same location with an appropriately sized and localized Doppler range gate, proper Doppler gain, and a precise (and low) Doppler angle should yield an adequate spectral time–velocity tracing that can be used for measuring the time-average mean velocity. The ultrasound equipment's computer is used to calculate this velocity, but unfortunately, it is extremely difficult to double-check the result.

COLOR FLOW MAP

The color Doppler flow map is a color-coded map of flow velocity information superimposed on the gray-scale ultrasound image. The color scale (on the side of the image) is the key to reading this map. The scale presents a spectrum of colors or shades of colors on each side of the base line. The color or spectrum above the base line is the code for vascular flow toward the transducer, whereas the color or spectrum below the base line indicates flow away from the transducer. At the base line, there is no color and no flow. With greater distance up or down the scale, away from the base line, the change in color denotes increasing velocity.[15] The maximum velocity measurement possible for a particular PRF is shown at the ends of the scale. Actually, however, color Doppler sonography measures mean velocity; therefore, a particular color scale may faithfully record vascular flow with a peak systolic velocity above the maximum listed on the scale as long as the mean velocity is within the appropriate range. When the mean velocity of blood flow is greater than the maximum on the scale, however, aliasing of the color coding occurs: The color portrayal of vascular flow is spuriously mapped on the other side of the base line (Fig. 13–11). It is imperative to set the color scale appropriately for accurate and useful vascular data. A scale set too high does not detect low-velocity flow, and a scale set too low produces aliasing.

Color Doppler sonography provides two types of information: primary and secondary. The primary information answers questions directly on the color map: Is there flow into a cardiac chamber? Is this anechoic structure a vessel with flow or a cystic mass? What is the direction of flow in this vessel? The secondary information is the detection and localization

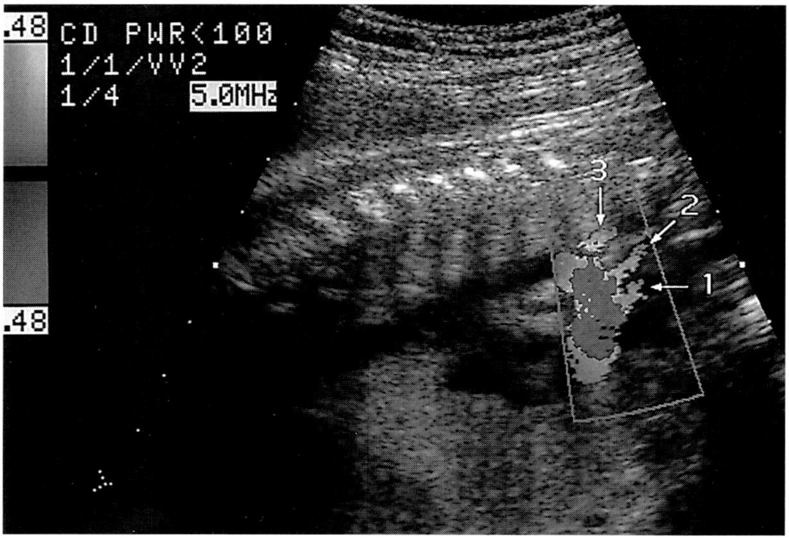

FIGURE 13–11.
(See Color Figure 13–11.) Sagittal color flow image of the fetal aortic arch demonstrating aliasing in the color coding of flow. Much of the arch is color coded blue, which incorrectly indicates retrograde flow. Higher pulse repetition frequency was not possible with this transducer at this distance between the transducer and the interrogated vessel. Solutions include lowering the base line of the color scale or changing to a lower-frequency transducer. The three head and neck branches—(1) the innominate artery, (2) the left carotid artery, and (3) the left subclavian artery—are clearly seen branching off the top of the arch.

of vascularity on the ultrasound image for the purpose of guiding pulsed Doppler interrogation. Color Doppler sonography is used most widely for this secondary role and is responsible for a shorter and more accurate pulsed Doppler examination.[19]

History

Vessels of the umbilical cord were the first components of the fetal circulation in which vascular flow was studied. The umbilical cord was described by Aristotle as the means for supplying nourishment from a woman to her fetus.[20] In 1884, Cohnstein and Zuntz first attempted to study the fetal lamb circulation through the umbilical cord using a flowmeter in an umbilical artery.[21] In 1949, Cooper and colleagues studied the umbilical flow in sheep using plethysmographic techniques.[22] Until about 25 years ago, most knowledge of fetal circulatory physiology had been based on animal studies. The first human fetal circulatory data were described about 30 years ago, but they were based on observations made either immediately after delivery[23, 24] or during abortion by hysterotomy.[25, 26] The various methods used to obtain these data included thermodilution, electromagnetic flowmeter, and radioactive microspheres.

One of the first descriptions of Doppler sonography in the human fetus circulation was reported in 1977 by Fitzgerald and associates, who used continuous wave Doppler in the fetoplacental circulation.[27] In 1978, Gill and colleagues described a Doppler ultrasound technique to study umbilical vein flow rates in the human fetus under normal conditions.[20] Many other investigators followed with descriptions of Doppler techniques to evaluate the fetal and maternoplacental circulations.[20,28,29] Among the various techniques used for analyzing the fetal Doppler circulatory data have been velocity ratios, determination of blood flow volume of specific vessels, and time–velocity waveform analysis. The latter approach, using indexes of resistance, became the standard technique because it is the easiest and least time-consuming to acquire and provides clinically useful information. Use of indexes of resistance proliferated also because of the availability of lower-cost, nonimaging continuous wave Doppler ultrasound machines that were incapable of providing flow volume measurements.[16,18]

Today, color Doppler sonography has advanced the cause of noninvasive fetal and maternoplacental circulatory investigation.[30] Small vessels that were not previously visible are now detectable with color flow mapping and are able to be interrogated with pulsed Doppler. Waveforms of these vessels are thus available for study and correlation with other test results and clinical outcomes. Although umbilical artery velocimetry remains the most widely used clinical Doppler test of the fetal circulation, a number of tests involving other fetal vessels are emerging.

Umbilical Arteries

The umbilical cord vessels are the most extensively Doppler-investigated vessels in the human fetus. The umbilical arteries and vein have been studied the most because they are large and easy to locate and have recognizable patterns with both continuous and pulsed wave Doppler. Continuous wave Doppler has been used extensively for the intracord umbilical arteries, particularly because the equipment is inexpensive and available and an umbilical artery is not a particularly challenging target. Furthermore, continuous wave Doppler produces a lower output of energy than does pulsed Doppler sonography.[9, 10] It is believed that index of resistance values within the umbilical artery are the same whether the measurements are taken with continuous wave or pulsed Doppler sonography.[1, 31] However, the inability to visualize the site of vascular sampling with continuous wave Doppler may lead to error in the interpretation of a specific fetal vessel, such as when differentiating an umbilical artery from the descending aorta or a uterine artery from an arcuate artery.[32–34]

Many studies have demonstrated falling umbilical artery S/D ratios during the course of gestation. S/D ratios fall from approximately 4.0 at 20 weeks to 2.0 at term in uncompromised fetuses.[35–37] S/D ratios may vary from one location to another in the umbilical artery.[37] Thus, the site as well as the length of the cord may cause differences in S/D ratios.[32] See Chapter 16.

Placental Vasculature

The placenta consists of maternal and fetal tissues that bring together maternal and fetal circulations in very close proximity in order to accomplish nutrient and waste transfer.[38, 39] The maternal side is supplied by the uterine arteries, which branch into the arcuate arteries and then the radial arteries. Ultimately, the placenta is supplied by a dense network of spiral arteries that connect to the intervillous space.[38]

The chorionic villi represent the major fetal component of the placenta. Fetal umbilical arteries branch at the insertion site of the cord into the placenta. These branches diverge throughout the chorionic plate and ultimately descend into the substance of the placenta, into the cores of the chorionic villi. Villus arteries branch further within the secondary and tertiary villi. Nutrient and waste exchange occurs between the maternal blood, within the intervillous space, and the fetal blood, within the chorionic villi.[38] Veins carrying newly oxygenated fetal blood leave the villi, ascend to the chorionic plate, and converge toward the umbilical cord, where the umbilical vein is formed.

The maternoplacental and fetoplacental circulations are critical to fetal growth and survival, performing essential renal, intestinal, and pulmonary functions. Dawes reported that fetoplacental flow in fetal lambs increases with gestational age.[40] This increased flow is secondary to a decrease in placental resistance, which has been recognized in human fetuses with Doppler sonography as a fall in the indexes of resistance within the umbilical artery during the course of gestation. The change results from an increase in umbilical artery diastolic velocity rather than from a change in the systolic velocity. The fall in placental resistance is believed to occur secondary to placental (actually, placental vascular bed) growth during gestation. A reduction in the fetoplacental blood flow (and an elevated umbilical artery resistance) has been shown to be associated with an increased risk of IUGR.[20, 36, 41–43] Umbilical artery resistance measurements should be obtained during fetal apnea, because fetal respiratory motion causes fluctuations in the velocity measurements.[42, 44, 45]

The uterine arteries are found medial to the iliac vessels and along the lateral aspects of the uterus (Fig. 13–12). Identification of each vessel with continuous wave Doppler is achieved by standardized transducer placement and recognition of a characteristic waveform. Using color flow Doppler, the bilateral uterine arteries can be directly visual-

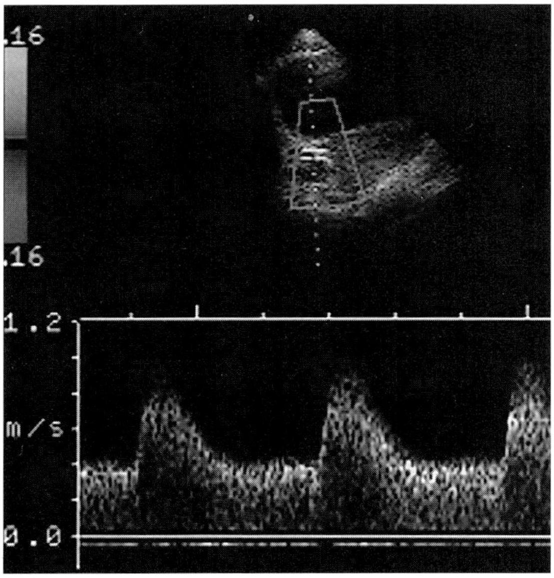

FIGURE 13–12.
Transverse image of the right uterine artery demonstrating normal high diastolic arterial flow.

ized as they course toward the cervix and then ascend the uterus along its lateral margins. The arcuate, radial, and spiral branches can be identified farther into the uterine substance. This direct visualization allows for precise localization of the pulsed Doppler sampling. The typical main uterine artery waveform of a gravid uterus has a characteristic diastolic notch (which is normally gone by 24 weeks) and a high systolic peak velocity.[35, 42, 46]

Fetal Circulation

The fetus receives oxygenated blood from the placenta via the umbilical vein. The umbilical vein enters the fetus in the midline through the anterior abdominal wall at the umbilical cord insertion. It then proceeds cephalad, entering the liver and continuing intrahepatically to terminate at the portal sinus, which ultimately becomes the left portal vein after birth. Umbilical venous blood flows into the portal sinus, several small left hepatic portal branches, and the ductus venosus. The ductus venosus travels cephalad into the confluence of hepatic veins and then on to the inferior vena cava (IVC). The ductus venosus thus provides a detour for umbilical venous blood to bypass the liver parenchyma. Umbilical venous blood entering the small branches to the left hepatic lobe and the portal sinus to the right hepatic lobe passes through hepatic sinusoids and is drained by the hepatic veins into the IVC, which continues on to the right atrium. The most highly oxygenated blood current arriving into the right atrium from the IVC passes through the physiological interatrial shunt, the foramen ovale, into the left atrium. The rest of the IVC blood mixes in the right atrium with deoxygenated superior vena cava (SVC) blood from the head and arms. The left atrium empties into the left ventricle and then into the ascending aorta. The coronary, carotid, and subclavian arteries are the first branches of the ascending aorta and receive highly oxygenated blood. Mixed right atrial blood passes through the tricuspid valve and into the right ventricle, then on into the pulmonary artery. The high resistance of the pulmonary vascular bed directs the major portion of pulmonary trunk blood through the ductus arteriosus into the descending thoracic and then the abdominal aorta. After supplying the celiac axis, the SMA, and renal arteries, the abdominal aorta bifurcates into left and right common iliac arteries. Internal iliac arteries branch off the common iliac arteries and continue on into the umbilical arteries. The umbilical arteries pass ventrally and cranially in the pelvis to enter the umbilical cord to return deoxygenated blood to the placenta. See also Figure 14–14.

Abdomen

Because it is so large and travels such a straight course, the umbilical vein is probably the most obvious fetal abdominal blood vessel visible with conventional real-time sonography. It is quite easy to detect with color Doppler sonography particularly because its anteroposterior and slightly craniad orientation often provides an optimal Doppler angle. Pulsed Doppler interrogation reveals a nonpulsatile venous type of waveform, with a slightly rising velocity during gestation and an overall mean velocity of approximately 15 cm/sec.[47]

The intrahepatic umbilical vein is a logical site for fetal flow calculations. Although volume flow calculations are subject to large errors due to even small errors in vessel diameter determination, the umbilical vein is a relatively large fetal vessel and is thus one of the fetal vessels least subject to this sort of error. The vein is straight, aiding accurate diameter measurement and correct determination of Doppler angle for greater accuracy of velocity calculation. Finally, umbilical venous flow provides an indication of complete fetoplacental blood flow because it carries all the returning blood from the placenta to the fetus. As such, umbilical flow can provide a useful look at placental and fetal physiological status.[20]

Gill and colleagues described normal human umbilical vein flow as increasing from 100 ml/min at 25 weeks to 300 ml/min at 37 weeks' menstrual age.[20] When normalized to fetal weight, however, flow remained constant at 100 ml/min/kg.[20] Another study, using color Doppler sonography, found weight-normalized umbilical venous flow to remain steady at 120 ml/min/kg from 22 to 35 weeks and then to fall to 90 ml/min/kg at term.[47]

As is the case in all vessels in which volume flow is calculated, certain precautions should be taken when studying umbilical venous flow. First, to obtain the most accurate vessel diameter, the vein should be measured with the transducer as nearly perpendicular to it as possible and measurements made from an enlarged image. The diameter should be measured with real-time gray-scale sonography. Color Doppler flow maps should not be used for this measurement because they may artifactually exaggerate the diameter of the vessel. Second, pulsed Doppler interrogation should be localized to the same site at which the diameter was measured. The Doppler angle should be maintained as low as possible, certainly at less than 60 degrees (Fig. 13–13).[16] Color Doppler sonography may assist accurate angle correction. Finally, the pulsed Doppler range gate should be enlarged to encompass the entire vessel.

The ductus venosus appears very narrow with sonography and is often not seen unless it is specifically sought. Nevertheless, animal studies using radiolabeled microspheres have shown that the ductus shunts 40% to 91% of umbilical venous flow past the liver.[26,48] Us-

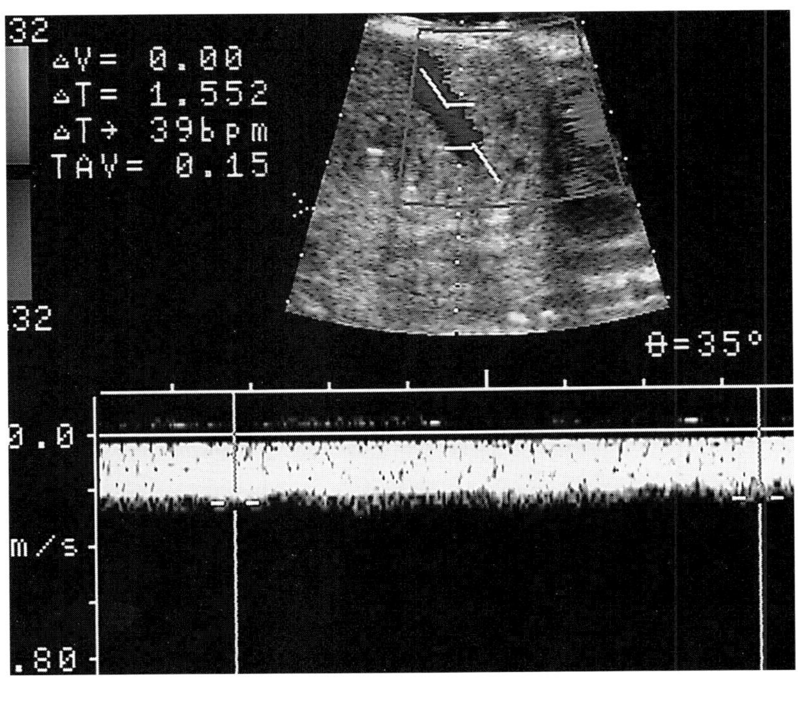

FIGURE 13–13.
(See Color Figure 13–13.) Calculation of mean umbilical flow in a 25-week fetus. Doppler angle is set at 35 degrees to minimize error in this calculation. Color Doppler flow map assists rapid and accurate determination of the Doppler angle. The pulsed Doppler spectral tracing demonstrates a venous waveform with a time-averaged mean velocity of 15 cm/sec. Unlike the time-averaged maximum velocity, which averages the peak velocities throughout the cycle (see Fig. 13–10), the time-averaged mean velocity averages the mean velocities throughout the cardiac cycle.

ing volume flow calculations via pulsed Doppler sonography, Emerson and coworkers calculated the percentage of normal human ductus venosus shunting to be only 24±13% (± 1 SD), with a range of 0 to 50%. One of the main sources of potential error in this study was in the accuracy of the ductus venosus diameter measurement (1.2±0.4 mm at 20 weeks to 1.6±0.6 mm at term).[47] Although shunting by the ductus venosus is greater than would be expected for the very small diameter of this vessel, it is accomplished by the very high-flow velocities within it (Fig. 13–14). The mean velocity was measured at 29.9±12.9 cm/sec in this study,[47] and the maximal velocity was measured from 65 to 75 cm/sec in another study.[49] Possibly, this high velocity is what propels the oxygenated blood as a coherent current through the IVC and right atrium and across the foramen ovale into the left atrium.[49]

Hepatic veins are seen in a transverse view of the abdomen at the level of the liver. The confluence of the right, middle, and left hepatic veins draining the lobes of the liver can be seen joining the IVC just caudad to the right atrium (Fig. 13–15*A*). These vessels may be imaged with color Doppler, but this is typically not necessary because their identity is readily obvious from their anatomical location. Pulsed Doppler interrogation of the hepatic veins reveals venous flow modulated by troughs due to raised atrial pressures during atrial systole (Fig. 13–15*B*). This is similar to what is seen in the ductus venosus, although the mean and peak velocities are typically less than in the ductus. Portal venous flow, however, is not characterized by these modulations.

The IVC courses cephalad anterior to the spine and to the right of the aorta. It travels through the posterior portion of the liver, extending ventrally to receive the confluence of hepatic veins and ductus venosus immediately before entering the right atrium (Fig. 13–16). The pulsed Doppler waveform reflects the changes in intracardiac pressures within the left atrium (Fig. 13–16).

Aside from these previously described vessels and the aorta, iliac arteries, and umbilical arteries, no other fetal abdominal vessels are readily visible with real-time conventional sonography. Color Doppler sonography, however, makes visible other vessels, particularly branches off the abdominal aorta and their venous counterparts. Color Doppler detection of these abdominal vessels can be accomplished as early as 16 weeks' menstrual age.[50]

The celiac trunk and the SMA are the first

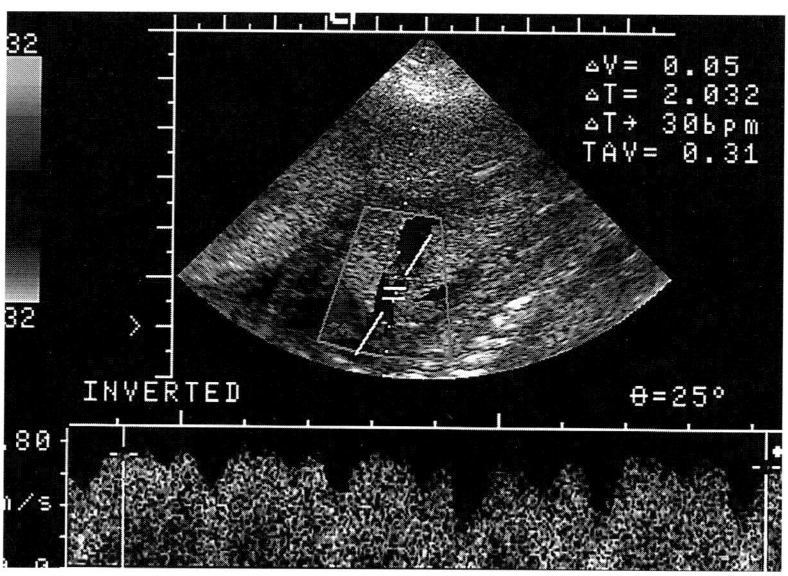

FIGURE 13–14.
(See Color Figure 13–14.) Flow through the ductus venosus (DV) with color and pulsed Doppler in a 20-week fetus. The color map indicates higher velocities through the DV than through the umbilical vein (UV). As demonstrated on the pulsed Doppler tracing, DV flow is pulsatile. This derives from pressures reflected down from the right atrium. The maximal velocity is 75 cm/sec, and the time-averaged mean velocity is 31 cm/sec.

FIGURE 13–15.
(See Color Figure 13–15.) *A*, Hepatic veins are coded blue on the color map as blood flow moves away from the transducer toward the inferior vena cava (red). *B*, The pulsed Doppler tracing demonstrates flow modulations in the hepatic veins. These variations in flow reflect changes in right atrial pressures. Flow alterations above the base line occur secondary to atrial pressures. Flow alterations above the base line occur secondary to atrial systole, which is responsible for flow reversal in the hepatic veins. Flow below the base line is antegrade and occurs during atrial diastole. These changes are more dramatic than those seen in the ductus venosus because the flow velocities are lower in the hepatic veins.

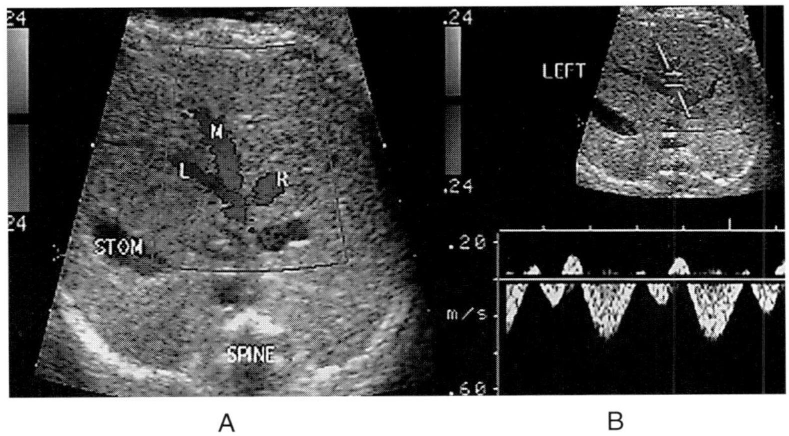

two major branches off the abdominal aorta, supplying the spleen, liver, stomach, pancreas, and small and large intestines. They are best seen with color Doppler sonography when a fetus is supine but may be identified even when a fetus is in other positions (Fig. 13–17). For optimal detection, the color scale and wall filter must be set for low-velocity flow (Fig. 13–17). With the color scale set even lower, color Doppler imaging also can demonstrate the smaller mesenteric branches of the SMA that feed the small intestines (Fig. 13–18). Color Doppler visualization of these vessels makes possible pulsed Doppler interrogation. Systolic peak velocity of the SMA increases as gestational age increases. The mean velocity of the SMA is 45 cm/sec (range 13 to 82 cm/sec).[50] The smaller mesenteric branches vary little with gestational age, and their mean velocities range from 7 to 22 cm/sec. There is a small difference in PI calculations between the SMA and its distal branches (SMA mean 2.1, branches 1.7). Although color and pulsed Doppler sonography of the SMA and its branches is not currently used as a clinical test, it may ultimately enhance our understanding of normal and abnormal fetal physiology.[50]

FIGURE 13–16.
(See Color Figure 13–16.) *A*, Inferior vena cava flow is seen traveling in a cranial direction through the liver and continuing into the right atrium. *B*, Modulations in venous waveform of the IVC due to changing atrial pressures during cardiac cycle. Additional changes in the waveform occur as a result of fetal breathing motion.

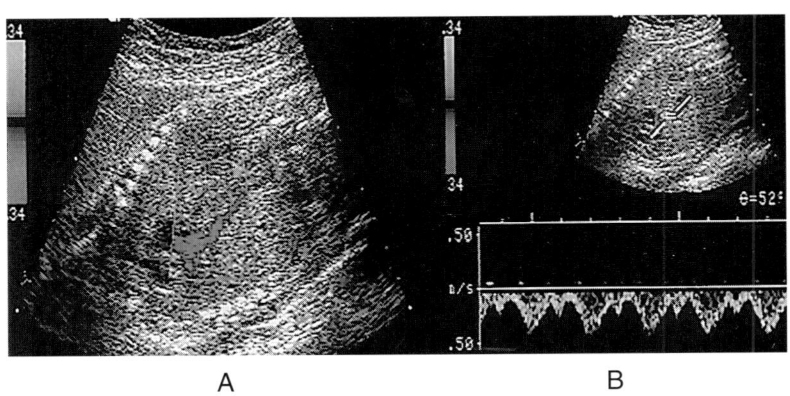

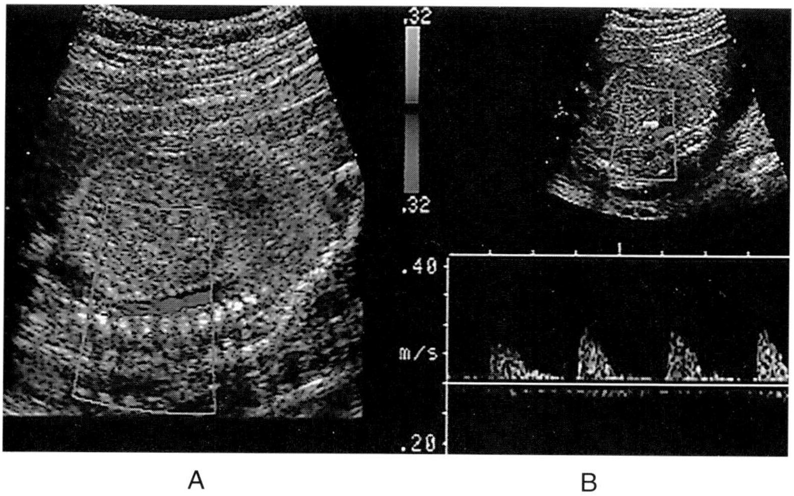

FIGURE 13–17.
(See Color Figure 13–17.) Superior mesenteric arterial flow in a 16-week fetus. *A*, Color Doppler flow map with a fetus in the sagittal plane demonstrates flow in the abdominal aorta (coded blue) and the superior mesenteric artery (coded red). *B*, Pulsed Doppler interrogation reveals low-velocity flow with minimal diastolic component in the superior mesenteric artery.

The next set of aortic branches recognizable with color Doppler sonography are the renal arteries (Fig. 13–19*A*). Arising laterally from the abdominal aorta, they are best visualized with Doppler interrogation from the lateral aspect of the fetus with the arteries coursing toward or away from the transducer. The color scale is set for low velocities, similar to that of the SMA. Color flow mapping permits optimal placement of the pulsed Doppler range gate close to the renal hilum to ensure that the main renal artery is evaluated without contamination from the aorta[7, 51] (Fig. 13–19*B*). Mean PI values decrease linearly with gestational age, from 4.0 at 16 weeks to 2.1 at 38 weeks, indicating a fall in renal arterial resistance from the middle of the second trimester to term.[7, 51] This fall in resistance may parallel increasing renal function as a fetus grows. Renal artery Doppler velocimetry may provide useful clinical information in small-for-gestational-age fetuses. Renal artery PI values have been shown to rise with fetal hypoxia, possibly a function of cardiac output redistribution in such fetuses.[7] Color Doppler flow maps may be used also to demonstrate intrarenal vasculature. The renal veins are seen with color Doppler sonography adjacent to the renal arteries but with flow in the opposite direction. The renal veins and arteries are so intimately related that they are often interrogated together with pulsed Doppler, with both waveforms appearing simultaneously on the spectral time–velocity tracing although on opposite sides of the base line (Fig. 13–19C).

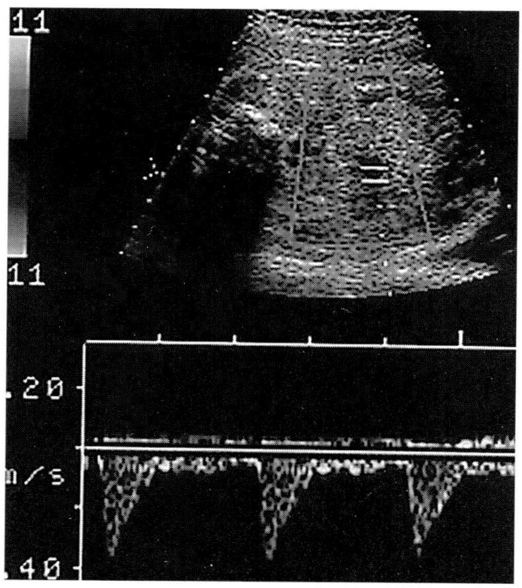

FIGURE 13–18.
(See Color Figure 13–18.) Doppler flow in the mesentery of fetal bowel seen in a 36-week fetus. The color Doppler flow map permits detection of this flow, and pulsed Doppler interrogation reveals the waveforms. The arterial signal is seen below the base line, and the venous signal is above the base line.

The color map may also demonstrate flow in the adrenal arteries and veins toward and away from the adrenal glands (Fig. 13–20). Color and pulsed Doppler velocity scales and filters should be set to detect minimal flow and then increased as necessary. Adrenal artery waveforms are similar to those of the mesenteric branches. Investigation is ongo-

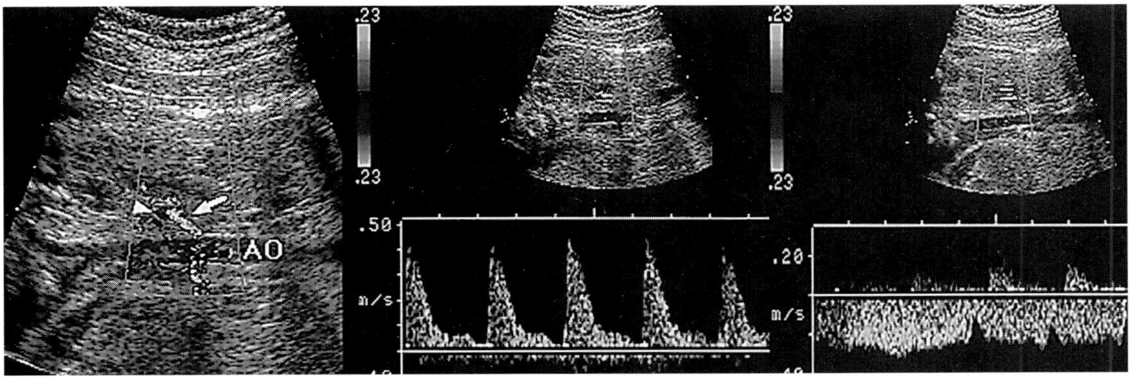

A B C

FIGURE 13–19.
(See Color Figure 13–19.) Color and pulsed Doppler sonography of fetal renal arteries and veins. *A*, The renal arteries and veins are clearly seen on the color Doppler flow map. The renal artery (large arrow), seen exiting the aorta (AO) and traveling toward the kidney, is color coded red because its flow is directed toward the transducer. The renal vein (coded blue, arrowhead) is seen next to the artery. *B*, The pulsed Doppler time–velocity tracing confirms the color Doppler information, revealing the renal artery waveform. *C*, Pulsed Doppler spectral tracing reveals venous waveform of the renal vein below the base line. Some renal arterial signal is seen above the base line, indicating oppositely directed flow.

ing, although no useful Doppler information is available at this time.

The common iliac arteries are demonstrable with conventional imaging sonography, although color flow imaging improves the ease of detection (Fig. 13–21). The color Doppler velocity scale should be set for higher velocities than for the branch arteries supplying abdominal organs. The umbilical arteries, representing the largest branches of the common iliac arteries, course ventrally along the lateral aspects of the urinary bladder. Color Doppler sonography easily demonstrates these vessels coursing around the bladder, providing a well-defined anatomical demarcation of bladder location. The arteries then course superiorly to the umbilicus, where they enter the umbilical cord and travel toward the placenta (Fig. 13–22). The umbilical arteries are the fetal vessels most commonly investigated with Doppler sonography. Doppler sampling is most often performed, however, within the umbilical cord.

Chest

Particular challenges associated with color and pulsed Doppler evaluation of fetal thoracic structures result from both cardiac mo-

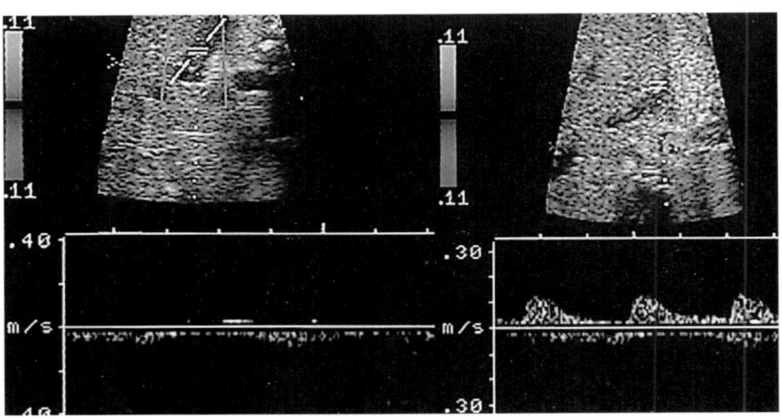

A B

FIGURE 13–20.
(See Color Figure 13–20.) Color and pulsed Doppler of a fetal adrenal artery and vein. *A*, Very low-velocity flow is seen in the adrenal vein. *B*, Adrenal arterial flow has a relatively low velocity, typically between 10 and 20 cm/sec, similar to that of mesenteric arterial branches.

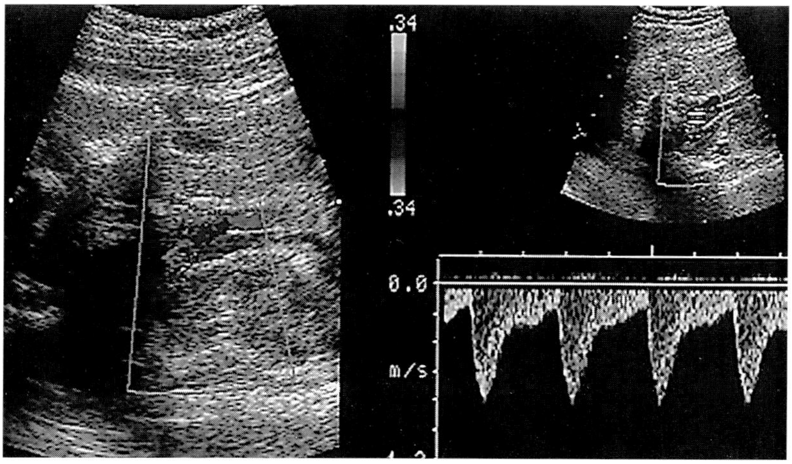

A B

FIGURE 13–21.
(See Color Figure 13–21.) *A,* The common iliac arteries are best visualized in the coronal plane, bifurcating from the long axis of the aorta. They are easily identified with color mapping. One of the arteries is heading toward the transducer, and the other is heading away. This is reflected in the color coding of flow. *B,* The pulsed Doppler spectrum reveals a high-velocity arterial waveform with low end-diastolic velocity in one of the common iliac arteries.

tion and high-velocity blood flow. Cardiac motion results in artifactual placement of flow information over nonflow regions such as myocardium and pulmonary parenchyma. This can be solved through the use of a high-pass filter with a higher-frequency cutoff set at a minimum of 400 Hz to reduce low flow velocities. Peak systolic velocities in the ascending aorta, pulmonary artery, and especially the ductus arteriosus are typically higher than anywhere else in a fetus. Because of these high velocities and the distance between these structures and the transducer, Doppler signal aliasing tends to occur, in both color and pulsed modes. Therefore, the color and Doppler range scales should be set appropriately, at approximately 50 cm/sec at the level of the atrioventricular valves and at 100 cm/sec or more at the outflow tracts and ductus. To reduce aliasing, it may be necessary to use a lower transducer frequency for Doppler interrogation than might otherwise be used for imaging. Transducers whose operating frequency can be altered during an examination offer the greatest flexibility in dealing with such conflicts between two-

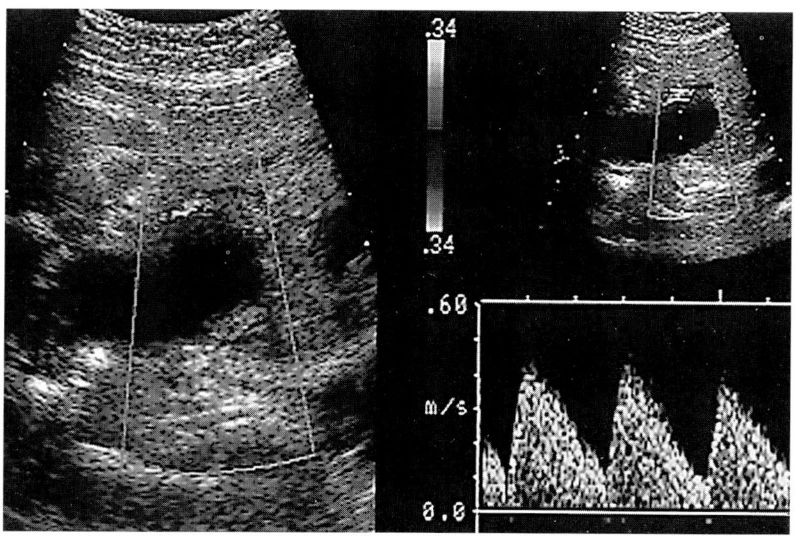

A B

FIGURE 13–22.
(See Color Figure 13–22.) *A,* Color flow map reveals umbilical arteries coursing around the bladder. They are very useful anatomical landmarks for identifying bladder location when visualization is poor and the bladder is empty. *B,* Pulsed Doppler demonstrates a typical umbilical artery waveform. Pulsed Doppler of the umbilical arteries for determination of placental resistance is generally performed at the umbilical cord.

dimensional image resolution and Doppler aliasing.

The SVC and IVC can be seen draining into the right atrium with conventional and color Doppler sonography, particularly when imaging in a longitudinal axis. SVC and IVC pulsed Doppler waveforms are similar and are characterized by venous flow modulated by troughs and peaks due to atrial contraction and relaxation (Fig. 13–23). This modulation grows in amplitude as vessel interrogation moves closer to the right atrium. Troughs may be so deep that they drop below the base line, representing brief periods of retrograde flow. SVC waveforms may be distinguished by a pattern of more abrupt peaks due to transmission of pulsations from the nearby ascending aorta.

Although direction of intracardiac blood flow currents may be deduced from motion of the atrioventricular valves and the septum primum, such flow can be visualized directly with color Doppler sonography (Fig. 13–24). Color Doppler demonstrates inflow into the right atrium, from the SVC and IVC, and into the left atrium, from the right atrium and pulmonary veins, as the atria begin to relax after atrial systole. The tricuspid and mitral valves open in early ventricular diastole as blood moves passively into the ventricles, which are beginning to relax. Atrioventricular blood flow slows down as the ventricles reach capacity. In atrial systole, blood is pushed forcefully through the atrioventricular valves by atrial contraction (the atrial kick), thereby emptying the atria and increasing ventricular volume. As the ventricles begin to contract in early systole, blood flow from the atria to the ventricles ceases abruptly and the atrioventricular valves rapidly close. This entire cycle can be monitored on the color Doppler flow map, particularly with the use of cine for reviewing these events in slower motion. The pulsed Doppler spectral velocity tracings of the tricuspid and mitral valves corresponds well to the events just described. The atrioventricular spectral waveform resembles an M. The first peak, called the *E point*, represents early passive flow into the ventricles. The middle trough represents slowing of this flow as the ventricles reach capacity. The second peak, called the *A point*, is produced by the forceful atrial contraction. The ratio of velocity and the A point divided by velocity at the E point, the A/E ratio, is greater in the fetus than after birth, denoting lower ventricular compliance prenatally.[52] The M-shaped waveform is best seen when the Doppler angle is less than 25 degrees (Fig. 13–25*A* and *B*). If fetal positioning prevents using such a Doppler angle, the sonographer should wait for the fetus to move or should move the transducer to a new location. The flow tracing across an atrioventricular valve is most accurately rendered when the Doppler range gate is located inside the ventricle in close proximity to the valve. Only forward flow should be seen in a normal fetus. However, it may be difficult to sample mitral valve flow without also including some aortic flow, because the size of the pulsed Doppler range gate may partially overlap the left ventricular inflow and outflow tracts of the fetus (Fig. 13–26). Placement of the range gate as close as possible to the left ventricular free wall may help to minimize the jet in the opposite direction.

Although the M-shaped flow velocity waveforms across each of the atrioventricular valves appear similar, differences have been noted. For instance, the A/E ratio of both valves falls during gestation, but the ratio

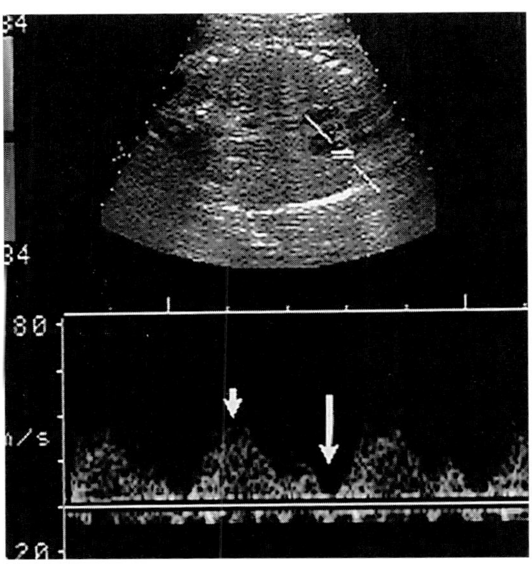

FIGURE 13–23.
(See Color Figure 13–23.) Pulsed Doppler tracing of flow in the superior vena cava (SVC). Arrows indicate modulations in the SVC due to atrial systole and diastole.

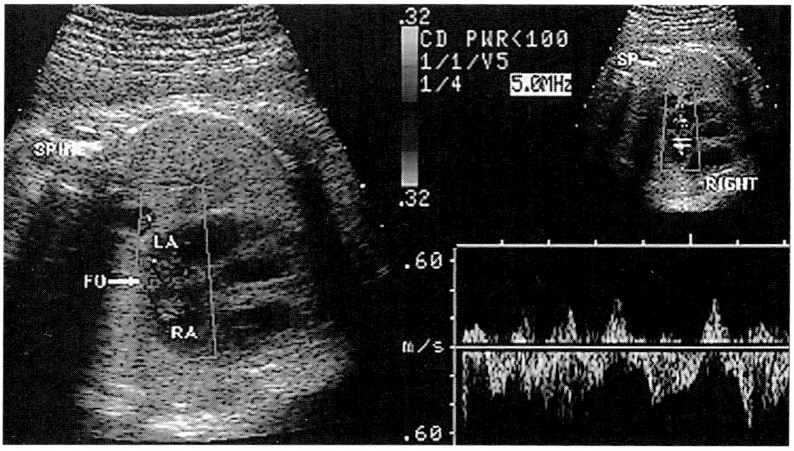

FIGURE 13–24.
(See Color Figure 13–24.) Color and pulsed Doppler sonography of interatrial flow via the foramen ovale (FO). The color flow map on the left shows flow between the left and right atrium (LA, RA) through the normally patent foramen ovale. Flow is coded blue, indicating movement away from the transducer. Although this suggests an abnormal left-to-right shunt at this level instead of the expected right-to-left shunt, it should be remembered that this image represents only one frame from a cine of the entire cardiac cycle. In reality, bidirectional flow often occurs at the FO, as can be seen on the pulsed Doppler spectral tracing on the right.

change at the tricuspid valve is due to *increasing* velocity in *early* diastole (E point) whereas at the mitral valve it is due to *falling* velocity in *late* diastole (A point).[52] Also, peak velocities across the tricuspid valve are higher than those across the mitral valve (51±1.2 cm/sec versus 47±1.1 cm/sec).[53] Both of these findings imply functional differences between both ventricles. Indeed, Doppler blood flow evidence indicates greater cardiac output from the right side of the heart than from the left side.[53] Thus, Doppler can be useful for

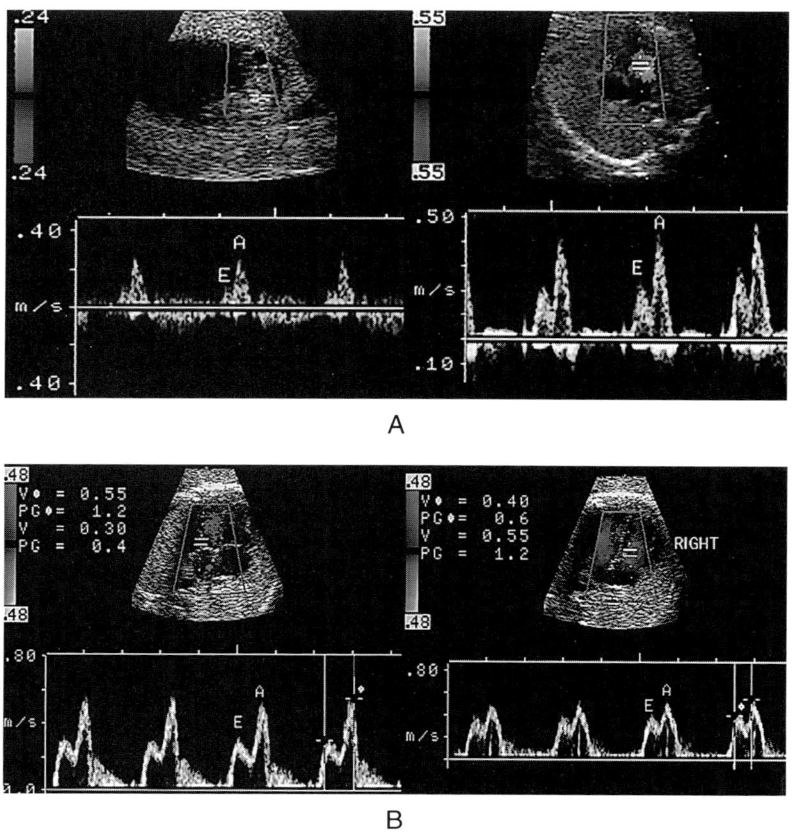

FIGURE 13–25.
(See Color Figure 13–25.) *A*, Pulsed Doppler waveforms across the atrioventricular valves. The typical M-shaped waveform is seen in both the 9.5-week fetus (left) and the 25-week fetus (right). A/E ratio represents peak velocity at atrial systole (A) divided by the peak velocity at early diastole (E). *B*, Although the M-shaped waveform is seen across both atrioventricular valves, there are differences in flow velocity and therefore in the A/E ratios. In this case, the peak velocity during atrial systole, 55 cm/sec, is the same for the mitral valve (left) and the tricuspid valve (right). The peak velocity at early diastole (E) is lower at the mitral valve (30 cm/sec) than at the tricuspid valve (40 cm/sec).

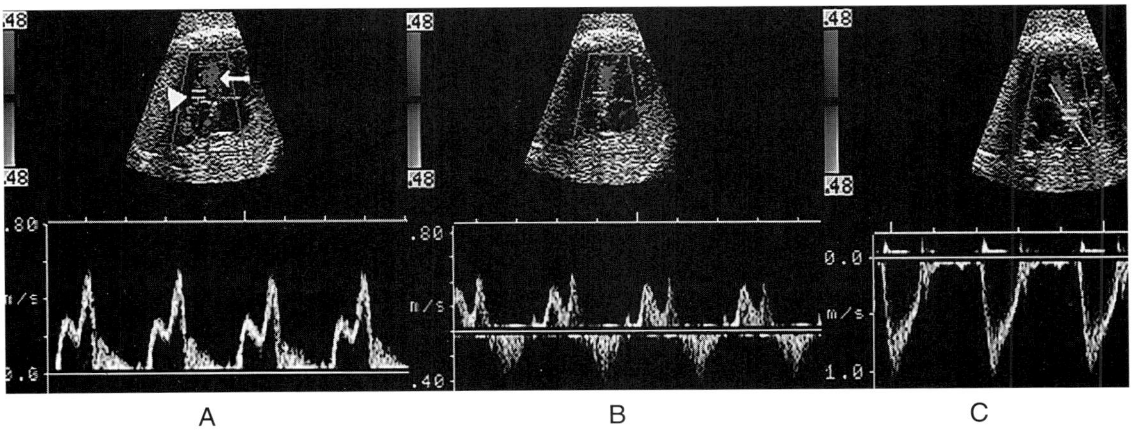

FIGURE 13–26.
(See Color Figure 13–26.) Pulsed Doppler sampling of mitral and aortic flow. *A*, The Doppler range gate (arrowhead) is appropriately placed for an accurate representation of mitral flow. *B*, Doppler range gate straddles both the inflow and outflow tracts of the left ventricle, yielding imperfect Doppler waveforms of both mitral and aortic flow on opposite sides of the base line. *C*, Further positioning of the range gate into the ascending aorta produces a clean and accurate aortic outflow waveform.

study of relative flows at the atrioventricular valves or at the aortic and pulmonary valves in health and disease.[53]

The pulmonary artery bears to the left as it courses cranially and dorsally from the right ventricular outflow tract. The main trunk gives rise to the right and left pulmonary arteries and terminates in the ductus arteriosus, which continues on to the descending aorta. The main pulmonary artery and the ductus arteriosus together form a continuous vascular arch called the *ductal arch*. The ductal arch and aortic arch are distinctly different in appearance on gray-scale imaging and demonstrate different flow parameters on color and pulsed Doppler sonography (Fig. 13–27). The ductus arteriosus shunts right ventricular output away from the high-resistance pulmonary circulation and toward the lower-resistance descending aorta.[52,54] The main pulmonary artery waveform has a low diastolic component, and the ductus arteriosus has relatively high diastolic flow. Pulmonary arterial branches, on the other hand, reveal minimal or no diastolic flow. Normal slight narrowing of the ductus arteriosus may explain the Doppler finding of high peak systolic velocity, the highest found in a fetus (50 to 140 cm/sec).[55]

The aortic arch courses from left to right then back to the left again as it joins the descending aorta. Systolic peak velocity is greater in the ascending aorta than the pulmonary artery (70±2.6 cm/sec versus 60±1.9 cm/sec).[53] The aorta and pulmonary arterial waveforms reveal some diastolic flow but less than in the ductus arteriosus. Volume flow (and cardiac outputs) can be calculated through diameter and Doppler flow measurements of the great vessels at the valvular level. Although mean velocities are higher in the aorta than in the pulmonary artery (18±0.7 cm/sec versus 16±0.6 cm sec), right ventricular volume flow is greater than on the left because of the greater pulmonary valve diameter.[53] Pulmonary artery weight-normalized volume flow is 312±11 ml/kg/min, and aortic flow is 250±9 ml/kg/min.[53]

The aortic arch is recognized through its connections with the left ventricular outflow tract and the branching head and neck vessels, the innominate, left carotid, and left subclavian arteries (see Fig. 13–11). The left subclavian artery can be seen branching off the aorta just before the entrance of the ductus arteriosus. The head and neck vessels are typically seen best with gray-scale sonography in the longitudinal view, with the vessels perpendicular to the transducer. Unfortunately, this is not the optimal orientation for Doppler sonography. Nevertheless, color Doppler sonography may be able to depict directional flow in these vessels despite a nearly perpendicular orientation if the velocity scale is set

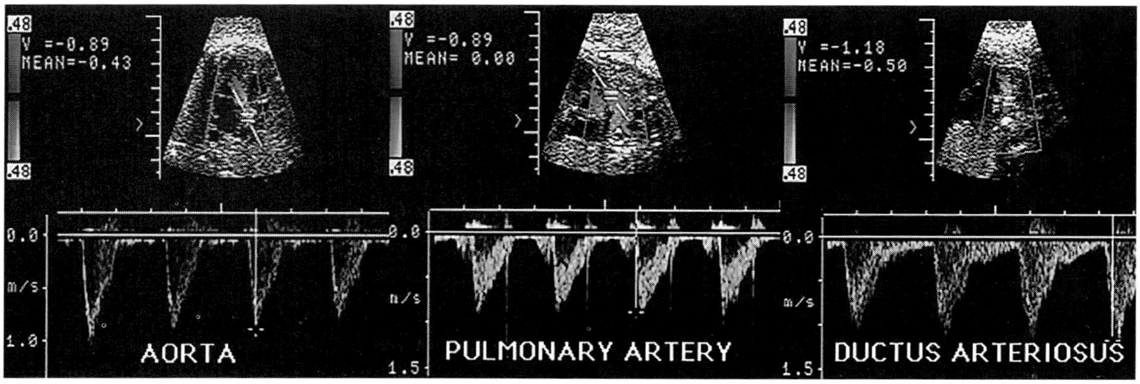

FIGURE 13–27.
(See Color Figure 13–27.) Pulsed Doppler waveforms of the aorta, pulmonary artery, and ductus arteriosus. The aorta and pulmonary artery have little diastolic flow compared with that of the ductus arteriosus. Peak velocities are lower in the aorta (89 cm/sec) and pulmonary artery (89 cm/sec) than in the ductus arteriosus (118 cm/sec). Color Doppler expedites accurate placement of the pulsed Doppler range gate and determination of the Doppler angle adjustment.

extremely low. Acquisition of meaningful pulsed Doppler flow data, however, requires a more parallel relationship between transducer and vessel.

The main, right, and left pulmonary arteries were investigated in fetuses using pulsed Doppler even before the use of color Doppler sonography (Fig. 13–28). Color Doppler, however, made it first possible to study distal pulmonary branch arteries and veins of the fetus noninvasively[56] (Fig. 13–29). Because of low-velocity flow in these vessels, color Doppler velocity scales must be lowered as interrogation proceeds from the mediastinum to the lung periphery. The color and pulsed Doppler wall filter, however, should be set higher to eliminate excess cardiac motion. Analysis of pulsed Doppler flow data in the distal branches demonstrates a high-resistance arterial circulation. The unique spectral waveform is characterized by a rapid needlelike systolic peak followed by rapid deceleration (possibly followed by a second brief systolic peak) and then a more gradual fall in flow velocity. There is little or no diastolic flow. This waveform occurs throughout the pulmonary arterial circulation, except that peak systolic velocities decrease as interrogation moves more peripherally[56] (see Fig. 13–29). Pulmonary veins may be seen with conventional sonography, but they are easier to see with color Doppler sonography. Pulsed Doppler interrogation of the pulmonary veins reveals changing atrial

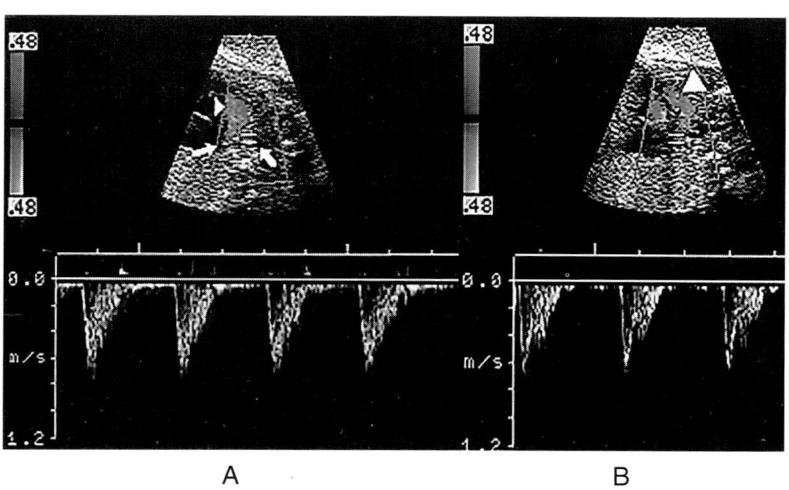

FIGURE 13–28.
(See Color Figure 13–28.) Although flow within right and left pulmonary artery branches (arrows) of the main pulmonary artery (arrowhead) is seen clearly on the color map, pulsed Doppler sampling can be performed even without color Doppler. *A*, Left pulmonary artery. *B*, Right pulmonary artery.

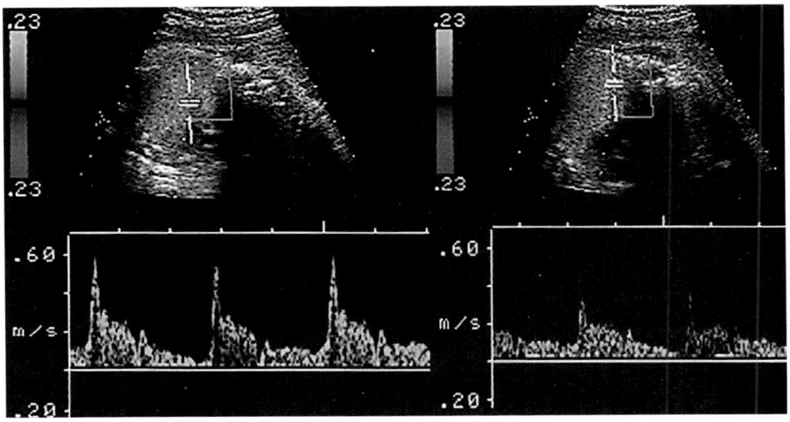

FIGURE 13–29.
(See Color Figure 13–29.) Waveforms of the distal pulmonary arterial branches of the lungs demonstrate an initial needlelike systolic peak and a rapid diastolic decay. This appearance suggests the effects of high vascular resistance in the pulmonary bed. The shape of the waveform remains unchanged as pulsed Doppler sampling moves farther into the periphery of the lungs, although peak systolic velocities decrease.

pressures during the cardiac cycle (Fig. 13–30).

The azygos vein is commonly seen coursing adjacent to the upper abdominal aorta. Color and pulsed Doppler demonstrate flow in this vessel in the opposite direction to that in the aorta (Fig. 13–31). The azygos vein continues into the chest to the right of the descending thoracic aorta. The azygos vein courses anteriorly to empty into the SVC just cranial to the right atrium.

Cerebral

The left and right internal carotid arteries and the vertebral arteries supply the circle of Willis. Sweeping the transducer superiorly, the internal carotid artery (ICA) can be seen dividing into the MCA and anterior cerebral artery (ACA). The circle of Willis is best visualized with conventional sonography on an axial plane that includes the cerebral peduncles. Real-time sonography demonstrates the MCA pulsating adjacent to the insula.[57–60]

There is high resistance in all cerebral arteries early in the first and second trimester, manifested on the time–velocity waveform by little or no diastolic flow (Fig. 13–32). RI in the cerebral vessels decreases somewhat toward the end of pregnancy.[61,62] The ICA and MCA flow velocity waveforms are similar in appearance, and thus, these vessels can be distinguished only on the basis of their location. Nevertheless, PI calculations for the ICA and ACA are slightly lower than for the

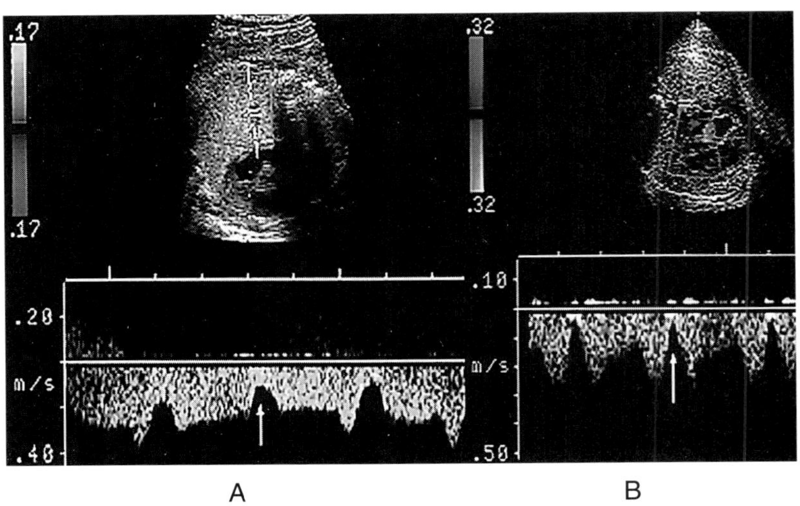

FIGURE 13–30.
(See Color Figure 13–30.) The pulmonary veins may be followed with color flow Doppler from the periphery of the lungs (*A*) to the left atrium (*B*). Similar modulations in the venous waveform due to changes in atrial pressures are seen in the pulmonary veins as in the inferior vena cava, hepatic veins, and ductus venosus. Arrows indicate slowing of forward flow due to atrial contraction.

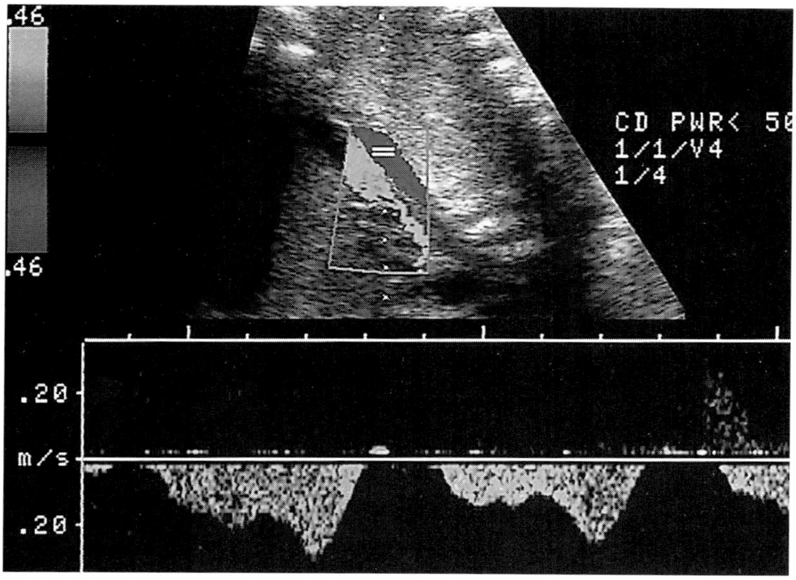

FIGURE 13–31.
(See Color Figure 13–31.) Color Doppler map demonstrates azygos vein coded blue, indicating opposite flow from that of the aorta, which is coded red-yellow because of aliasing. Pulsed Doppler interrogation reveals the venous waveform with low-frequency modulations produced by fetal breathing.

MCA. The mean PI value for the ICA is 1.5, for the ACA, 1.8, and for the MCA approximately 2.2.[59,60] Cerebral PI calculations may be clinically useful, because in fetuses with IUGR, intracranial arterial resistance decreases as descending aortic resistance rises.[62,63] (See Figure 16–26.) The jugular veins drain the intracerebral vessels into the SVC. Returning blood flow may be demonstrated with color Doppler sonography in these vessels as well as in the subclavian and brachiocephalic veins.

Extremities

Each leg is supplied by its femoral artery, which is the major branch of the external iliac artery. The superficial femoral artery, the major branch of the common femoral artery, courses toward the knee, where it travels posteriorly, continuing as the popliteal artery. The popliteal artery travels a short distance in the upper calf before it trifurcates into the anterior tibial, posterior tibial, and peroneal ar-

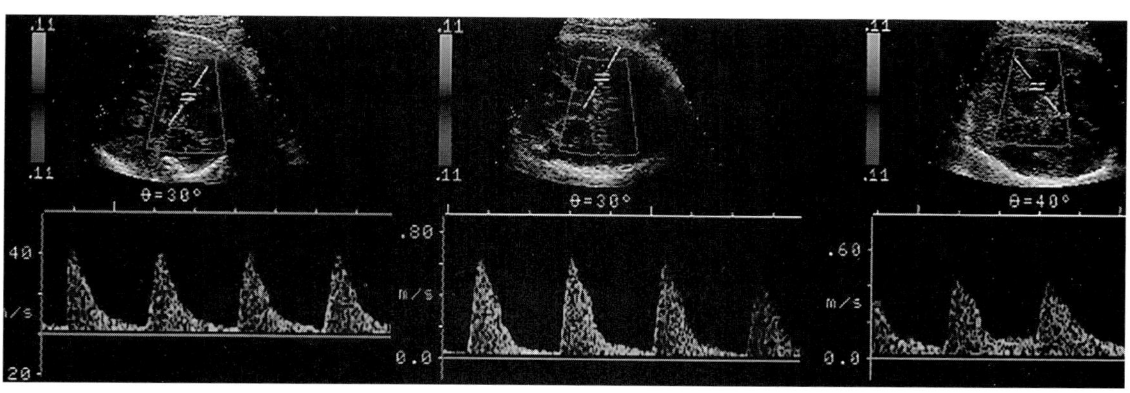

A B C

FIGURE 13–32.
Color and pulsed Doppler of the cerebral arteries. *A*, Anterior cerebral (ACA). *B*, Middle cerebral (MCA). *C*, Posterior cerebral (PCA). The flow velocity waveforms of the ACA and the MCA are similar, although their pulsatility index values differ. The PCA has more diastolic flow than both the ACA and MCA, denoting lower resistance to flow.

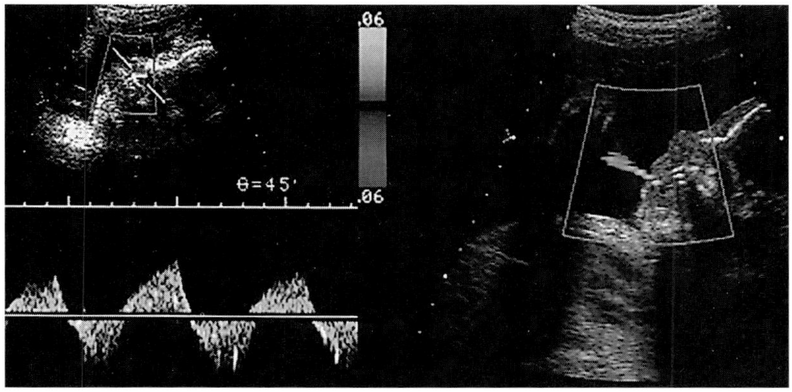

A B

FIGURE 13–33.
(See Color Figure 13–33.) Fetal breathing motion on Doppler in a 32-week fetus. *A*, Sagittal view of a fetal face with a color Doppler map demonstrating movement of amniotic fluid during breathing motion. *B*, Pulsed Doppler demonstrates a waveform of the amniotic fluid movement in the nasopharynx. Inspiration is plotted below the base line, and expiration is plotted above the base line.changes in atrial pressures are seen in the pulmonary veins as in the inferior vena cava, hepatic veins, and ductus venosus. Arrows indicate slowing of forward flow due to atrial contraction.

teries, supplying the lower calf, ankle, and foot. Flow in a fetus can be demonstrated within each of these vessels with color Doppler sonography. The veins of the thigh and calf are seen in parallel with the arteries. Color and pulsed Doppler interrogation confirms oppositely directed flow. Color and pulsed Doppler sonography similarly demonstrates flow within the vessels of the arms.

Miscellaneous Uses

Doppler evaluation need not be limited to measuring flow within blood vessels. Both color and pulsed Doppler can evaluate flow involving fetal respiration, swallowing, and urination. Color Doppler imaging quickly demonstrates this flow and aids in the efficient placement of the pulsed Doppler range gate for analysis of velocity of flow, flow velocity waveforms, and frequency of occurrence. Fetal breathing is virtually nonexistent in the early second trimester but generally increases in frequency with gestation. This rhythmic activity is usually monitored by observing abdominal movements with conventional real-time sonography. It has been suggested that use of color and pulsed Doppler sonography results in more sensitive detection of this activity.[64, 65] Furthermore, it is possible that analysis of the time–velocity waveform of amniotic fluid movement associated with breathing motion may yield clinically important diagnostic information. These waveforms can be obtained by Doppler interrogation over the respiratory tract of a fetus[64, 65] (Fig. 13–33).

REFERENCES

1. Brar H, Medearis A, Devore G, et al: Fetal umbilical velocimetry using continuous wave and pulsed wave Doppler ultrasound in high risk pregnancies: A comparison of systolic to diastolic ratios. Obstet Gynecol 1988;72:607–610.
2. Schulman H, Winter D, Farmakides G, et al: Pregnancy surveillance with Doppler velocimetry of uterine and umbilical arteries. Am J Obstet Gynecol 1989;160:192–196.
3. Jauniaux E, Jurkovic D, Campbell S, et al: Investigation of placental circulations by color Doppler ultrasonography. Am J Obstet Gynecol 1991;164: 486–488.
4. Jouppila P: Studies of uteroplacental and fetal hemodynamics by Doppler ultrasonography. Curr Opin Obstet Gynecol 1991;3:248–254.
5. Jauniaux E, Jurkovic D, Campbell S: In vivo investigations of the anatomy and the physiology of early human placental circulations. Obstet Gynecol 1991; 1:435–445.
6. Hseih F, Kuo P, Ko T, et al: Doppler velocimetry of intraplacental fetal arteries. Obstet Gynecol 1991;77: 478–482.
7. Vyas S, Nicolaides K, Campbell S: Renal artery flow-velocity waveforms in normal and hypoxemic fetuses. Am J Obstet Gynecol 1989;161:168–172.
8. Copel JA, Morotti R, Hobbins JC, et al: The antenatal diagnosis of congenital heart disease using fetal echocardiography: Is color flow mapping necessary? Obstet Gynecol 1991;78(1):1–8.
9. Zweibel W: Introduction to Vascular Anatomy, 2nd ed. Grune & Stratton, New York, 1986.
10. Miller D: Update on safety of diagnostic ultrasonography. J Clin Ultrasound 1991;19:531–540.
11. United States Food and Drug Administration: Guideline for measuring and reporting acoustic output of diagnostic ultrasound medical devices. Ultrasound Medical Devices. US Government Printing Office, Washington, DC, 1987; FDA/CDRH 510K.
12. American Institute of Ultrasound in Medicine: Bioeffects Considerations for the Safety of Diagnostic Ul-

trasound. American Institute of Ultrasound in Medicine, Bethesda, MD, 1988.
13. Nyborg W, Ziskin M: Biological Effects of Ultrasound, vol 13. Churchill Livingstone, New York, 1985, pp 167–186.
14. Stewart H, Stewart H, Moore R, et al: Compilation of reported biological effects data and ultrasound exposure levels. J Clin Ultrasound 1985;13:167–186.
15. Mitchell D: Color Doppler imaging: Principles, limitations, and artifacts. Radiology 1990;177:1–10.
16. Kremkau F: Diagnostic Ultrasound: Principles, Instruments, and Excercises, vol 7. WB Saunders, Philadelphia, 1989, pp 131–133.
17. Taylor K, Holland S: Doppler U.S. I. Basic principles, instrumentation, and pitfalls. Radiology 1990;174: 297–307.
18. Kremkau F: Seeing and hearing blood flow noninvasively using the Doppler shift. Diagn Imag 1985; 7:131–133.
19. Arduini D, Rizzo G, Buccolini M, et al: Functional assessment of uteroplacental and fetal circulations by means of color Doppler ultrasonography. J Ultrasound Med 1990;9:249–253.
20. Gill R, Kossoff G, Warren P, et al: Umbilical venous flow in normal and complicated pregnancy. Ultrasound Med Biol 1984;10:349–363.
21. Cohnstein J, Zuntz N: Untersuchungen uber das Blut, den Kreislauf und die Athmung beim Saugethier-Fotus. Pflugers Arch Ges Physiol 1884;34:173–233.
22. Cooper K, Greenfield A, Huggett, A. St. G. The umbilical blood flow in the sheep. J Physiol 1949; 108:160–166.
23. Stembera C, Hodr J, Janda J: Umbilical blood flow in healthy newborn infants during the first minutes after birth. Am J Obstet Gynecol 1965;91:568–574.
24. McCallum W: Thermodilution measurement of human umbilical blood flow at delivery. Am J Obstet Gynecol 1977;127:491–496.
25. Assali N, Rauramo L, Peltonen T: Measurement of uterine blood flow and uterine metabolism. VIII. Uterine and fetal blood flow and oxygen consumption in early human pregnancy. Am J Obstet Gynecol 1960;79:86–98.
26. Rudoph A, Heymann M, Teramo K, et al: Studies on the circulation of the previable human fetus. Pediatr Res 1971;5:452–465.
27. FitzGerald D, Stuart B, Drumm J, et al: The assessment of feto-placental circulation with continuous wave Doppler ultrasound. Ultrasound Med Biol 1984;10:371–376.
28. Eik-Nes S, Brubakk A, Ulstein M: Measurement of human fetal blood flow. Br Med J 1980;280:283–284.
29. Kurjak A, Rajhvajn B: Ultrasonic measurements of umbilical blood flow in normal and complicated pregnancies. J Perinat Med 1982;10:3–16.
30. Fleischer A, Emerson D: Color Doppler Sonography in Obstetrics and Gynecology. Churchill Livingstone, New York, 1993, p 333.
31. Mehalek K, Berkowitz G, Chitkara U, et al: Comparison of continuous wave and pulsed Doppler S/D ratios of umbilical and uterine arteries. Am J Obstet Gynecol 1988;72(4):603–606.
32. Kofinas A, Penry M, Greiss F, et al: The effect of placental location on uterine artery flow velocity waveforms. Am J Obstet Gynecol 1988;159(6): 1504–1508.
33. Trudinger B, Cook C, Giles W, et al: Fetal umbilical artery flow velocity waveforms and placental resistance: Clinical significance. Br J Obstet Gynaecol 1985;92:23.
34. Stuart B, Drumm J, FitzGerald D, et al: Fetal blood velocity waveforms in normal pregnancy. Br J Obstet Gynaecol 1980;87:780.
35. Giles W, Lingman G, Marsal K, et al: Fetal volume blood flow and umbilical artery flow velocity waveform analysis: A comparison. Br J Obstet Gynecol 1986;93:461.
36. Erskine R, Ritchie J: Quantitative measurement of fetal blood flow using Doppler ultrasound. Br J Obstet Gynaecol 1985;92:600.
37. Abramowicz J, Warsof S, Arrington J, et al: Doppler analysis of the umbilical artery: The importance of choosing the placental end of the cord. J Ultrasound Med 1989;8:219–221.
38. Sadler T: Langman's Medical Embryology. 5th ed. Williams & Wilkins, Baltimore, 1985.
39. Pansky B: Review of Medical Embryology. Macmillan, New York, 1982, p 527.
40. Dawes G: The umbilical circulation. Am J Obstet Gynecol 1962;84:1634.
41. Jouppila P, Kirkinen P: Umbilical vein blood flow as an indicator of fetal hypoxia. Br J Obstet Gynecol 1984;91:107.
42. Cohen-Overbeek T, Pearce J, Campbell S: The antenatal assessment of utero-placental and feto-placental blood flow using Doppler ultrasound. Ultrasound Med Biol 1985;11(329).
43. Griffin D, Cohen-Overbeek T, Campbell S: Fetal utero-placental blood flow. Clin Obstet Gynecol 1983;10:565.
44. Maulik D, Yarlagadda P, Downing G: Doppler velocimetry in obstetrics. Obstet Gynecol Clin North Am 1990;17:163–186.
45. Gill R: Measurement of blood flow by ultrasound: Accuracy and sources of error. Ultrasound Med Biol 1985;11:625.
46. Giles W, Trudinger B, Baird P: Fetal umbilical artery flow velocity waveforms and placental resistance: Pathological correlation. Br J Obstet Gynecol 1985; 92:31.
47. Emerson D, Cartier M, Brown D, et al: Shunting of umbilical vein blood via the ductus venosus: Fetal Doppler study. Radiology 1989;(173):249.
48. Edelstone D, Rudolph A, Heymann M: Liver and ductus venosus blood flows in fetal limbs in utero. Circ Res 1978;42:426–433.
49. Kiserud T, Eik-Nes S, Blaas H, et al: Ultrasonographic velocimetry of the fetal ductus venosus. Lancet 1991;338:1412–1414.
50. Cartier M, Emerson D, Felker R, et al: Color and pulsed Doppler of the fetal superior mesenteric artery. J Ultrasound Med 1992;11(Suppl):531.
51. Cartier M, Emerson D, Felker R, et al: Pulsed Doppler waveforms of renal arteries in the fetus. J Ultrasound Med 1990;9(Suppl):S32.
52. Reed K, Sahn D, Scagnelli S, et al: Doppler echocardiographic studies of diastolic function in the human fetal heart: Changes during gestation. J Am Coll Cardiol 1986;8:391–395.
53. Reed K, Meijboom E, Shan D, et al: Cardiac Doppler flow velocities in human fetuses. Circulation 1986;73: 41–46.
54. Van Praagh R, Weinberg P, Matsuoka R, et al: Malpositions of the heart. In: Adams F, Emmanuoilides G, eds: Moss' Heart Disease in Infants, Children, and Adolescents, 3rd ed. Williams & Wilkins, Baltimore, 1984, pp 422–458.
55. Huhta J, Moise K, Fisher D, et al: Detection and quantitation of constriction of the fetal ductus arteriosus by Doppler echocardiography. Circulation 1987;75: 406–412.
56. Emerson D, Cartier M, DeVore G, et al: Distal pul-

monary artery branches in the fetus: New observations with color flow and pulsed Doppler. J Ultrasound Med 1991;10(S):S19.

57. Arbeille P, Tranquart F, Berson M, et al: Visualization of the fetal circle of Willis and intra-cerebral arteries by color-coded Doppler. Eur J Obstet Gynecol Reprod Biol 1989;32:195–198.
58. Arbeille P, Body G, Fignon A, et al: Doppler assessment of the intracerebral circulation of the fetus. Clin Phys Physiol Meas 1989;10:51–57.
59. Woo J, Liang S, Roxy L, et al: Middle cerebral artery Doppler flow velocity waveforms. Obstet Gynecol 1987;4:613–616.
60. Mari G, Moise KJ, Deter RL, et al: Doppler assessment of the pulsatility index in the cerebral circulation of the human fetus. Am J Obstet Gynecol 1989;160:698–703.
61. Kirkinen P, Muller R, Huch R, et al: Blood flow velocity waveforms in human fetal intracranial arteries. Obstet Gynecol 1987;4:617–621.
62. Griffin D, Bilardo K, Masini L, et al: Doppler blood flow waveforms in the descending thoracic aorta of the human fetus. Br J Obstet Gynaecol 1984;94: 997–1006.
63. Wladimiroff JW, Tonge HM, Stewart PA: Doppler ultrasound assessment of cerebral blood flow in the human fetus. Br J Obstet Gynaecol 1986;93: 471–475.
64. Birnholz J, Isaacson G: Fetal nose breathing. Radiology 1990;177:194.
65. Isaacson G, Birnholz JC: Human fetal upper respiratory tract function as revealed by ultrasonography. Ann Otol Rhinol Laryngol 1991;100: 743–747.

CHAPTER 14

ABDOMEN

Marcus L. Lines, M.D.
Robert M. Milman, M.D.

First Trimester

The fetal abdomen is best seen after 14 to 16 weeks' gestation; however, improved sonographic techniques and equipment have allowed for better visualization in first-trimester pregnancies. Several key events in abdominal development occur in the first trimester. Of particular interest to sonographers are changes involving the abdominal wall and gut. The umbilical cord forms during the first 5 weeks of gestation as a result of fusion of the omphalomesenteric duct and the allantoic duct. It eventually becomes enveloped by the amniotic membranes as the amniotic cavity enlarges. The yolk sac is connected to the embryo by the omphalomesenteric duct. A portion of the yolk sac becomes incorporated into the primitive gut, and the remainder of the yolk sac and duct separates from the developing primitive gut by the eighth week of gestation. During the sixth week, the midgut begins to elongate faster than the embryo's body. Because of its rapid growth, the midgut herniates or projects into the umbilical cord, resulting in a normal herniation (Figs. 14–1 and 14–2). It may be visualized as a bulge or thickening of the umbilical cord near the anterior fetal abdominal wall. This pseudoherniation of the midgut is seen at the sixth to ninth week of gestation. The bowel undergoes a 90-degree rotation around the axis of the superior mesenteric artery. During the 10th week, it rapidly returns to the abdomen and rotates another 180 degrees counterclockwise to complete normal bowel migration (Figs. 14–3 and 14–4). This return is likely the result of enlargement of the abdominal cavity and the relative decrease in size of the liver and kidneys.[1] This pseudoherniation is usually reduced by 11 weeks or slightly later in some cases. Therefore, it is important that the diagnosis of abdominal wall defects, such as omphalocele or gastroschisis, should not be made before the 14th week of gestation.[2] A pseudo-omphalocele may also be seen when the fetal abdomen is compressed transversely between the walls of the uterus or placenta, causing a compensating protrusion of the anterior abdomen. This may be a transient compression in a normal fetus and can change with fetal movement, or it may be seen in association with oligohydramnios.[3]

Second and Third Trimesters

By the beginning of the second trimester, the abdominal organs have attained their normal adult positions. The liver, kidneys, and

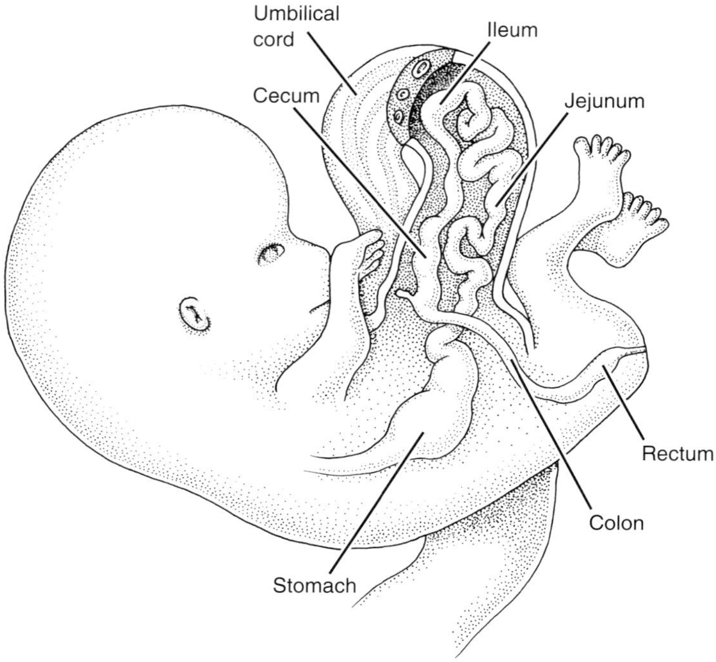

FIGURE 14–1.
PSEUDO-OMPHALOCELE: UMBILICAL HERNIATION.
Schematic drawing of the fetal gut herniating into the umbilical cord before 14 LMP weeks (see Fig. 14–2 for the corresponding sonogram).

stomach are easily identified, but visualization of the pancreas and spleen is much more variable. The large bowel is better seen in the third trimester as it becomes fluid filled, and the small bowel is often seen.

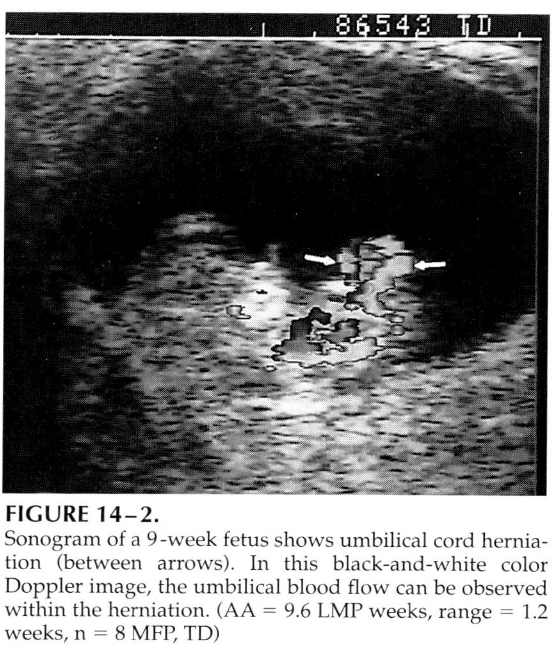

FIGURE 14–2.
Sonogram of a 9-week fetus shows umbilical cord herniation (between arrows). In this black-and-white color Doppler image, the umbilical blood flow can be observed within the herniation. (AA = 9.6 LMP weeks, range = 1.2 weeks, n = 8 MFP, TD)

ABDOMINAL WALL

The anterior abdominal wall is well visualized by the 14th week of gestation, because the midgut has returned to the abdominal cavity by that time. Only the umbilical cord interrupts the smooth outward convexity of the abdominal wall. The abdominal wall muscles are hypoechoic, with occasional thin echogenic lines representing fascial planes between the three main muscle groups: the internal oblique, transverse abdominis, and external oblique muscles. The sonolucent band representing normal muscle should not be mistaken for ascites. This pseudoascites is always confined to the anterior abdominal wall and is not seen within the peritoneal recesses[4] or surrounding bowel loops within the abdomen (Figs. 14–5 to 14–7).

The skin thickness should be observed and should be less than 5 mm. Skin thickness greater than 5 mm may reflect the presence of skin edema or anasarca, and the fetus may have hydrops fetalis. Hydrops fetalis may be immune and secondary to Rh incompatibility between the mother and fetus or may be nonimmune. Nonimmune hydrops fetalis is often idiopathic, but causes include hematological, infectious, cardiac, or metabolic abnormali-

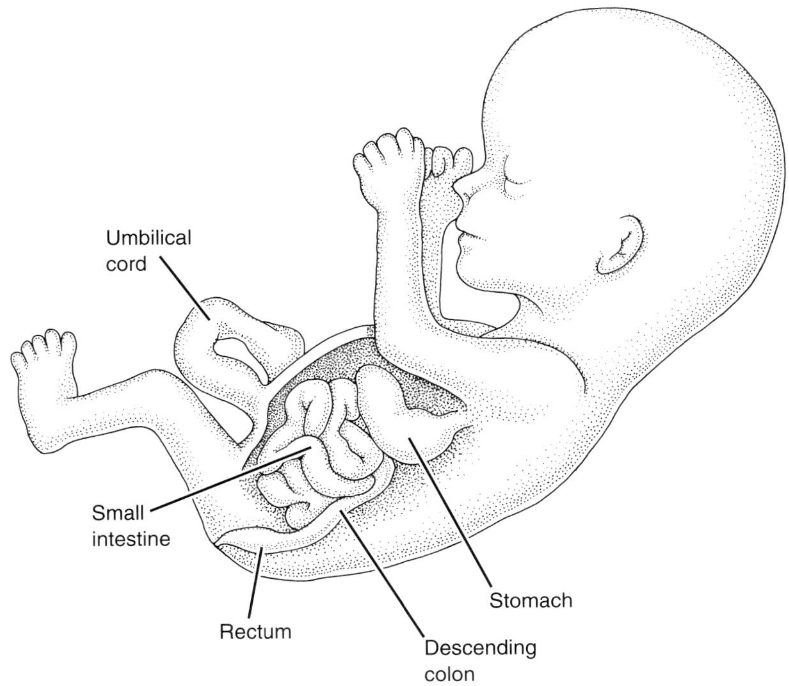

FIGURE 14–3. UMBILICAL HERNIATION RESOLVED. The normal umbilical cord insertion into the fetal abdominal wall and bowel is shown after the 14th LMP week. This drawing corresponds to the sonogram in Figure 14–4.

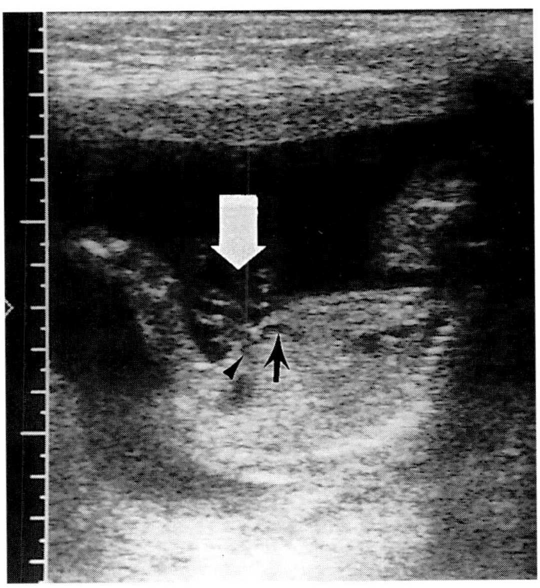

FIGURE 14–4.
The umbilical insertion into the anterior abdominal wall of a 17-LMP-week fetus is shown. The umbilical vein (black arrow) can be seen coursing cephalad, and an umbilical artery (black arrowhead) is seen coursing caudad. The loops of umbilical cord (large white arrow) anterior to the abdominal wall should not be mistaken for a gastroschisis or omphalocele. (AA = 17.6 LMP weeks, range = 1.2 weeks, n = 10 MFP, TD)

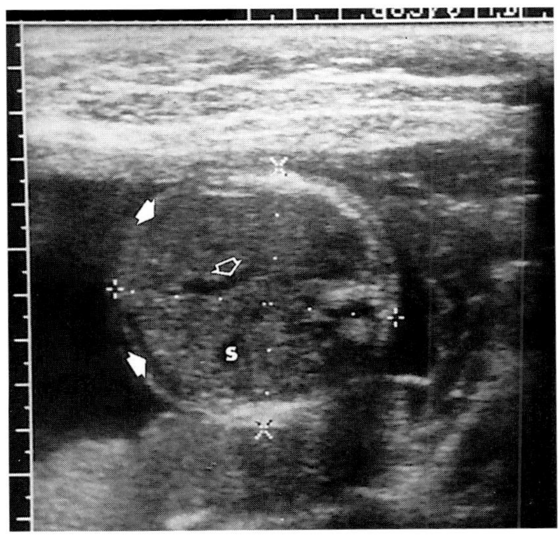

FIGURE 14–5. ABDOMINAL WALL WITH PSEUDOASCITES.
The correct plane for the abdominal circumference measurement is shown. The anteroposterior abdominal diameter, between the + cursors, measures 63.5 mm from the outer skin line at the anterior abdominal wall to the outer skin line just behind the spine. The transverse abdominal diameter is measured at the outer skin lines at the fetal sides. The sonographer should make sure to measure to the skin and not to the more obvious rib or peritoneal echoes. The hypoechoic pseudoascites (solid arrows) can be observed just inside the anterior abdominal wall. The curve of the umbilical vein (open arrow) to the fetal right and into the liver is also shown, as is the stomach (s). This image is illustrated in Figure 14–6. (AA = 24.8 LMP, range = 1.2 weeks, n = 9 MFP, TD)

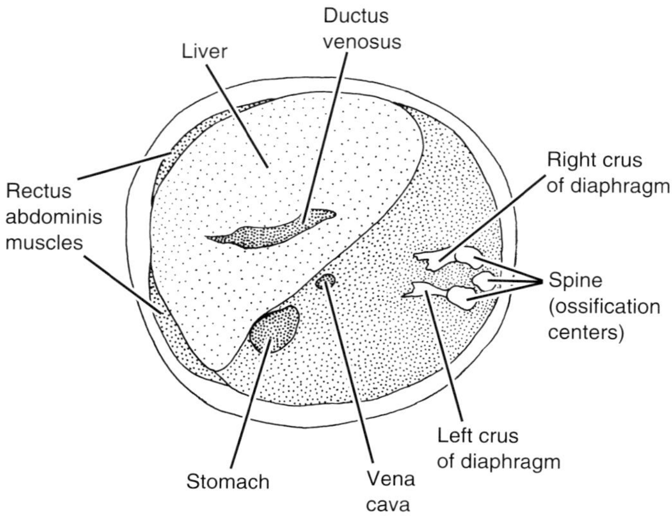

FIGURE 14–6.
Illustration of the anatomy shown in Figure 14–5. The correct level for the abdominal circumference measurement is perpendicular to the fetal spine and at the level where the umbilical vein curves right, joining the left portal sinus and vein. The hypoechoic rectus abdominis muscles (arrows in Fig. 14–5) should not be mistaken for fetal ascites.

ties.[5,6] Although skin thickness is often increased in this condition, accumulation of fluid is usually noted in the pleural, pericardial, and peritoneal spaces.[5]

The thickness of the subcutaneous tissue is not a reliable indicator of fetal growth abnormalities, although tissue thickness less than or equal to 2 mm or greater than or equal to 8 mm beyond 34 weeks' gestation may be an indicator of fetal growth disturbances.[7]

Evaluation of the anterior abdominal wall also helps to determine the location for measurement of the abdominal circumference (AC). Once the umbilical cord insertion is located in a transverse image through the fetal abdomen, the umbilical vein is followed into the fetal liver to the point where it empties into the ductus venosus at the level of the left portal vein. This is the level used for AC measurement[8] (see Figs. 14–5 to 14–7). The AC measurement should also be perpendicular to the fetal spine (see Chapter 7 for the use of the AC for fetal size and age analysis).

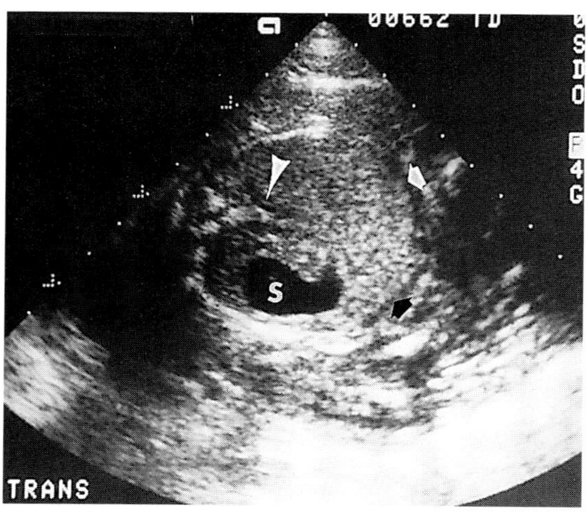

FIGURE 14–7.
Transverse image of the fetal abdomen also demonstrates the pseudoascites of the abdominal muscles (black and white arrows) and stomach (S). The umbilical vein is not visualized in this image and therefore should not be used for abdominal circumference measurements. The right adrenal gland (white arrowhead) is seen. (AA = 21.9 LMP, range = 2.8 weeks, n = 9 MFP, TD)

The two most common ventral wall defects are omphaloceles and gastroschisis. Both are associated with exteriorization of abdominal contents. An omphalocele is a true midline defect at the level of the umbilicus, with the abdominal contents covered by a thin peritoneal membrane. Gastroschisis is a paraumbilical defect usually to the right of midline, with no associated covering membrane (Fig 14–8). Prognostically, gastroschisis is usually an isolated defect, whereas omphaloceles are often associated with other congenital anomalies including cardiac, genitourinary, gastrointestinal, and neural tube defects.[9]

THE FETAL GASTROINTESTINAL TRACT

Sonographically, the stomach appears as an anechoic bubble as early as 10 weeks and becomes more visible as fetal swallowing improves (Fig. 14–9). It is seen in the left upper quadrant and may be noted to empty and fill during the course of an examination. Al-

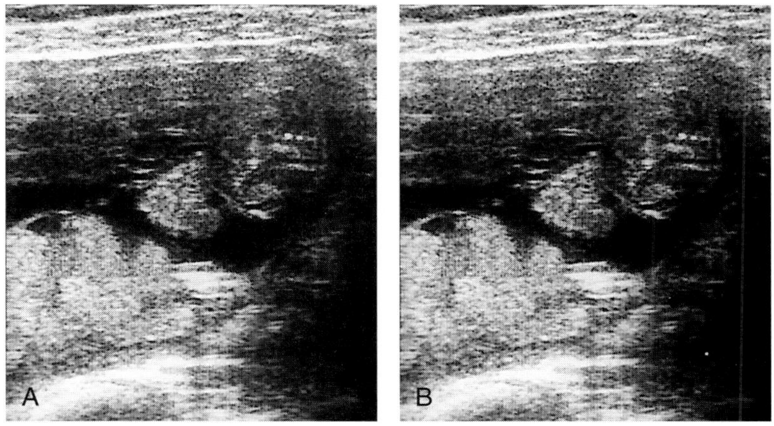

FIGURE 14–8.
Gastroschisis is demonstrated in *A* and *B* by echogenic bowel lying anterior to the fetal abdominal wall. *B*, Free loops of umbilical cord can also be seen adjacent to the echogenic bowel. Color Doppler interrogation can be helpful to differentiate between loops of cord and loops of fluid-filled bowel. (AA = 19.3 LMP, range = 2.3 weeks, n = 9 MFP, DKD)

though typically sonolucent, the intraluminal contents of the stomach may contain echogenic debris or a pseudomass. This may be the result of aggregates of swallowed cells and cell fragments.[10] It is important to visualize the stomach, because its absence on fetal sonograms obtained after 14 weeks' gestational age is highly suggestive of a fetal gastrointestinal abnormality, and sonography should be repeated in those patients.[11] The coronal view of the abdomen may allow visualization of three fluid cavities—the heart, stomach, and urinary bladder. Figure 14–9*B* shows these fluid cavities in normal relationship. The stomach should be between the heart and bladder and near the left lateral abdominal wall. In cases of diaphragmatic hernia, the stomach may be found in the thorax,

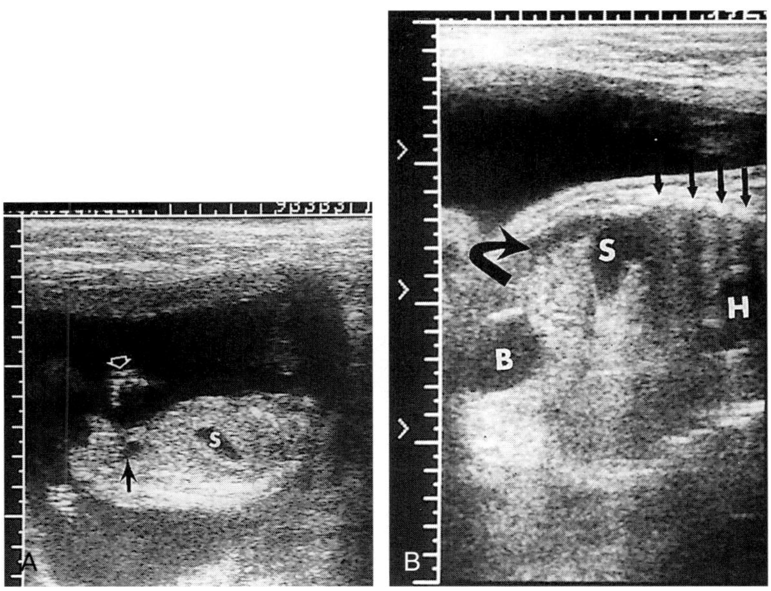

FIGURE 14–9.
A, Parasagittal plane through the fetal stomach (S). The fetal bladder (black arrow) can be observed in the pelvis. The fetal hand (open arrow) was observed to be touching the umbilical cord just anterior to the abdominal wall. The amniotic fluid was considered to be in excess of normal in this case. (AA = 17.6 LMP, range = 1.2 weeks, n = 10 MFP, TD) *B*, Coronal view of the fetal abdomen shows the three fluid cavities, heart (H), stomach (S), and urinary bladder (B) in normal relationships. Ribs (straight arrows) cast acoustic shadows across the heart. The echogenicity of the small bowel can be observed between the stomach and bladder, and a short portion of the descending colon (curved arrow) is seen adjacent to the stomach. (AA = 37.7 LMP, range = 3.7 weeks, n = 9 MFP, TD)

next to the heart. Although in some cases the stomach or bladder may be empty at the time of the examination, a few minutes' wait usually allows enough filling to determine their location in a normal fetus.

Small Intestine

The small bowel is centrally located and changes its appearance with peristalsis. In Figure 14–10*A*, the small bowel can be observed adjacent to the urinary bladder. Peristaltic waves may be seen in the second trimester, characterized by vigorous fleeting movements that become more prolonged in the third trimester. Normal small bowel is less than 7 mm in diameter and 15 mm in length, and small bowel loops are normally transient. Segments that have a fixed position should also suggest small bowel pathology.[12] The small bowel may be seen as an increased echogenicity in the fetal abdomen in the second trimester.[13] The hyperechoic appearance may be due to collapsed loops of small bowel or mesenteric fat between collapsed loops.[14] Other causes of increased echogenicity are reported to be meconium peritonitis, meconium ileus, infections, neoplasms, and cystic fibrosis.[13–17] As pregnancy progresses and more amniotic fluid is swallowed, the bowel loops become more sonolucent with rounded hypoechoic areas.[18]

Small bowel dilatation may be seen secondary to atresia, malrotation, or meconium ileus. Duodenal atresia is recognized sonographically by the fluid-filled double bubble in the fetal abdomen, secondary to an overdistended stomach in the left upper quadrant and an enlarged duodenum on the right. Duodenal atresia is associated with a high incidence of other congenital anomalies, and its presence should prompt careful sonographic evaluation of the fetus. The double-bubble sign may be associated with other forms of obstruction such as Ladd's bands, midgut volvulus, annular pancreas, and duodenal web.[9]

Small bowel obstruction distal to the duodenum results in increasing numbers of dilated small bowel loops, often associated with polyhydramnios. These obstructions are most commonly due to atresias secondary to in utero vascular accidents.[18]

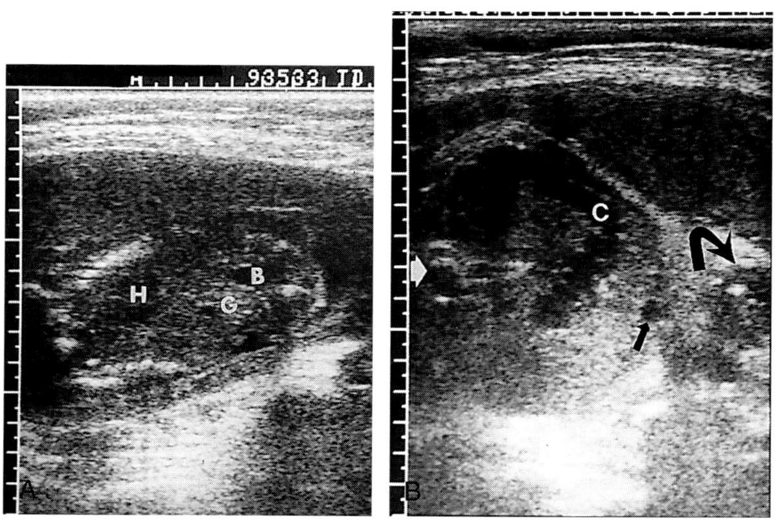

FIGURE 14–10. SMALL BOWEL. *A*, WEEK 21 BOWEL.
Coronal view of the fetal trunk shows the fetal heart (H), gut (G), and urinary bladder (B). The stomach and colon are not seen in this image. The echogenicity of the bowel can be observed adjacent to the bladder. (AA = 21.1 LMP, range = 1.4 weeks, n = 9 MFP, TD)
B, WEEK 35 BOWEL.
The colon (C) is obvious in the third trimester. Because the fetus was noted to be in a cephalic presentation, we can infer that the fetal left side is anterior by conventional sonographic presentation; thus, portions of the transverse and descending colon are visualized. The umbilical cord insertion (small black arrow) is seen, as is a portion of the transverse spine (white arrow). A fetal extremity (curved black arrow), most likely the knee, is seen at the edge of the image anterior to the abdominal wall. (AA = 34.8 LMP, range = 1.4 weeks, n = 9 MFP, TD)

Large Intestine

The colon is a hypoechoic tubular structure at the periphery of the abdomen. It may be seen as early as 22 weeks but typically is seen after 28 weeks. Figure 14–10*B* shows a normal colon in a 34.8-week fetus. The diameter of the colon, measured from the inner walls, progressively enlarges from 4 to 6 mm up to 10 to 18 mm at term.[12] No significant peristalsis of the colon is seen, and meconium is routinely visualized. Meconium accumulation fills the colon and is hypoechoic as compared with the bowel wall. Colonic segments greater than 18 mm in diameter are considered abnormal. Obstructions may be secondary anorectal malformations, meconium plug syndrome, or Hirschsprung's disease. Anal agenesis, imperforate anus, and rectal atresias are anorectal malformations that are usually associated with other complex abnormalities. In the meconium plug syndrome, a collection of meconium causes a transient obstruction in the distal colon. Hirschsprung's disease is a result of the congenital absence of ganglion cells in the colonic wall, which precludes normal peristalsis, and functional obstruction develops. These different causes are difficult to distinguish until after birth, however.

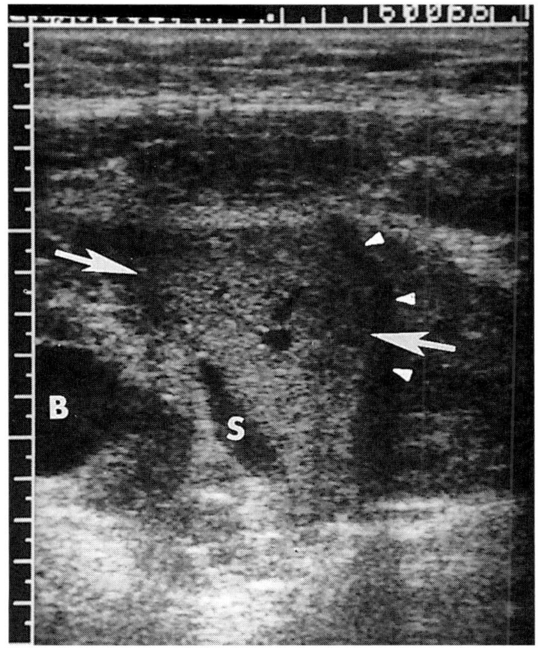

FIGURE 14–12. WEEK 40 CORONAL LIVER.
In this term fetus, the liver is well visualized. The liver length (between long arrows) is approximately 57 mm and normal for this age. The diaphragm is a hypoechoic curve (arrowheads) and marks the dome of the liver. The stomach (S) and urinary bladder (B) are also seen. (AA = 39.9 LMP, range = 3.6 weeks, n = 9 MFP, TD)

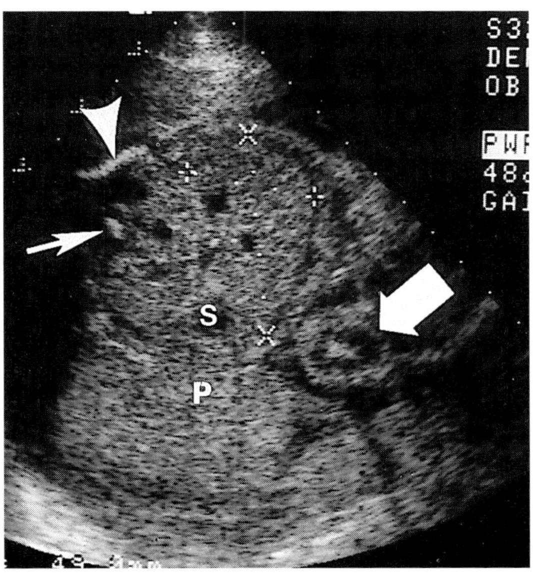

FIGURE 14–11. WEEK 21 LIVER.
Oblique longitudinal view of the fetal abdomen with liver measurements. The X cursors measure the transverse liver diameter (49 mm), and the + cursors the length (31.8 mm), which is normal for the fetal age. The fetal spine (thin arrow) is not well visualized in this image because of shadowing from an iliac bone (arrowhead). The stomach (S) is adjacent the left lobe of the liver. A cross section of one fetal extremity (wide arrow) is seen anterior to the abdominal wall. The placenta (P) is posterior to the fetus. (AA = 24.6 LMP, range = 1.3 weeks, n = 9 MFP, TD)

Liver

The fetal liver occupies the right upper portion of the abdomen and extends across the midline to the left lateral abdominal wall. The liver is a large organ representing 10% of the fetal weight at 11 weeks' gestation and 5% at term.[19] The relative sizes of the right and left lobes differ in a fetus and an adult. In a fetus, the left lobe is larger than the right. Gross and colleagues compared the size of the lateral segment of the fetal left lobe with the remainder of the liver and found a mean ratio of 1.04, which was constant regardless of fetal age.[20] In adults, this ratio measured 0.76. The disproportionate fetal left lobe size presumably is due to a greater percentage of oxygenated blood reaching the left lobe. The length of the liver is determined by measuring in the longitudinal plane from the right hemidiaphragm to the inferior liver margin (Figs. 14–11 and 14–12). Table 14–1 shows nor-

TABLE 14–1. ABDOMINAL ORGANS: SIZE/AGE

AGE (LMP WEEKS)	LIVER Long Axis (mm)			AGE (LMP WEEKS)	KIDNEY Long Axis (mm)			KIDNEY Anteroposterior (mm)			AGE (LMP WEEKS)	SPLEEN Long Axis (mm)			SPLEEN Transverse Axis (mm)		
	Mean	*−2 SD*	*+2 SD*		*Mean*	*−2 SD*	*+2 SD*	*Mean*	*−2 SD*	*+2 SD*		*Mean*	*−2 SD*	*+2 SD*	*Mean*	*−2 SD*	*+2 SD*
18				18							18	14	7	21	9	4	13
19				19							19	16	12	23	9	4	14
20	27.3	20.9	33.7	20							20	18	11	26	10	5	15
21	28	26.5	29.5	21							21	20	12	27	11	6	16
22	30.6	23.9	37.3	22				11.1	8.7	13.5	22	22	15	29	12	7	16
23	30.9	26.4	35.4	23				11.5	9.1	13.9	23	23	16	31	12	8	17
24	32.9	26.2	39.6	24	24.4	22.0	26.8	11.9	9.5	14.3	24	25	19	32	13	8	18
25	33.6	28.3	38.9	25	25.0	22.6	27.4	12.4	10.0	14.8	25	26	19	33	14	9	19
26	35.7	29.4	42.0	26	25.7	23.3	28.1	13.0	10.6	15.4	26	27	20	34	15	10	19
27	36.6	33.3	39.9	27	26.4	24.0	28.8	13.5	11.1	15.9	27	29	22	37	15	10	20
28	38.4	34.4	42.4	28	27.2	24.8	29.6	14.2	11.8	16.6	28	31	24	38	16	11	21
29	39.1	34.1	44.1	29	28.0	25.6	30.4	14.8	12.4	17.2	29	33	25	40	17	12	21
30	38.7	33.7	43.7	30	28.8	26.4	31.2	15.5	13.1	17.9	30	34	27	41	17	13	22
31	39.6	33.9	45.3	31	29.6	27.2	32.0	16.3	13.9	18.7	31	36	30	43	18	13	23
32	42.7	35.2	50.2	32	30.4	28.0	32.8	17.1	14.7	19.5	32	38	31	45	19	14	24
33	43.8	37.2	50.4	33	31.3	28.9	33.7	18.0	15.6	20.4	33	40	33	47	20	15	24
34	44.8	37.7	51.9	34	32.2	29.8	34.6	18.9	16.5	21.3	34	43	35	50	20	16	25
35	47.8	38.7	56.9	35	33.1	30.8	35.4	19.9	17.5	22.3	35	45	38	52	21	16	26
36	49.0	41.4	57.4	36	34.1	31.8	36.4	20.9	18.5	23.3	36	48	41	55	22	17	27
37	52.0	45.2	58.8	37	35.1	32.8	37.4	22.0	19.6	24.4	37	51	44	58	23	18	27
38	52.9	48.7	57.1	38	36.1	33.8	38.4	23.2	20.8	25.6	38	54	47	62	23	18	28
39	55.4	48.7	62.1	39	37.1	34.8	39.4	24.4	22.0	26.8	39	58	51	65	24	19	29
40	59.0			40	38.2	35.9	40.5	25.7	23.3	28.1	40	62	55	70	25	20	29
41				41	39.3	37.0	41.6										
42				42	40.4	38.1	42.7										

This table was adapted from three different references for the size/age of the fetal liver, kidneys, and spleen. The liver and kidney data are from the original publication. The splenic measurements were treated with a locally weighted smoothing (LOWESS) algorithm (see Chapter 7 for an explanation of LOWESS).

Liver from Vintzileos AM, Neckles S, Campbell WA, et al: Fetal liver ultrasound measurements during normal pregnancy. Obstet Gynecol 1985;66:477–480. The above liver table is a LOWESS smoothing of the original data.

Kidney from Bertagnoli L, Gallicchio R, et al: Quantitative characterization of the growth of the fetal kidney. J Clin Ultrasound 1983;11:349–356.

Spleen from Schmidt W, Yarkoni S, Jeanty P, et al: Sonographic measurements of the fetal spleen: Clinical implications. J Ultrasound Med 1985;4:667–672. Note that the above spleen table shows measurements in millimeters. The original article reported measurements in centimeters, which were erroneously labeled *mm*. This error was reproduced in Romero R, Pilu G, Jeanty P, et al: Prenatal Diagnosis of Congenital Anomalies. Appleton & Lange, Norwalk, CT, 1988, p 247.

mal values for gestational age (see also Fig. 14–9*A*). The liver length increases proportionately to the AC from 20 weeks to term.[21] Liver size decreases with intrauterine growth retardation. Common causes of fetal hepatomegaly are listed in Table 14–2.[22]

The echotexture of the liver is uniform. Sonographically, the portal and hepatic veins are visualized but the normal hepatic arteries and bile ducts are not seen. The fetal intrahepatic circulation is seen routinely on sonographic imaging of the fetal abdomen (Figs. 14–13 and 14–14). Oxygenated placental blood containing necessary nutrients returns to the fetus via a single umbilical vein in the umbilical cord. At the cord insertion, the umbilical vein enters the fetal abdomen and makes a sharp cephalad turn (Figs. 14–15 and 14–16). The umbilical vein courses superiorly and to the right, entering the liver, and two umbilical arteries course inferiorly around the bladder and connect to the internal iliac arteries. No umbilical venous branches are present proximal to the liver. Passing into the liver, the umbilical vein becomes the umbilical portion of the left portal vein. Blood flow continues through the left portal vein and portal sinus and either into the liver or directly into the systemic circulation via the ductus venosus to the inferior vena cava (IVC). Branches of the left portal vein supply the left lobe. The right lobe receives most of its blood supply from the main portal vein and a limited volume from the portal sinus. Flow within the portal system accounts for 40% to 60% of umbilical venous blood, with the bulk going to the left lobe.[23, 24] Within the liver, blood from the portal system reaches the hepatic microcirculation and is drained by the hepatic veins into the IVC. The remainder of the umbilical venous blood flow bypasses the liver parenchyma through the ductus venosus, a fetal conduit from the portal sinus to the left hepatic vein or IVC (Figs. 14–14 to 14–16). The ductus venosus is narrow relative to the umbilical and left portal veins.[25] A sphincter at the origin of the ductus venosus regulates flow, preventing fetal cardiac volume overload.[26] Fetal compromise due to placental insufficiency causes the sphincter to relax and the ductus venosus to dilate, increasing blood flow.[27] The ductus venosus lies within the hepatogastric ligament between the left lobe and the caudate lobe of the liver. In the neonatal period, the ductus venosus closes and becomes the ligamentum venosum. The umbilical vein becomes the ligamentum teres, which in an adult is routinely imaged as an echogenic focus within the left lobe.

TABLE 14–2. COMMON CAUSES OF HEPATOMEGALY

- Infectious causes
  - Hepatitis
  - Cytomegalovirus infection
  - Rubella
  - Toxoplasmosis
  - Syphilis
  - Varicella
  - Coxsackievirus infection
- Congenital anemia
  - Congenital hemolytic anemias, such as spherocytosis
  - Isoimmunization
- Congestive heart failure
- Hepatic tumors
  - Mesenchymal hamartoma
  - Hemangioma
  - Metastatic neuroblastoma
  - Hepatoblastoma
  - Hemangiopericytoma
- Metabolic disorders
  - Galactosemia (AR)
  - Tyrosinemia (probably AR)
  - Alpha$_1$-antitrypsin deficiency (AR)
  - Disorders of the urea cycle (AR)
  - Methylmalonic acidemia (probably AR)
  - Infantile sialidosis (AR)
- Genetic disorders
  - Beckwith-Wiedemann syndrome (sporadic, some familial cases)
  - Zellweger's syndrome (AR)
- Hepatic cysts
  - Adult polycystic disease of liver and kidneys
  - Solitary cyst

AR, Autosomal recessive.
From Romero R, Pilu G, Jeanty P, et al: Prenatal Diagnosis of Congenital Anomalies. Appleton & Lange, Norwalk, CT, 1988, p 250.

Gallbladder

The fetal gallbladder is an anechoic ovoid structure located between the right and left lobes of the liver. The gallbladder is best imaged on transverse scans of the fetal abdomen

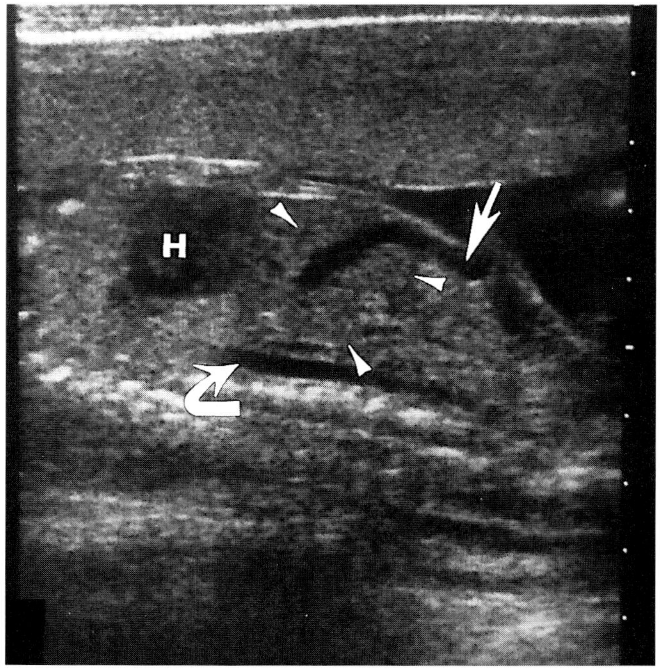

FIGURE 14–13.
WEEK 21 PARASAGITTAL.
Oblique parasagittal view of the fetal trunk shows the umbilical vein (long arrow) coursing cephalad into the liver (arrowheads). A portion of an umbilical artery is also visualized. The fetal aorta (curved arrow) is anterior to the fetal spine. The heart (H) is also seen. (AA = 21.0 LMP, range = 1.6 weeks, n = 8 MFP, SG)

and is routinely identified by the third trimester (Figs. 14–17 and 14–18). The portal-umbilical vein can be mistaken for the gallbladder (see Fig. 14–17), but the two structures can be differentiated by appearance and location. The portal-umbilical vein is tubular and can be traced back to the umbilical cord, whereas the gallbladder maintains its ovoid shape along the inferior surface of the liver. When a fatty meal or large glucose challenge is administered to a pregnant woman, no significant volume changes are seen within the fetal gallbladder.[28] Echogenic foci may be detected within the gallbladder lumen in the third trimester and are of uncertain clinical significance. In many of these cases, the echogenic foci resolve on subsequent prenatal or postnatal sonograms.[29]

Normal measurements for the fetal gallbladder have been published.[30] This research provided only a limited table for five periods between 15 and 19 weeks and term. By applying a robust LOWESS smoothing function to Wei and colleagues' table, Table 14–3 and Figure 14–29*D* were constructed. Although this graph is based on limited data, it is currently the only graph of fetal gallbladder size available.

Spleen

The fetal spleen is often difficult to visualize sonographically. When seen, the spleen has a homogeneous, slightly hypoechoic echotexture similar to the kidneys. The presence of ascites makes visualization of the spleen easier. The spleen is located in the left upper quadrant of the abdomen, lateral and posterior to the stomach and superior and lateral to the left kidney. The key to imaging the fetal spleen is locating the stomach and kidney. Splenic size is determined by measuring the longitudinal, transverse, and vertical diameters of the spleen. The longitudinal diameter is the length from the portion of the spleen closest to the anterior abdominal wall to the portion closest to the spine. Transverse diameter is the longest measurement perpendicular to the longitudinal diameter, and the vertical diameter is the longest measurement in the coronal plane. Figures 14–19 and 14–20 show normal spleens in the 39th and 31st weeks, respectively. Nomograms have been established for normal splenic size based on gestation age (see Table 14–1). (Mean splenic length is shown in Fig. 14–29*C*.)

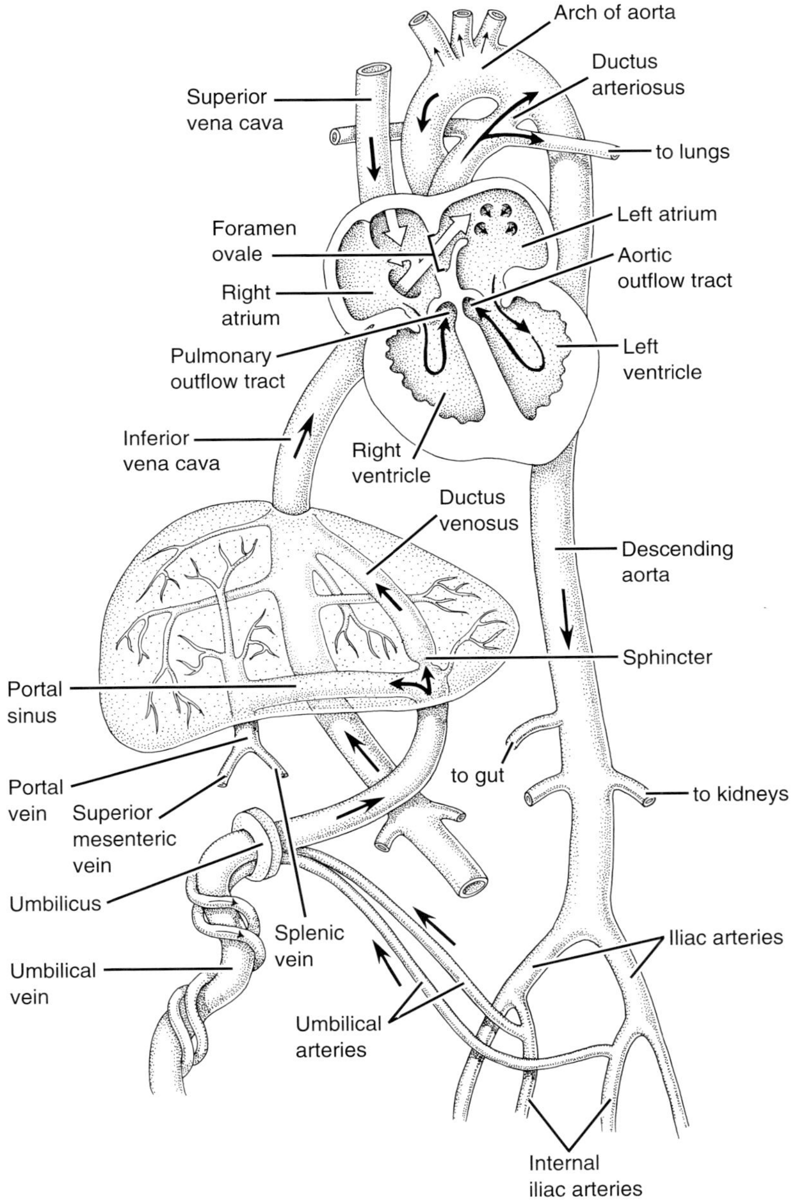

FIGURE 14–14.
Schematic showing the normal fetal circulation. (Adapted from Moore KL, Persaud TVN: The Developing Human: Clinically Oriented Embryology, 5th ed. WB Saunders, Philadelphia, 1993, p 344.)

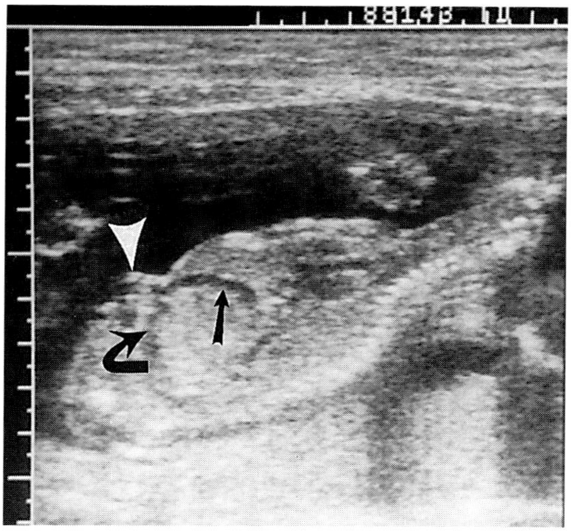

FIGURE 14–15.
SONOGRAM OF FETAL CIRCULATION.
Parasagittal image showing the umbilical vein (straight black arrow) and one umbilical artery (curved black arrow) just below the umbilical insertion (white arrowhead). The vein enters the fetal liver. (AA = 19.8 LMP, range = 2.5 weeks, n = 9 MFP, TD)

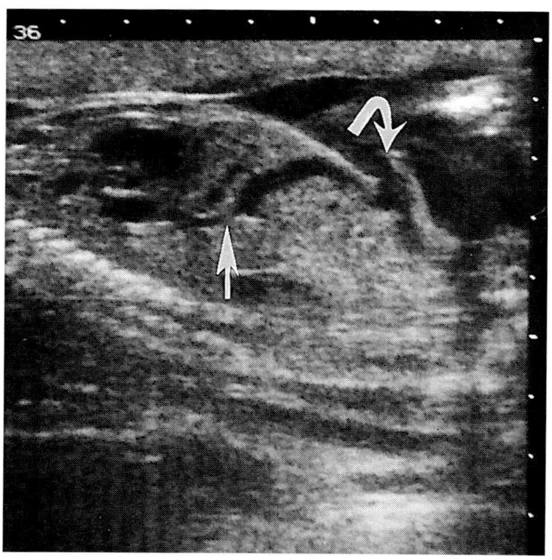

FIGURE 14–16.
SONOGRAM OF FETAL CIRCULATION.
Sagittal image of the fetal trunk showing the umbilical cord insertion (curved arrow). The umbilical vein can be observed coursing from the cord insertion into the liver and joining the ductus venosus at the sphincter (straight arrow) (see Fig. 14–14 for comparative anatomy). The portal sinus and left portal vein are not in this plane of view. (AA = 21.0 LMP, range = 1.6 weeks, n = 8 MFP, SG)

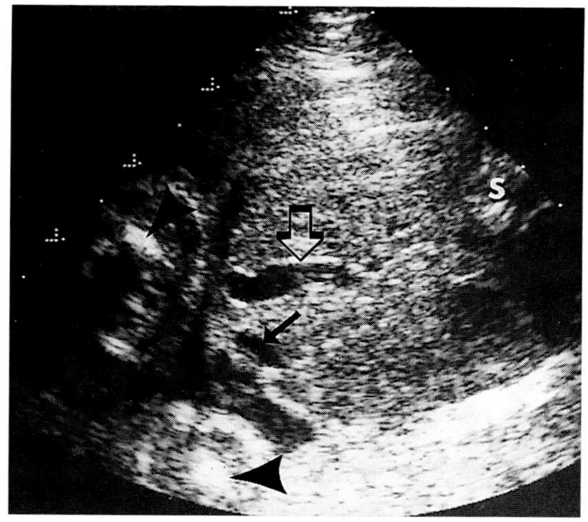

FIGURE 14–17.
FETAL GALLBLADDER AT 24 WEEKS.
The fetal gallbladder (open arrow) is well demonstrated. It appears that this gallbladder may be developing a phrygian cap, or a small fold of the gallbladder fundus. The umbilical vein (thin black arrow) is often confused with the gallbladder but can be traced back to the cord insertion. The fetal spine (S) is at the edge of the image, and both thighs (black arrowheads point to femurs) are seen in cross section against the anterior abdominal wall. (AA = 24.6 LMP, range = 1.3 weeks, n = 9 MFP, TD)

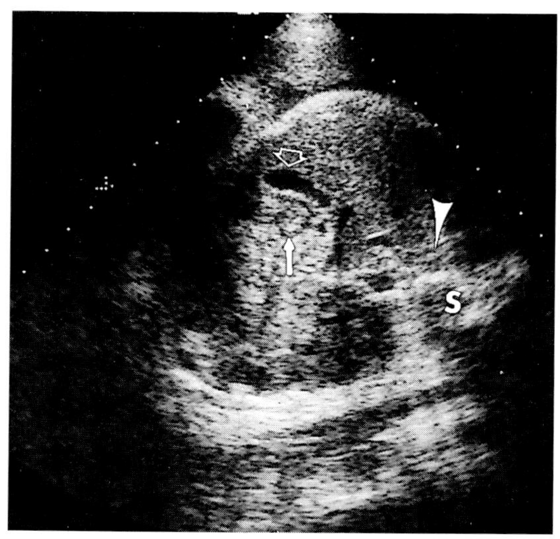

FIGURE 14–18.
FETAL GALLBLADDER AT 34 WEEKS.
A normal teardrop-shaped gallbladder (open arrow) is shown. The gallbladder is adjacent to the hypoechoic muscle ring of the fetal pyloris (thin white arrow). It was thought that this was particularly obvious (in all images) and might indicate an early pyloric stenosis; however, the woman was unavailable for follow-up. The spine (S) and right adrenal gland (white arrowhead) are also shown. (AA = 34.5 LMP, range = 3.1 weeks, n = 9 MFP, TD)

TABLE 14–3. GALLBLADDER SIZE/AGE

WEEK (RANGE)	GB LENGTH (mm) + 1 SD	GB WIDTH (mm) + 1 SD	WEEK (LMP)	LENGTH (mm)	+2 SD (mm)	−2 SD (mm)	WIDTH (mm)	+2 SD (mm)	−2 SD (mm)
15–19	9.59 + 2.98	3.51 + 1.33	17	9.59	15.55	3.63	3.51	6.17	.85
			18	11.21	18.22	4.20	3.76	6.34	1.17
			19	12.18	19.82	4.54	3.90	6.44	1.36
			20	13.48	21.96	5.00	4.10	6.58	1.62
			21	14.77	24.09	5.45	4.29	6.71	1.87
20–24	16.07 + 5.08	4.49 + 1.18	22	16.07	26.23	5.91	4.49	6.85	2.13
			23	17.32	27.41	7.23	4.76	7.16	2.36
			24	18.57	28.59	8.55	5.02	7.46	2.58
			25	19.82	29.78	9.86	5.29	7.77	2.81
			26	21.07	30.96	11.18	5.55	8.07	3.03
25–29	22.32 + 4.91	5.82 + 1.28	27	22.32	32.14	12.50	5.82	8.38	3.26
			28	22.87	32.66	13.08	6.03	8.56	3.49
			29	23.42	33.19	13.66	6.23	8.74	3.73
			30	23.98	33.71	14.24	6.44	8.91	3.96
			31	24.53	34.24	14.82	6.64	9.09	4.20
30–34	25.08 + 4.84	6.85 + 1.21	32	25.08	34.76	15.40	6.85	9.27	4.43
			33	27.21	37.43	16.99	6.99	9.94	4.03
			34	29.34	40.09	18.59	7.12	10.61	3.64
			35	31.47	42.76	20.18	7.26	11.27	3.24
			36	33.07	44.76	21.38	7.36	11.78	2.95
35–39	35.73 + 6.18	7.53 + 2.54	37	35.73	48.09	23.37	7.53	12.61	2.45

The originally published gallbladder (GB) size/age table is shown in the three columns on the left. These show the weeks range for the measurements, the mean GB length +1 SD, and the mean width +1 SD. The seven columns on the right are derived from the original data by a robust LOWESS smoothing algorithm (see Chapter 7 for an explanation of LOWESS). These seven columns show the LMP weeks ages and the mean GB length ±2 SD and the mean width ±2 SD.

Adapted from Wei JMC, Haller JO, Rachlin S, et al: Sonographic evaluation of the fetal gallbladder in utero: Incidence of visualization and morphology. J Diagn Med Sonogr 1993;9:291–296.

Kidneys

The kidneys develop in three stages: pronephros, mesonephros, and metanephros. The initial stages are rudimentary and brief. The metanephros (permanent kidney) starts to form in the fetal pelvis in the seventh menstrual week. For the metanephros to develop, the ureteric bud and metanephric blastema must interact. The ureteric bud originates from the mesonephric (wolffian) duct and undergoes multiple branching.[31] When the growing and dividing ends of the ureteric bud, the ampullae, contact the mesodermal cells of the metanephric blastema, metanephric differentiation begins, and nephrons (glomeruli, proximal and distal convoluted tubules, and Henle's loop) develop.[32, 33] The ureteric bud branches become the collecting system (ureter, renal pelvis, calyces, infundibula and tubules)[32] (Fig. 14–21). During this process, the metanephros migrates cephalad from the fetal pelvis, reaching its permanent paraspinal location by 11 weeks.[31] An ectopic kidney develops when the ascent is interrupted (Figs. 14–22*A* and *B*). Figure 14–22*A* shows a left pelvic kidney that was found in utero and confirmed neonatally by sonography; the right kidney was normal (Fig. 14–22*B*). The subtleness of this finding can be appreciated from these images. By 13 to 15 weeks, urine production begins.[27] Fetal urine is the major component of amniotic fluid after 16 to 18 weeks.[34]

Sonographic visualization of the kidneys in their paraspinal location is dependent on fetal position, with both kidneys best seen in a prone fetus (Figs. 14–23 and 14–24). In images oblique to the spine, posterior acoustical shadowing from the fetal spine often obscures the kidney farthest from the transducer. The kidneys appear round on transverse images

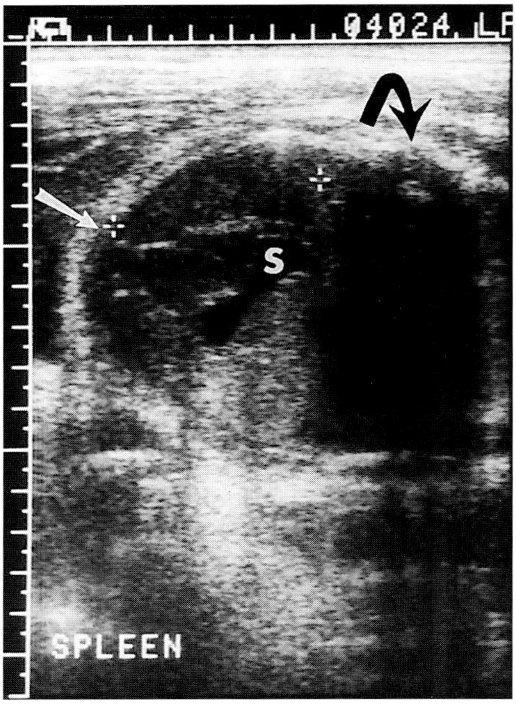

FIGURE 14–19.
The long axis of the spleen (between + cursors) runs from the anterior abdominal wall (white arrow) toward the fetal spine (curved arrow) and is posterolateral to the stomach (S). This spleen measured 52.2 mm in longest axis and was large for age. The spleen is often difficult to image and measure because it is generally isoechoic with the surrounding tissues. The fluid-filled stomach, spine, and abdominal wall are the best landmarks for locating it. (AA = 39.0 LMP, range = 4.1 weeks, n = 9 MFP, LP)

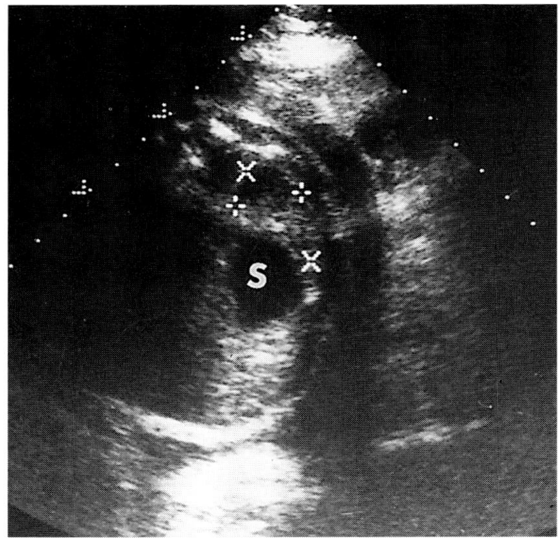

FIGURE 14–20.
In this transverse view of a term fetal abdomen, the spleen is measured in anteroposterior axis (X cursors = 30.3 mm) and thickness (+ cursors = 18 mm). The thickness was slightly small for age according to Table 14–2. Because the spleen is usually isoechoic to the surrounding tissues, it can be difficult to visualize and measure. Note the relationships of the stomach (S), spine, and abdominal wall to the spleen. (AA = 31.5 LMP, range = 4.0 weeks, n = 9 MFP, TD)

and ovoid on longitudinal images. With transabdominal sonography, the kidneys are routinely seen at 17 weeks but can be seen as early as 14 to 15 weeks.[19, 27, 34] Bronshtein and colleagues[35] report reliable identification of both kidneys with transvaginal sonography at 12 weeks.

Between 16 and 26 weeks, the kidneys are hypoechoic structures difficult to distinguish from surrounding retroperitoneal soft tissue. In the third trimester, the kidneys become easy to image because of an echogenic border produced by perinephric fat. The central renal sinus becomes hyperechoic as a result of deposition of fat, which distinguishes it from the peripheral relatively hypoechoic cortex[36] (Figs. 14–23 to 14–25). In Figure 14–25, the renal pyramids are clearly seen as hypoechoic structures surrounding the renal sinus. On high-contrast images, the pyramids should not be mistaken for renal cysts.

The renal pelvis typically is not imaged, but not uncommonly, a small amount of fluid can be seen in the renal pelvis. This mild pyelectasis is considered physiological if it measures less than 10 mm in anteroposterior (AP) diameter,[37] and the AP pelvis/AP kidney ratio is less than 0.5[34] (Figs. 14–26 and 14–27). Proposed causes of this physiological pyelectasis include transient reflux,[38, 39] stasis secondary to a full urinary bladder (Fig. 14–28), fetal diuresis,[37] or an extrarenal pelvis.[38] Degree of maternal hydration does not appear to be a factor.[37, 40]

Normal growth of the kidneys parallels normal abdominal growth, with the ratio of renal circumference to AC remaining constant at 0.27 to 0.30 throughout gestation.[41] The renal length has an approximate linear relationship to gestational age, with the renal length in millimeters approximately the same as the menstrual age in weeks[42] (see Table 14–1 and Fig. 14–29*B*). Bertagnoli and colleagues report that at 32 weeks, the average length is 30 mm and at 40 weeks, 38 mm.[42] The ureters are not routinely imaged.

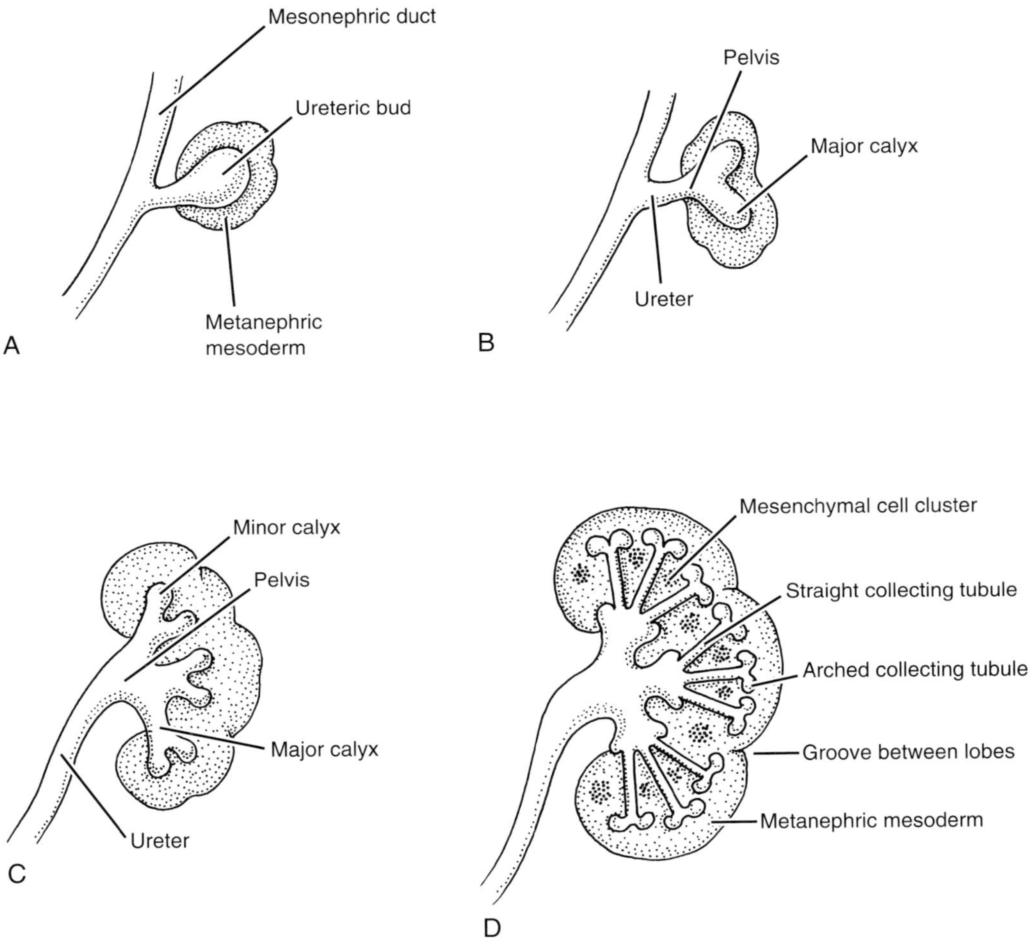

FIGURE 14–21. KIDNEY EMBRYOGENESIS.
The stages of human kidney development from the 7th to 10th LMP weeks. (Adapted from Moore KL, Persaud TVN: The Developing Human: Clinically Oriented Embryology, 5th ed. WB Saunders, Philadelphia, 1993, p 269.)

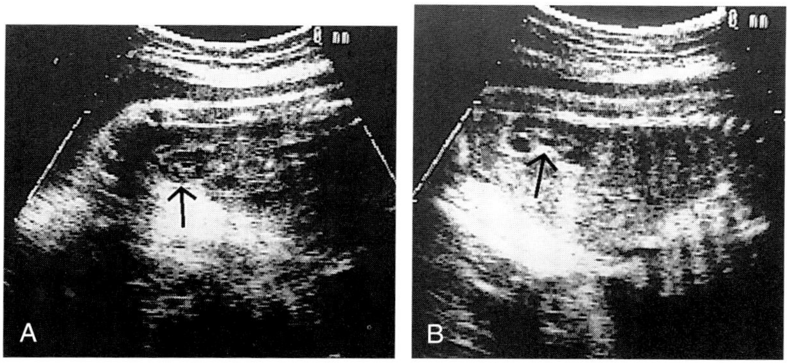

FIGURE 14–22. *A,* PELVIC LEFT KIDNEY AT 34 WEEKS.
A left fetal pelvic kidney (arrow) found in utero and confirmed neonatally by sonography. Ectopic kidneys occur most often on the left. (AA = 34.1 LMP, range = 3.1 weeks, n = 5 MFP, SL)
B, NORMAL RIGHT KIDNEY AT 34 WEEKS.
Normal right kidney (arrow) in the same fetus shown in *A*. This kidney was in a normal location. (AA = 34.1 LMP, range = 3.1 weeks, n = 5 MFP, SL)

Bladder

The fetal urinary bladder is first imaged at 13 to 15 weeks, the time when fetal urine production begins. The bladder is visualized in more than 90% of fetuses older than 14 weeks.[43]

The bladder is identified as a midline anechoic rounded structure within the pelvis; it has an imperceptible wall (see Fig. 14–28). Normal bladder filling and emptying occurs every 30 to 45 minutes.[43] Bladder capacity at 32 weeks is 10 ml and at term is 40 ml.[44] Occasionally seen is a quite prominent, dilated bladder, which is most often normal, and

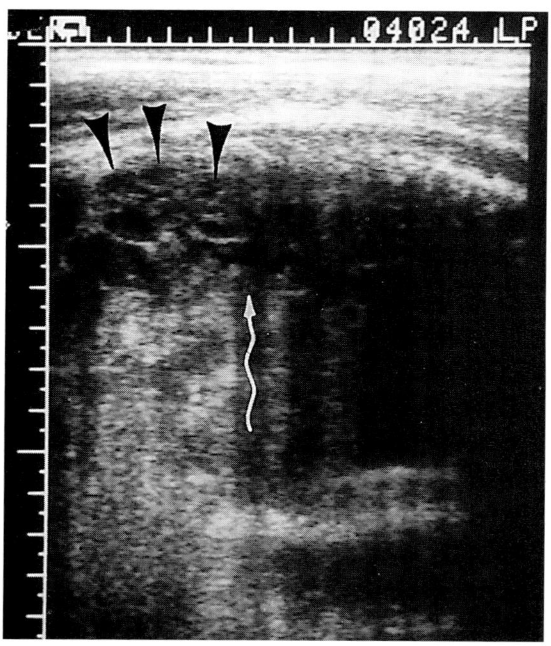

FIGURE 14–23. LONGITUDINAL KIDNEY.
Near term, the fetal kidneys are more easily observed. Here the long axis of the kidney is shown with normal hypoechoic pyramids (arrowheads). The echogenic bowel can be seen distal to the kidney, and a rib shadow (wavy arrow) lies across the upper pole of the kidney. (AA = 39.0 LMP, range = 4.1 weeks, n = 8 MFP, LP)

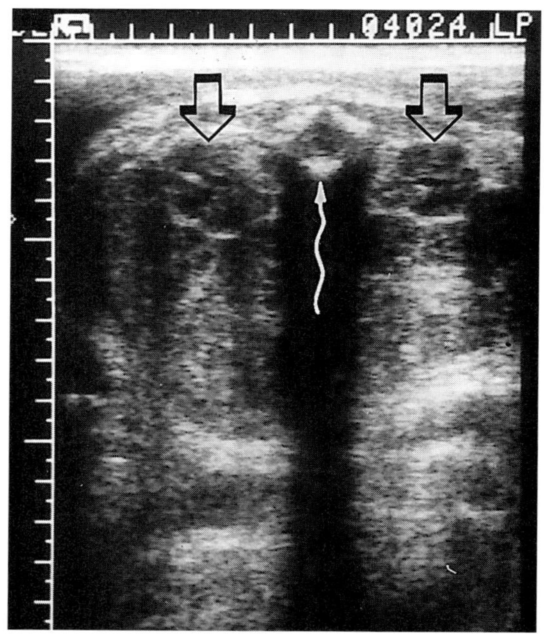

FIGURE 14–24.
In this transverse section (same examination as Fig. 14–23) through the fetal abdomen, the kidneys (open arrows) are observed bilaterally on either side of the spine (wavy arrow in spine shadow). There is a very small amount of fluid centrally in the renal pelves. The pyramids are faintly seen as hypoechoic areas around the renal sinus. This is the appearance of normal term kidneys. (AA = 39.0 LMP, range = 4.1 weeks, n = 8 MFP, LP)

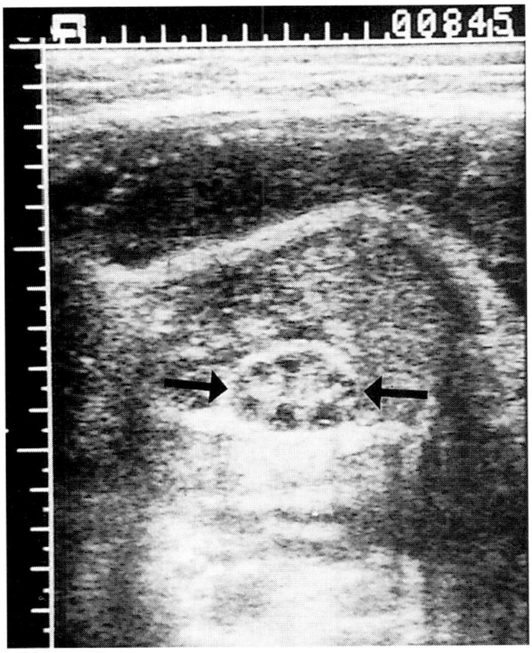

FIGURE 14–25. RENAL PYRAMIDS AT 35 WEEKS. In this high-contrast sonographic image, the fetal kidney (between arrows) and renal pyramids are easily observed. The pyramids should not be confused with renal cysts in images such as this. (AA = 35.3 LMP, range = 2.5 weeks, n = 9 MFP, LP)

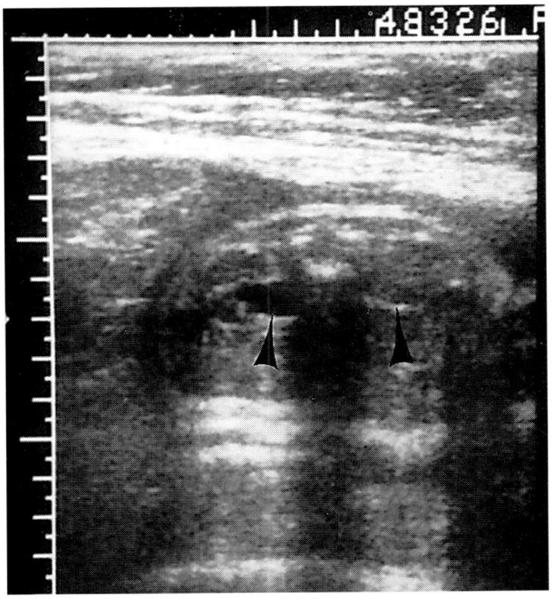

FIGURE 14–26. TRANSVERSE PYELECTASIS. This sonogram demonstrates mild physiological renal pyelectasis (arrowheads). (AA = 30.7 LMP, range = 3.1 weeks, n = 9 MFP, PC)

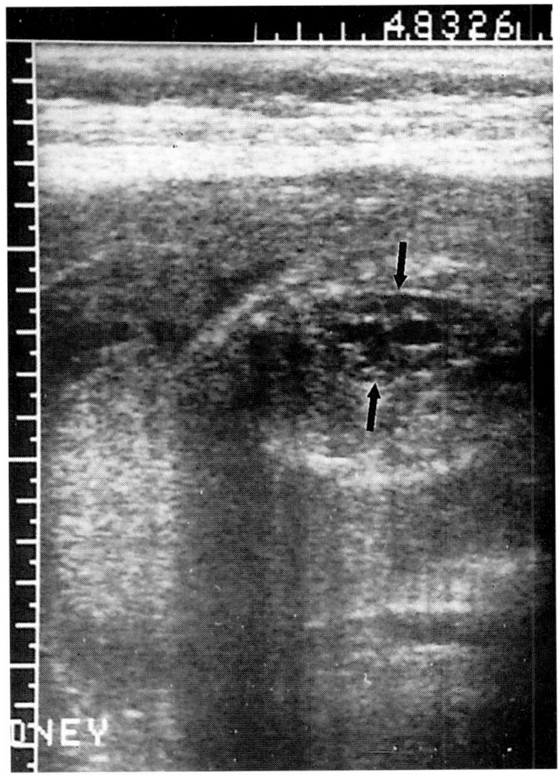

FIGURE 14–27. LONGITUDINAL PYELECTASIS. Long axis of a kidney (short axis between arrows) shown in Figure 14–26. Here the pyelectasis is shown to fill the upper and lower poles of the renal collecting system. This is not considered abnormal as long as the anteroposterior diameter of the pelvis is less than 1 cm. (AA = 30.7 LMP, range = 3.1 weeks, n = 9 MFP, PC)

reimaging after 30 minutes usually shows a decrease in bladder size due to interval fetal micturition.[45] Conversely, with nonvisualization of the bladder, delayed imaging often shows filling. Clautice-Engle and colleagues[43] report that in their series, nonvisualization of the bladder with normal-appearing kidneys, adequate volume of amniotic fluid, and an otherwise normal sonogram was of no clinical concern and did not require follow-up.

Adrenals

The adrenal glands are prominent in a fetus. The fetal adrenal weight is 10 to 20 times greater relative to body mass than the adult

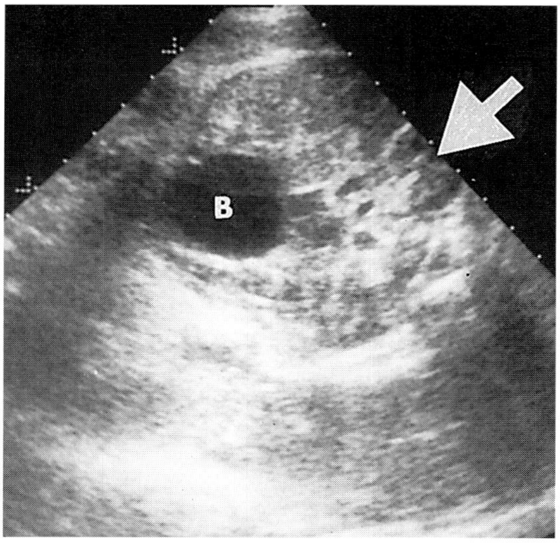

FIGURE 14–28.
The fetal bladder most often appears spherical, although it can have a pyramidal or triangular shape. This relatively large bladder (B) was shown to empty before the end of the examination. The fetal kidney (arrow) is shown at the edge of this obliquely transverse image low in the fetal abdomen. (AA = 33.5 LMP, range = 2.1 weeks, n = 9 MFP, TD)

adrenal.[46] Ovoid, triangular, or curvilinear in shape, depending on the plane, the adrenals have a hyperechoic central medulla (ectoderm) and a peripheral hypoechoic cortex (mesoderm) (see Figs. 14–7 and 14–18). This appearance may be similar to the kidneys, and one must avoid the pitfall of identifying an adrenal gland as a kidney, especially in cases of renal agenesis. Visualization of the adrenals can be hindered by shadowing from overlying ribs or spine.

Genitalia

Fetal gender is routinely determined with accuracy after 18 weeks.[34] Coronal and transverse images of the perineum best demonstrate the genitalia. In females, the labia majora are seen as paired structures of intermediate echogenicity separated by the central linear echo of the labia minora (Fig. 14–30). The uterus and ovaries are not identifiable. The

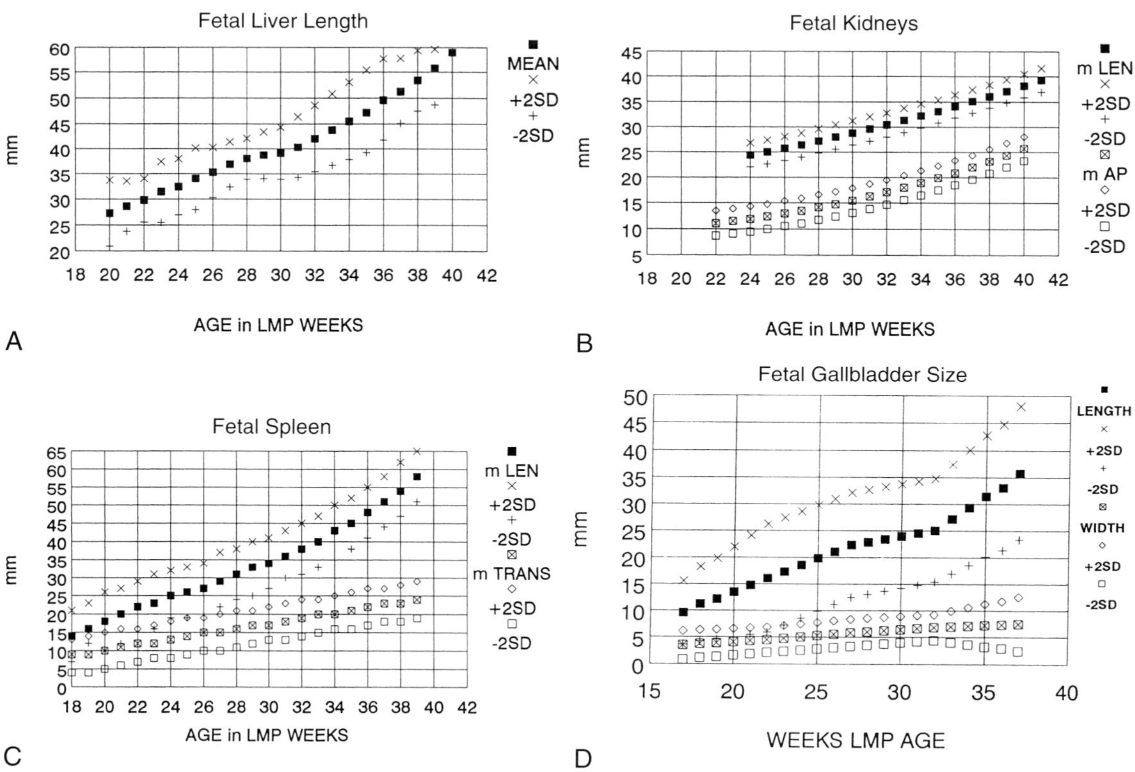

FIGURE 14–29 *See legend on opposite page*

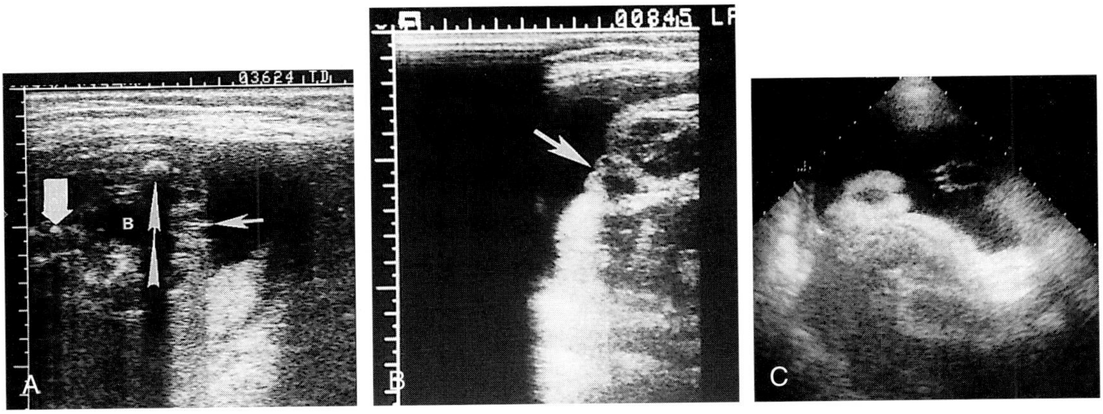

FIGURE 14–30. FEMALE GENITALIA.
A, This image of a female fetus is transverse through the lower pelvis, showing the female genitalia. The labia are hypoechoic structures on either side of the vaginal tract, which appears as an echogenic line (thin arrow). The urinary bladder (B) is observed posterior to the vagina, and the fetal spine (wide arrow) posterior to the bladder. The femur nearest the transducer casts a shadow across the anterior bladder wall (long arrow). (AA = 27.2 LMP, range = 1.9 weeks, n = 9 MFP, TD) *B*, In this transverse view, slightly swollen labia (arrow) are shown as two bumps. The slight swelling is due to the hormones of pregnancy and can be mistaken for the more prominent scrotum of a male fetus. (AA = 35.3 LMP, range = 2.5 weeks, n = 9 MFP, LP) *C*, The labia are quite swollen by the hormones of pregnancy and are shown in a tangential section. This appearance could easily be mistaken by the less experienced for the scrotum of a male fetus. The labia minora are seen as a slightly hypoechoic area between the two labia majora. Note that the three-vessel umbilical cord is in close proximity, between the legs. Because the legs tend to funnel the cord near the genitalia, this is a common observation. (AA = 34.5 LMP, range = 3.1 weeks, n = 9 MFP, TD)

labia may appear swollen owing to the hormones of pregnancy and may be mistaken for the scrotum of a male fetus (Fig. 14–30*B* and *C*). A tangential view of the swollen labia (Fig. 14–30*C*) demonstrates this normal appearance.

In males, the scrotum and penis are visualized (Fig. 14–31). Pitfalls include swollen labia or a loop of umbilical cord between the fetal thighs.[34] The legs often act as a funnel, bringing the umbilical cord between the thighs (Figs. 14–30*C* and 14–31*B*). Erections are occasionally seen. The testicles descend into the scrotum during the third trimester; 62% descend by 30 weeks and 93% by 32 weeks.[47]

Hydroceles are not uncommonly seen, especially near term, and are usually of no clinical significance if the amount of fluid remains

FIGURE 14–29. FETAL ABDOMINAL ORGAN SIZE/AGE GRAPHS. *A*, FETAL LIVER GRAPH.
This XY graph shows the growth of the fetal liver length from the 20th LMP week to term. The solid squares are the mean liver lengths, the X plots show +2 SD, and the + are −2 SD for length. This measurement is made in the coronal or sagittal fetal abdomen from the dome of the liver to the tip of the right lobe. This graph was plotted from the liver data in Table 14–1.
B, FETAL KIDNEY GRAPH.
The mean kidney length (m LEN = solid squares) and +2 SD (X) and − 2 SD (+) are shown. The mean anteroposterior kidney diameter (m AP = boxed X) and +2 SD (diamonds) and −2 SD (open squares) are shown also. This graph is from the kidney data in Table 14–1 and shows the growth of the fetal kidneys from 22 LMP weeks until term.
C, FETAL SPLEEN GRAPH.
The mean spleen length (m LEN = solid squares) and +2 SD (X) and −2 SD (+) for growth are shown from 18 LMP weeks until term. The mean splenic transverse diameter (m TRANS = boxed X) and +2 SD (diamonds) and −2 SD (open squares) are also shown. This graph was plotted from the splenic data (LOWESS smoothing) in Table 14–1.
D, FETAL GALLBLADDER GRAPH.
This graph shows the length and width of the fetal gallbladder from the 17th LMP week until term. It was constructed from the LOWESS smoothed data in Table 14–3.

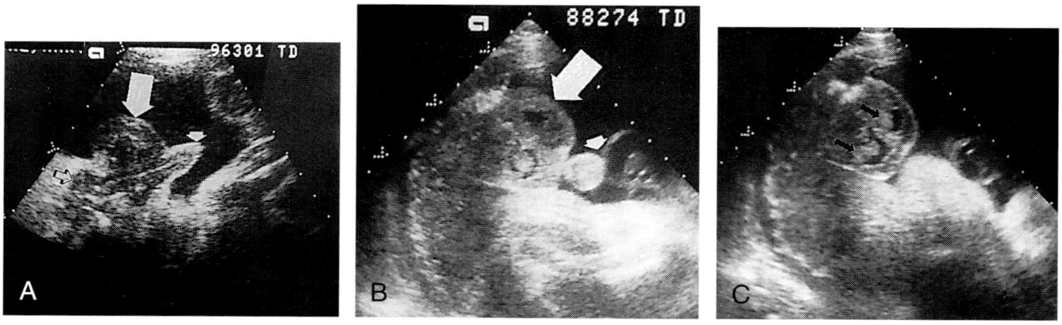

FIGURE 14–31. MALE GENITALIA.
A, Normal male genitalia in a sagittal section. The scrotum (large white arrow) can be observed to bulge toward the transducer, anterior to the shaft of the penis. The foreskin (small white arrow) can be seen as hyperechoic tissue surrounding the glans or head of the penis. The urethra is seen as an echogenic line along the central penile shaft, which originates at a bulge (open arrow). (AA = 30.5 LMP, range = 2.1 weeks, n = 9 MFP, TD) *B*, The male genitalia in a coronal section. The scrotum (large arrow) can be seen containing hypoechoic rings of the fluid of a hydrocele; the testes are within the rings. The penis is seen pressed against the three-vessel umbilical cord (small arrow). Hydroceles are not considered unusual if small, and they generally resolve before or at birth. (AA = 38.4 LMP, range = 4.1 weeks, n = 9 MFP, TD) *C*, Transverse section of the scrotum shown in *B*. The bilateral hydroceles are obvious and contain the testes (arrows).

stable (Fig. 14–31*B* and *C*). An enlarging hydrocele can be associated with an inguinal hernia, and appropriate clinical examination after birth is warranted.[48]

Determination of fetal gender is rarely of medical interest but can be important in certain conditions such as X-linked genetic diseases. Expectant parents often wish to know the sex of the fetus. With modern real-time sonography and experience, a sonographer can usually satisfy parents' request.

REFERENCES

1. Moore KL, Persaud TVN: The Developing Human: Clinically Oriented Embryology, 5th ed. WB Saunders, Philadelphia, 1993, pp 248–251.
2. Cyr DR, Mack LA, Schoenecker SA, et al: Bowel migration in the normal fetus: Ultrasound detection. Radiology 1986;161:119–121.
3. Salzman L, Kuligowska E, Semine A: Pseudoomphalocele: Pitfall in fetal sonography. AJR 1986; 146:1283–1285.
4. Hashimoto BE, Filly RA, Callen PW: Fetal pseudoascites: Further anatomic observations. J Ultrasound Med 1986;5:151–152.
5. Samuels P, Ludmir J: Nonimmune hydrops fetalis: A heterogeneous disorder and therapeutic challenge. Semin Roentgenol 1990;25:353–360.
6. Williamson MR, Williamson SL: Gamuts in Ultrasound. WB Saunders, Philadelphia, 1992, pp 168–169.
7. Hill LM, Guzick D, Gmitter P: Subcutaneous tissue thickness cannot be used to distinguish abnormalities of fetal growth. J Ultrasound Med 1992;11:512.
8. Higginbottom J, Slater J, Porter G, et al: Estimation of fetal weight from ultrasonic measurement of trunk circumference. Br J Obstet Gynaecol 1975;82:698–701.
9. Hertzberg BS, Bowie JD: Fetal gastrointestinal abnormalities. Radiol Clin North Am 1990;28:101–114.
10. Fakhry J, Shapiro LR, Schechter A, et al: Fetal gastric pseudomasses. J Ultrasound Med 1987;6:177–180.
11. Pretorius DH, Gosink BB, Clautice-Engle T, et al: Sonographic evaluation of the fetal stomach: Significance of nonvisualization. AJR 1988;151:987–989.
12. Nyberg DA, Mack LA, Patten RM, et al: Fetal bowel: Normal sonographic findings. J Ultrasound Med 1987;6:3–6.
13. Fakhry J, Reiser M, Shapiro LR, et al: Increased echogenicity in the lower fetal abdomen: A common normal variant in the second trimester. J Ultrasound Med 1986;5:489–492.
14. Parulelcar SG: Sonography of normal fetal bowel. J Ultrasound Med 1991;10:211–220.
15. Lince DM, Pretorius DH, Mamco-Johnson ML, et al: The clinical significance of increased echogenicity in the fetal abdomen. AJR 1985;145:683–686.
16. Caspi B, Elchalal U, et al: Echogenicity of the fetal bowel due to gas accumulation. J Ultrasound Med 1993;12:231–233.
17. Hogge WA, Hogge JS, Boehm CD, et al: Increased echogenicity in the fetal abdomen: Use of DNA analysis to establish a diagnosis of cystic fibrosis. J Ultrasound Med 1993;12:451–454.
18. Dinsmore BJ, Grumbach K: Disorders of the fetal thorax and abdomen. Semin Roentgenol 1990; 25:334–341.
19. Callen PW. Ultrasonography in Obstetrics and Gynecology, 2nd ed. WB Saunders, Philadelphia, 1993, p 351.
20. Gross BH, Harter LP, Filly RA: Disproportionate left hepatic lobe size in the fetus: Ultrasonic demonstration. J Ultrasound Med 1982;1:79–81.
21. Vintzileos AM, Neckles S, Campbell WA, et al: Fetal liver ultrasound measurements during normal pregnancy. Obstet Gynecol 1985;66:477–479.
22. Romero R, Pilu G, Jeanty P, et al: Prenatal Diagnosis

of Congenital Anomalies. Appleton & Lange, Norwalk, CT, 1988, p 250.
23. Harrison MR, Golbus MS, Filly RA, eds: The Unborn Patient: Prenatal Diagnosis and Treatment. WB Saunders, Philadelphia, 1984, p 110.
24. Rudolph AM: Hepatic and ductus venosus blood flows during fetal life. Hepatology 1983;3:254–258.
25. Chinn DH, Filly RA, Callen PW: Ultrasonic evaluation of fetal umbilical and hepatic vascular anatomy. Radiology 1982;144:153–157.
26. Callen PW, ed: Symposium on ultrasonography in obstetrics and gynecology. Radiol Clin North Am 1982;20:277.
27. Benacerraf BR, ed: Fetal ultrasound. Radiol Clin North Am 1990;28:184.
28. Jouppila P, Heikklnen J, Kirkinen P: Contractility of maternal and fetal gallbladder: An ultrasonic study. J Clin Ultrasound 1985;13:461.
29. Brown DL, Teele RL, Doubilet PM, et al: Echogenic material in the fetal gallbladder: Sonographic and clinical observations. Radiology 1992;182:73–76.
30. Wei JMC, Haller JO, Rachlin S, et al: Sonographic evaluation of the fetal gallbladder in utero: Incidence of visualization and morphology. J Diagn Med Sonogr 1993;9:291–296.
31. Moore KL, Persaud TVN: The Developing Human: Clinically Oriented Embryology, 5th ed. WB Saunders, Philadelphia, 1993, p 269.
32. Fleisher AC, Romero R, Manning FA, et al: Ultrasonography in Obstetrics and Gynecology, 4th ed. Appleton & Lange, Norwalk, CT, 1991, pp 251–252.
33. Pansky B: Review of Medical Embryology. Macmillan, New York, 1982, pp 244–247.
34. Louie A, Arger PH: Fetal genitourinary tract. Semin Roentgenol 1990;25:342–352.
35. Bronshtein M, Kushnir O, Ben-Rafael Z, et al: Transvaginal sonographic measurement of fetal kidneys in the first trimester of pregnancy. J Clin Ultrasound 1990;18:299–301.
36. Bowie JD, Rosenberg ER, Andreotti RF, et al: The changing sonographic appearance of fetal kidneys during pregnancy. J Ultrasound Med 1983;2:505–507.
37. Hoddick WK, Filly RA, Mahony BS, et al: Minimal fetal renal pyelectasis. J Ultrasound Med 1985;4:85–89.
38. Kurtz AB, Goldberg BB: Obstetrical Measurements in Ultrasound: A Reference Manual. Year Book Medical Publishers, Chicago, 1988, pp 88–92.
39. Cohen HL, Atwood R, Newelt M: Ultrasound of the normal fetal chest, abdomen, and pelvis. In: Berman MC, ed: Diagnostic Medical Sonography: A Guide to Clinical Practice, vol 1. JB Lippincott, Philadelphia, 1991, p 243.
40. Cohen HL, Atwood R, Newelt M: Ultrasound of the normal fetal chest, abdomen, and pelvis. In: Berman MC, ed: Diagnostic Medical Sonography: A Guide to Clinical Practice, vol I. JB Lippincott, Philadelphia, 1991, p 243.
41. Grannum P, Bracken M, Silverman R, et al: Assessment of fetal kidney size in normal gestation by comparison of ratio of kidney circumference to abdominal circumference. Am J Obstet Gynecol 1980;136:249.
42. Bertagnoli L, Lalatta F, Gallicchio R, et al: Quantitative characteristics of the growth of the kidneys. J Clin Ultrasound 1983;11:349–356.
43. Clautice-Engle T, Pretorius D, Budorick NE: Significance of nonvisualization of the fetal urinary bladder. J Ultrasound Med 1991;10:615–618.
44. Campbell S, Wladimiroff JW, Dewhurst CJ: The antenatal measurement of fetal urine production. J Obstet Gynaecol Br Commonw 1973;80:680–686.
45. Kurjak A: CRC Handbook of Ultrasound in Obstetrics and Gynecology, vol 1. CRC Press, Boca Raton, FL, 1990, pp 175–177.
46. Chervenak FA, Isaacson GC, Campbell S, eds: Ultrasound in Obstetrics and Gynecology. Little, Brown & Co, Boston, 1993, p 725.
47. Birnholz JC: Determination of fetal sex. N Engl J Med 1983;309:942–944.
48. Romero R, Pilu G, Jeanty P, et al: Prenatal Diagnosis of Congenital Anomalies. Appleton & Lange, Norwalk, CT, 1988, p 304.

CHAPTER 15

EXTREMITIES

Terry J. DuBose

Six extremity bones of the fetus are well documented in the sonographic literature. The distal extremity long bones, the ulna and radius in the forearm, and the tibia and fibula in the leg are less often measured.[1] The most commonly measured long bone is the femur in the thigh, followed by the humerus in the arm.[1-5] This is because the long bones are usually accessible and fairly straightforward to measure. These measurements are considered *fairly* straightforward because some concepts must be understood by novice sonographers.

First, in much sonographic literature, the humerus and femur measurements are referred to as the "length" of the respective bones. This is a misnomer, however, because the humerus (Figs. 15–1*A* and 15–3 to 15–6) and femur (Figs. 15–1*B* and 15–15*A* to 15–20) lengths are actually the length of the diaphysis of the bone and do not include the heads or condyles of the respective bones.[6,7] These ends of the humerus and femur do not calcify completely until well after birth and in a fetus are cartilaginous tissues that are hypoechoic sonographically. The diaphysis becomes echogenic very early in pregnancy and is easily observed. Figure 15–1*A* and *B* demonstrates both the humeral (Fig. 15–1*A*) and femoral (Fig. 15–1*B*) lengths at 10.5 LMP weeks for the same fetus. For simplicity's sake, however, the femoral and humeral diaphyseal lengths are referred to here as the femoral length (FemL) and the humeral length (HumL). This is the conventional nomenclature used in most sonographic literature for these measurements.

At the distal end of both the humerus and femur are condyles, which affect the measurements of these bones. The condyles of the humerus and femur calcify at different times. The specifics of the measurements of these bones are discussed later in their respective sections.

The upper portion of a fetus develops slightly sooner than the lower portion.[8] The humerus tends to be as long as or slightly longer than the femur until about the 16th week after the last menstrual period (16th LMP week). This is only a tendency and certainly not absolute. Early in pregnancy, the bones are approximately equal in length, but either may be longer than the other. The XY scattergram in Figure 15–2*A* shows the growth curves for the HumL and FemL. Note that after the 25th LMP week, the femur is almost always the longer bone. This is a little easier to appreciate as a ratio of the humerus to the femur (HumL/FemL). Figure 15–2*B* shows HumL/FemL ratios throughout pregnancy. The wide variation early in pregnancy is most likely due to the fact that the bones

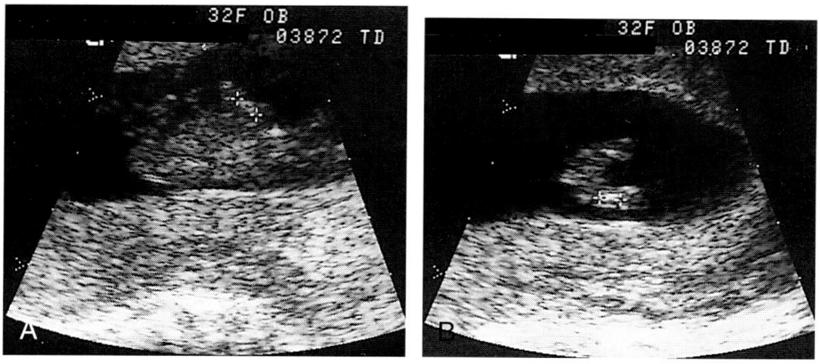

FIGURE 15–1.
A, Early humerus. Humerus length measured at 10.5 LMP weeks by average of 10 parameter ages. This humerus measured 3.9 mm. Good fetal motion could be observed with real-time sonography. *B,* Early femur. Femur measurement for the same 10.5-LMP-week fetus as in *A.* This femoral diaphysis measured 3.5 mm. (AA = 10.5, n = 10, range = 1.7 weeks, TD)

are very small then and any variation in cursor placement produces relatively larger percent errors (see the other discussion of the long bones' relationship to age in Chapter 7, the section on embryo and fetal size/age analysis).

Another consideration in the measurement of the long bones is their locations. The leg and thigh have a smaller range of motion than the arm. This is true in a fetus just as it is after birth. The thighs' range of motion is more or less limited to flexion (drawing the knee toward the chest) and downward extension, and lateral adduction and abduction are limited. The arms can be moved in a wider range of motion: across the chest, toward the back, down the side, up beside the head, and to all intermediate positions. The bones of the arms thus are slightly more difficult to locate than the bones of the thighs. This difficulty is increased in the distal extremities. The ulna and radius are more difficult to locate than the humerus, and the tibia and fibula are more difficult to locate than the femur. This variability in difficulty of location is directly related to the range of motion of the respective extremity bones. Distal extremity measurements of an active fetus may be time-consuming.

In general, the measurement of any extremity long bone should begin with a survey of the uterus and the fetal position. By locating the fetal head and spine and forming a mental image of the fetal lie, it is easier to predict where the extremities might be located. If the fetal spine is to the woman's right and the fetus is facing the woman's left side, then the extremities are usually also on the woman's left. Once the fetal head and spine are located, it is fairly simple to follow the spine to the level of the shoulders to locate the arms or to follow the spine all the way down to the pelvis to locate the hips and legs. In the words of the African-American folk spiritual "Dry Bones":

> *"Head bone connected from de neck bone,*
> *neck bone connected from de shoulder bone,*
> *shoulder bone connected from de back bone,*
> *back bone connected from de hip bone,*
> *hip bone connected from de thigh bone,*
> *thigh bone connected from de knee bone,*
> *knee bone connected from de leg bone,*
> *leg bone connected from de ankle bone,*
> *ankle bone connected from de foot bone,*
> *foot bone connected from de toe bone. . . ."*[9]

Although a sonographer does not necessarily have to follow the sequence described in this primitive musical piece, this is the system of thinking that makes sonographic location of the various fetal parts logical. The transducer is slid over the woman's abdomen, using in-plane and cross-plane sliding to follow the fetal anatomy to the specific structures sought. For readers who are new to sonography and who have not yet read Chapter 5, it is suggested that they read that chapter before this one. An understanding of transducer manipulation is necessary for success in lining up on linear structures such as the long bones of the extremities.

For the most part, a sonographer takes linear measurements of the bone diaphysis. The ability to locate the long bones quickly and then orient the sonographic field of view to demonstrate the longest axis of these bones is one mark of an experienced sonographer. Lining up on linear structures is one of the first difficulties encountered by novice sonographers. This technique, which involves the cybernetic nature of sonography, is discussed in detail in Chapter 5.

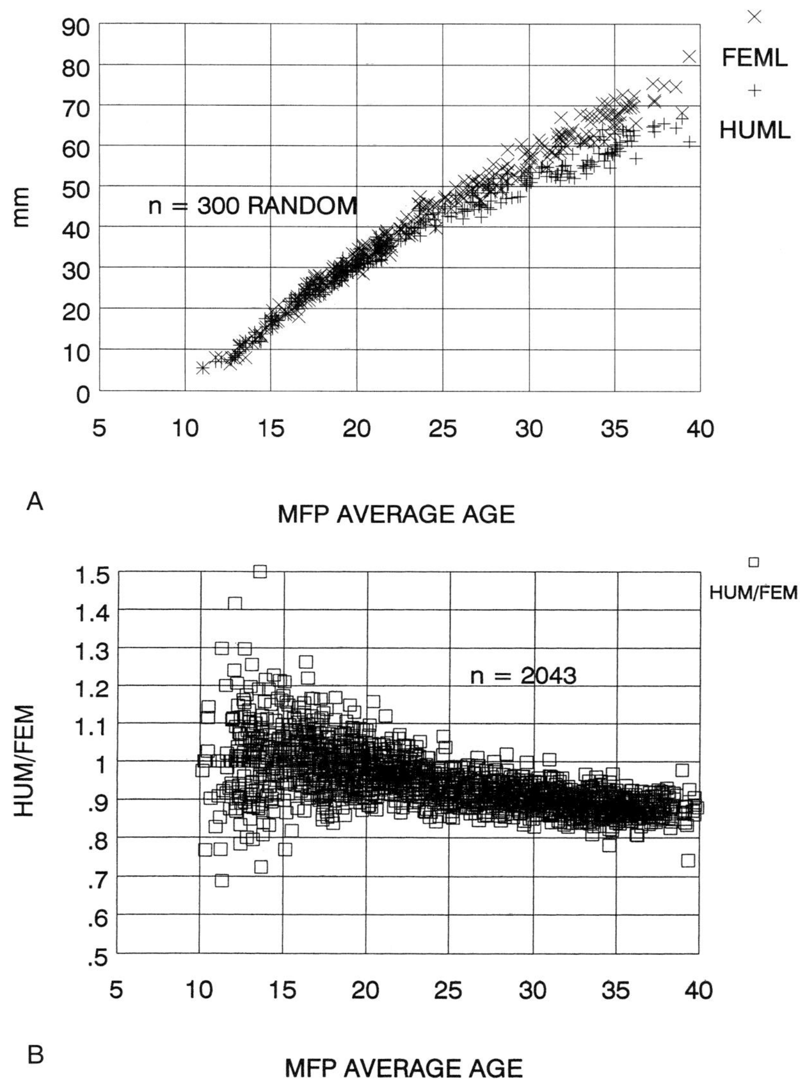

FIGURE 15–2.
A, Growth curves for femoral (FemL = X) and humeral (HumL = +) lengths. Note that the humerus is not clearly less than the femur in length until after the 25th LMP week. A random sample of 300 fetuses was used so that the plot density would not completely obscure individuals. *B,* Ratios of humeri to femurs for all fetuses in which both bones were measured in 1993. Note that the ratios are fairly evenly distributed about 1 until the 20th LMP week and not clearly below 1 until after the 25th week. After 30 weeks, the FemL should exceed the HumL.

Moore and Persaud state, "Ossification begins in the long bones by the eighth week of embryonic development and initially occurs in the diaphyses of the bones from primary centers of ossification."[10] This places ossification in the 10th LMP week. At this early age, the humerus or femur is really just a bright dot in the proximal extremity, but it is distinct from the surrounding soft tissues and with good resolution may be measured by the 10th LMP week. In my group's study population of 10,336 consecutive referred obstetrical examinations performed between the beginning of 1984 and the end of 1993, in eight cases measured by three sonographers (DKD, SG, and TD), the femur or humerus was measured before the 10th LMP week, using the crown-rump length (CRL) to estimate age by the Hadlock and colleagues' method for dating.[11] In all cases, the bones measured between 2 and 4.5 mm and the CRLs were between 19.4 and 30 mm, or between 8.5 and 9.9 LMP weeks.

Most authorities have advocated measuring one long bone because these bones are usually symmetrical. However, because large anomalous differences in the lengths can occur, an attempt to observe the morphology of all extremities is advised. I measured one fetus in which the right femur length was only 21.7 mm but the left was more normal for age (35.3 LMP weeks), at approximately 66 mm.[12]

The relative lengths of the extremity long bones have also been related to certain skeletal dysplasias.[6] A discussion of the particulars that are applicable to the sonographic study of the specific bones of the extremities follows.

Jeanty and colleagues published a widely used table for estimating the fetal age from four long bones, the femur, humerus, ulna, and tibia.[1] This research showed all long bone measurements to have coefficients of determination (r^2) of 0.92 or greater. Table 15–1 gives the polynomial regression formulas for fetal age estimates from these measurements.

Some attempts have been made to research the calculation of extremity volumes; however, these have not been widely accepted for routine examination.[13–15] This is most likely because of the small size of the extremities' cross-sectional diameters and circumferences.[16] Any error in cursor placement during measurements of small structures causes relatively larger percent errors. The measurement of the diameter and circumference of the extremities is also prone to exaggeration owing to planes that are slightly oblique to the true transverse. Another consideration is that extremities are not perfect cylinders, and the location of the cross section can affect the circumference measurement (see Figs. 15–7*B* and 15–20*B*).

TABLE 15–1. **LONG BONE POLYNOMIAL REGRESSION FORMULAS***

Age in LMP weeks = a + (b)X + (c)X^2

PARAMETER X IN MM	CONSTANTS a	b	c	r^2
Femur	9.54	0.298	0.00109	0.935
Humerus	9.65	0.262	0.00261	0.921
Tibia	10.06	0.313	0.00168	0.937
Ulna	10.03	0.286	0.00291	0.933

*Family of four polynomial regressions. To estimate age, substitute parameter measurement in millimeters for X and corresponding variables a, b, and c into the formula. Fetal age from LMP is estimated to tenths of a week. Coefficients of determination (r^2) all are greater than 0.92.

Adapted from Jeanty P, Rodesch F, Delbeke D, et al: Estimation of gestation age from measurements of fetal long bones. J Ultrasound Med 1984;3:75–79.

Anomalies

Although the purpose of this book is to describe the normal fetus from a sonographic perspective, it is wise to remember that one of the main reasons for knowing what normal anatomy looks like is to be able to recognize abnormalities. Wide variations are observed in the abnormalities of the extremities. These may include all the extremities, only one, or only a part of an extremity. Sonographically, anomalies of the extremities are generally recognized by evaluating for changes of bone brightness (echogenicity), bone deformities of shape, and length appropriate to age.[6]

Sonography is the preferred method for evaluating skeletal anomalies in utero. A study by Kurtz and Wapner[6] found that neither radiographs nor amniograms of a gravid uterus provided as much information as was provided by obstetrical sonography. Both FemL and HumL abnormalities have been associated with certain syndromes such as Down's. However, this was not found to be a strong association, and these measurements are not recommended for routine use in screening for genetic abnormalities.[17–19] Although sonography does not always give specific diagnoses for pathology, it is highly accurate for identifying many fetuses with skeletal dysplasias.[6] Kurtz and Wapner gave four cautions when evaluating skeletal dysplasia sonographically[6]:

"1. It is possible that certain dysplasias may not manifest themselves during the second or early third trimester. Therefore, normal fetal ultrasonographic examination during that period might not totally rule out abnormality.
2. It is possible that subtle deossification or deformity may not be appreciated on ultrasonographic examination.
3. Skeletal dysplasias consisting predominantly of abnormalities of the ilia, ribs, foot and ankle, or hand and wrist, are less likely to be routinely detected.
4. The analysis of the fetal skeleton for dysplasias is technically difficult, requiring additional time and considerable experience" on the part of the sonographer.

They further stated that detailed study for dysplasias should be limited to patients at risk for skeletal anomalies. This does not mean that sonographers do not need to be observant and to measure certain bones. Measurement of FemL is so common now that it could be considered as a part of the standard of care along with the biparietal diameter and abdominal circumference. Routine measurement of at least one femur and one humerus in each examination is recommended because one of each of these usually is relatively easy to locate. An attempt to visualize the other, more distal extremities is also recommended because anomalies may affect only one extremity bone. The difficulty and time involved in measuring all of the long bones of the extremities, 12 in all, are probably not cost-effective at this time. Jeanty and colleagues have investigated automated, computerized extremity measurement, a worthy endeavor.[20]

Absence or shortening of the bones of the extremities is generally classified using combining forms of Greek words: *melos* for "limb," *podos* for "foot," *dactyl* for "fingers" and "toes," and *cheir* for "hands." These are combined with the Greek *a-* for "absence," *hemi-* for "half," and *phoke* for "seal-like."

Amelia	Congenital absence of one or more limbs
Phocomelia	Congenital absence of the proximal extremities
Hemimelia	Congenital absence of the distal extremities
Acheiria	Congenital absence of one or more hand(s)
Apodia	Congenital absence of one or more feet
Adactyly	Congenital absence of fingers or toes

Numerous books describe the sonographic appearance of various anomalies in detail.[21-24] A very useful reference that does not show sonographic images but does provide a comprehensive, organized listing is Williamson and Williamson's *Gamuts in Ultrasound*.[25] This handy little book can help narrow the possible differential diagnoses when specific anomalies or pathologies are located with sonography, not only in a fetus but in an adult as well.

Upper Extremities

HUMERUS AND UPPER ARM

Methods

The fetal humerus has been less often researched and measured with sonography than the femur. This is probably because of the greater range of motion that the humerus exhibits and the resulting greater difficulty in locating this bone. The humerus can be rotated through most of the 360 degrees of motion around the shoulder. Sonographers can find themselves chasing the humerus about a woman's abdomen as an active fetus changes position. With experience and resulting speed in acquiring images, one humerus can be measured in almost 100% of cases after the first trimester.

The humerus that is in the near field of the sonographic image is usually easier to find in relationship to the head and spine. The humerus that is away from the transducer in the far field is often shadowed by other fetal parts such as the head, spine, or ribs. The humerus nearer to the transducer thus is the one that is usually measured. In the vast majority of fetuses, the two humeri are about the same length, so it really makes little difference which one is used for measurements. The caution is again offered that both humeri should be observed to ensure at least visual symmetry, even if both are not measured.

The humeral diaphysis appears linear (Figs. 15–1*A* and 15–3 to 15–7). The surfaces of the humerus may have some slight curvature but not as much as is seen in the medial and posterior aspects of the femur (see the femur discussion later).

It is usually easiest to locate the humerus by first locating the fetal head and spine; then it is fairly easy to locate the shoulder. Once the shoulder is located, the sonographer must follow the arm distally and determine the lie of the humerus. The humerus is easiest to follow using a cross-plane slide. Once the position of the humerus is determined, the transducer can then be rotated to view the bone in the long axis.

The sonographer should use a small degree of cross-plane rocking or angling to be sure that only one bone is being viewed. This is

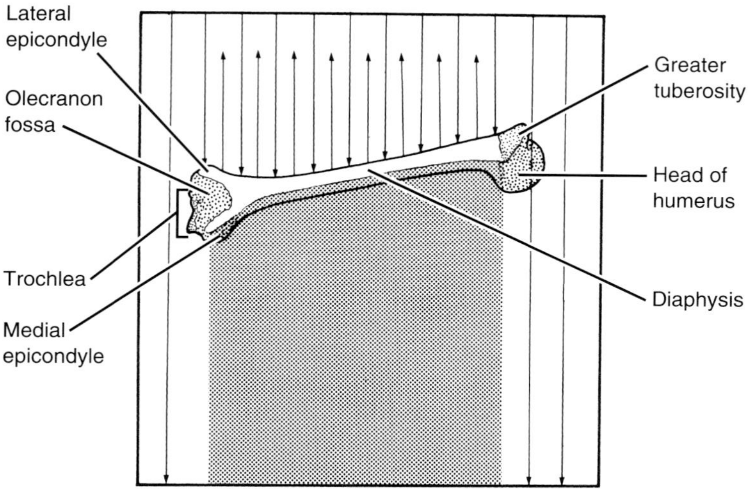

FIGURE 15–3.
Schematic of a humeral sonogram showing the source of the apparent Y shape of the distal humerus. The two epicondyles, which calcify relatively early in pregnancy, and the fossae between cause this apparent Y or split end (see also Figs. 15–4 and 15–5). The lateral epicondyle is slightly longer. The trochlea may be observed and measured in late pregnancy (see Fig. 15–6*A*). The differences in the lengths of the two epicondyles and the trochlea are a source of variation in humeral measurements. The edges of the distal acoustical shadow may help locate the true ends of the epicondyles.

because it can be easy to confuse the ulna or radius of the forearm with the humerus, especially if the fetus has the elbow tightly flexed with the hand at its mouth or ear, a common activity, so that the forearm is nearly parallel to the humerus.

The humeral head is not completely calcified until the third and fourth years after birth.[26] The cartilaginous tissue of the humeral head is hypoechoic or anechoic and often exhibits posterior enhancement (see Figs. 15–6 and 15–7). The cartilaginous humeral head has a smooth surface and often produces specular echoes from the surface nearest to the transducer. These specular echoes appear as a point extending from the proximal end of the humeral diaphysis but are not part of the diaphysis (see Figs. 15–6*A* and 15–7*A*). These are referred to in this text as the proximal humeral point (PHP) following

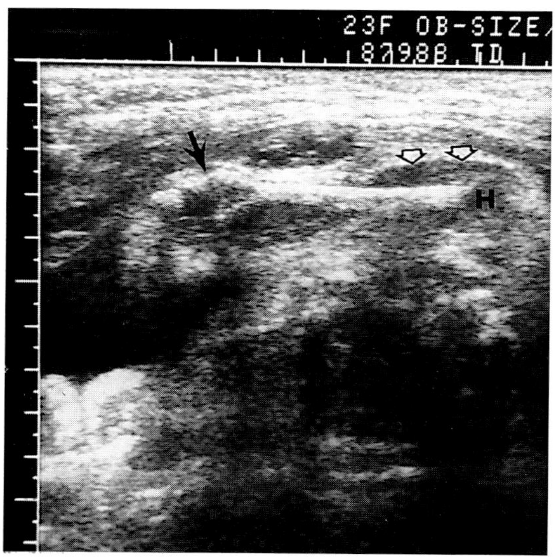

FIGURE 15–4.
Lateral approach to the humerus. Note the Y or split end of the distal humerus (solid arrow). This Y shape is due to the epicondyles and the fossae between. The solid arrow points to the lateral epicondyle. The hypoechoic, cartilaginous humeral head is marked by the H. The open arrows lie on the echogenic skin and subcutaneous fat and point to the hypoechoic deltoid muscle. (AA = 33.5 LMP weeks, n = 9, HumL = 58 mm, TD)

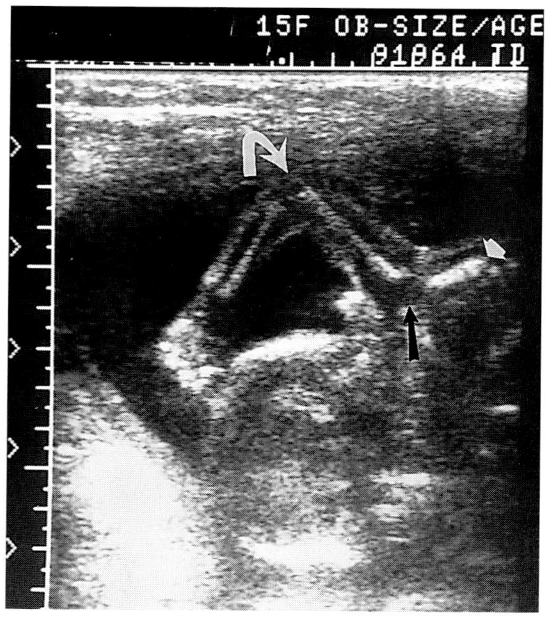

FIGURE 15–5.
The fetal elbow is bent, with the hand touching the head. The humerus is between the elbow (curved white arrow) and hypoechoic humeral head (black arrow). The ulna and radius can be observed between the elbow and hand. The short white arrow points to the end of a section of the scapula. (AA = 20.8 LMP, n = 9, range = 1.7 weeks, TD)

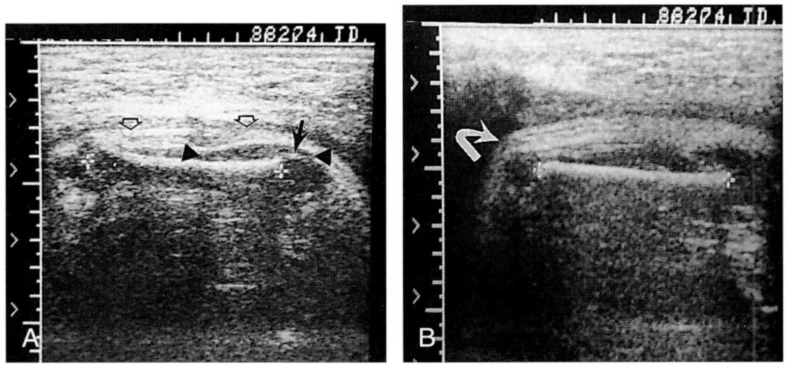

FIGURE 15–6. *A,* Lateral approach to the humerus with measurement to the end of the trochlea; HumL = 69.5 mm in this image. A more correct measurement would have been to the end of the lateral epicondyle. The HumL measurement of record in this case was 68 mm. The open arrows point to the skin line; the deltoid muscle is between the two black triangles. The thin black arrow points to the proximal humeral point (PHP), which should not be included in the HumL measurement. The PHP is the result of specular echoes from the near surface of the hypoechoic, cartilaginous humeral head. (AA = 38.4 LMP, n = 9, range = 4.1 weeks, TD) *B,* Posterior approach to the same humerus demonstrated in *A.* The humerus here appears straight, and the slight anterior clubbing of the distal humeral capitulum can be appreciated at the elbow + cursor. The curved arrow points to the elbow. In this image, the humerus measured 66.5 mm.

the precedent of Goldstein and colleagues, who first described the distal femoral point (DFP, discussed later).[27]

The distal end of the humerus has two condyles, the medial and lateral condyles. These can be observed in a true coronal plane of the arm, which can make the distal end of the humerus appear split or Y shaped. This Y shape is caused by the two divergent epicondyles and the coronoid and the olecranon fossae between them (see Figs. 15–3 and 15–4). The coronoid fossa is on the anterior surface, and the olecranon fossa is on the posterior surface between the condyles.

Measurements

The measurements are from the proximal end of the calcified humeral diaphysis, excluding the proximal humeral point, to the ends of the condyles. If both condyles are observed closely, it may be seen that the medial condyle tends to be slightly longer than the lateral one. A search of the sonographic literature did not find any discussion of which epicondyle was measured. Most articles simply measured "the longest dimension of the bone"[17] or "to the humeral condyle."[28] It has been suggested that the measurement be taken "to the middle of an imaginary line across the ends of the epicondyles."[20] The differences in measurements to either condyle or to a line across their ends are very small.

When the sonographic image is aligned with the long axis of the humerus, the bone often causes shadowing distally. If poor resolution or beam-width artifacts are a concern, the edges of these shadows can be used to help judge where the greatest extents of the humeral diaphyses are located[28] (see Fig. 15–6).

Figure 15–1*A* is an example of an early HumL measurement in the 10th LMP week. The smallest HumL obtained in my group's study population of 10,000+ obstetrical examinations was 2.1 mm. In this case, the LNMP age was 8.6 weeks and the average age of multiple fetal parameters (MFPs n = 8) was

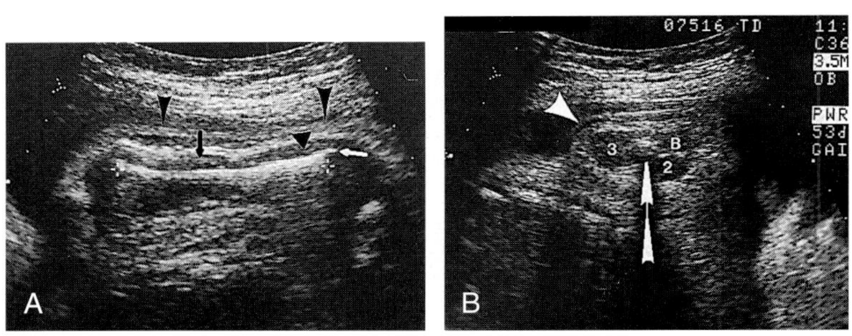

FIGURE 15–7. THREE-DIMENSIONAL UPPER ARM. *A,* Long axis of upper arm. Humeral diaphysis is measured between + cursors at 55.7 mm. Note that the measurement excludes the proximal humeral point (white arrow). The black arrowheads point to the lateral skin line. The black triangle points to the center of the deltoid muscle, and the black arrow points to the brachialis muscle. (AA = 35.7, n = 9, range = 4.8 weeks, TD) *B,* Tranverse section of upper arm. Cross section near the middle of the same upper arm shown in *A.* The long arrow points to the femur and lies in its acoustical shadow. The arrowhead points to the arm skin line. The muscles shown are the triceps (3), biceps (2), and brachialis (B).

8.1 weeks, range = 0.8 week. The CRL was 19.4 mm, or the equivalent of 8.3 weeks, and the embryonic heart rate was appropriate at 163 B/M, which evaluated to 7.8 LMP weeks.

Jeanty and colleagues[1] found the HumL normally to be approximately 69 mm at a mean age of 40.1 weeks or term. In my group's study population, the longest HumL was 78 mm, but the LNMP was unknown, and because many of the fetal parameters were off the charts, an age could not be estimated in the case beyond "postterm pregnancy." The next longest HumL in this population was 76 mm at 42 LMP weeks. A total of 30 fetuses had HumL measurements of 70 mm or greater. These HumL data are given as examples of extremes.

Table 7–7 shows Jeanty and colleagues' widely used fetal ages for the fetal long bones.[1] My published table of MFP ages is similar and lists the HumL as 68 mm at 40 weeks and 71 mm at 42 weeks.[7] A more recent version of this table can be found elsewhere (see Chapter 7).

ULNA, RADIUS, AND FOREARM

The distal long bones of the arms can be difficult to locate because of the diverse positions in which they may be found. This difficulty can be compounded for measurements in an active fetus. For this reason, the ulna and radius are not routinely measured in most sonographic laboratories.

In the arm, the radius is on the true anatomical lateral side, nearest the thumb, and the ulna is on the medial side of the arm, nearest the fifth or smallest finger. The ulna is the longer of the two bones. The longer length of the ulna compared with the radius is most obvious at the proximal or elbow end of the bones (Fig. 15–8*A*). The olecranon process of the ulna is responsible for most of the greater length. If the fetal wrist and hand are rotated, the ulna and radius appear crossed rather than parallel (Fig. 15–8*B*).

The ulna may be used for measurements if a disparity of the more common fetal parameters raises questions. Tables 15–1 and 7–7 can be used to estimate the fetal age in LMP weeks from the ulna in millimeters.[1]

HANDS

The fetal hands have received sonographic attention during the past few years (Figs. 15–9 and 15–10). Most of the discussion has been on the study of hand morphology to diagnose genetic syndromes. Although some features such as simian creases have been identified sonographically,[30] a search for such anomalies does not seem useful in routine screening. The fetal hand can be difficult to isolate and view in its open position. Most of the time when the palm of the hand is well seen, it is by chance. This is not to say that observations of the

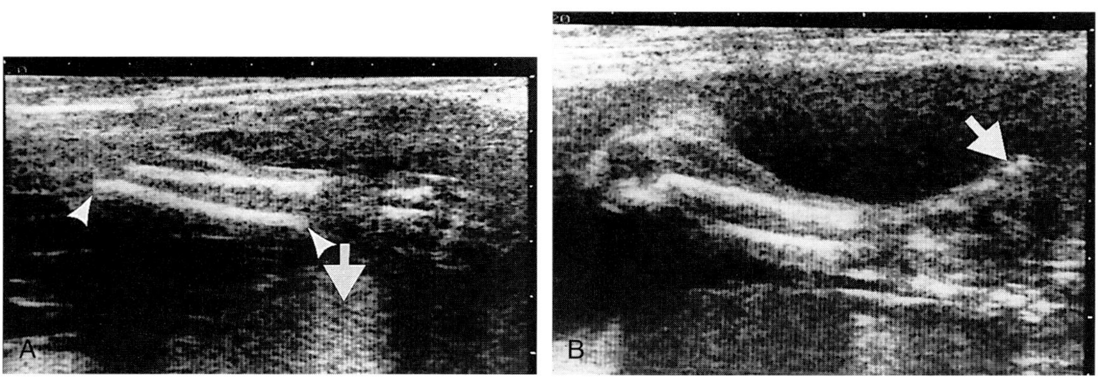

FIGURE 15–8. FOREARM. *A*, Coronal view of ulna and radius. Forearm showing the parallel ulna (between arrowheads) and radius. Note the greater length of the ulna, with most of the excess length being at the proximal end. The second and third metacarpal bones can be seen distal to the hypoechoic wrist bones. The arrow points to the artifactitious through transition or posterior enhancement of the echoes passing through the wrist. (AA = 25.0, n = 9, range = 1.4 weeks, TD) *B*, Coronal view with rotation of arm. This is the same forearm and hand as shown in *A*, with a slight twist of the fetal wrist. Note that the ulna and radius are no longer parallel, and the proximal end of the ulna is out of the plane of view. The arrow points to the distal phalanx of the thumb.

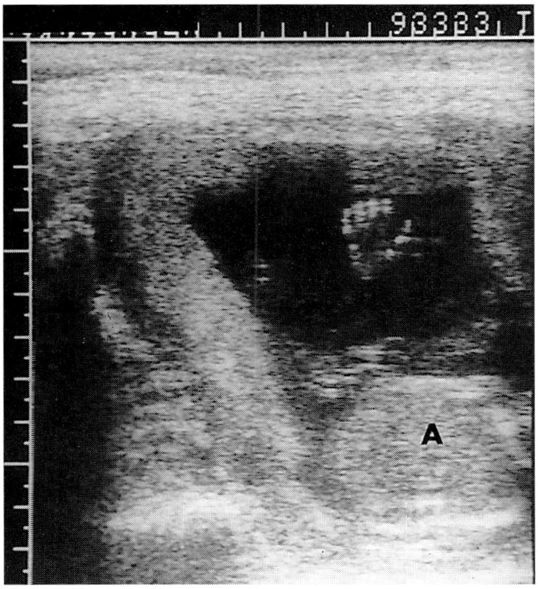

FIGURE 15–9. HAND IN 17th WEEK.
The fetal hand anterior to the cross section of the supine abdomen (A). Echoes from the umbilical cord are seen across the anterior abdominal wall. (AA = 17.6, n = 10, range = 1.2 weeks, TD)

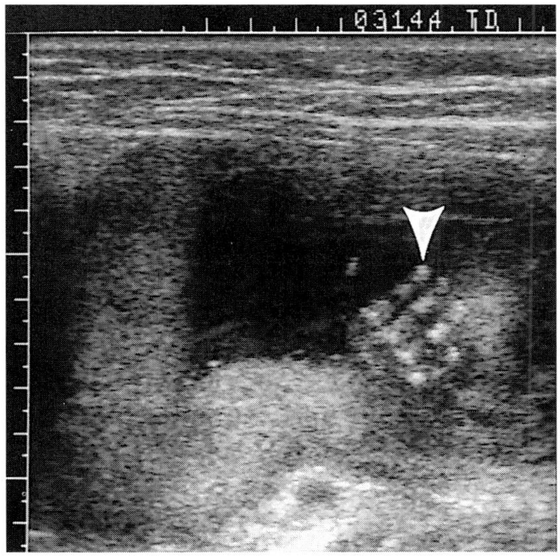

FIGURE 15–10.
A hand in the 24th LMP week. The arrowhead points to the distal phalanx of the second digit (index finger). The proximal, middle, and distal phalanges of the second, third, and fourth digits can be seen. Portions of the fifth digit (little finger) can be seen. The thumb is out of the plane of view, and its tip appears as an echo in the amniotic fluid. With real-time sonography, slight back-and-forth cross-plane rocking provides a look at the complete hand. (AA = 24.6, n = 9, range = 1.3 weeks, TD)

hands are not helpful when certain problems are encountered. Benacerraf and colleagues have used sonography extensively to study fetal hands and the relationship to various anomalies, particularly Down's syndrome.[31, 32] Anomalous development of the hand often correlates with genetic defects.

Because of the importance that physical anthropologists have placed on the hands and tool making in the evolution of the human species,[33, 34] it seems worthwhile to observe a few normal fetal hands. The possible value of these observations was reinforced by a statement in a book about evolution: "It has been said that 'Man's [and woman's] place in nature is largely writ upon the hand.' Any evidence bearing on the evolution of the human hand would be extremely interesting."[35]

In the uterine environment, fetal hand use is completely controlled by genetics, without external visual cues to show a fetus what to do with its hand. In the early 1980s, two sonographers (TD and LP) recorded their observations on use of fetal hands during the last half of pregnancy (after 20 LMP weeks). At the start of each obstetrical sonographic examination, a survey is normally performed to ascertain the fetal and placental positions. In this study, during the initial survey, one hand was located and the sonographers recorded what the hand was touching. This generally took less than 1 minute. These observations were recorded for approximately 100 fetuses. It was found that 50% of fetal hand activities were head and face touching. This included thumb sucking, nose and ear grasping, eye poking, and scalp and hair rubbing (Fig. 15–11).

The second most common activity was umbilical cord touching, grasping, or manipulating (Figs. 15–12 to 15–14). This was at first surprising, although the umbilical cord attaches to the abdomen at the level of the elbows, right between the hands. Obviously, umbilical cord touching and grasping is not only common but is probably unavoidable. This observation runs contrary to others or at least to the suggestion that fetal asphyxia might be attributable to a fetus's occluding its own blood supply.[36–39] It appears probable that if fetal grasping of the umbilical cord could pose a danger to a fetus, the opposing thumb would never have evolved.

The remaining 15% of the time, the fetuses were observed to be touching other objects

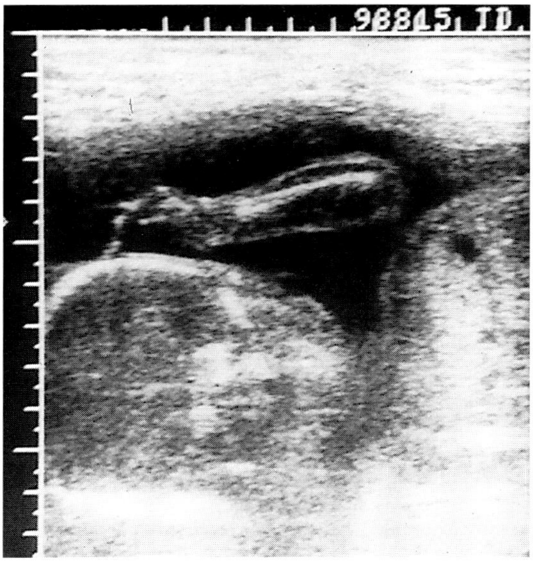

FIGURE 15–11.
The most frequent activity of a fetus is face and head touching (found approximately 50% of the time). Here a fetus is shown touching the side of its head. (AA = 24.0, n = 9, range = 2.1 weeks, TD)

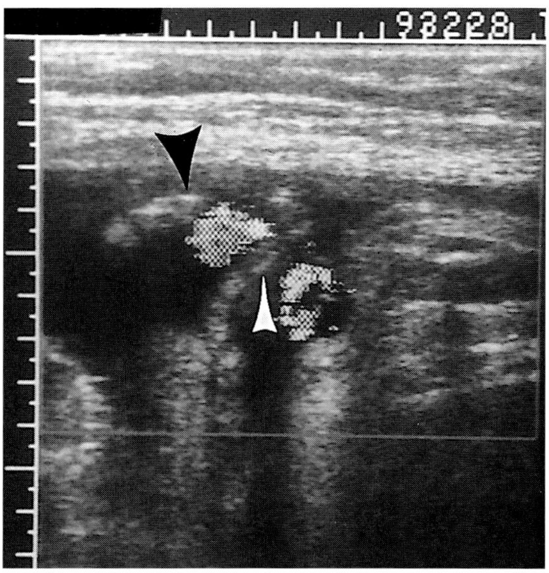

FIGURE 15–12.
The second most frequent activity of a fetus is umbilical cord touching and grasping, found in approximately 35% of cases in one study of 100 brief looks. This 35% occurrence is thought to translate to a universal activity at one time or another during pregnancy. Here a 39-LMP-week fetus is palpating its cord between its thumb (white arrowhead) and index finger (black arrowhead). This black-and-white color Doppler shows the flow in the umbilical cord as a checkered display. (AA = 39.4, n = 9, range = 5.5 weeks, TD)

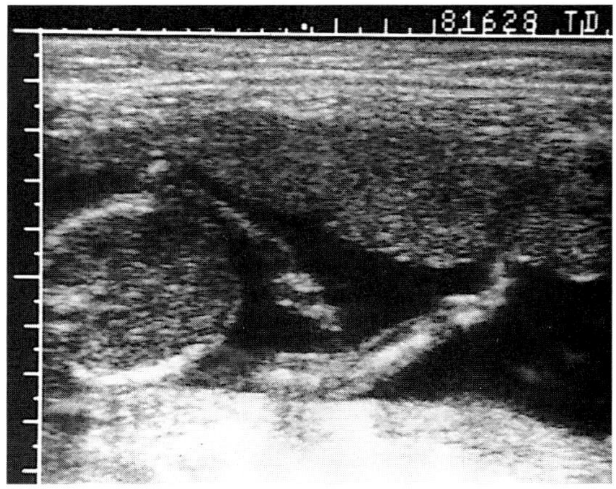

FIGURE 15–13.
Here a fetus is seen to touch the placenta with its right hand while the left hand touches the inside of the right elbow. This type of touching activity was observed in only about 15% of cases. In approximately 85% of cases, the fetus touched its face or head (50%) and the umbilical cord (35%). (AA = 18.4, n = 9, range = 1.2 weeks, TD)

(see Fig. 15–13). This included random touching of the uterine wall and placenta, as well as its own feet, knees, genitalia, and body parts other than the face and head or umbilical cord. At least one discussion of fetal masturbation has been published.[40] However, the application of the term *masturbation* to what may be

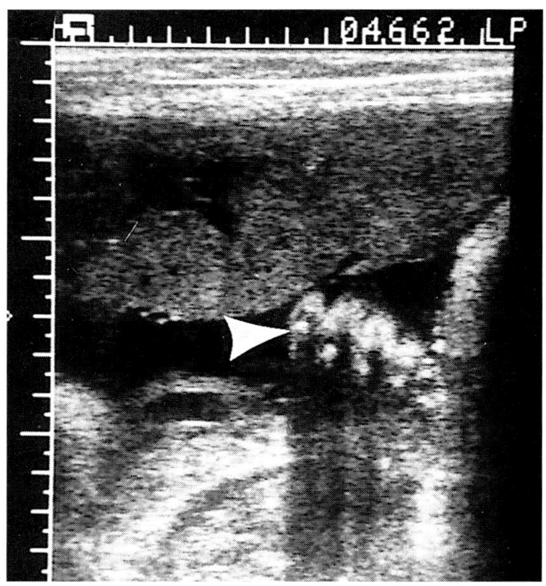

FIGURE 15–14.
The fingernails can sometimes be observed with modern sonographic equipment. The arrowhead points to the fingernail of the fifth digit. The nails of the fourth, third, and second digits can also be seen as bright echogenic dots. This fetus was grasping its umbilical cord, which is seen just below the arrowhead. (AA = 35.6, n = 9, range = 4.2 weeks, LP)

random grasping by a fetus seems rather extreme. A fetus grasps and sucks on anything that is convenient. Two sonographers (TD and DKD) have actually observed one twin sucking the other's penis, but to describe this in utero act as "oral sex" seems to take the definition out of the social context. On another occasion, a fetus was observed to appear to be playing "patty-cake" by gently patting its open hands, finger against finger, one against the other. It is not uncommon to see one hand grasping the other (see Fig. 19–2*L*).

It must be emphasized that the foregoing observations of fetal hand use were an informal study, without peer review. They are offered here only for their interest and possible inspiration to others to pursue this intriguing topic. Clinically, the current information on fetal hand activities is of little significance other than to point out that umbilical cord grasping is common and to dispel the fear that a fetus might commit suicide by squeezing its umbilical cord.

Sonographers should not forget that the actions of a fetus must not be interpreted in a social context. It is only the fetal activities that seem universal or routine that may shed light on the evolution of the hand and its possible genetic control and use. One discussion of hand control points out that hand use moved from the pure power grip required for tree swinging to the more refined precision touch. "In the so called precision grip, the grip you use in such delicate work as starting to insert and turn a small screw in its socket, the tool handle is held between thumb and fingertips. . . . Precision grip has evolved to its highest form in man, and the trend can be deduced from studies of tools and toolmaking."[41] Figure 15–12 shows a fetal hand (39.4 weeks by average of nine parameters) using a precision grip to palpate its cord between the pads of the fingertips and thumb. Is it possible that this sort of gentle, precision grip develops only very near term? Perhaps this is a way of looking at ontogeny recapitulating phylogeny.

In conversations on the topic of fetal umbilical cord grasping, others have pointed out the importance of hand movements and oral activity in understanding psychological development in utero.[42] This importance is emphasized by Graves, who discusses some of the contributions of sonography to the study of the fetus and motility and concludes with a quote from the poet Samuel Coleridge (1885): "Yes,—the history of a man for the nine months preceding his birth, would, probably, be far more interesting, and contain events of greater moment, than all the three score and ten years that follow."[43]

Carrying this line of thought to a logical conclusion, it is possible to imagine some sort of intelligence quotient that could be based on the time of onset of certain activities, similar to the observation of the various "blink–startle responses" to acoustical stimulation that have been suggested as a measure of psychological habituation. Habituation has something to do with being able to focus mentally and correlates with intelligence,[44] a subject that is beyond this discussion.

Will a fetus that invents a game of patty-cake to occupy itself while waiting for delivery be more creative as an adult than a 2-year-old who has to be taught the game to avoid boredom while waiting to see the pediatrician? Although appearing frivolous, this idea should not be taken lightly. Sonography opens a window on human development that is very interesting, from both a physiological and psychological standpoint.

Lower Extremities

FEMUR AND UPPER LEG

Methods

The fetal FemL is a useful, dependable parameter for sonographic measurement. The femur does not have the range of motion that the humerus does, and FemL is a relatively long linear measurement. The longer linear measurement means that variations in cursor placement produce relatively smaller percent errors, and the femur grows at a relatively rapid pace, which makes it a fairly reliable predictor of fetal age.

FemL has been found to correlate with the crown-heel length at birth.[45] Therefore, longer fetuses tend to have longer femurs, thus overestimating fetal age, and shorter fetuses have shorter femurs, resulting in an underestimation of age. This variation in FemL results in greater variation in the estimated ages but should produce more accurate fetal weight estimates from regressions that use this parameter.[46] This assumes that all other parameters being equal, longer fetuses weigh more than shorter fetuses.

The data from the Routine Antenatal Diagnostic Imaging with Ultrasound Study (RADIUS) showed a difference in FemL between white and black fetuses, with the latter having persistently longer femurs.[47] This large and controversial study included pregnancies from six states in the United States. The authors of this report state, "Perhaps the biological variation within a race or gender accounts in part for these differences." Another finding was that FemL values were similar for both females and males.

All published sonographic measurements of the fetal femur are actually the length of the diaphysis and not the complete femur. The diaphyseal length includes only the calcified shaft of the bone and excludes the femoral head and distal condyles of the epiphysis. The measurement should also exclude the specular echoes from the near side of the cartilaginous condyles, the DFP[27] (Figs. 15–15 and 15–16).

The femur often appears curved when viewed sonographically.[48] The degree of this apparent curving depends on the approach. From the anterior and lateral approach, the femoral diaphysis appears relatively straight (see Figs. 15–15*A* and 15–16) but from the posterior and medial aspects it appears noticeably curved (Figs. 15–15*B*, 15–17, and 15–18*B*). In each approach, the side of the diaphysis nearest the transducer is well visualized; however, the side away from the trans-

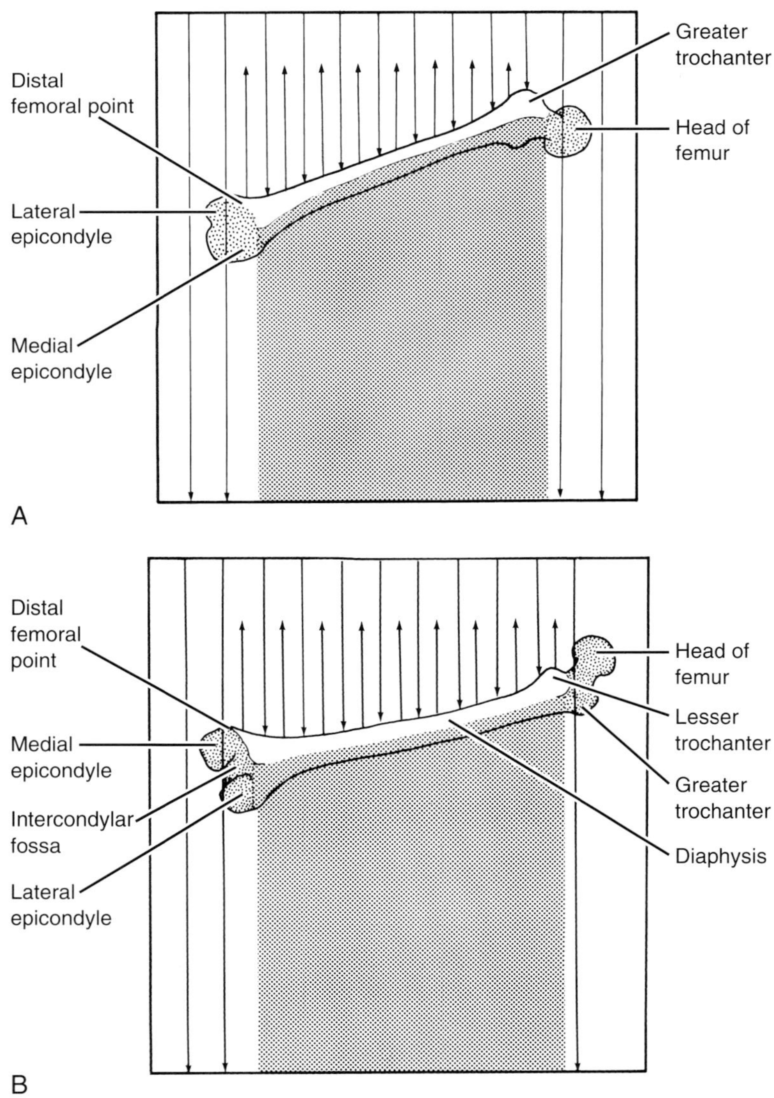

FIGURE 15–15.
A, The femur appears relatively straight from the anterolateral approach. The distal femoral point is not actually calcified but is caused by specular echoes from the nearest surface of the cartilaginous condyles. The edges of the acoustical shadow can help identify the ends of the diaphysis. Compare this drawing with Figure 15–16. *B*, From the posteromedial approach, the femur appears markedly curved. This is because of the shape of the bone. The more linear side of the bone is lost in the acoustical shadows. This apparent curvature is normal and does not affect the FemL measurement. Again, the edges of the acoustical shadows may help locate the true ends of the diaphysis. Compare this image with the more distal femur in Figures 15–17 and 15–18*B*.

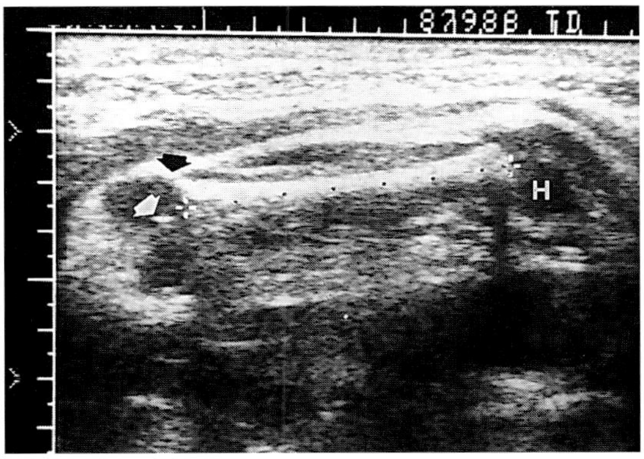

FIGURE 15–16.
Lateral approach to the thigh showing the measurement of the femoral diaphysis (+ cursors = 65.8 mm). Note the relatively linear appearance of the diaphysis in this view. The hypoechoic femoral head (H) and distal condyles are easily seen. The white arrow is in the lateral condyle and points to the distal femoral ossification center. The distal femoral point can be faintly seen around the near edge of the lateral condyle. (AA = 33.5, n = 9, range = 2.1 weeks, TD)

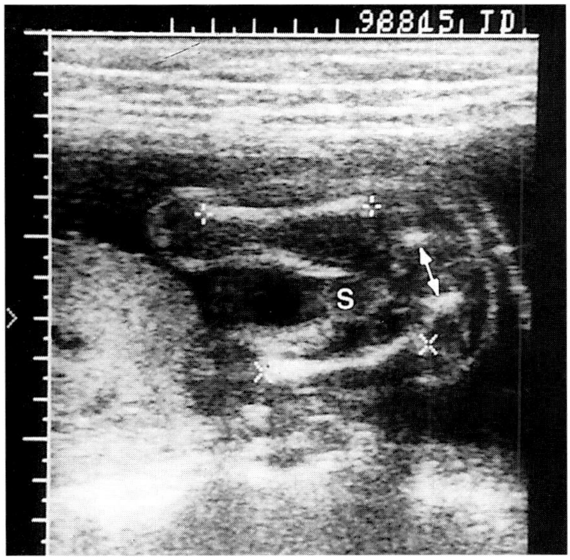

FIGURE 15–17. LATERAL AND MEDIAL VIEWS OF BOTH FEMURS. Both femurs can often be measured in a single image. Note that the top femur appears less curved than the more distal femur. This is because of the shape of the bone surfaces, which reflect the echoes. These femurs measured 41.1 mm (+) and 41.0 mm (×), only 0.1 mm difference. The scrotum (S) is between the thighs. The bright echoes of the pelvic ischial ossification centers are at either end of the double arrow. The gluteus maximus muscles are seen around the posterior of these echoes. (AA = 24.0, n = 9, range = 2.1 weeks, TD)

ducer is not visualized owing to acoustical shadowing. At least one study has looked at the effect of this apparent curvature on sonographic measurements.[49] This study did not find a significant difference in ages predicted from straight or curved FemL. This normal curvature of the medial and posterior surfaces of the femur should not be confused with pathological processes or fractures.

Often the anatomy of the fetal knee is visualized sonographically. Figure 15–19*A* shows the measurement of the FemL, which should not include the ossification center in the cartilaginous femoral condyles. The echogenic distal femoral ossification center normally is pres-ent by the 36th LMP week and should not be confused with the patella. In a plane slightly posterior to Figure 15–19*A*, Figure 15–19*B* shows the hypoechoic cartilaginous fetal patella. The patella does not calcify until after birth.

Measurements

As stated earlier, Moore and Persaud report that the extremity bones begin calcifying about the 10th LNMP week.[49] At this early age, the femur, similar to the humerus, is just a bright dot in the lower extremity, but it also is distinct from the surrounding soft tissues, and with good resolution, we found it may be measured after the eighth LMP week. Figure 15–1*B* is an example of an early FemL measurement.

The smallest FemL measurement obtained in my group's study population of 10,000+ obstetrical examinations was 2.0 mm. In this case, the LNMP age was 8.9 weeks and the average age of six MFPs was 8.1 weeks, range = 1.6 weeks. The CRL was 20 mm for an equivalent age of 8.4 weeks, and embryonic heart rate was appropriate at 177, which also evaluated to 8.4 LNMP weeks (see Chapter 12 for estimating the fetal age embryonic heart rate).

The longest femur measured in my group's study population was 87 mm at 41.3 LNMP age, and the average of eight MFP ages was 40.2 weeks. The population included a total of 26 fetuses with femurs measuring 80 mm or greater. Again, these are examples of extreme cases. These wide variations of fetal parameter sizes at any given time, most particularly near term, are the reason why fetal age dating charts usually provide a range of ages rather than a single specific age.[50]

FemL is one of the most often measured parameters for estimation of fetal age. Jeanty and colleagues' table of long bone size age es-

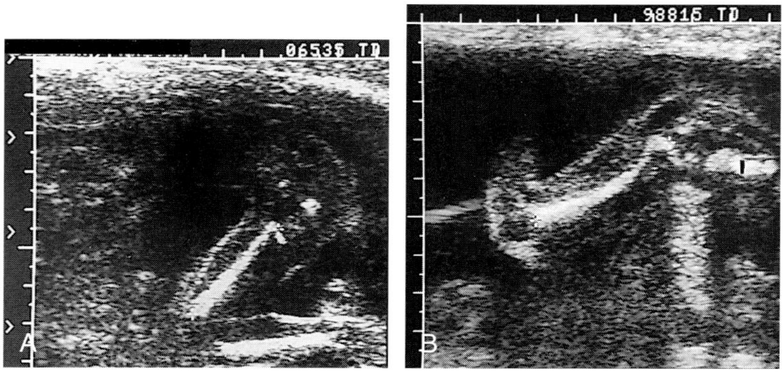

FIGURE 15–18. ANTERIOR AND POSTERIOR FEMUR. *A*, The anterior surface of the femur is very straight (+ cursors = 31.9 mm). Here the fetus is in a kneeling position with its lower leg at the bottom of the image. A section of umbilical cord is across the leg. (AA = 20.0, n = 9, range = 1.8 weeks, TD) *B*, The posterior surface of the femur (nearest the transducer) is quite curved (+ cursors = 40.6 mm). The knee is bent, with the lower leg passing out of the plane of view toward the transducer. A section through the ilium (I) of the pelvis is also seen. (AA = 24.0, n = 9, range = 2.1 weeks, TD)

timates is in common use.[1] Table 15–1 gives the polynomial regression formulas that may be used in computer spreadsheets for age estimations, and Table 7–7 is Jeanty and colleagues' nomogram for ages from long bones.

By the end or term of a pregnancy, FemL normally is slightly less than 80 mm. Jeanty and colleagues reported a FemL of 80 mm for a mean age of 40 weeks (±2 SD = 37.9 to 40.1 weeks). In my group's study population, the mean FemL was 78 mm at 40 weeks and 82 mm at 42 LNMP weeks (see Tables 7–7 and 7–1). In a study by the group at the Baylor College of Medicine in Houston, the 39.9-week femur was found to be approximately 78 mm and 80 mm at 40.8 weeks[51] (see Chapter 7 for the actual use of fetal age tables for the various measurements including the FemL).

With modern sonographic equipment, it is possible to study the muscle groups of the extremities. Figure 15–20 shows some of the more prominent muscles in long axis and a transverse section of the thigh.

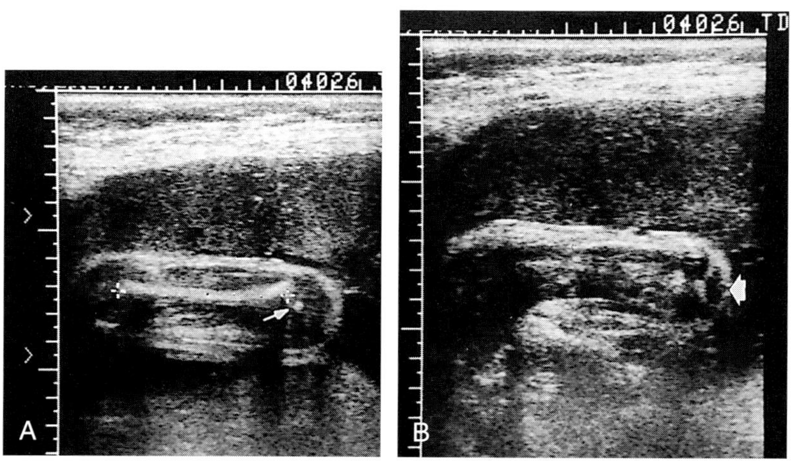

FIGURE 15–19. KNEE IN 31st WEEK. *A*, The distal femoral ossification center (arrow) can often be seen by the 32nd LMP week and always by the 36th week. This bright echo is near the center of the cartilaginous condyles and should not be included in the measurement of the FemL (+ cursors = 62.1 mm). Note the faint acoustical shadow distal to the ossification center. *B*, The patella or kneecap (arrow) is seen in this image, which is slightly posterior to the plane shown in *A*. The patella is cartilaginous and does not calcify until after birth. The ovoid hypoechoic condyles can be seen just proximal to the patella; the diaphysis is not seen in this plane. (AA = 31.5, n = 9, range = 4.0 weeks, TD)

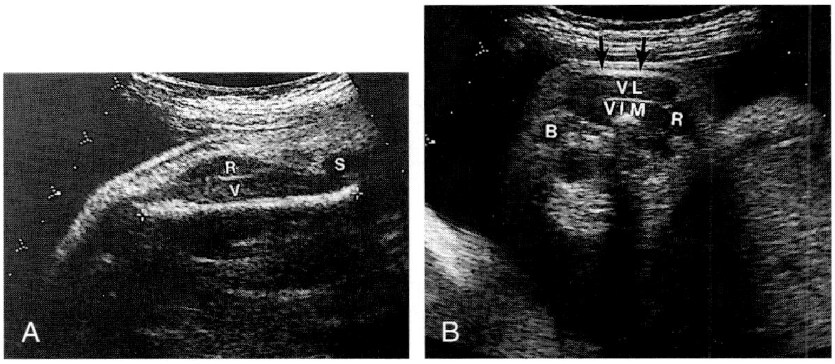

FIGURE 15–20. THREE-DIMENSIONAL THIGH. *A*, Long axis of thigh. Measurement of the femur diaphysis from the anterior approach. Muscles observed are the vastus intermedius (V), rectus femoris (R), and a portion of the sartorius (S), which crosses the upper rectus femoris. Overlying the rectus femoris are the echogenic subcutaneous fat and the skin line over the fat. (AA = 35.7, n = 9, range = 4.8 weeks, TD) *B*, Transverse section of thigh. Cross section of the midthigh from a lateral approach. This shows the same extremity as in *A*. The echogenic iliotibial tract (black arrows) lies just beneath the skin line. The iliotibial tract is over the vastus lateralis muscle (VL), which overlies the vastus intermedius muscle (VIM). The femoral diaphysis is seen beneath the VIM as a bright echo producing distal shadowing. The biceps femoris (B) is in the posterior thigh, and the rectus femoris (R) is in the anterior thigh. The adductor canal is an echogenic area between the biceps femoris and the shadow from the femur. The canal extends into the shadow.

TIBIA, FIBULA, AND LOWER LEG

The shin bones are also valid long bones for measurement and fetal age estimation. However, because of the range of motion of the leg, these are somewhat more difficult to measure than is the femur. For this reason, they are less often used.

The tibia is the larger of the two bones. The fibula is the smaller and more lateral in the lower leg. Figure 15–21 demonstrates the fibula and tibia sonographically. Tables 15–1 and 7–7 show fetal age estimation from the tibia.

FEET

The fetal foot has also been measured and the dimensions have been correlated to age (see Table 15–2). The foot may be difficult to measure in an active fetus. The feet are more often studied for anomalies such as clubfoot or polydactyly. These anomalies are associated with many syndromes and genetic problems.[52]

The growth of the fetal foot was first sonographically measured and the findings published in 1987.[53] This research studied the foot from the 12th LMP week through term and found good correlation with Streeter's fetal specimen measurements of 1920. The dating nomogram from this study (Table 15–2) seems to correlate fairly well with our observations. However, the polynomial regression formulas given in the original article do not appear to produce the results shown in the nomogram. For this reason, the regression formulas are not recommended for use and are not provided here.

The ±2 SD for age in Mercer and col-

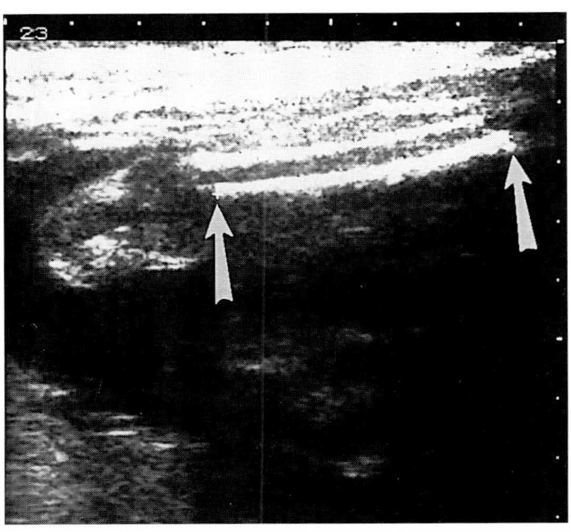

FIGURE 15–21.
The fibula and tibia (arrows) are bright echogenic lines. The hypoechoic cartilaginous ankle bones (medial and lateral malleolus) and the calcaneus can be seen adjacent to the distal ends of the two bones. (AA = 29.5, n = 9, range = 2.9 weeks, TD)

TABLE 15–2. **FOOT LENGTH GROWTH AND DATING CURVES BASED ON POLYNOMIAL REGRESSION ±2 SD**

GROWTH CURVE OF FOOT LENGTH				DATING CURVE OF GESTATIONAL AGE			
Gestational Week	Lower Limit (mm)	Predicted Value (mm)	Upper Limit (mm)	Foot Length (mm)	Lower Limit (wk)	Predicted Value (wk)	Upper Limit (wk)
12	7	8	9	10	11.5	12.5	13.5
13	10	11	12	12	12.1	13.1	14.2
14	13	15	16	14	12.7	13.8	14.9
15	16	18	20	16	13.3	14.4	15.5
16	19	21	23	18	13.9	15.1	16.3
17	22	24	27	20	14.5	15.7	17
18	24	27	30	22	15.1	16.4	17.7
19	27	30	34	24	15.7	17.1	18.4
20	30	33	37	26	16.3	17.7	19.1
21	32	36	40	28	16.9	18.4	19.9
22	35	39	43	30	17.6	19.1	20.6
23	37	42	46	32	18.2	19.8	21.4
24	40	45	50	34	18.9	20.5	22.1
25	42	47	53	36	19.5	21.2	22.9
26	45	50	55	38	20.2	21.9	23.7
27	47	53	58	40	20.8	22.7	24.5
28	49	55	61	42	21.5	23.4	25.2
29	51	58	64	44	22.2	24.1	26
30	54	60	67	46	22.9	24.9	26.8
31	56	62	68	48	23.6	25.6	27.6
32	58	65	72	50	24.3	26.4	28.4
33	60	67	74	52	24.9	27.1	29.3
34	62	69	77	54	25.7	27.9	30.1
35	64	71	79	56	26.4	28.4	30.9
36	66	74	82	58	27.1	29.4	31.8
37	67	76	84	60	27.8	30.2	32.6
38	69	78	86	62	28.5	31	33.5
39	71	80	88	64	29.3	31.8	34.3
40	72	81	90	66	30	32.6	35.2
				68	30.7	33.4	36.1
				70	31.5	34.2	36.9
				72	32.2	35	37.8
				74	33	35.9	38.7
				76	33.8	36.8	39.6
				78	34.5	37.5	40.5
				80	35.3	38.4	41.4
				82	36.1	39.2	42.4
				84	36.9	40.1	43.3
				86	37.7	41	44.2

From Mercer BM, Sklar S, Shariatmadar A, et al: Fetal foot length as a predictor of gestational age. Am J Obstet Gynecol 1987;156:350–355.

leagues' study calculates to approximately 16% (±8%) of the mean age, which is similar to findings in other studies.[53] Hadlock and coworkers found ±8% for the head circumference and FemL in the second and third trimesters.[54] It has been hypothesized that all fetal parameters will have a ±2 SD for age of less than ±10% of the mean age.[12]

Figures 15–22 to 15–24 show the measurement of foot length from the great toe to the heel. Figure 15–23 is a transverse view, and the third is a sagittal section of the foot. In this transverse view, it is easy to distinguish the location of the great toe. In the sagittal view, however, it is less obvious whether the section is through the great toe or one of the other toes. This determination must be made with real-time ultrasound during the examination.

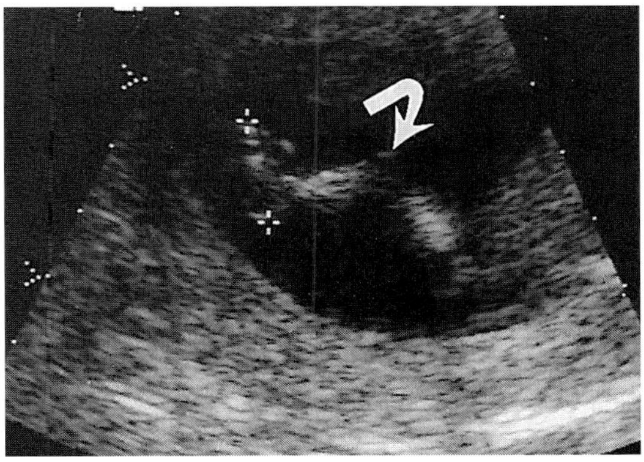

FIGURE 15–22. FOOT IN 13TH WEEK.
Anterior, sagittal fetal foot measurement of 14.2 mm between + cursors. The knee (curved arrow) is slightly flexed. (AA = 13.5, n = 10, range = 1.3 weeks, TD)

The calcaneous bone in the heel is cartilaginous and appears hypoechoic. The calcaneous ossification center may be observed in the late second trimester. This bone does not completely calcify until after birth.[55]

REFERENCES

1. Jeanty P, Rodesch F, Delbekd D, et al: Estimation of gestational age from measurements of the fetal long bones. J Ultrasound Med 1984;3:75–79.

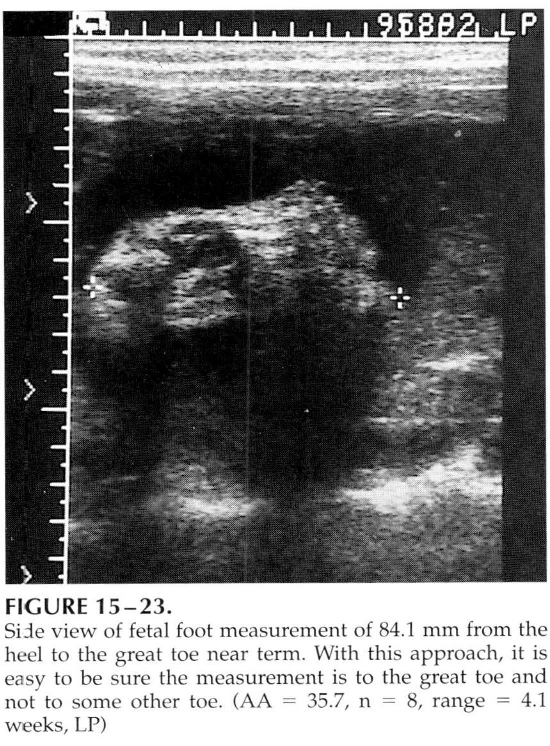

FIGURE 15–23.
Side view of fetal foot measurement of 84.1 mm from the heel to the great toe near term. With this approach, it is easy to be sure the measurement is to the great toe and not to some other toe. (AA = 35.7, n = 8, range = 4.1 weeks, LP)

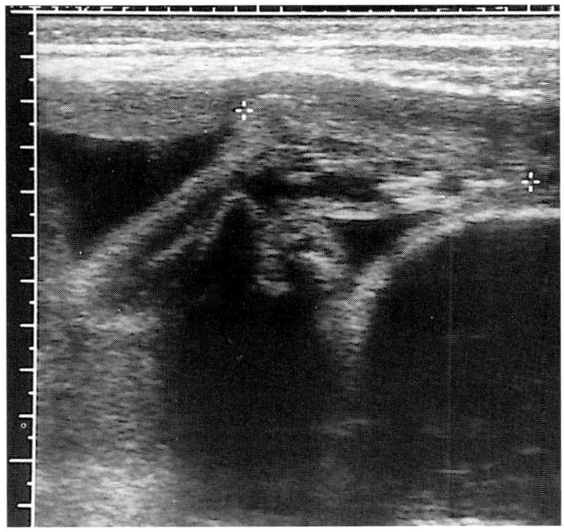

FIGURE 15–24.
Posterior, sagittal fetal foot measurement of 66.0 mm. In this view it is more difficult to ascertain that the measurement is to the great toe and not to some other toe. (AA = 33.0, n = 9, range = 1.4 weeks, TD)

2. O'Brien GD, Queenan JT, Campbell S: Assessment of gestational age in the second trimester by real-time ultrasound measurement of the femur length. Am J Obstet Gynecol 1981;139:540–545.
3. Hohler CW, Ouetel TA: Fetal femur length: Equations for computer calculation of gestational age from ultrasound measurements. Am J Obstet Gynecol 1982; 143:479.
4. Hadlock FP, Harrist RB, Deter RL, et al: Ultrasonically measured fetal femur length as a predictor of menstrual age. AJR 1982;183:875.
5. Wolfson RN, Peisner DB, Chik LL, et al: Comparison of biparietal diameter and femur length in the third trimester: Effects of gestational age and variation in fetal growth. J Ultrasound Med 1986;5:145.
6. Kurtz AB, Wapner RJ: Ultrasonographic diagnosis of second-trimester skeletal dysplasias: A prospective analysis in a high-risk population. J Ultrasound Med 1983;2:99–106.
7. DuBose TJ: Assessment of fetal age and size: Techniques and criteria. In: Berman MC, ed: Obstetrics & Gynecology: Diagnostic Medical Sonography. A Guide to Clinical Practice, vol 1. JB Lippincott, Philadelphia, 1991, p 291.
8. Moore KL, Persaud TVN: The Developing Human: Clinically Oriented Embryology, 5th ed. WB Saunders, Philadelphia, 1993, pp 93–94.
9. Chambers HA, editor and arrangement: Dry Bones: The Treasury of Negro Spirituals. Blandford Press, London, 1953, pp 26–30.
10. Moore KL, Persaud TVN: The Developing Human: Clinically Oriented Embryology, 5th ed. WB Saunders, Philadelphia, 1993, p 365.
11. Hadlock FP, Shah YP, Kanon DJ, et al: Fetal crown-rump length: Reevaluation of relation to menstrual age (5–18 weeks) with high-resolution real-time US. Radiology 1992;182:501–505.
12. DuBose TJ, Poole EK, Butschek C, et al: Range of multiple fetal parameters. J Ultrasound Med 1988; AIUM Proceedings Abstract 1508; 7:205.
13. Thompson TR, Manning FA: Estimation of volume and weight of the perinate: Relationship to morpho-

metric measurement by ultrasonography. J Ultrasound Med 1983;2:113–116.
14. Jeanty P, Romero R, Hobbins JC: Fetal limb volume: A new parameter to assess fetal growth and nutrition. J Ultrasound Med 1985;4:273–282.
15. Hills D, Baim R: Fetal thigh diameter unreliable as a predictor of birth weight percentile (abstract 518). Official Proceedings: Annual AIUM/SDMS Convention. J Ultrasound Med 1984;3:220.
16. Vinzileos AM, Neckles S, Campbell WA, et al: Ultrasound fetal thigh-calf circumferences and gestational age, independent fetal ratios in normal pregnancy. J Ultrasound Med 1985;4:287–292.
17. Rotmensch S, Luo JS, Liberati M, et al: Fetal humeral length to detect Down syndrome. Am J Obstet Gynecol 1992;166:1330–1334.
18. Platt LD, Mederaris AL, Carlson DE, et al: Screening for Down syndrome with the femur length/biparietal diameter ratio: A new twist of the data. Am J Obstet Gynecol 1992;167:124–128.
19. Winston YE, Horger OE III: Down syndrome and femur length. Am J Obstet Gynecol 1988;159:1018.
20. Thomas JG, Jeanty P, Peters RA, et al: Automatic measurements of fetal long bones. J Ultrasound Med 1991;10:381–385.
21. Romero R, Pilu G, Jeanty P, et al: Prenatal Diagnosis of Congenital Anomalies. Appleton & Lange, Norwalk, CT, 1988.
22. Crane JP: Ultrasound evaluation of fetal chromosome disorders. In: Callen P: Ultrasonography in Obstetrics and Gynecology. WB Saunders, Philadelphia, 1993, pp 35–51.
23. Mahony BS: Ultrasound evaluation of the fetal musculoskeletal system. In Callen P: Ultrasonography in Obstetrics and Gynecology. WB Saunders, Philadelphia, 1993, pp 254–290.
24. Sabbagha RE: Diagnostic Ultrasound: Applied to Obstetrics and Gynecology, 2nd ed. JP Lippincott, Philadelphia, 1987, pp 229–412.
25. Williamson MR, Williamson SL: Gamuts in Ultrasound. WB Saunders, Philadelphia, 1992.
26. Hamilton WJ, Simon G, Hamilton SG, eds: Surface and Radiological Anatomy for Students and General Practitioners, 5th ed. Williams & Wilkins, Baltimore, 1971, pp 58–60.
27. Goldstein RB, Filly RA, Simpson G: Pitfalls in femur length measurements. J Ultrasound Med 1987;6: 203–207.
28. Jeanty P, Kirkpatric C, Dramaix-Wilmet M, et al: Ultrasonic evaluation of fetal limb growth. Radiology 1981;140:165.
29. DuBose TJ: Assessment of fetal age and size: Techniques and criteria. In: Berman MC, ed: Obstetrics & Gynecology: Diagnostic Medical Sonography, A Guide to Clinical Practice, vol 1. JB Lippincott, Philadelphia, 1991, pp 292–293.
30. Jeanty P: Prenatal detection of simian crease. J Ultrasound Med 1990;9:131–136.
31. Benacerraf BR, Osathanondh R, Frigoletto FD: Sonographic demonstration of hypoplasia of the middle phalanx of the fifth digit: A finding associated with Down syndrome. Am J Obstet Gynecol 1988;159:181.
32. Benacerraf BR, Harlow BL, Frigoletto FD Jr: Hypoplasia of the middle phalanx of the fifth digit. J Ultrasound Med 1990;9:389–394.
33. Campbell BG: Humankind Emerging, 5th ed. Scott, Foresman & Co, Boston, 1988, pp 49–50.
34. Jolly A: The Evolution of Primate Behavior. Macmillan, New York, 1972, pp 279–294.
35. Oakley KP: Skill as a human possession. In: Korn N, Thompson F, eds: Human Evolution. Holt, Rinehart & Winston, New York, 1967, p 250.
36. Sherer DM, Hearn B, Woods JR: Possible intermittent umbilical cord occlusion. J Ultrasound Med 1990; 9:182.
37. Petrikovsky B, Kaplan G: Fetal grasping of the umbilical cord causing variable fetal heart rate decelerations. J Clinical Ultrasound 1993;21:642–644.
38. Collins JH: Fetal grasping of the umbilical cord with simultaneous fetal heart rate monitoring. Am J Obstet Gynecol 1994;170:1836.
39. Petrikovsky B, Collins JH: Grasping of the umbilical cord (Letter and Reply). Am J Obstet Gynecol 1995;172:1071.
40. Meizner I: Sonographic observation of in utero fetal masturbation. J Ultrasound Med 1987;6:111.
41. Pfeiffer JE: The Emergence of Man. Harper & Row, New York, 1969, pp 412–413.
42. Bieri J: Personal communications, University of Texas at Austin, Dept. of Psychology, 1986–1993.
43. Graves PL: The functioning fetus. In: Greenspan SI, Pollock GH, eds: The Course of Life: Psychoanalytic Contributions Toward Understanding Personality Development. Mental Health Study Center, Division of Mental Health Service Programs, National Institute of Mental Health, U.S. Department of Health and Human Services, Washington, D.C., 1980, pp 235–256.
44. Khulman KA: Fetal behavior. In: Sabbagha RE, ed: Diagnostic Ultrasound: Applied to Obstetrics and Gynecology, 2nd ed. JB Lippincott, Philadelphia, 1987, pp 186–190.
45. Hadlock FP, Deter RL, Roecker E, et al: Relation of fetal femur length to neonatal crown-heel length. J Ultrasound Med 1984;3:1–3.
46. Hadlock FP, Harrist RB, Sharman RS, et al: Estimation of fetal weight with the use of head, body and femur measurements: A prospective study. Am J Obstet Gynecol 1985;151:333–337.
47. Bromley B, Frigoletto FD, Harlow BL, et al: Biometric measurements in fetuses of different race and gender. Ultrasound Obstet Gynecol 1993;3:395–402.
48. Abrams SL, Filly RA: Curvature of the fetal femur: A normal sonographic finding. Radiology 1985;156:490.
49. Warda A, Deter R, Rossavik I, et al: Femur length; Effect of bone curvature on its measurement and its relationship to menstrual age. (abstract 518).Official Proceedings: Annual AIUM/SDMS Convention. J Ultrasound Med 1984;3:222.
50. Kurtz AB, Wapner RJ, Kurtz RJ, et al: Analysis of biparietal diameter as an accurate indicator of gestational age. J Clin Ultrasound 1980;8:321–325.
51. Warda AH, Deter RL, Rossavik IK, et al: Fetal femur length: A critical reevaluation of the relationship to menstrual age. Obstet Gynecol 1985;66:69–75.
52. Williamson MR, Williamson SL: Gamuts in Ultrasound. WB Saunders, Philadelphia, 1992, pp 159–162.
53. Mercer BM, Sklar S, Shariatmadar A, et al: Fetal foot length as a predictor of gestational age. Am J Obstet Gynecol 1987;156:350–355.
54. Callen PW: Ultrasound in Obstetrics and Gynecology. WB Saunders, Philadelphia, 1993, p 719.
55. Callen PW: Ultrasound in Obstetrics and Gynecology. WB Saunders, Philadelphia, 1993, p 154.

CHAPTER 16

EXTRAFETAL STRUCTURES OF PREGNANCY

Terry J. DuBose

The objective of this textbook is to describe the sonographic study of the developing embryo and fetus, but the book would be incomplete without a discussion of the extrafetal structures (female reproductive system) that support the fetus. The changes in the uterus and its blood supply before, during, and after pregnancy are an amazing process of profound alterations in size and perfusion. This chapter offers a brief generalized discussion of the normal female reproductive system from the viewpoint of sonography.

Until the advent of sonography, most direct study of the tissues of pregnancy was limited to animals. The early research by Markee went so far as to implant uterine tissue in place of the rhesus monkey's eye so that the process of menstruation could be observed directly.[1,2] Clearly, experiments of this nature on humans were unacceptable and could not be performed. Indeed, in all probability the original experiment could not be repeated today in most developed countries.

Sonography has opened a window into the fascinating world of human reproduction. The uterus, ovaries, and fetus were among the first structures to be studied using this modality, partly because Ian Donald discovered that the full urinary bladder provided a clear acoustic window into the pelvis (see Chapter 2). As equipment provided better views of the menstrual cycle, including noticeable textural changes of the uterine tissues and ovarian follicles, sonographers around the world were captivated.

Uterus

NONGRAVID

Menstrual Cycle

Days 1 to 5

The first day of bleeding during menses is considered the start of the menstrual cycle. In reality, bleeding is the terminal event of the proceeding cycle, but historically, pregnancy and the cycle have been dated from the menstrual period because in ancient times menstruation was the only empirical date to document these events. It is noteworthy that veterinarians use ovulation as the start of the fertility cycle in animals, a much more logical approach. Sonographers use the standard human approach of dating the fertility cycle and pregnancy from the start of the last menstrual period (LMP). The complete, normal fertility cycle usually is 28 days from period to period.

During a woman's fertile period, midcycle, the reproductive hormones, primarily estrogen, cause a dramatic increase in the blood vessel sizes and blood supply to the reproductive tissues. This rich blood supply in turn causes proliferation of the soft endometrial lining of the uterine cavity (cavum). At the end of the fertile period, the blood vessels constrict, and as a result, the blood supply is diminished. "The mechanisms regulating changes in blood flow to the uterus are not thoroughly understood."[3] The endometrium appears to be very sensitive to this reduction in blood supply and begins to shed, with concomitant bleeding. This is the start of menses and is the date (LMP) from which most events of pregnancy are timed. A normal menstrual period, in timing and blood flow, is often referred to as the *reported last normal menstrual period* (LNMP).

Menses or menstrual periods usually last from 3 to 5 days, but wide variations occur from individual to individual and occasionally from period to period. During menses, the uterus appears relatively homogeneous sonographically, with a thin endometrial stripe of echoes. This stripe should measure about 1 mm thick (including anterior and posterior layers) at the end of menses.[4] The ovaries normally appear ovoid in shape and have a relatively echogenic center. No cysts or only very small follicular cysts are seen about the periphery (Fig. 16–1*A*).

Days 6 to 9

The menses is followed by the early and midfollicular phases (6 to 9 LMP days).[4,5] Sonographically, this is often referred to as the *early proliferative phase* because the endometrium can be observed to begin to thicken, causing the endometrial stripe to become more obvious. The double-layer (anterior and posterior) thickness at this time is 2 to 4 mm.

The myometrium, which is primarily a mass of muscle containing a vascular network, becomes more coarsely echogenic and heterogeneous during midcycle and more homogeneous during menses. It is probable that the coarse textural changes that occur in the proliferative phases are due to the echoes from the walls of the dilating blood vessels under the influence of the fertility hormones.[3,6,7]

The ovaries begin to develop follicular cysts in the early proliferative (follicular) phase. By the midproliferative phase, a larger follicle, which will develop into the dominant follicle, may be detected. It is this dominant follicle that carries the ovum (egg), which may be fertilized later in the cycle.

Days 10 to 13

The late proliferative or follicular phase lasts from 10 to 13 days after the LMP. The endometrium becomes thick and takes on a layered appearance. The endometrium should measure approximately 4 to 8 mm at this time.[4] Each ovary contains several follicular cysts. The dominant follicle reaches approximately 20+ mm toward the end of this phase.

At the very end of the follicular phase, the dominant cyst bursts, releasing the egg, thus beginning the secretory or fertile phase.

Days 14 to 28

The secretory phase is also called the *luteal phase*. This is the fertile period in women, and it normally lasts from the release of the egg on day 14 after the LMP until approximately the 25th or 26th LMP day. After the dominant follicle releases the egg, the area of the follicle on the ovary develops into a corpus luteum (yellow body), which is instrumental in production of the hormones of the early pregnancy if fertilization occurs. Fertilization occurs in the fallopian tube within 3 days after ovulation. Mitotic division produces a mass of cells called a *morula* in days after fertilization. Cell division continues, forming a blastocyst, which implants 6 to 7 days after fertilization.[8,9]

The endometrium thickens from approximately 10 mm to about 14 to 15 mm during the secretory phase.[4] Both layers of the endometrium should be obvious sonographi-

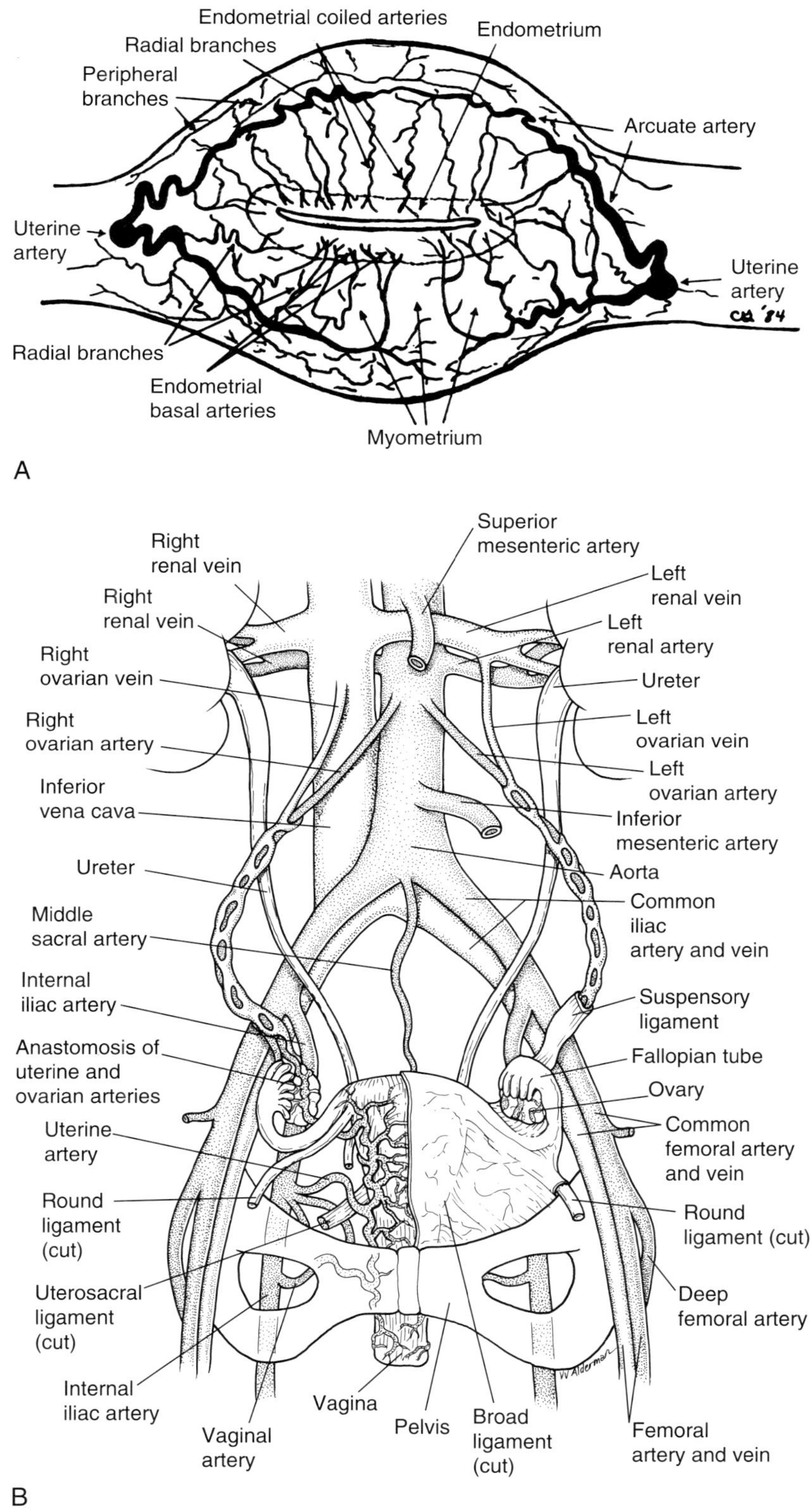

FIGURE 16–1.
A, Cross section of the uterus showing the myometrium, endometrium, and arterial system. For simplicity, the approximately parallel venous system is not shown. (Adapted from Sampson JA: The escape of foreign material form the uterine cavity into the uterine veins. Am J Obstet 1918; 78:161–175. From DuBose TJ, Hill LW, Cunyus JA, et al: Sonography of menstrual changes in arcuate uterine blood vessel diameters. J Cardiovasc Ultrasonogr 1985;4:243–251.) *B*, Female reproductive blood supply. The origin of the ovarian vessels high in the abdomen facilitates uterine growth. Note the ample collateral paths for blood supply to the uterus.

cally. The endometrium is very vascular, spongy, succulent, and rich with glycogen, ready to receive the blastocyst for implantation.[10] In the myometrium, individual arcuate blood vessels may be seen to course around the anterior and posterior periphery of the uterus (Figs. 16–1 to 16–3). The myometrium takes on a coarse, echogenic texture as a result of dilation of the vessels under the influence of the hormones (Figs. 16–2 to 16–4). All female reproductive tissues have a tendency to swell or .enlarge slightly under the influence of the reproductive hormones. Even the breasts appreciably change volume through the phases of the menstrual cycle.[11]

If pregnancy does not occur, the last 2 or 3 days of this phase are sometimes called the *premenstrual phase,* when the corpus luteum regresses and secretion of the fertility hormones (estrogen and progesterone) declines.[10]

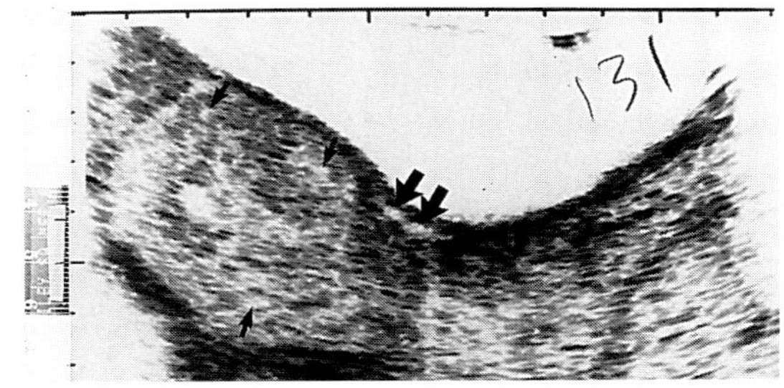

FIGURE 16–3.
Sagittal section through uterus showing myometrial arcuate vessels in a primigravida. Most obvious vessels (largest arrows) are in the uterine isthmus in this case. Smaller arrows point out other vessels. The uterus is a mass of muscle containing a network of vessels that give it the characteristic sonographic texture in early pregnancy. Vessels can be found throughout the myometrium. This was case 131 in a double-blind study (see Table 16–1) using an articulated arm B-scanner to produce black echoes on a white background (4.8 LMP weeks, DKD)

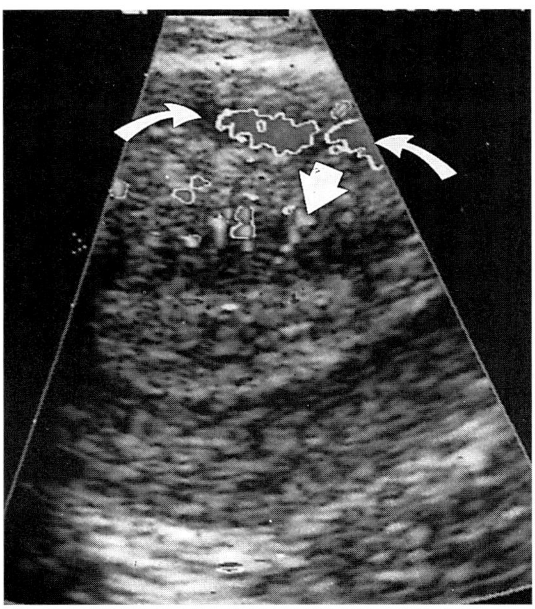

FIGURE 16–2.
Transvaginal sonogram of uterine cross section. (See Color Figure 16–2.) Arcuate myometrial vessels are blue (curved arrows) around the periphery of uterus. The spiral artery, shown spiraling toward the endometrium (large arrow), is unusually well demonstrated. Compare the anatomy with Figure 16–1*A*. In this case, a left ectopic pregnancy was diagnosed in the fifth LMP week; therefore, it is hypothesized that the hormones of pregnancy were dilating the vessels, making them easier to visualize. (LNMP 5.1 weeks, TD)

PERFUSION AND DOPPLER

Ovarian Vessels

During the early embryonic period, the kidneys are actually in the pelvis and the gonads are higher. As the kidneys ascend out of the pelvis to their eventual bilateral location in midabdomen, they receive their blood supply from a succession of vessels.[12] Because of this complex process, the gonadal vessels that supply the testes and ovaries actually originate from or near the renal vessels. The ovarian vessels thus are quite long and can therefore accommodate the great expansion of the gravid uterus (see Figs. 16–1*B* and 16–4).

In midpregnancy, between approximately 20 and 24 LMP weeks, large, septated, bilateral masses are often located at the sides of the uterine body. Doppler study has proved these to be very large, kinked gonadal (ovarian) vessels and anastomoses to the uterine vessels (Fig. 16–5). It is hypothesized that as the uterus expands out of the pelvis (see Fig. 16–4*A*), the gonadal vessels are carried superiorly and often coil up as the fundus approaches the level of the maternal kidneys near the origin of these vessels (see Fig. 16–4*B*). As the uterus continues to expand toward term, the vessels again are stretched out, around the uterus (see Fig. 16–4*C*). This

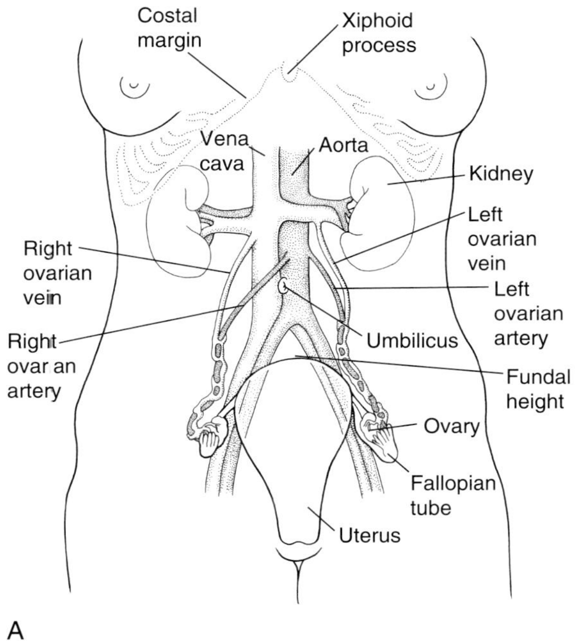

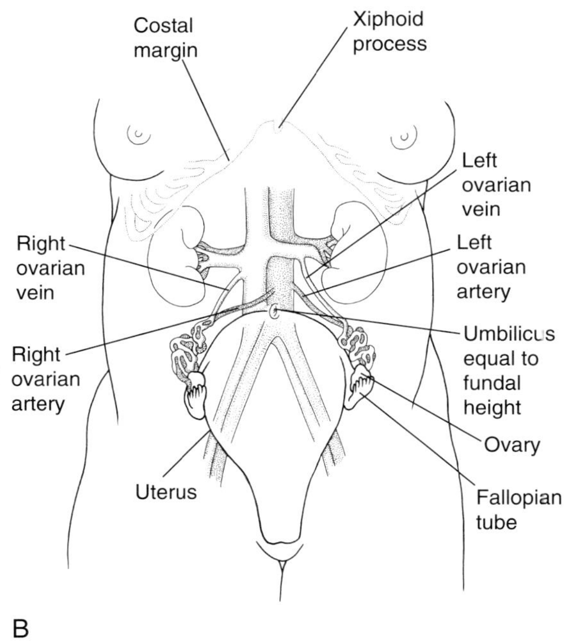

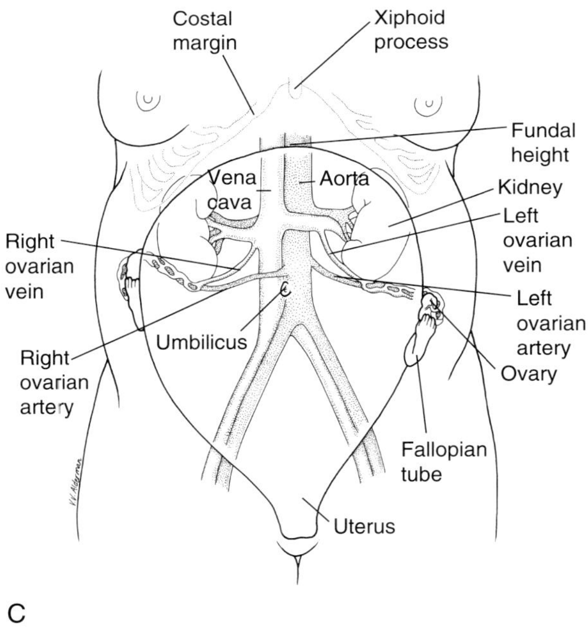

FIGURE 16–4. UTERINE GROWTH.
A, Uterine fundal height at approximately 10 LMP weeks. Note the ovarian vessels. *B*, Uterine fundal height at approximately 20 LMP weeks (midpregnancy). Note ovarian vessel kinking at each side of the uterus. These may appear as septated cystic masses from about 18 to 24 LMP weeks. Doppler can distinguish between these vessels and cystic masses. Overlying bowel may obscure the vessels. *C*, Fundal height at term. The ovarian vessels again stretch out, and the cystic mass effect is lost.

explains why these vessel masses are most obvious at midpregnancy. The gonadal vessel coils occasionally are difficult to see because they may form a long loop, hidden by surrounding bowel rather than kinking into a mass. This gonadal looping is illustrated in Figure 16–5*C*, where a left gonadal vein is observed to loop anterior to the linear psoas muscle.

Uterine Vessels

After the ovarian vessels attach to the ovaries, they connect (anastomose) with the uterine vessels, which network bilaterally along the length of the uterus (see Fig. 16–1*B*). Other vessels that anastomose with the ovarian and uterine vessels are the uterine and vaginal branches of the internal iliac (hypogas-

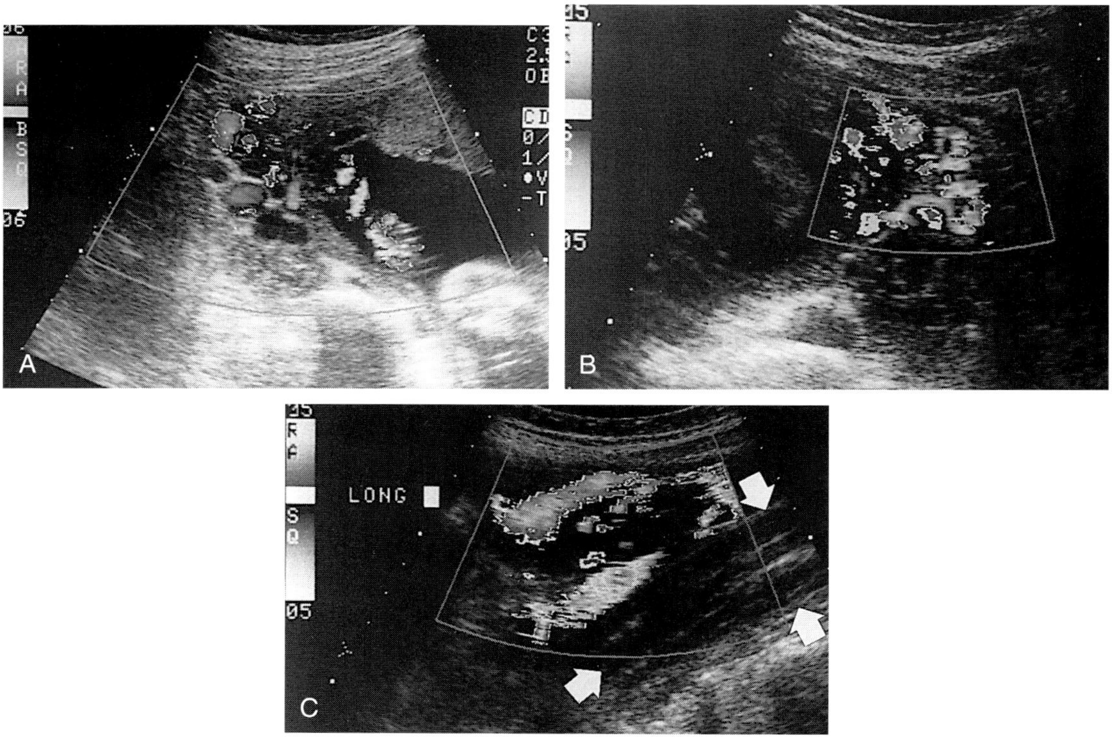

FIGURE 16–5.
A, Transverse right lateral section of the uterus showing a mass of vessels. (See Color Figure 16–5*A*.) Color Doppler proves these to be vessels and not cysts. In this case, a slow-flow velocity tag was used to outline blood flowing toward the transducer so that direction can be distinguished in black-and-white images. The free-floating umbilical cord is seen within the amniotic fluid. (AA = 25.1 LMP weeks, range = 3.1 weeks, n = 9, TD) *B*, Transverse left lateral section of the uterus showing a vessel mass in black and white. Flow toward the transducer is outlined in white by a slow-flow tag. (AA = 18.2 LMP weeks, range = 0.9 weeks, n = 10, TD) *C*, Parasagittal section lateral to the left side of the uterus from the same case shown in *B*. Real-time Doppler demonstrated flow toward the transducer (white slow-flow tag) looping away from the transducer anterior to linear echoes of the psoas muscle (arrows).

tric) (see Fig. 16–1*B*).[13] All these form a complex network along the sides of the uterus and provide the gravid uterus with a rich supply of blood. As the uterine vessels course along the length of the uterus, numerous branches enter the myometrium and arch around the anterior and posterior margins of the uterus. Because these vessels form arches in the uterine cross section, they are called the *myometrial arcuate arteries* and *veins* or *uterine arcuate vessels* (see Fig. 16–1).[6,14] The uterine arcuate veins were first described sonographically by a transabdominal, articulated arm B-scanner in 1985.[15] The arcuate arteries have branches into the endometrial radial arteries, which extend into the myometrium along the radii of the uterine cross section, thus the name *radial*. The radial arteries become the endometrial spiral or coiled arteries, which in turn become the endometrial basal arteries (see Figs. 16–1 and 16–2). It is to these basal arteries that an implanted blastocyst and its chorionic villus and trophoblastic lacunar network first join to form the maternofetal placental perfusion. The venous system is approximately parallel.

Under the influence of the hormones of fertility and pregnancy, all the reproductive vessels begin to dilate to accommodate the requirements of the growing pregnancy. During the mid-1980s my group conducted a double-blind study of a cross-sectional population in an attempt to measure the changes in the diameters of the myometrial arcuate vessels.[6] Figure 16–3 is case number 131 of 319 cases in the study. The average measurements from this study are summarized in Table 16–1. The

TABLE 16–1. **MYOMETRIAL ARCUATE VESSEL MEASUREMENTS AND LMP**

DAYS SINCE LAST MENSTRUAL PERIOD	NUMBER OF EXAMS	MEAN VESSEL DIAMETERS (mm)	± 2 SD (mm)	RANGE (mm)
0–10 days (menstrual and postmenstrual)	70	2.03	2.1	0.0–8.0
11–17 days (ovulation)	61	2.73	2.2	1.0–7.0
18–30 days (premenstrual)	52	1.90	1.26	1.0–3.3
Over 30 days (nonpregnant)	45	2.01	2.35	0.0–5.0
First trimester pregnancy	91	2.65	1.91	1.0–7.0

± 2 SD = 2 standard deviations (in millimeters).

This table demonstrates that vessel diameters are greatest during ovulation (fertile period) and pregnancy; both are times during which fertility hormones are increased. The table was developed from a double-blind study of 319 consecutive cases. The two largest mean vessel diameters were measured in the sagittal section and averaged for the measurement of record by the sonographer without prior knowledge of LMP or history. Each image was photographed to scale (see Fig. 16–3), and the 319 images were then measured by two experienced sonologists. All measurements were grouped by LMP and averaged for this table. The averaging has an obtundant effect on the extremes. Longitudinal studies should yield significant results.

From DuBose TJ, Hill LW, Cunyus JA, et al: Sonography of menstrual changes in arcuate uterine blood vessel diameters. J Cardiovasc Ultrasonogr 1985;4:243–281.

arcuate vessels were found to dilate at midcycle and during the first trimester, but their diameters were constricted during the menses and before menstrual periods. This finding was expected, based on the earlier nonsonographic research by others.[3,16,17] The use of average measurements from a cross-sectional population has an obtundant effect on the final diameters, however, and the changes were not statistically significant.

It was believed that longitudinal studies would show significant changes in the sizes of these vessels. In the longitudinal study, through a single menstrual cycle, my group found that the same arcuate vessel increased from a diameter of 3 mm on the LMP day 7 to just greater than 5 mm on LMP day 13 and constricted to less than 2 mm in the premenstrual period on day 24.[6] This represents a change in diameter of approximately 250% from smallest to largest, or an increase of about 625% in vessel lumen cross-sectional area or blood flow, assuming constant flow velocity (volume flow = velocity × lumen cross-sectional area).[18,19] This very large potential increase of flow is less than that found by Greiss and Anderson in sheep.[3,20] They found a 10-fold (1000%) increased flow in sheep uterine arteries from the lowest flow to the greatest flow at estrus.

The location and size of the largest arcuate vessels, therefore the most obvious sonographically, vary somewhat from individual to individual; however, in an individual, the same vessel can be found and measured throughout the menstrual cycle.[6] In a nulliparous or primiparous woman, the largest arcuate vessels in the midsagittal plane normally are in the anterior arc of the isthmus or lower uterine body (see Fig. 16–3). After two or three pregnancies, a cesarean section, or severe episodes of pelvic inflammatory disease, the largest arcuate vessels appear to be nearer the fundus of the uterus. It should be emphasized, however, that between pregnancies, it is possible to find and measure the same arcuate vessel throughout the menstrual cycle. This research was conducted during the time of development of transvaginal transducers,[21] which were not then available but should facilitate the study of uterine perfusion and its relationship to infertility.

With pregnancy, the arcuate vessels become quite large. They are often observed around the periphery of the gravid uterus, particularly in the lower segments posterior to the bladder (Fig. 16–6).

Placental Texture

The placenta is the tissue through which oxygen, nutrition, and waste products (as well as drugs and other substances) are ex-

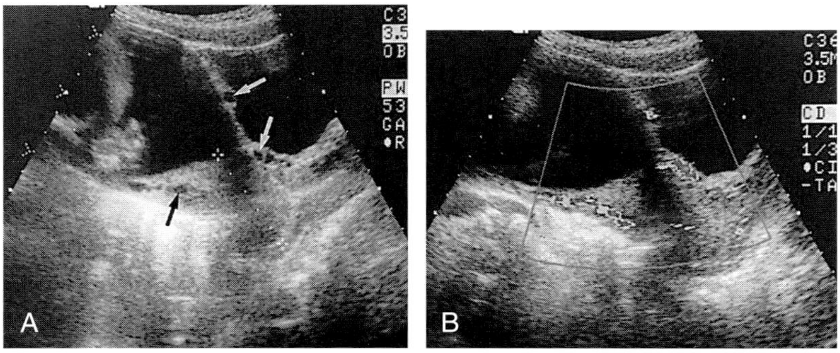

FIGURE 16–6.
Midsagittal view of lower uterine segment showing many myometrial arcuate vessels in a dilated state as a result of the hormones of pregnancy. *A*, Without color Doppler. Vessels in anterior (white arrows) and posterior (black arrow) uterine walls are seen. *B*, Black-and-white color Doppler with white slow-flow tag showing blood flow throughout the uterine walls. (AA = 25.7 LMP weeks, range = 1.8 weeks, n 9, TD)

changed between a woman and her fetus (Fig. 16–7). One of the first reports of the normal sonographic appearance of the placenta was by Spirt and colleagues in 1979.[22] They reported observing the placenta as early as 8 LMP weeks in some cases and clearly viewing the placenta by the end of the first trimester (10 to 12 LMP weeks). This report also described the hypoechoic band now referred to as the *subplacental complex*[23] or the *anechoic retroplacental clear area* (Fig. 16–8). The subplacental complex was described as providing venous drainage through basal veins. This venous drainage was confirmed by Smith and Foley[25] using sonographic Doppler (Figs. 16–9 and 16–10).

Figure 16–9*A* is a color and spectral Doppler of this area illustrating low-resistance arterial flow in the subplacental band. Figure 16–9*B* shows a coiled appearance or a

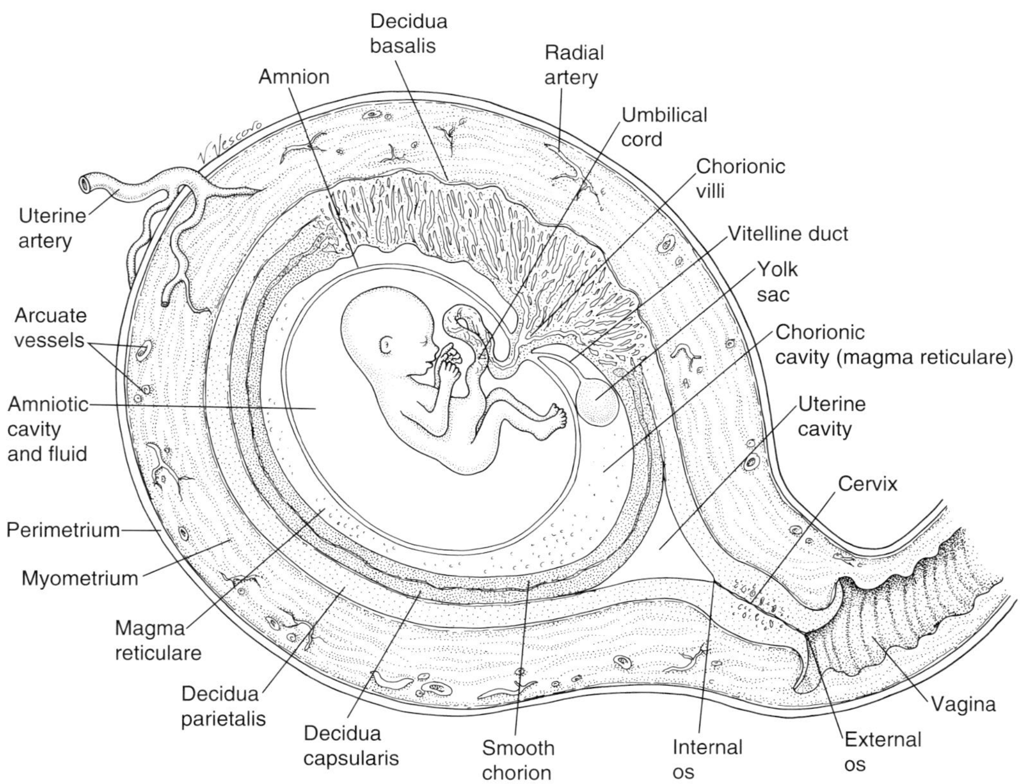

FIGURE 16–7.
Stylized rendering of uterine anatomy (longitudinal section) at about 10 LMP weeks in pregnancy. Compare with Figure 16–12C.

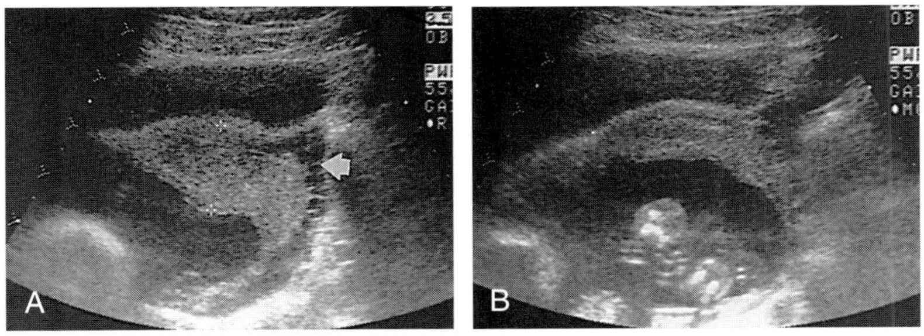

FIGURE 16–8.
Focal uterine contraction and uterine vessels. *A,* A structure that was at first thought to be placenta (between + cursors). Uterine vessels are hypoechoic (arrow). *B,* Sonogram made 18 minutes later at the same location as *A.* Note that localized contraction has resolved.

regular spiral flow, which also proved to be arterial. This appearance may mean that the subplacental complex includes the endometrial coiled vessels as well as the radial and arcuates. A hypothesis that would explain this is that as the gravid uterus expands, the radial and spiral vessels stretch from their perpendicular, penetrating branching from the arcuate vessels to orientations more parallel to the arcuates. Thus, all vessels would be passing more parallel to the uterine wall, forming the subplacental complex (clear area). The exact composition of the subplacental complex will undoubtedly receive more attention in the near future with advances in color Doppler sonography (see Fig. 16–10). Subplacental waveforms that are similar to these have now been identified as spiral arterial flow.[26]

Normal placenta undergoes a maturation process that affects its appearance throughout gestation.[27] When this was first noticed sonographically and a grading system was established, the hope was that the advancing placental grades might be an indicator of fetal lung development. However, although some correlation between placental and lung maturity is noted, placental grading cannot always predict the maturity of the pulmonary system.[28] This is because of the wide variation in the progression of placental maturation from pregnancy to pregnancy. It is not uncommon to see most grades at any time during the second and third trimesters. The textural changes on which grading is based involve the development of echogenic areas of calcification, divisions which define the placental cotyledons, and hypoechoic areas that are often called *maternal lakes.* Various diseases can also affect the placental texture. Maternal dia-

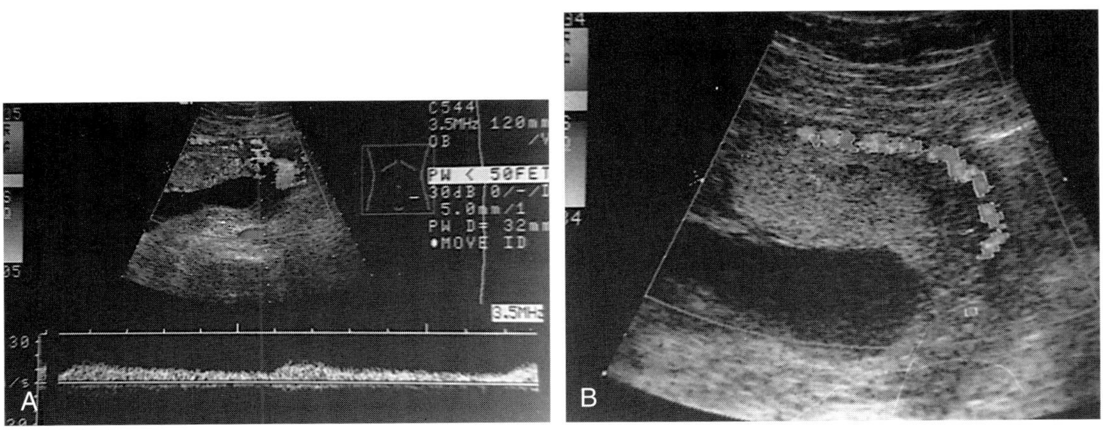

FIGURE 16–9.
Subplacental complex of vessels. (See Color Figure 16–9.) *A,* Color and spectral Doppler show this to be a low-resistance arterial flow. This type of flow has been documented as originating from spiral arteries.[26] *B,* Color Doppler from the same region of the uterus as in *A.* Note the spiraling effect of color flow It is believed that these are spiral myometrial arteries, which are stretched from their normal penetrating angle before pregnancy to more horizontal positions with uterine growth. (AA = 17.7 LMP weeks, range = 1.3 weeks, n = 9, TD)

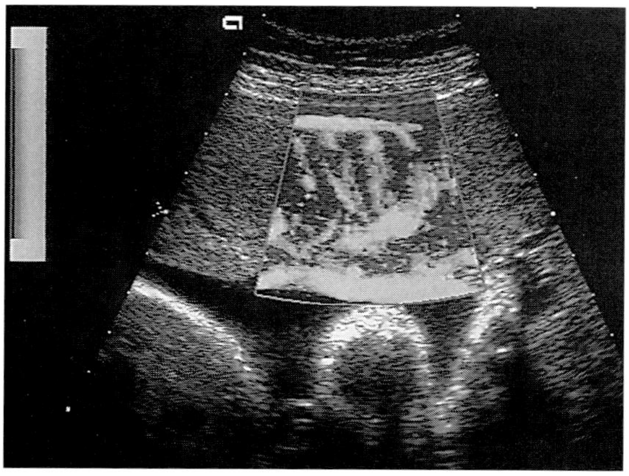

FIGURE 16–10.
This image demonstrates the use of Doppler energy or amplitude imaging. (See Color Figure 16–10.) This new modality does not show direction or velocity of blood flow, only the amplitude of the Doppler echoes. With more research, this type of Doppler should provide more information about placental perfusion. (Image courtesy of ACUSON Corp.)

betes usually causes the placenta to retain a homogeneous sonographic texture throughout pregnancy.

Because the placental maturation process is gradual, the grading system at some point becomes subjective. Between each grade is a placental texture that may be given one of either the less or more mature grades, depending on the plane of view, the gain settings, and the experience and opinion of the observer. Figure 16–11 graphs placenta grades against gestational age and demonstrates how 13 sonographers graded placentas in 2145 referral examinations in 1993 (Grannum's method). Table 16–2 is a statistical summary of the LMP ages for the placental grades for the graphs. The following is a discussion of two placental grading systems. The first, by Grannum and associates, was proposed in 1979.[27] The second, by Kazzi and associates, was proposed in 1985.[28, 29] Both are very similar.

Grades

Grannum's Grading System

Grade 0. In Grannum's system, a placental grade of 0 is a placenta that is completely homogeneous without calcifications and with a smooth chorionic plate on the fetal side. Figure 16–12 demonstrates grade 0.

This grade is always seen in the first trimester and frequently in the early second (see Fig. 16–11).

As mentioned earlier, maternal diabetes may cause this grade to continue until term. Usually, even with diabetes, some placental textural changes develop and cause most observers to assign it a grade I or higher after the first trimester.

Grade I. With grade I, some areas of calcifications may start developing, and these appear as bright, echogenic spots scattered through the placenta. The chorionic surface remains smooth but becomes undulating. Figures 16–13 and possibly 16–14 demonstrate a grade I placenta. Notice the coarser placental texture in comparison with the prior images.

In our group's study population, grade I was observed after the embryonic period until term (see Fig. 16–11).

Grade II. A grade II placenta has a more irregular surface with rounded areas. Some divisions of the cotyledons are seen starting at the chorionic surface but not extending to the base plate or retroplacental vascular complex of the myometrium.[30] Figure 16–15 illustrates a grade II placenta. In our population, grade II was only rarely seen in the first half of pregnancy and most often in the late second and early third trimesters.

Figure 16–14 presents a dilemma. Is this a grade I or II? It has relatively rounded areas of the chorionic plate and some cotyledon development but no obvious echogenic calcium. This placenta could be classified either as grade I or II, depending on the appearance of the remainder of the placenta with a real-time survey and the opinion of the observer. Early textural changes are very subtle.

Grade III. Placental grade III has a heterogeneous texture. Lines of calcifications divide the cotyledons, and many maternal lakes are seen, often at the center of the cotyledons or placental divisions (Fig. 16–16). No placentas in our population were graded III before the 27th LMP week. Most were in the late third trimester (see Fig. 16–11).

Kazzi's Grading System

Kazzi and associates proposed a new placental classification that is both similar to and slightly simpler than Grannum's system.

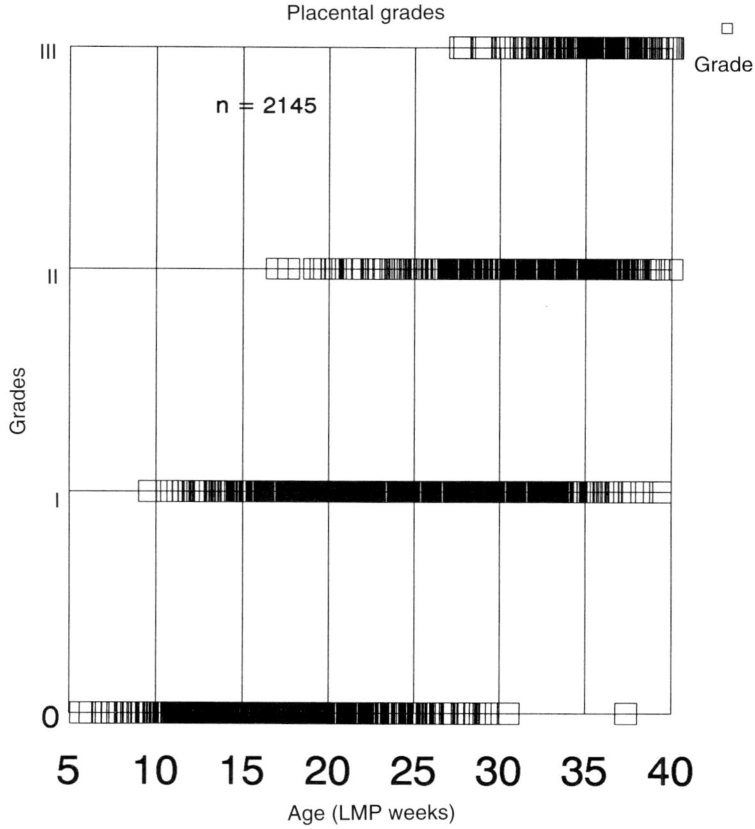

A

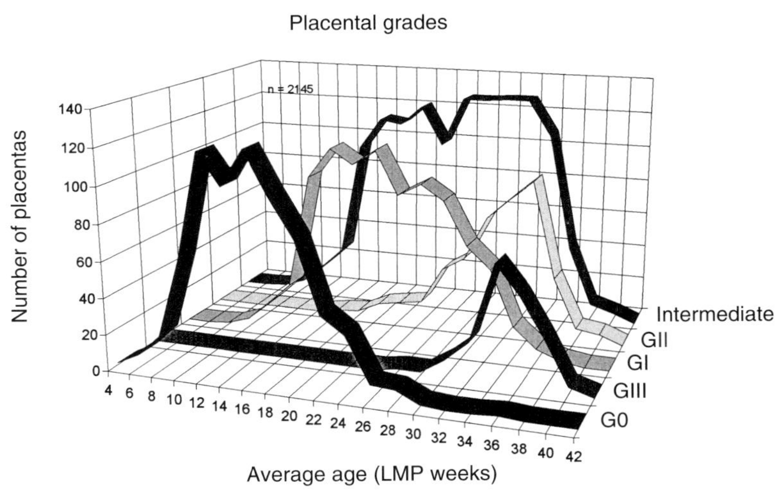

B

FIGURE 16–11.
A, A plot of placental grades 0, I, II and III for 2145 pregnancies. The placental grading was subjective and performed by 13 sonographers (ARDMS) using machines by various manufacturers in four different sonographic laboratories. Only slight overlap is noted between grades 0 and III, whereas more overlap occurs between grades I, II, and other grades. *B*, Ribbon graph of the data in *A*. Grades 0 and III (G0 and GIII) are placed together for easier comparison. Grades I and II are added together to form the intermediate grade at the rear (see the discussion of placental grades for rationale of this method).

TABLE 16–2. **SUMMARY: PLACENTAL GRADES**

AVERAGE AGE STATISTICS	AVERAGE AGE GRADE 0	AVERAGE AGE GRADE I	AVERAGE AGE GRADE II	AVERAGE AGE GRADE III	POPULATION AVERAGE AGE
Mean	16.9	23.9	31.8	35.7	24.0
1 SD	4.5	5.6	4.3	2.5	7.9
Mean + 2 SD	**25.8**	35.1	40.3	40.7	39.8
Mean − 2 SD	7.9	12.6	23.2	**30.7**	8.2
Count (n)	704	863	397	181	2145

Descriptive statistics for the placental grades shown in Figure 16–11*A* and *B*. Columns show statistics for the average age of multiple fetal parameters. Note that the average age mean + 2 SD for grade 0 is 25.8 LMP weeks and the average age mean − 2 SD for grade III is 30.7 LMP weeks. This means that between about 26 and 30.5 LMP weeks the extreme placental grades 0 and III are rarely observed.

Kazzi's system has only three placental classifications: immature, intermediate, and mature.[28,29]

Immature Grade. Immature in Kazzi's system of placental classifications equates to grades 0, I, and II in Grannum's system. It is defined as nongrade III.[28]

Intermediate Grade. Kazzi's intermediate grade means that only a portion qualifies as grade III. The placenta often has one portion that is heterogeneous, as in grade III, but other portions are more homogeneous.

Mature Grade. In Kazzi's system of grading, the mature placenta must be completely inhomogeneous—that is, a grade III in *all* parts of the placenta. Using this system of classifying placentas has resulted in better correlation with the lecithin/sphingomyelin ratio and absence of hyaline membrane disease.[31]

Combining Grannum's and Kazzi's Classifications

I tend to think of the intermediate classification as the combination of grades I and II, whereas grade 0 is the same as immature and grade III is mature. Although Kazzi and colleagues[28] and others[32,33] have found that extremely mature placentas were significant

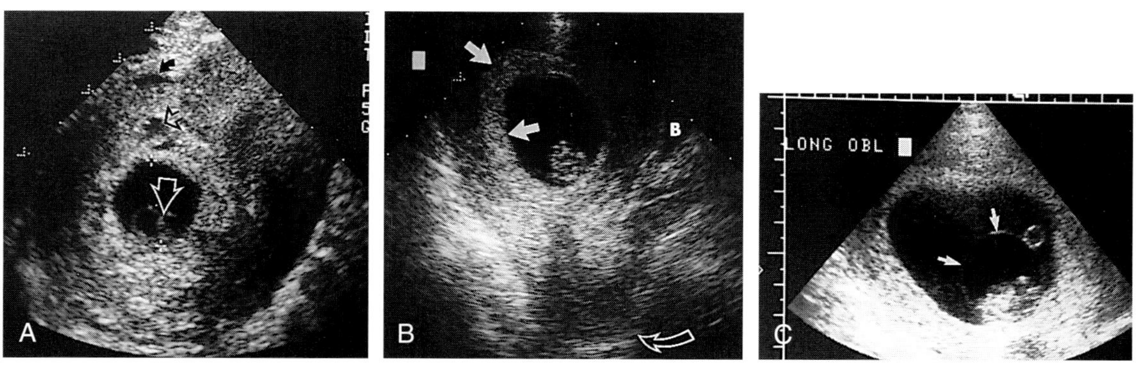

FIGURE 16–12.
A, Early intrauterine pregnancy, placental grade 0, with a double bleb inside the chorionic cavity. One sphere (bleb) is the amnion and the other is the yolk sac, but they cannot be distinguished in this image. The embryonic heartbeat (84 B/M), observed at the center of the blebs (open white arrow), was slower than normal for age. The myometrial arcuate vessel (MAV, curved black arrow) is seen, with lacunae (open black arrow) between the MAV and chorionic sac. Other lacunae are around the anterior fundal edge of the sac. (AA = 6.1 LMP weeks, range = 0.4 weeks, n = 2, TD) *B*, Intrauterine pregnancy with definite placental (white arrows) grade 0 in the posterior uterus. The cervix (open arrow) and maternal bladder (B) are seen. (AA = 9.6 LMP weeks, range = 0.2 weeks, n = 2, LG) *C*, Amniotic fluid is clear inside the amniotic membrane (arrows). The embryo is in the inferior amniotic sac. The chorionic cavity around the amnion is filled by the slightly echoic magma reticulare. The small circle outside the amniotic sac is the yolk sac. The placenta is grade 0 and appears to be rather circumferential at this time. (AA = 9.2 LMP weeks, range = 1.2 weeks, n = 2.) (Image courtesy ACUSON Corp.)

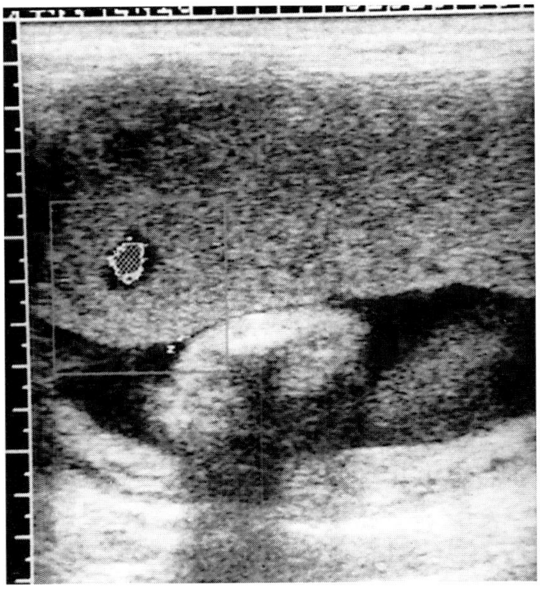

FIGURE 16–13.
This placenta might be considered to be a I or 0, depending on the appearance of the remainder, but more likely is a I. A venous lake shows flow with a slow-flow tag, and textural changes are very subtle. (AA = 31.5, range = 2.5, n = 9, TD)

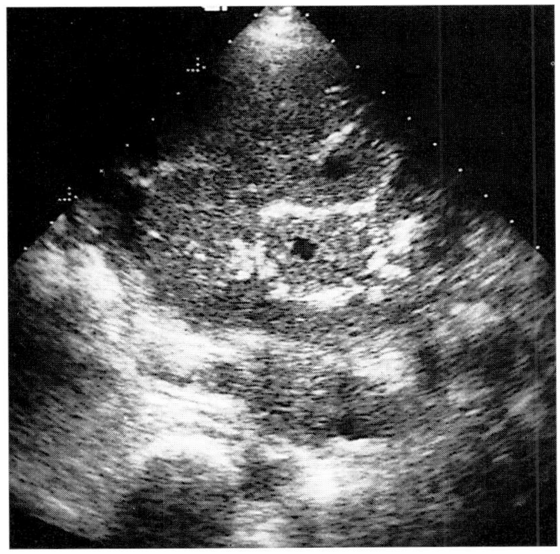

FIGURE 16–15.
This placenta was considered to be a grade II because the cotyledon divisions were not spread throughout. Areas of more homogeneous texture are shown in the near field. Hypoechoic centers have formed at the center of two cotyledons. (AA = 35.9 range = 3.9, n = 9, TD).

indicators of lung maturity and had a relationship with intrauterine growth retardation (IUGR), it seems that an extremely immature placenta (grade 0) very late in pregnancy is also remarkable. It may be that this finding only raises a question of maternal diabetes; however, if sonographers develop the habit of looking for only completely mature placentas, this question may be overlooked.

Table 16–2 summarizes the data in Figure

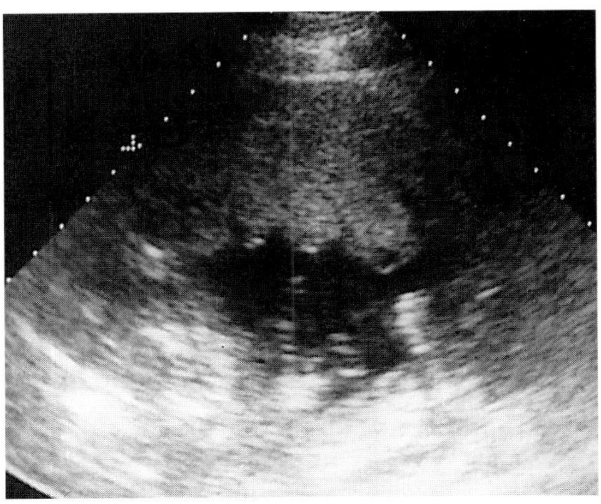

FIGURE 16–14.
This placenta, grade I or II, has beginnings of cotyledon divisions. The rounded bulges of the placental surface and chorionic plate are over the developing cotyledons. It might be considered a grade II by some but more likely is a grade I because of its overall homogeneity and the lack of echogenic calcium. (AA = 15.0 LMP weeks, range = 1.0 weeks, n = 10, TD)

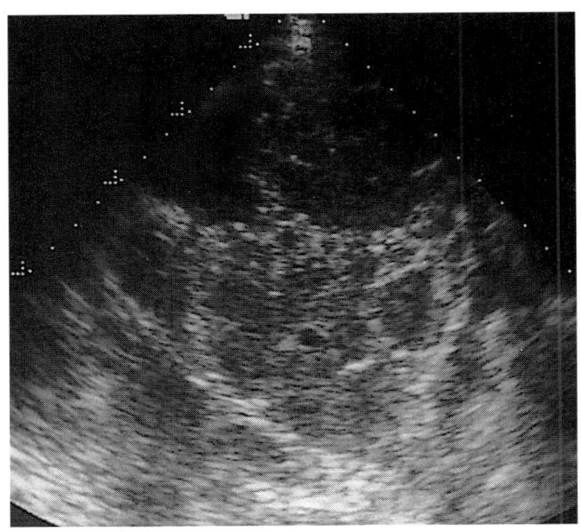

FIGURE 16–16.
This placenta was considered to be a definitely mature grade III. The cotyledon divisions were apparent throughout. (AA = 39.4, range = 5.5, n = 9, TD)

16–11, which represents 2145 placentas, graded by 13 different sonographers in four laboratories, using 7 different sonographic machines. Two important numbers are the multiple fetal parameter (MFP) average age mean +2 SD for grade 0 and the MFP average age mean −2 SD for grade III. The mean +2 SD for grade 0 was 25.8 LMP weeks. The grade III mean −2 SD average age was 30.7 LMP weeks. This means that 95% of the grade 0 placentas were found before 26 LMP weeks and 95% of the grade III placentas were after 30 LMP weeks. Very few extreme placental grades were noted between 26 and 30 LMP weeks.

Figure 16–11*B* is a three-dimensional ribbon graph of the data in Figure 16–11*A*. Placing immature grade 0 and mature grade III in the forefront of the graph makes them easy to compare. Grades I and II are added together to form the intermediate grade at the rear of the graph. This is essentially the same as Kazzi's system, except that it retains grade 0 as a distinct grade. This classification system may help sonographers to avoid missing a markedly homogeneous placenta near term.

Uterine Fibroids and Braxton Hicks Contractions

Changes in the uterine myometrium may have an effect on the appearance of the placenta. Both myomas (fibroids, leiomyomas) and Braxton Hicks–type contractions cause the uterine wall to appear thick. In most cases, myomas cause the outer uterine wall to bulge, whereas localized contractions cause the wall to bulge inward. Uterine contractions can appear very much like placental tissue (see Fig. 16–8). If one suspects that a contraction is causing confusion about the thickness or location of the placenta, continuing with other parts of the examination and reassessing after 30 minutes or so usually answers the question.[34] Local contractions should disappear in that time.

Abruption and Abnormalities

Abruption

The placenta can have a remarkably variable texture on sonographic examination and deserves close scrutiny. Most textural changes are benign, but some can have a detrimental effect on a fetus. Abruption and related hematomas may occur almost anywhere around the placenta or beneath the chorion or amnion. As with all hematomas, their sonographic appearance changes with the age of the bleed. Early, before coagulation, blood appears sonographically as a fluid. With clotting, the sonographic appearance becomes more echodense and homogeneous. Old clot can take on a varied appearance, from very echodense fibrotic-appearing tissues to complex with areas of reliquefaction. Placental bleeding is often associated with maternal hypertension and may present with vaginal bleeding and pain.[35]

The most dangerous form of hematoma is the subplacental or retroplacental hematoma. In these cases, the placenta is separated from the base plate by the hematoma. Some hematomas have been found to have a sonographic texture very similar to placenta and cause the misdiagnosis of thickened placenta[36] (see the later discussion of placental size). Hematomas that involve as much as 30% to 40% of the base plate of the placenta may result in fetal hypoxia. Others have found that if the hematoma separates more than 50% of the maternal surface of the placenta from the base plate, the fetal mortality rate can be approximately 75%. Less than a 20% separation resulted in only a 13% mortality rate.[37]

Other forms of placental bleeding are marginal hematomas that exist at the edge of the placenta and may extend beneath the chorion and may or may not lift the edge of the placenta from the base plate. Hematomas can also be subamniotic (between the amniotic membrane and the chorionic plate) or subchorionic thrombus on the surface of the placenta.[37] Massive subchorionic thrombus may be called a *Breus mole*, first described in 1892 by Breus.[38] Hypoechoic areas within the tissue of the placenta are often intervillous thrombosis.

Abnormalities

The placental tissue frequently has hypoechoic spaces. Besides the intervillous thrombosis mentioned earlier, vascular spaces or channels connect with the umbilical cord and usually show flow with color Doppler. Placental cysts or avillous areas may also be noted at the center of mature cotyledons.[39]

A hydatidiform mole or molar pregnancy contains many small cystic structures (Fig. 16–17). These may fill the uterus or may be coexistent with a fetus. Although some reports have described a normal fetuses with a coexistent mole, a high correlation with abnormalities is possible. Elevated human chorionic gonadatropin levels and theca-lutein cysts of the ovaries are associated with molar pregnancies.[40]

Chorangiomas (hemangiomas) are solid and may be quite large. These can protrude from the fetal surface of the placenta. Although chorangiomas may appear ominous, they are generally benign unless large enough to affect placental perfusion.[37]

Choriocarcinoma, although relatively rare, is highly malignant. These dangerous tumors have some association with molar pregnancies.[40]

Placenta Accreta

Placenta accreta is a condition in which the placental villi invade the uterine myometrium. The word *accrete* means to "adhere" or to "grow together." In the least severe cases, the placenta accreta may attach to only small portions of the myometrium. In more severe cases, the villi may invade the myometrium (placenta increta) or actually penetrate the myometrium (placenta percreta).[41] In very severe placenta percreta, the penetration may involve extrauterine tissues such as the urinary bladder.[42]

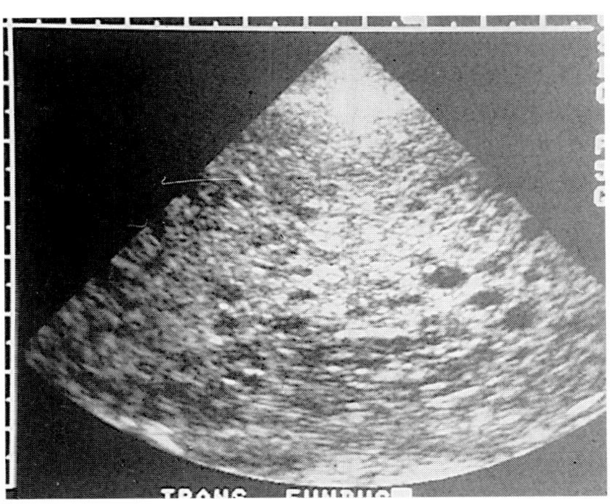

FIGURE 16–17.
In this case, the entire uterus was filled by a hydatidiform mole. Although the contrast of this image is suboptimal, the general appearance is characteristic of molar pregnancies.

In cases of placenta accreta, the placental villi extend through the decidua basalis (see Fig. 16–7). Because these deep attachments disrupt the placental base plate, complications at delivery may ensue and can be fatal to the mother.[42]

Although these abnormally deep placental attachments may occur anywhere within the uterus, they are most often in the lower, anterior uterine segment in association with prior cesarean sections. The prevalence of placenta accreta increases with the number of prior cesarean sections.[43]

Four distinct sonographic appearances and associations with placenta accreta have been noted[41–46]:

1. Placenta previa, or low-lying placenta, in association with previous cesarean section(s) or other uterine scarring
2. Loss of the hypoechoic retroplacental zone (vascular bed)
3. Thinning or disruption of the hyperechoic uterine serosa-bladder interface
4. Presence of unusually numerous intraplacental lakes, venous channels, or lacunae in the region of the accreta

Other entities that have been associated with abnormal placental attachments are increased maternal parity and age, previous dilatation and curettage, submucosal fibroids, uterine synechia, and therapeutic abortions. All of these may increase the chances of some sort of uterine wall damage or scarring. One report suggested that Doppler examination of the subplacental complex could rule out obliteration of the retroplacental vasculature in severe cases.[42]

The retroplacental vascular area has been called the *retroplacental clear area*[24,25] and the *subplacental complex*.[23] This area has been shown to be primarily dilated veins. It appears that the retroplacental complex is the myometrial spiral, radial, arcuate, and decidual vascular network under the dilating effects of the hormones of pregnancy[3,6,25] (see Figs. 16–1 to 16–3 and 16–5 to 16–10). In addition, cesarean sections and other scarring may disrupt the normal path of the low uterine vessels in the area of the isthmus. It may be that "obliteration" of these vessels, as described by Pasto, Kurtz, and others, is due to scarring, which prevents the formation of the subplacental complex and results in chorionic villus attachments directly to the myometrial tissue.[45]

PLACENTAL SIZE

Normal Placenta

Placental thickness normally varies slightly from pregnancy to pregnancy but also varies as a result of disease processes. A well-conducted study by Hoddick and colleagues found an increase in thickness with advancing menstrual age and decreasing area covered by the placental insertion.[47] In a sonogram, the area under the placenta is a curvilinear measurement and in this research was referred to as long or short insertions.

Hoddick and associates found that the mean perpendicular thickness of the placenta normally increases from approximately 12 mm at 10 LMP weeks to a mean of 34 mm at 40 LMP weeks. Table 16–3 was adapted from a graph in the report and gives the approximated values found for placental thicknesses throughout pregnancy. The edge of the placenta normally approached the uterine wall at a relatively low (or narrow) angle. As the angle at the edge of the placenta increased toward 90 degrees, the area beneath the placenta decreased and the thickness increased. Therefore, a widely implanted placenta with a large base area normally is thinner and has a smaller angle at the edges. This study also found that placental thickness did not vary as a result of placental location.[47]

TABLE 16–3. **PLACENTAL THICKNESS**

LMP WEEK	− 2 SD (mm)	MEAN (mm)	+ 2 SD (mm)
10	7	12	16
15	12	18	25
20	12	21	29
25	17	25	33
30	23	30	37
35	25	32	40
40	25	35	40

Columns show average (mean) placental thickness for every 5 LMP weeks of pregnancy. Normal ranges of placental thicknesses are between − 2 SD (thinnest) and + 2 SD (thickest).

Adapted from Hoddick WK, Mahony BS, Callen PW, et al: Placental thickness. J Ultrasound Med 1985;4:479–482.

Thick Placenta

A placenta may be thicker owing to a small base area. However, Hoddick and colleagues found no normal placenta exceeding 40 mm. Diseases associated with enlarged, thickened placentas are maternal diabetes, Rh disease, infection, triploidy, maternal heart failure, and hydrops fetalis.[48] In many cases of disease-caused placental thickening, the echotexture appears homogeneous and immature, even at term.

Local uterine contractions (Braxton Hicks), uterine leiomyomas (fibroids), subplacental hematomas, and abruption may cause a normal placenta to appear thickened. Sonographic study of the subplacental complex of vessels may help identify these events (see Fig. 16–8).

Thin Placenta

Normal thinning of the placenta can be observed in cases in which the placental base is wide and covers a large area of the uterine wall. However, polyhydramnios causes an increase in uterine volume and therefore stretches the surface area of the uterus and placenta. This stretching of the placenta can result in a dramatic thinning of the placenta.[47] It is also possible that the hydrostatic pressure of polyhydramnios may compress the placenta, contributing to this thinning.

PLACENTAL LOCATION

Normal Locations

The placenta normally implants away from the birth canal. However, advanced maternal age, multiparity, prior cesarean sections, and cigarette smoking may increase the chances of a low-lying placenta.[49] Implantation at any site within the uterus, except over the birth canal, is considered normal. In general, these normal locations are described as fundal, anterior, posterior, left, or right. These descriptions are often used in combinations to describe intermediate locations, such as fundal, anterior, and right.

An anterior placenta in a normal patient (not obese) results in better fetal sonographic imaging and occasionally exquisite images. To date, no discussion or explanation has been offered for this phenomenon. It might be logically assumed that any tissue in the path of the beam would have an attenuating, deleterious effect, but this is not the case. It is hypothesized that scanning through the placenta must have one or two effects on the beam. One is that the placenta acts as a succulent offset pad not unlike those used for "small-parts" sonography of the thyroid, breasts, or testicles. Another possibility is that the intervening placenta acts as a sort of acoustic filter to remove unwanted scatter, reverberation, and noise, thus improving the noise-to-signal ratio of the image. Readers are encouraged to test this observation. When the placenta covers only part of the anterior uterus, it is occasionally possible to observe the same structure through a window containing placenta and from another angle without the intervening placenta. The image that is obtained through the placenta almost always exhibits better detail and less reverberation. Of course, a woman's umbilicus is not an acceptable location for scanning (see Chapter 5).

Placenta Previa

Placenta previa is a placenta that covers the internal os of the cervix, the birth canal. This is an important condition to diagnose because it can be fatal to both a woman and her fetus if it is not discovered before the onset of labor.

A placenta previa is considered complete or central when it completely covers the internal os. A placenta that is truly central to the internal os is a symmetrical complete previa. If one edge of the placenta crosses and completely covers the os, asymmetrical complete previa is diagnosed. When the edge of the placenta just touches the internal os but does not cross, the condition is marginal previa. In a simple low-lying placenta, the placenta approaches near the os but does not touch it.[50] An anterior, low-lying placenta is illustrated in Figure 16–18.

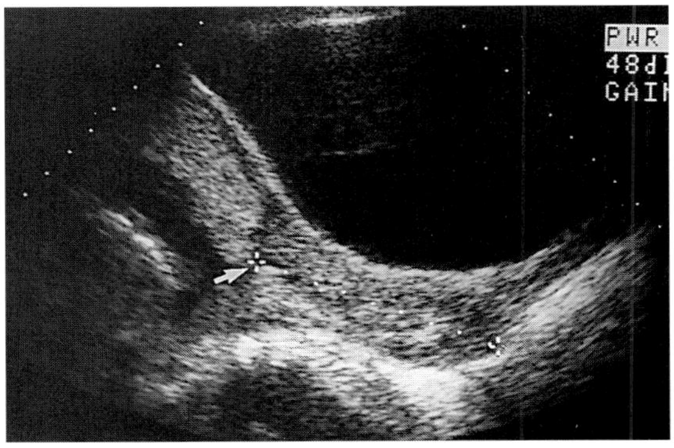

FIGURE 16–18.
Example of a low anterior placenta that does not cross the internal os (arrow). The cervical length was measured at 83 mm. (AA = 19.5 LMP weeks, range = 1.5 weeks, n = 9 TD)

Whenever a pregnant woman presents with painless bleeding, placenta previa must be considered. Figure 16–19 illustrates an interesting case in which the sonographic diagnosis was made of impending spontaneous abortion because of the large, unusual fluid collection surrounding the chorionic (gestational) sac at 7.4 LNMP weeks. Follow-up on this case found that the pregnancy progressed normally until the 30th week, at which time the patient presented with heavy vaginal bleeding. Sonography at that time demonstrated a complete placenta previa, and a

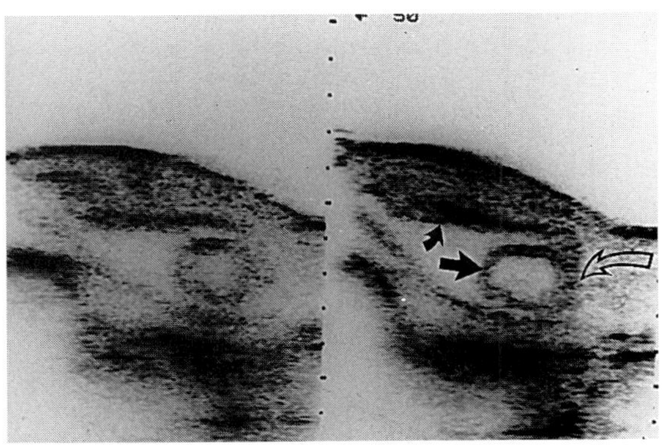

FIGURE 16–19. EARLY PREVIA.
This older (1988) image shows black echoes on a white background. The decidua capsularis (large black arrow) of the chorionic sac is separated from the uterine wall (decidua parietalis, curved black arrow) by fluid (blood). The decidua basalis was implanted over the internal os (curved open arrow). The embryonic heart rate was appropriate for age at 151 B/M. This woman had a complete placental previa in the 30th LMP week. (LNMP = 7.4 weeks, AA = 7.1 LMP weeks, range = 0.4 weeks, n = 2, EHR = 151 B/M = 7.3 LMP weeks, TD)

normal (1265 g) male was delivered by emergency cesarean section. Mother and child fared well.

Placental Migration and Trophotrophism

In the sonographic literature, one occasionally sees a reference to placental migration. This phenomenon was first reported by King in 1973.[51] In King's study, placenta previa was observed in early sonographic examinations but the follow-up scans later in the pregnancies found that the placentas appeared to have moved away from the internal os. This observation is now common in obstetrical sonography.[49] Although no one has proposed that the placenta actually slides or moves its attachments to the uterus, no satisfactory explanation has been offered for the migrating placenta until recently.

Finberg proposed that trophotropism explains this apparent placental migration.[52] The term *trophotropism* is defined as the "attraction and repulsion of cells to nutritive substances; positive and negative trophotropism respectively."[53] In the context of placental migration, Finberg says:

> "Trophotropism is defined as the preferential proliferation of trophoblastic villi of the placenta into regions of better endometrial blood supply, along with atrophy of villi in areas of poorer blood supply. This phenomenon allows a placenta to change its position and remodel its shape within the uterus as the pregnancy progresses."[52]

This simple and elegant explanation for the perplexing and logic defying placental migration also explains a number of placental oddities. Finberg also proposes trophotropism as an explanation for succenturiate placental lobes, marginal and velamentous cord insertions, vasa previa, and obligate cord presentation. Figure 16–20 demonstrates a succenturiate placenta.

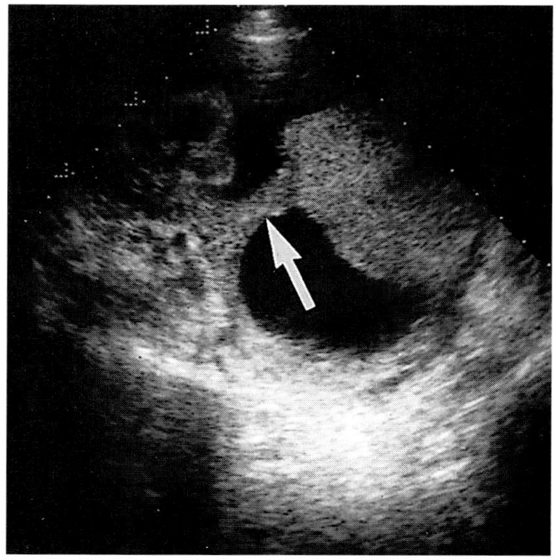

FIGURE 16–20.
This image tangential to the uterine wall shows a bridge (arrow) of placenta to a succenturiate lobe. Real-time observation showed this bridge to be attached to the uterine wall. (LNMP = 20.0 weeks, AA = 19.7 LMP weeks, range = 1.7 weeks, n = 9, TD)

MULTIPLE GESTATIONS

Identification of the placenta and the number of placentas in multiple gestations can help to define the type of gestation. A single placenta indicates monoamniotic, monozygotic twinning. Monozygotic twins, from a single egg, have a higher incidence of anomalies. Two placentas indicate dizygotic, diamniotic twinning. Diamniotic twins may be monochoronic or dichorionic. Every effort should be made to define the number and location of placentas in multiple gestations. This information assists the obstetrician in the management of the case.[54]

In some pregnancies with twins, the two placentas are abutting each other. This situation may make identifying the two placentas difficult. One particular observation that may help is the twin peak sign,[55] in which a slight peak of placenta on the fetal surface lies adjacent to the amniotic membrane between the two placentas.

Umbilical Cord

NORMAL AND ABNORMAL SONOGRAPHIC FINDINGS

In early embryonic life (approximately 6 LMP weeks), two arteries and paired allantoic veins form the umbilical cord. Also present are vitelline veins, which drain the yolk sac and primitive midgut. This early anatomy is not visible sonographically. The right vein normally disappears early, leaving only the two arteries and one vein that are sonographically visible in a normal umbilical cord.[56]

A few reports have described persistent right umbilical veins, which are often associated with other fetal anomalies. In an important report of this unusual finding, Jeanty proposes that persistent right umbilical veins are underreported. He points out that the right vein is lateral to the gallbladder and curves toward the stomach rather than away from it. Jeanty's report categorizes numerous anomalies that are associated with persistent right umbilical veins, including gastrointestinal, cardiovascular, musculoskeletal, genitourinary, and several miscellaneous anomalies. Both the right and left umbilical veins occasionally are present. If a sonographer suspects an anomalous umbilical vein in a fetus, this short (four pages) but in-depth report is recommended reading.[57]

The umbilical cord extends from the placental surface to the anterior fetal abdominal wall and ranges in length from 30 to 100 cm but usually is about 50 cm.[58] Its diameter usually is 1 to 2 cm. The umbilical vein carries blood from the placenta to the fetal liver by way of the ductus venosus and portal sinus.[59] The two umbilical arteries carry blood to the placenta from the fetal left and right internal iliac arteries (see Figs. 16–21 and 14–14). Cords larger than 2 cm in diameter have been reported and are normal in some fetuses.[60] Abnormally large cords are also associated with a patent urachus and omphalomesenteric ducts, tumors, allantoic cysts, hemangiomas, hematoma, excess Wharton's jelly, and both false and true umbilical cord knots.[61,62]

It is important to ascertain that the umbilical cord contains three vessels because a two-vessel cord (single artery) is associated with an increased incidence of other fetal anomalies. The arteries anastomose within 2 cm of the insertion in most normal placentas[58] and may fuse just before placental insertion. For this reason, it is preferable to count the number of cord vessels at the fetal abdominal insertion rather than at the placental end.[63] Observation at the fetal end has the advantage of ruling out gastroschisis and omphaloceles of the abdomen without increased scanning time. The two umbilical arteries can be seen to pass on either side of the fetal urinary bladder (Fig. 16–21).

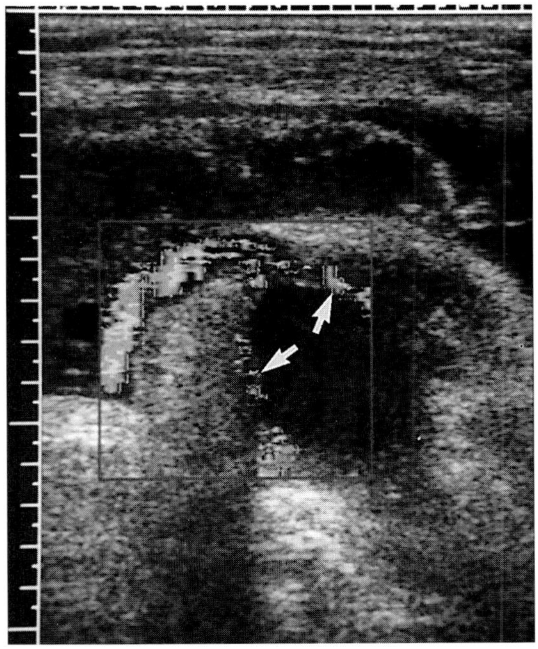

FIGURE 16–21.
Color Doppler of umbilical attachment to the fetal abdomen. The two umbilical arteries (arrows) can be seen passing from the attachment around either side of the fetal bladder. (LNMP = 40.7 weeks, AA = 39.9 LMP weeks, range = 3.6, n = 9, TD)

The umbilical cord normally inserts near the center of the placental disk. However, owing to trophotropism or placental migration (discussed earlier), the placenta may grow away from the original implantation site, resulting in a marginal or velamentous cord insertion or a succenturiate lobe of the placenta. A velum is a veil-like or curtainlike membrane. A succenturiate lobe is a separate placental lobe connected by velamentous vessels (see Fig. 16–20). These succenturiate lobes or marginal or velamentous cord insertions tend to be more common in low-lying placentas and in twin (or multiple) gestations. Low-lying velamentous cords are associated with an increased risk of vasa previa, in which the vessels cross the internal os of the birth canal. Rupture of the vasa previa poses a risk that the fetus might exsanguinate in minutes. Color Doppler offers the best chance of identifying vasa previa, which can be difficult to diagnose.[46]

Because the umbilical cord attaches to the anterior abdomen at the level of the fetal elbows, it is common to observe a fetus grasping or manipulating the cord. Umbilical cord grasping is observed in such a high percentage (35%) of short sonographic observation periods that this activity must be universal from time to time in all normal pregnancies (Figs. 16–22 and 16–23). (See Chapter 15 for more discussion of fetal hand activities.) Another observed fetal activity is sucking on the cord (Fig. 16–24).[64]

In about 25% of cases, the umbilical cord can be observed to be across or around the fetal neck, a nuchal cord. However, unless the cord clearly makes two complete loops around the neck or is tight enough to indent the skin or to flatten the umbilical vein, there is usually little to worry about.[65]

Figure 16–25 shows the umbilical cord indenting the fetal abdominal wall. When first noticed (Fig. 16–25*A*), this image was perplexing. Real-time and color Doppler (Fig. 16–25*B*) proved that the defect in the abdominal wall was the cord pressed between the fetus and the placenta. Observation after fetal movement found a normal fetal abdominal wall.

The normal umbilical cord coils in a helix; a left counterclockwise twist is seven times more common than a right twist (see Fig. 16–22). The twist is determined by pathological inspection: "With the cord held vertically, vessels along the anterior surface that spiral downward from high left to low right, angled like the left side of the letter V, indicate a left helix. Those angled like the right side of the V form a right helix."[66] The cause of the umbilical cord coiling, left or right, is not known but is suspected to arise from fetal activity. The direction of twist has not been found to relate to the handedness of the mother or child. It also does not relate to the Earth's hemispheres, such as the "bathtub vortex" theory. It is notable that right-hand twists or no twist (straight cords) are found more often with two-vessel cords. Straight cords have been related to fetal demise, poor outcomes, and anomalies.[67]

DOPPLER

Doppler study of the umbilical arteries has caused considerable excitement in the past 10 years. Several studies have found that increased resistance to arterial blood flow return to the placenta from the fetus is associated with IUGR.[68–74] However, other research has not completely supported this conclusion.[75,76] This is currently a very popular topic in the field of fetal sonography, and many more references are available than listed here. Because the umbilical cord is the source of fetal nourishment and oxygen as well as the route of waste riddance, it is logical that any impediment to blood flow would have a detrimental effect on fetal growth and well-being. It has been suggested that some fluid and electrolyte transfer occurs across the amniotic-chorionic plate, but most occurs through the umbilical cord as maternofetal placental perfusion.[77]

The current thinking is that placental resistance to blood flow is indicative of poor fetal outcomes and is most obvious as a reduction of umbilical artery diastolic velocity (Table 16–4). Therefore, when the diastolic umbilical

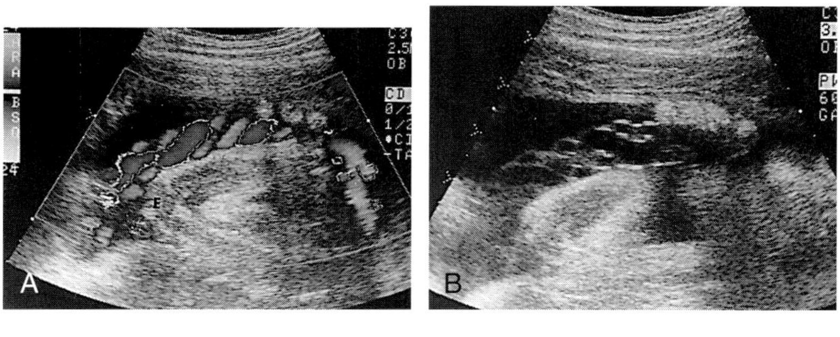

FIGURE 16–22.
Normal umbilical cord. (See Color Figure 16–22*A*.) The two arteries and vein. Where flow is toward the transducer, the shorter Doppler shift is shown as blue, and flow away as red. Three fetal fingers can be seen to grasp and press the cord against the other wrist, with the cord passing along the forearm to the elbow (E). (LNMP = 31.9, AA = 31.6 LMP weeks, range = 2.5 weeks, n = 9, TD) *B*, The same umbilical cord as in *A* but without color Doppler. The two arteries can be observed to be smaller than the single vein. This is a normal cord.

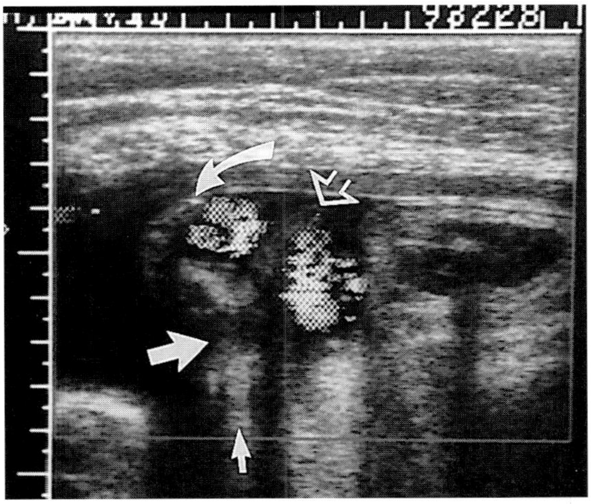

FIGURE 16–23.
Cross section of umbilical cord in grasp of fetal hand. Open arrow, thumb; curved arrow, finger; large arrow, wrist; small arrow, distal radius. A loop of cord wraps around the thumb. (AA = 28.2 LMP weeks, range = 2.8 weeks, n = 9, TD)

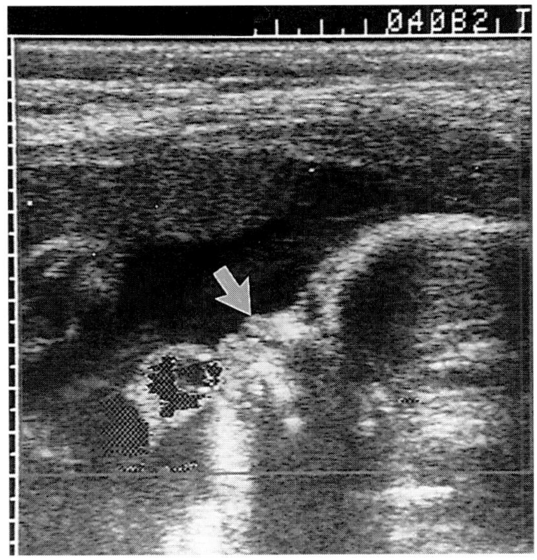

FIGURE 16–24.
Profile of fetal face sucking umbilical cord (Doppler). Arrow, nose. The umbilical cord seems to occupy much of the fetal attention in the last half of pregnancy. (AA = 28.2 LMP weeks, range = 2.8 weeks, n = 9, TD)

artery flow is compared with the systolic flow in a ratio or index, reduced diastolic velocity relative to systolic velocity indicates greater resistance to flow. If the diastolic flow is not present (zero velocity) or reversed, more severe resistance is indicated. The most common indexes or ratios used are the S/D or A/B ratio, the pulsatility index (PI), and the resistive index (RI) or Pourcelot's index.

S/D or A/B ratio = maximum systolic velocity/minimum diastolic velocity

PI = (maximum systolic velocity − end-diastolic velocity)/mean velocity

RI = (maximum systolic velocity − end-diastolic velocity)/maximum systolic velocity[78]

All these indexes (S/D, PI, and RI) correlate with resistance; as the index increases, so does the resistance to flow downstream from the fetus (i.e., toward the placenta). The RI is relatively simple to calculate and widely used (see Chapter 13).

FIGURE 16–25.
A, The umbilical cord is compressed between the placenta and fetal abdominal wall, causing a depression (arrows) in the abdominal wall. In the initial image (*A*), the cord appeared to be a septated cystic structure. *B*, Color Doppler revealed it to be a normal three-vessel cord. In images subsequent to fetal motion, the abdominal wall appeared normal. (AA = 31.2 LMP weeks, range = 2.5 weeks, n = 9, TD)

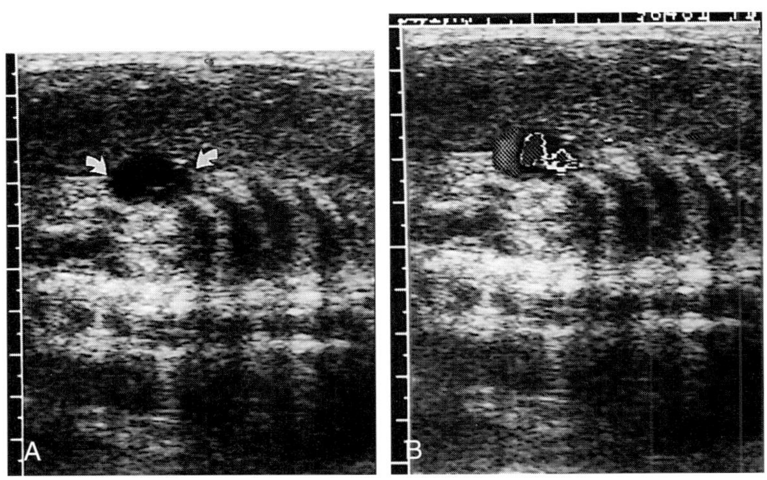

TABLE 16–4. UMBILICAL DOPPLER REGRESSIONS

STUDY	ESTIMATED VARIABLE (y)	GIVEN VARIABLE (x)	INTERCEPT CONSTANT (I)	SLOPE CONSTANT (S)	STANDARD ERROR OF ESTIMATE	r2	SIGNIFICANCE	n
Umbilical Resistive Index (RI) Regressions								
DeVore et al	Umbilical/artery RI	LMP age	89.743	−0.904	5.659	0.457	$P < 0.001$	228
DuBose et al	Umbilical/artery RI	LMP age	95.24	−0.958	7.517	0.425	$P < 0.001$	144
Umbilical Systolic/Diastolic (S/D ratio) Regressions								
DeVore et al	Umbilical artery S/D	LMP age	4.91979	−0.07101	0.40849	0.499	$P < 0.001$	228
DuBose et al	Umbilical artery S/D	LMP age	6.846	−0.117	1.176	0.311	$P < 0.001$	144
Gerson et al	Umbilical artery S/D	LMP age	6.46	−0.12	0.79	0.347	Significant	209
Schulman et al	Umbilical artery S/D	LMP age	3.58	−0.029	0.002	0.096	$P < 0.001$	127
Umbilical Venous Flow Regressions								
Gerson et al	Umbilical/venous	LMP age	−187.02	12.7	66.07	0.46	Significant	209
Gerson et al	Umbilical/venous	ml/min/kg	198.629	−2.24	41.89	0.06	Significant	209

The variables above are used in the following linear regression formula:

$$y = I + (Sx)$$

The eight sets of variables in this table use the fetal age in LMP weeks to estimate the umbilical artery resistive index (RI), the systolic/diastolic (S/D) ratios, and umbilical venous flow in milliliters/minute/kilogram weight. The variables are inserted into the regression formula given at the bottom of the table. Note the similar magnitude of all variables and statistics. These regressions are compared graphically in Figures 16–27 and 16–28. DeVore's and DuBose's dates are from 16 to 40 LMP weeks, and Gerson's dates were between 20 and 40 LMP weeks. It is noted that DeVore and colleagues' umbilical S/D slope constant was given as −0.7101 in the original publication. This yields absurd results, and observation of the other constants led to the conclusion that the constant should have been −0.07101, as given here.

DeVore and colleagues' data adapted from DeVore GR, Medearis AL, Platt LD: The effect of altitude on the umbilical artery Doppler resistance. J Ultrasound Med 1992;11:317–320.

Gerson and colleagues' data adapted from Gerson AG, Wallace DM, Stiller RJ, et al: Doppler evaluation of umbilical venous and arterial blood flow in the second and third trimesters of normal pregnancy. Obstet Gynecol 1987;70:622–626.

Schulman and colleagues' data adapted from Schulman H, Fleischer A, Stern W, et al: Umbilical velocity wave ratios in human pregnancy. Am J Obstet Gynecol 1984;148:985–990.

It is thought that as placental resistance to blood flow increases, the exchange of nutrients, oxygen, and wastes is impeded. As a result of this decrease in nutrients and oxygen supplied to the fetus, a natural system of priorities causes more of the blood to flow toward the fetal brain and heart at the expense of much of the rest of the body.[79-83] This condition, which results in a relatively small abdomen compared with the head, is often referred to as *head-sparing* or *asymmetrical IUGR*. However, a small fetus with normal umbilical flow may be simply a normal small-for-gestational-age (SGA) fetus rather than a fetus with IUGR. Doppler may provide a method for distinguishing between fetuses with IUGR and normal SGA fetuses.[84] Chronic reduction of blood flow to the body results in a decrease in fetal renal function and urine output and consequently decreased amniotic fluid, oligohydramnios.[85] This is the primary basis for using amniotic fluid volumes as one indicator of fetal well-being in the Biophysical profile (see Chapter 17).

The precise relationships of the various maternofetal blood flow and resistive relationships constitute a new and exciting area of research. Figure 16–26 contains XY scatterplots for the RIs for a free loop of the umbilical cord artery (Fig. 16–26*A*), the fetal aorta (Fig. 16–26*B*), the middle cerebral artery (Fig. 16–26*C*), and the ratio of the cerebral artery RI to the aortic RI (Fig. 16–26*D*). Although the latter three graphs do not represent extrafetal

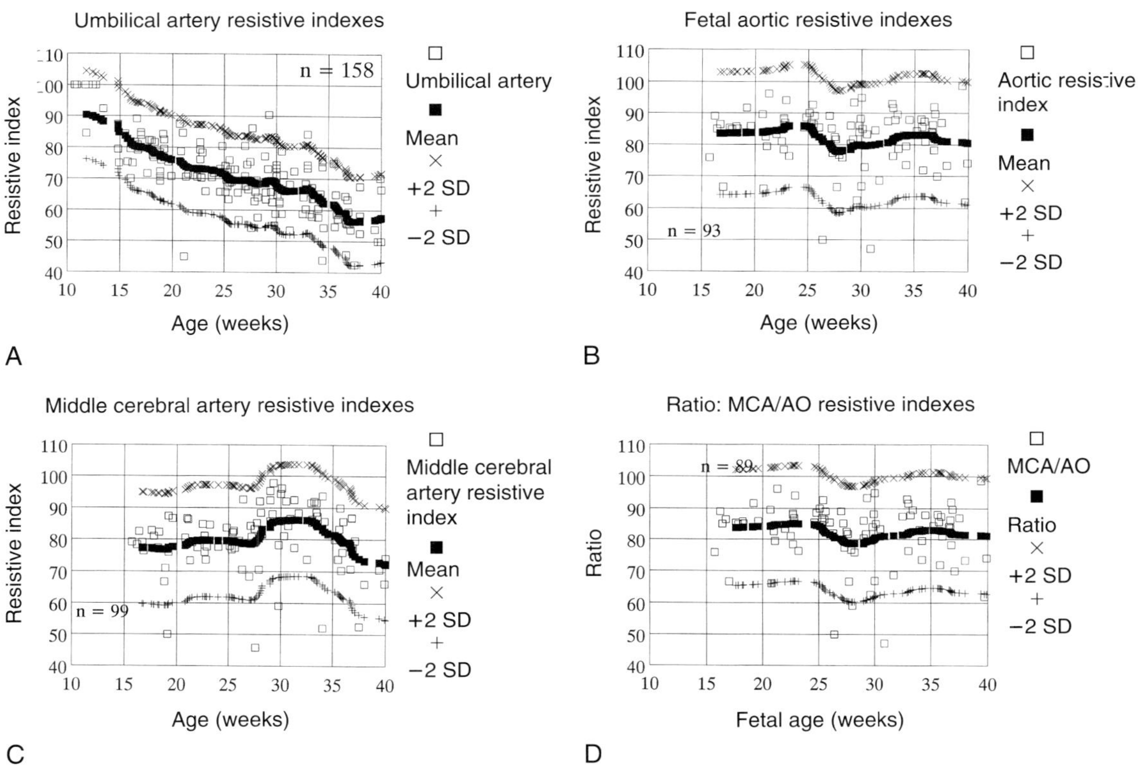

FIGURE 16–26. OBSTETRICAL DOPPLER RESISTIVE INDEXES.
A, Resistive indexes (RIs) for free loops of umbilical arteries in 158 cases. LOWESS smoothed means of RIs (solid black squares) decline in a relatively linear fashion. Open squares are actual RIs. High resistance to flow (> +2 SD, X) may indicate resistive placental perfusion, which may be associated with intrauterine growth retardation (IUGR). *B*, RIs for 93 fetal aortas above the renal branches. The LOWESS means remain relatively horizontal, with a slight reduction between 25 and 28 weeks. *C*, RIs for 99 fetal middle cerebral arteries. These RIs also remain relatively horizontal, with a slight increase after about 28 LMP weeks. Compare these increased RI means with the decrease in the RI for the aorta. The significance of these inverse changes in RIs is not understood at this time. *D*, The LOWESS smoothed means of ratios of the middle cerebral artery/aorta (MCA/AO) RIs are also relatively horizontal. Our group has found IUGR and low biophysical profile scores in association with low MCA/AO RI ratios. Although these data are from a referral population and do not represent a random normal population, this phenomenon deserves more study with a larger, controlled data set.

structures, they are included here because changes in them may theoretically be in response to changes in the umbilical artery RI.

Note that the umbilical artery RI exhibits a steady decrease from approximately 100 (high resistance, little or no end-diastolic flow)[86,87] in the late first trimester to lower resistance at term.[88-90] This is a relatively linear relationship. The mean and ± 2 SD for Figure 16–26*A* were estimated using a LOWESS (locally weighted scatterplot smoother) technique rather than regression.[91] The LOWESS technique is more sensitive to small, subtle changes in the mean than regression. However, a linear regression appears to serve as well in this case (Fig. 16–27).

The fetal aortic and middle cerebral artery RIs are less linear in their LOWESS graphs (see Fig. 16–26*B* and *C*). It was noted that between the 25th and 30th weeks, both exhibit a change that is inverse, one to the other. For this reason, the ratio of these two RIs was calculated and plotted (Fig. 16–26*D*). This is from data collected from referral diagnostic examinations and most likely includes more abnormal cases than formal randomized research should. However, fetuses that exhibit tendencies toward asymmetrical IUGR and a few with low biophysical profile scores also tend to have elevated umbilical artery and aortic RIs on these graphs but lower middle cerebral artery RIs and low middle cerebral artery to aorta ratios. Again, it is emphasized that this is not a formal randomized study and is included here only for interest to readers.

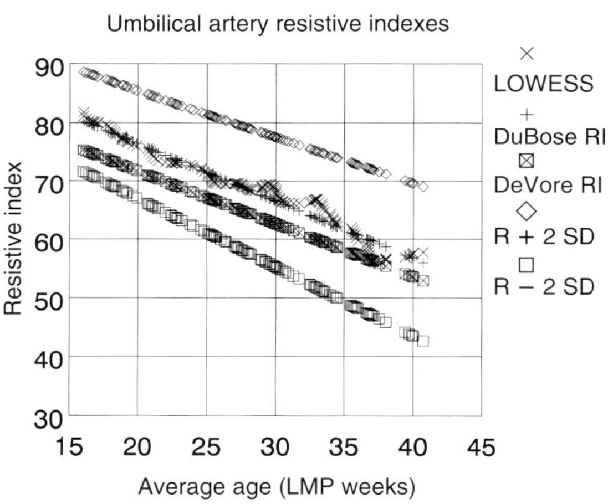

FIGURE 16–27.
This XY scattergram compares two regression formulas for the estimation of the umbilical artery resistive index (RI) from the fetal age in LMP weeks (see Table 16–2 for the formulas). Also included for comparison is the LOWESS smoothed means (X) from Figure 16–26*A*. The DuBose RI regression (+) was calculated using the same unpublished data (free loops of cord) as the LOWESS means, thus explaining the good fit. The R + 2 SD (open diamonds) and R − 2 SD (open squares) are the two standard deviations for the DuBose regression. Note that the DeVore formula (boxed X) results are parallel but slightly lower than the DuBose regression. (DeVore from composite regression in DeVore GR, Medearis AL, Platt LD: The effect of altitude on the umbilical artery Doppler resistance. J Ultrasound Med 1992;11:317–320.)

The foregoing data on umbilical artery RIs and S/D ratios were compared with regression formulas from published studies that were conducted with more rigorous scientific methods (Table 16–4).[88,92] Figure 16–27 shows the robust LOWESS and regression means (DuBose and colleagues' data) with ± 2 SD for the regression, and the regression mean from DeVore and coworkers. The LOWESS and regression lines fit very well, as expected, because they are from the same data, but they are slightly above DeVore's regression. Again, this may be because DuBose's data are from a population referred for medical indications and may have more abnormal RIs. It is possible to observe that both regressions lie between the ±2 SD lines and have a similar slope. DeVore and colleagues' study compared two groups of pregnancies, one at sea level and one group from between 4200 and 4500 feet above sea level, and found no significant difference in these groups. The regression used for comparison here is from the composite of both groups.

Four umbilical artery S/D regressions are compared in Figure 16–28. All four regression formulas were applied to the previous data. They have similar magnitude, but one has a slightly different slope, causing them to cross, and the other is again higher. Others have cautioned that the S/D ratio varies depending on the location of the Doppler interrogation. Kay and colleagues found that the lowest S/D ratios were at the placental end of the cord and the highest were at the fetal end.[93] Most reports use a free loop somewhere between these two locations or do not specify where the Doppler readings were taken.

Gerson and associates' report also included the umbilical venous flow volume and found it to have a statistically significant relation-

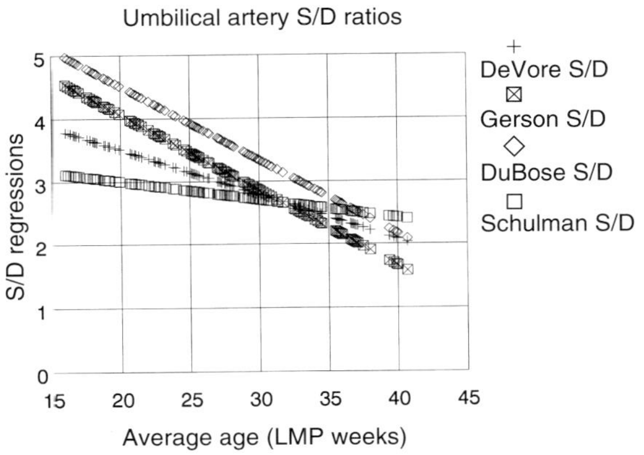

FIGURE 16–28.
This XY scattergram compares four regression formulas for the umbilical artery systolic/diastolic ratios (S/D) using the same data shown in Figures 16–26 and 16–27. Although the regressions produce results of the same order of magnitude, better correlation would be expected. The DeVore regression (+) may be judged the most accurate because of its more intermediate location; however, this observation needs to be confirmed with a large controlled population. (DuBose S/D from the previously used unpublished data. DeVore from composite S/D regression in DeVore GR, Medearis AL, Platt LD: The effect of altitude on the umbilical artery Doppler resistance. J Ultrasound Med 1992;11:317–320. Gerson from Gerson AG, Wallace DM, Stiller RJ, et al: Doppler evaluation of umbilical venous and arterial blood flow in the second and third trimesters of normal pregnancy. Obstet Gynecol 1987;70:622–626. Schulman from average-for-gestational age [AGA] fetuses regression in Schulman H, Fleischer A, Stern W, et al: Umbilical velocity wave ratios in human pregnancy. Am J Obstet Gynecol 1984;148:985–990. This reference also contained a regression for small-for-gestational age [SGA] fetuses [SGA S/D = 5.897 − 0.077 age]).

ship to both fetal age and fetal size. Those researchers point out several questions about Doppler investigation of the umbilical vein: How do fetal breathing movements affect venous flow? How accurate are angle corrections in the venous study? Can it be assumed that venous flow is laminar? They conclude that the usefulness of this Doppler is unproven.[88] An association between maternal hypertensive disease and reduced uterine artery diastolic flow has also been found.[94] Another report described increased fetal cerebrovascular resistance during increased glucose levels.[95]

Research has found that umbilical venous pulsations are a generic sign of fetal congestive heart failure and in combination with fetal nonimmune hydrops are a dismal sign.[96] Others point out that "fetuses may have umbilical venous pulsations with absent end-diastolic velocities in the umbilical artery, or with growth retardation, multiple anomalies, chromosomal abnormalities, urethral atresia, or cardiac hypertrophy, among other conditions."[97,98] This complex topic—maternal/fetal/placental Doppler study—is deserving of more research.

Gestational Sac and Contents

CHORION AND AMNION

A fetus normally lives in a bath of fluid inside three concentric containers. The outer container is the uterus. The two inner containers are generally referred to as sacs; the chorionic sac contains the amniotic sac (see Figs. 16–7 and 16–12C). In most cases, the amniotic sac fuses with the chorionic by the 16th LMP week. The chorionic sac is more obvious sonographically. Its dimensions are useful in early pregnancy to estimate dates and are called the *gestational sac diameter* (GSD) (discussed later).

Not all the underlying causes of GSDs that are too large or small are completely understood at this time. It can be cautioned that early abnormal sonographic appearances of pregnancy warrant follow-up to confirm viability.[99] It is known that in the second and third trimesters, oligohydramnios is associated with decreased fetal urine output and polyhydramnios is associated with reduced fetal swallowing. Other conditions such as infection and congenital anomalies can also either increase or decrease the amniotic fluid quantities.[100,101]

AMNIOTIC FLUID

First Trimester

In the very early embryonic stages, in the fifth or early sixth LMP week, the amniotic membrane appears on sonography to be rather spherical next to the spherical yolk sac. These two circular structures have been called the *double bleb* (see Fig. 16–12*A*).[102] The embryonic heartbeat is usually first observed between the double blebs when viewed with transvaginal transducers. Once the embryonic heart rate (EHR) is observed, the crown-rump length (CRL) can be measured as the greatest dimension of the echogenic structure between the double blebs.

As pregnancy progresses, the thin amniotic membrane enlarges and contains the embryo; the yolk sac remains outside the amnion (see Fig. 16–12C). The amniotic sac and its embryo, as well as the yolk sac, all are found within the so-called gestational sac. This gestational sac is actually the chorionic cavity. The chorionic space around the amniotic sac is filled "by a gel that liquefies upon touching, the magma reticulare."[103] This magma reticulare has a slightly echogenic appearance when compared with the very clear amniotic fluid (see Fig. 16–12C). The magma reticulare, also called the *chorioamniotic accumulation*, is a normal finding before the amnion and chorion fuse.[104] This fusion of the two membranes should be complete by about the 16th LMP week, but this timing may vary.

The dimensions of the gestational sac are used in early pregnancy to estimate the dates of the pregnancy. Three perpendicular diameters are usually taken and averaged, although in early studies only the greatest GSD was used. Nyberg and colleagues found that the GSD grows linearly at about 1.1 mm per day from the 5th to the 11th LMP weeks, and GSD growth less than 0.6 mm per day is abnormal during this period.[105] This study also concluded that it is abnormal not to detect a yolk sac after the GSD reaches 20 mm or not to detect an embryo after the GSD is greater than 25 mm. The planes and locations for obtaining the most accurate GSD measurements may be relatively subjective in cases of sac distortion by uterine masses or external pressures. The GSD is less useful for estimating gestational age after CRL or other fetal structures can be measured.

A study by Nazari and colleagues, using an infertility population with known dates of ovulation, found that small-for-dates GSDs and CRLs are predictive of first-trimester spontaneous abortion.[106] This observation may corroborate that of Schats and associates, who found a window of 5 days in which the EHR was first detected after follicle aspiration (25 to 30 days, or approximately 5.5 to 6.3 LMP weeks).[107] The later in this 5-day window of time that the EHR was first detected, the greater the chance of a first-trimester spontaneous abortion. It may be that small GSDs and CRLs and late EHRs all are related to late or abnormal implantation. The difficulty with using this information is that extremely accurate dates of conception or ovulation are required, and the LNMP is not very useful for this purpose (see Chapters 12 and 7).

Second and Third Trimesters

Amniotic Fluid Cycle

Early in pregnancy, before fetal renal function begins, the formation of amniotic fluid is not completely understood, and although it is "virtually unexplored, the most likely mechanism is an active transport of solute by the amnion into the amniotic space with water moving passively down the chemical potential gradient."[108] It is possible, although not explored, that this active transport of water across the membrane into the amniotic sac removes water from the magma reticulare in the chorionic cavity around the amnion. This reduction of volume from the magma reticulare, along with the enlargement of the spaces, must have a role in the fusion of the amnion and chorion. To date, the sonographic measurements of the amniotic sac have not been published, nor has its relative size in comparison with the chorionic space. If this process is controlled by active transport or osmosis, abnormal relationships in the sizes of the amniotic and chorionic sacs might indicate abnormal chemistry of these compartments. This is another interesting area for research.

Later in pregnancy, the major pathways of amniotic fluid control are fetal urination and swallowing. Fluid is also secreted by the fetal respiratory tract. It is assumed that some transport of fluid may occur across the fetal skin, the umbilical cord surface, and the chorionic plate; however, the degree of transport in these latter processes has not been proved conclusively.[109]

Normal amniotic fluid should be clear, and only fetal parts and umbilical cord should be seen during the first and second trimesters. In the third trimester, echogenic particles may be observed swirling in the fluid. In a normal pregnancy, these particles are vernix caseosa or just vernix, which is exfoliative skin and secretions of the sebaceous glands. Unfortunately, the normal swirling vernix cannot be distinguished sonographically from abnormal blood or meconium in the fluid.[110]

Quantity

The normal volume of amniotic fluid increases throughout pregnancy until about the 26th LMP week[111] and then declines slightly until term. During the second and third trimesters, the quantity of fluid normally is between 0.5 and 1.5 to 2.0 liters.[110]

Because the amniotic fluid is spread throughout the expanding uterus, around the growing fetus, its extremities, and the umbilical cord, absolute measurement of the quantity is not possible. Several methods of sonographically evaluating the amniotic quantities have been proposed.

One of the first attempts to quantitate the amniotic fluid with sonography measured total intrauterine volume.[112] This method used the three greatest perpendicular diameters in a formula for an ellipsoidal volume. The method was ultimately abandoned by most owing to large variations in results both between other researchers and between observers.[113] Others attempted parallel planimetric area measurements of the uterus, but the method was cumbersome, produced variable results, and was useful only with articulated arm static sonographic machines that could scan entire sections of the uterus in a single image.[114]

Two methods for evaluating amniotic fluid quantities are currently in general use. The most simple method, subjective visual assessment, requires experience on the part of the observer. The subjective method requires the observer to judge the amniotic fluid to be normal, less than normal, or more than normal. Figure 16–29 contains graphs of more than 2000 subjective evaluations of amniotic fluid quantities.

The other method is based on various measurements of pockets of amniotic fluid. Several ways to measure these pockets have been proposed. Both the subjective evaluation and the pocket measurements work well with the limited fields of view of real-time machines, and both have been shown to produce similar results.[115] As stated, the subjective method requires only that the sonographer have sufficient experience with obstetrical examinations to be able to judge when the amniotic fluid is normal to abnormal in quantity.

To measure fluid pockets, the dimensions of single pockets or pockets found in the four quadrants of the uterus have been used. Single-pocket methods have measured the vertical depth of the largest pocket[116] or two diameters of the largest pocket.[117–119] The vertical depth method found that a depth of greater than 1 cm was considered relatively normal. If no pocket of amniotic fluid with at least 1 cm was found, the diagnosis of oligohydramnios could be made. The two-diameter method was found to have similar results to the single-pocket 1-cm rule in normal pregnancies and in those with polyhydraminos; however, the investigators found the two-diameter method slightly more accurate for predicting oligohydramnios. This two-diameter method multiplied the perpendicular diameters of the largest pocket and defined normal quantities as 15.1 to 50 cm^2. Less than 15 cm^2 was defined as oligohydramnios, and greater than 50 cm^2 indicated hydramnios (polyhydramnios).

Currently, the most commonly used method is the four-quadrant method or amniotic fluid index (AFI), which was defined by Phelan, Rutherford, and others.[111,120] With this method, the uterus (amniotic cavity) is divided into four quadrants by the sagittal and transverse planes. The vertical diameter of the largest pocket of fluid in each quadrant is measured, and the sum of these four diameters is the AFI. The researchers define vertical diameter as being perpendicular to the transducer surface (i.e., along the axis of the sonic beam travel).[120] In general, Phelan and colleagues found that the AFI should not exceed 22 cm after the 25th LMP week. The minimum AFI declines from 15 cm at 26 LMP weeks to about 10 cm at term. Figure 16–30 is a modification of Phelan's data using a robust LOWESS (smoothing) technique.[91] The LOWESS means and ±SD are given, as well as the actual Phelan means. It is believed that a LOWESS treatment of the data is justified because the original data often had fewer than five data points to represent a given

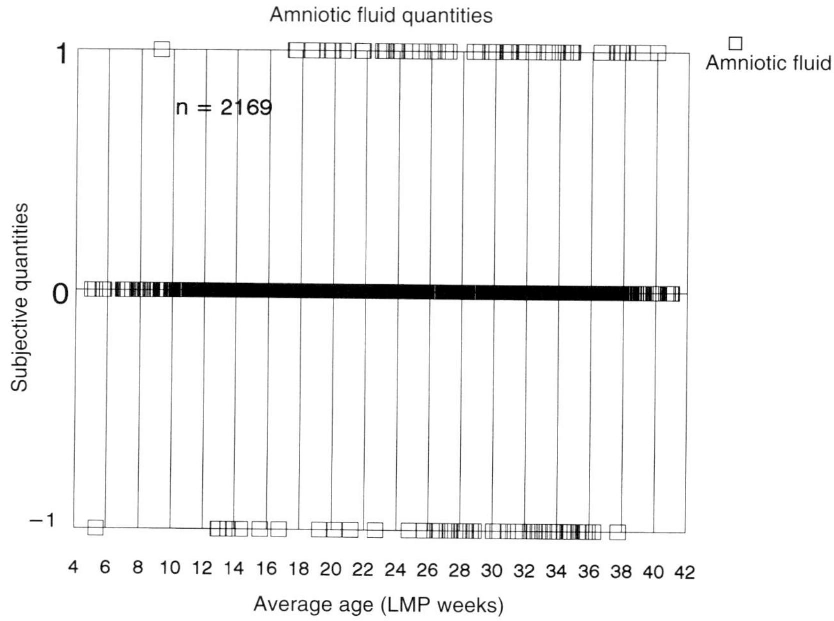

A

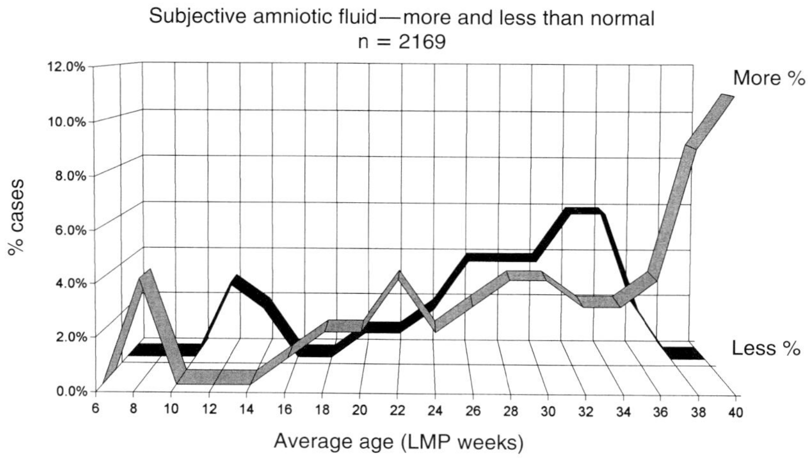

B

FIGURE 16–29.
A, Plots of subjective amniotic fluid quantities as discrete or meristic variables. Amniotic fluid quantities judged to be normal are 0, more than normal are 1, and less than normal are − 1. Data are from all cases in 1993 by 13 sonographers using machines by various manufacturers in four seperate laboratories. The sonographers in this study noticed in earlier studies (1984–1990) that there is a tendency toward slightly increased fluid between 20 and 30 weeks, and they may have compensated by judging slight increases at that time more normal in this population. *B*, Histographic ribbon graphs of the more-than and less-than normal amniotic fluid quantities shown in *A* as a percentage of the total cases.

week, and no week was represented by more than 24 measurements until the 32nd week. Observe that after the 32nd week, with the larger numbers of measurements, the Phelan means become less erratic and correlate well with the LOWESS means (see Fig. 16–30).

The AFI method of amniotic fluid evaluation was confirmed by an interesting study of pregnancies with severe oligohydramnios or anhydramnios.[121] These uteri were infused with a known volume of normal saline. The AFI and single-deepest-pool measurements were made and compared. The AFI

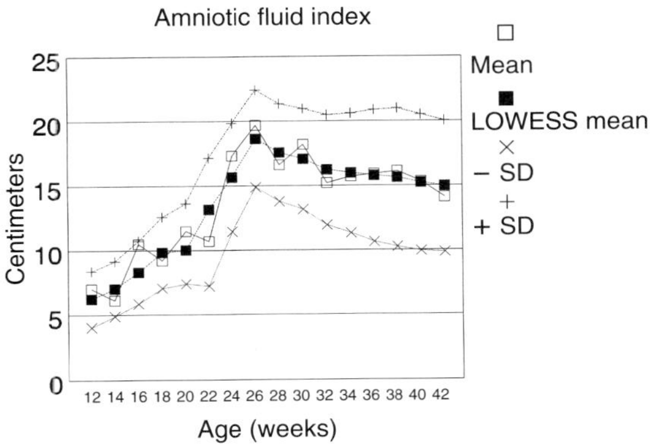

FIGURE 16–30.
Line graph of the amniotic fluid index (AFI) as described by Phelan and colleagues. The AFI means reported by Phelan's group are open squares, and the solid squares are the LOWESS smoothed means of those means. The LOWESS smoothed normal limits of ±SD are also shown. In the original study, small numbers of data points were used to calculate each mean before 32 weeks. Notice the smoother line and close correlation of LOWESS means after 32 weeks when 24 to 60 data points were used to calculate the means for each biweekly group. Also notice the tendency toward increased fluid between 20 and 30 weeks. (Adapted from Table II in Phelan JP, Ahn MO, Smith CV, et al: Amniotic fluid index measurements during pregnancy. J Reprod Med 1987; 23:601–604.)

had a statistically significant relationship to the infused volumes ($P < 0.05$), but the single-pool method did not ($P > 0.05$). The researchers concluded, "Amniotic fluid index is preferable to deepest pool measurement in assessing amniotic fluid volume in the second trimester of pregnancy. The low variance (30%) suggests that better predictors of amniotic fluid volume are still required."

Echogenicity

The amnion can occasionally remain or can become unfused from the chorion. If a fetus becomes entangled and attached to the free amnion, amniotic band syndrome can result, with severe fetal anomalies and demise. Any thin sheets of echoes that appear to be associated with the fetus and its extremities require close examination. One report described a sonographically detected extra-amniotic fetus that progressed to a normal delivery by cesarean section.[122]

Adnexa

The adnexa of the pelvis contains those structures on either side of the uterus, including the ovaries; fallopian tubes; uterine, ovarian, and other vessels; and bowel (see Fig. 16–1). The adnexa should be interrogated sonographically for abnormal masses. This is particularly true in early pregnancy, when corpus luteum and theca-lutein cysts (Fig. 16–31) may develop or an ectopic pregnancy may exist (Fig. 16–32). From the late first trimester to term, the ovaries and related structures are usually difficult to observe sonographically because of overlying bowel.

A corpus luteum (yellow body) or cyst forms in the place of the ruptured primary or dominate follicular cyst and, if pregnancy occurs, persists into the early second trimester. This luteal body appears as a hypoechoic area or cyst on a slightly enlarged ovary. A corpus luteum cyst most often is a simple cyst that resembles a mature ovarian follicle. These structures secrete the hormones of pregnancy until the fetal and placental tissues take over production, in the early second trimester.

In cases of multiple gestations or trophoblastic hydatidiform moles, the corpus lu-

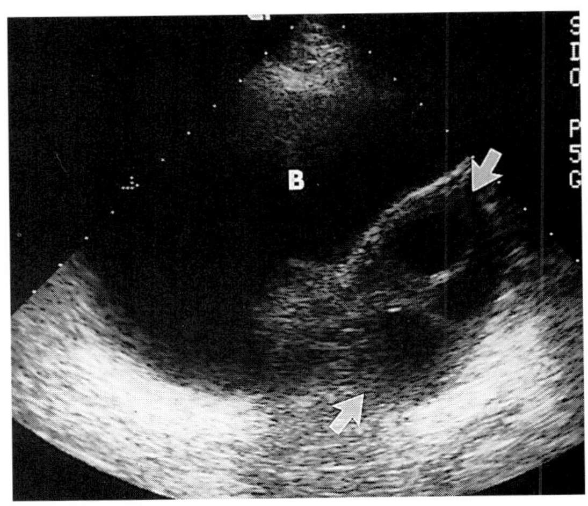

FIGURE 16–31.
Transverse, transabdominal sonogram showing left adnexal luteal cysts (between arrows) during the ninth LMP week of a singleton pregnancy. The cysts resolved by the 16th week. Multiple cysts of this nature are more common in multiple gestations and trophoblastic disease (hydatidiform moles) and are called *theca-lutein* cysts. Single, simple cysts that are more common in singleton pregnancies are corpus luteum cysts. *B*, full maternal bladder. (LNMP = 9.6 weeks, AA = 9.1 LMP weeks, range = 0.8, n = 8, TD)

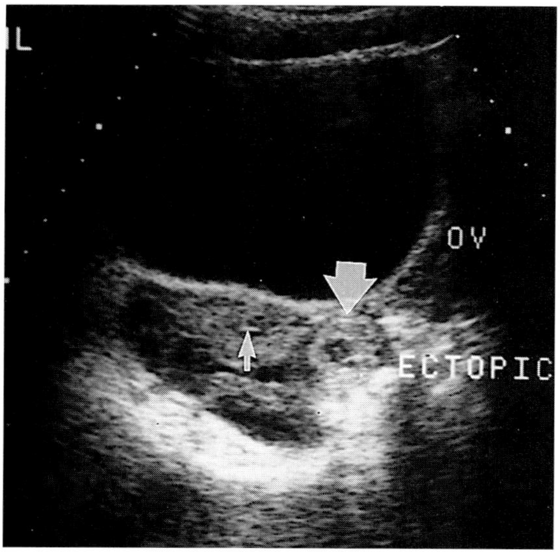

FIGURE 16–32.
Transverse, transabdominal sonogram of left ectopic pregnancy. A beating embryonic heart could be observed by real-time sonography at the center of the adnexal mass (large arrow) between the ovary (OV) and the uterus. The small arrow points to the endometrial/cervical canal. Notice the small quantity of fluid (blood) outlining the posterior margins of the uterus and mass (SH).

teum cyst may develop septa and is then referred to as a theca-lutein cyst. Theca-lutein cysts may become large and painful, occasionally larger than the uterus and rarely extending out of the pelvis to the level of the maternal kidneys. Septa may also develop in singleton pregnancies (see Fig. 16–31).

Other structures that are commonly observed in the adnexal region are the normal uterine and ovarian blood vessels, which dilate under the influence of the hormones of pregnancy. These masses of vessels should not be mistaken for cysts or vascular tumors. Doppler sonography can be useful for these distinctions. These vessels were discussed earlier (see Figs. 16–5 to 16–9).

Maternal Urinary Bladder and Vagina

When the full-bladder technique is used with transabdominal sonography, very clear views of the maternal bladder and vagina may be obtained. A sonographer occasionally finds abnormalities in the maternal bladder, such as bladder wall masses or ureteroceles. Figure 16–33 shows views of a normal, full maternal bladder at 10.8 LMP weeks of pregnancy.

The maternal urethra can normally be imaged suprapubically by angling the transducer caudally. The urethra is a muscular sphincter that forms a slight bulge in the inferior bladder wall anterior to the vagina (see Fig. 16–24). It should not be mistaken for a bladder tumor or other pathological process.[123,124] The trigone is a triangular area on the floor of the bladder; the urethra is at the apex of the inverted triangle, and the two ureteral orifices are at the base angles of the triangle.[125] The trigone thickens slightly under the influence of the hormones of pregnancy. The location and function of the adult ureteral orifices may be investigated by the use of color Doppler sonography to observe ureteral jets into the bladder.[126] Sonographers should remain observant of the entire image and not just focus on a single area of interest. Later in pregnancy, the fetal parts may press down and obscure this anatomy.

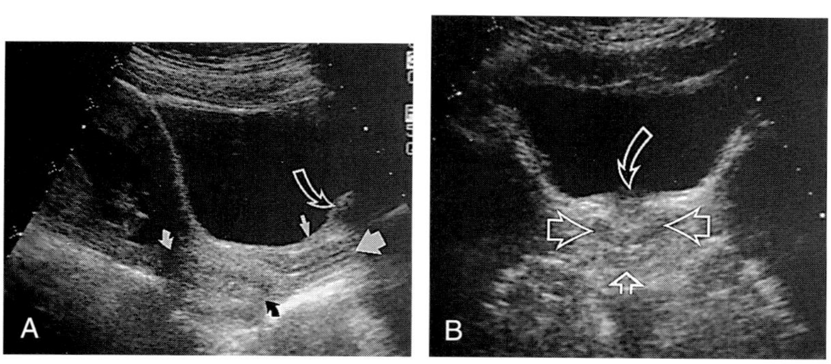

FIGURE 16–33.
A, Sagittal, transabdominal sonogram using the full-bladder technique to show maternal anatomy. Black curved arrow, cervix external os; white curved arrow, internal os; large white arrow, vaginal stripe; curved open arrow, internal urethra; small arrow, trigone. *B*, Transverse during same examination. Transverse of maternal urethra (curved open arrow). The vagina is between the large open arrows, and the rectum (small open arrow) is below the vagina. (LNMP = 12.4 weeks, AA = 10.8 LMP weeks, range = 1.4 weeks, n = 11, TD)

REFERENCES

1. Markee JE: Rhythmic uterine vascular changes. Am J Physiol 1932;100:32.
2. Markee JE: Menstruation in intra-ocular endometrial transplants in the rhesus monkey. Embryology 1940;28:221.
3. Resnik R: Anatomic alterations in the reproductive tract. In: Creasy RK, Resnik R, eds: Maternal-Fetal Medicine: Principles and Practice, 2nd ed, WB Saunders, Philadelphia, 1989, pp 137–140.
4. Waldrop L, Liu JB: Sonographic anatomy of the female pelvis. In: Berman MC, ed: Diagnostic Medical Sonography, vol 1: Obstetrics and Gynecology. JB Lippincott, Philadelphia, 1991, pp 46–48.
5. Cunningham FG, Mac Donald PC, Gant NF, eds: Williams Obstetrics, 18th ed. Appleton & Lange, Norwalk, CT, 1989, p 26.
6. DuBose TJ, Hill LW, Cunyus JA, et al: Sonography of menstrual changes in arcuate uterine blood vessel diameters. J Cardiovasc Ultrasonogr 1985;4: 243–251.
7. Sabbagha RE, Minogue JP: Altered fetal growth. In: Sabbagha RE, ed: Diagnostic Ultrasound: Applied to Obstetrics and Gynecology, 3rd ed. JB Lippincott, Philadelphia, 1994, p 197.
8. Moore KL, Persaud TVN: The Developing Human: Clinically Oriented Embryology. WB Saunders, Philadelphia, 1993, p 14–38.
9. Goldstein SR: Fertilization and Embryology. In: Berman MC, ed: Diagnostic Medical Sonography, vol 1: Obstetrics and Gynecology. JB Lippincott, Philadelphia, 1991, pp 195–198.
10. Cunningham FG, MacDonald PC, Gant NF, eds: Williams Obstetrics, 18th ed. Appleton & Lange, Norwalk, CT, 1989, p 27.
11. Malini S, Smith O, Goldzieher JW: Measurement of breast volume by ultrasound during normal menstrual cycles and with oral contraceptive use. Obstet Gynecol 1985;66:538–541.
12. Moore KL, Persaud TVN: The Developing Human: Clinically Oriented Embryology, WB Saunders, Philadelphia, 1993, p 269.
13. Anthony CP, Thibodeau GA: Textbook of Anatomy and Physiology. CV Mosby, St Louis, 1979, pp 622–624.
14. DuBose TJ, Hill LW, Hennigan HW: Sonography of arcuate uterine blood vessels. J Ultrasound Med 1985;4:229–233.
15. Hall DA, Yoder IC: Ultrasound evaluation of the uterus. In: Callen PW, ed: Ultrasonography in Obstetrics and Gynecology, 3rd ed. WB Saunders, Philadelphia, 1993, p 590.
16. Speroff L, Glass RH, Kase NG: Clinical Gynecologic Endocrinology and Infertility, 3rd ed. Williams & Wilkins, Baltimore, 1983, pp 231–232, 285–287.
17. Resnik R: The endocrine regulation of uterine blood flow in the nonpregnant uterus: A review. Am J Obstet Gynecol 1981;140:151–156.
18. Campbell S, Diaz-Recasens J, Griffin DR, et al: New Doppler technique for assessing uteroplacental blood flow. Lancet 1983; 675–677.
19. Griffen D, Choen-Overbeek T, Campbell S: Fetal and utero-placental blood flow. Clin Obstet Gynecol 1983;10:574.
20. Greiss FC, Anderson SG: Uterine vascular changes during the ovarian cycle. Am J Obstet Gynecol 1969;103:629.
21. Nyberg DA, Hill LM, Bohm-Velez M, et al: Transvaginal Ultrasound. Mosby/Year Book, St Louis, 1992, p 1.
22. Spirt BA, Kagan EH, Rozanski RM: Sonographic anatomy of the normal placenta. J Clin Ultrasound 1979;7:204–207.
23. Callen PW, Filly RA: The placental-subplacental complex: A specific indicator of placental position on ultrasound. J Clin Ultrasound 1980;8:21–26.
24. McGahan JP, Phillips HE, Reid MH: The anechoic retroplacental clear area: A pitfall in diagnosis of placental-endometrial abnormalities during pregnancy. Radiology 1980;134:475.
25. Smith DF, Foley WD: Real-time ultrasound and pulsed doppler evaluation of the retroplacental clear area. J Clin Ultrasound 1982;10:215–219.
26. van Zalen-Sprock MM, van Vugt JMG, Colenbrander GJ, et al: First-trimester uteroplacental and fetal blood flow velocity waveforms in normally developing fetuses: A longitudinal study. Ultrasound Obstet Gynecol 1994;4:284–288.
27. Grannum P, Berkowitz RL, Hobbins JC: The ultrasonic changes in the maturing placenta and their relation to fetal pulmonic maturity. Am J Obstet Gynecol 1979;133:915.
28. Kazzi GM, Evans MI, Sokol RJ, et al: Placental maturation and thickness. In: Sabbagha RE, ed: Diagnostic Ultrasound: Applied to Obstetrics and Gynecology, 3rd ed. JB Lippincott, Philadelphia, 1994, pp 290–297.
29. Kazzi GM, Gross TL, Sokol RJ, et al: Noninvasive prediction of hyaline membrane disease: An optimized classification of sonographic placenta maturation. Am J Obstet Gynecol 1985;152:213.
30. Chase LM, Cayea PD: The placenta and umbilical cord. In: Berman MC, ed: Diagnostic Medical Sonography, vol 1: Obstetrics and Gynecology, JB Lippincott, Philadelphia, 1991, pp 304–305.
31. Kazzi GM, Evans MI, Sokol RJ, et al: Placental maturation and thickness. In: Sabbagha RE, ed: Diagnostic Ultrasound: Applied to Obstetrics and Gynecology, 3rd ed. JB Lippincott, Philadelphia, 1994, p 294.
32. Hills D, Irwin GAL, Tuck S, et al: Distribution of placental grade in high-risk gravidas. AJR 1984; 143:1011.
33. Patterson RM, Hayashi RH, Cavazos D; Ultrasonographically observed early placental mtauration and perinatal outcome. Am J Obstet Gynecol 1983; 147:773.
34. Benson CB, Warneke LA: Sonographic appearance of milestones of pregnancy. In: Berman MC, ed: Diagnostic Medical Sonography, vol 1: Obstetrics and Gynecology. JB Lippincott, Philadelphia, 1991, pp 212–216.
35. Chase LM, Cayea PD: The placenta and umbilical cord. In: Berman MC, ed: Diagnostic Medical Sonography, vol 1: Obstetrics and Gynecology. JB Lippincott, Philadelphia, 1991, p 317.
36. Mintz MC, Kurtz AB, Arenson R, et al: Abrupto placentae: Apparent thickening of the placenta caused by hyperechoic retroplacental clot. J Ultrasound Med 1986;5:411–413.
37. Townsend RR: Ultrasound evaluation of the placenta and umbilical cord. In: Callen PW. ed: Ultrasonography in Obstetrics and Gynecology, 3rd ed. WB Saunders, Philadelphia, 1993, pp 453–455.
38. Hill LM: Placental maturation and thickness. In: Sabbagha RE, ed: Diagnostic Ultrasound: Applied to Obstetrics and Gynecology, 3rd ed. JB Lippincott, Philadelphia, 1994, p 304.
39. Hill LM: Placental maturation and thickness. In: Sabbagha RE, ed: Diagnostic Ultrasound: Applied to Obstetrics and Gynecology, 3rd ed. JB Lippincott, Philadelphia, 1994, pp 299–307.

40. Hill LM: Placental maturation and thickness. In: Sabbagha RE, ed: Diagnostic Ultrasound: Applied to Obstetrics and Gynecology, 3rd ed. JB Lippincott, Philadelphia, 1994, pp 308–310.
41. Tabsh KMA, Brinkman CR, King W: Ultrasound diagnosis of placenta increta. J Clin Ultrasound 1982; 10:288–290.
42. Pasto ME, Kurtz AB, Rifkin MD, et al: Ultrasonographic findings in placenta increta. J Ultrasound Med 1983;2:155–159.
43. Finberg HJ, Williams JW: Placenta accreta: Prospective sonographic diagnosis in patients with placenta previa and prior cesarean section. J Ultrasound Med 1992;11:333–343.
44. Guy GP, Peisner DB, Timor-Tritsch IE: Ultrasonographic evaluation of uteroplacental blood flow patterns of abnormally located and adherent placentas. Am J Obstet Gynecol 1990;163:723.
45. Hoffman-Tretin JC, Koenigsberg M, Rabin A, et al: Placenta accreta: Additional sonographic observations. J Ultrasound Med 1992;11:29–34.
46. Finberg HJ: The placenta and umbilical cord: Recent observations. Lecture and SDMS Official Proceedings: 10th Annual SDMS Conference, Anaheim, CA, Sept 16–19, 1993, pp 243–244.
47. Hoddick WK, Mahony BS, Callen PW, et al: Placental thickness. J Ultrasound Med 1985;4:479–482.
48. Williamson MR, Williamson SL: Gamuts in Ultrasound. WB Saunders, Philadelphia, 1992, p 175.
49. Scholl JS: Placenta position: Abdominal approach. In: Sabbagha RE, ed: Diagnostic ultrasound: Applied to Obstetrics and Gynecology, 3rd ed. JB Lippincott, Philadelphia, 1994, pp 271–279.
50. Townsend RR: Ultrasound evaluation of the placenta and umbilical cord. In: Callen PW, ed: Ultrasonography in Obstetrics and Gynecology, 3rd ed. WB Saunders, Philadelphia, 1993, p 447.
51. King DL: Placental migration demonstrated by ultrasonography. Radiology 1973;109:163.
52. Finberg HJ: The placenta and umbilical cord: Recent observations. Lecture and SDMS Official Proceedings: 10th Annual SDMS Conference, Anaheim, CA, Sept 16–19, 1993, p 241.
53. Thomas CL, ed: Taber's Cyclopedic Medical Dictionary, 16th ed. FA Davis, Philadelphia, 1989, p 1913.
54. Drose JA, Dennis MA: Multiple gestations. In: Berman MC, ed: Diagnostic Medical Sonography, Vol 1: Obstetrics and Gynecology. JB Lippincott, Philadelphia, 1991, p 508.
55. Finberg HJ: The "twin peak sign"—reliable evidence of dichorionic twinning. Official Proceedings, AIUM 36th Annual Convention, San Diego, 1992. J Ultrasound Med 1992;11:S53.
56. Cunningham FG, Mac Donald PC, Gant NF, eds: Williams Obstetrics, 18th ed. Appleton & Lange, Norwalk, CT, 1989, p 64.
57. Jeanty P: Persistent right umbilical vein: An ominous prenatal finding? Radiology 1990;177:735–738.
58. Resnik R: Anatomic alterations in the reproductive tract. In: Creasy RK, Resnik R, eds: Maternal-Fetal Medicine: Principles and Practice, 2nd ed. WB Saunders, Philadelphia, 1989, p 120.
59. Chinn DH, Filly RA, Callen PW: Ultrasonic evaluation of fetal umbilical and hepatic vascular anatomy. Radiology 1982;144:153–157.
60. Casola G, Scheible W, Leopold GR: Large umbilical cord: A normal finding in some fetuses. Radiology 1985;156:181–182.
61. Sachs L, Fourcroy JL, Wenzel DJ, et al: Prenatal detection of umbilical cord allantoic cysts. Radiology 1982;154:445–446.
62. Williamson MR, Williamson SL: Gamuts in Ultrasound. WB Saunders, Philadelphia, 1992, p 173.
63. Townsend RR: Ultrasound evaluation of the placenta and umbilical cord. In: Callen PW, ed: Ultrasonography in Obstetrics and Gynecology, 3rd ed. WB Saunders, Philadelphia, 1993, pp 458–463.
64. Sherer DM, Eggers PC, Smith SA, et al: Fetal sucking of the umbilical cord. J Ultrasound Med 1991;10:300.
65. Finberg HJ: The placenta and umbilical cord: Recent observations. Lecture and SDMS Official Proceedings: 10th Annual SDMS Conference, Anaheim, CA, Sept 16–19, 1993, p 246.
66. Finberg HJ: Avoiding ambiguity in the sonographic determination of the direction of umbilical cord twists. J Ultrasound Med 1992;11:185–187.
67. Lacro RV, Jones KL, Benirschke K: The umbilical cord twist: Origin, direction and relevance. Am J Obstet Gynecol 1987;157:833.
68. Fleischer A, Schulman H, Farmakides G, et al: Umbilical artery velocity waveforms and intrauterine growth retardation. Am J Obstet Gynecol 1985; 151:502.
69. Roechelson BL, Schulman H, Fleisher A, et al: The clinical significance of Doppler umbilical artery velocimetry in the small for gestational age fetus. Am J Obstet Gynecol 1987;156:1223.
70. Arduini D, Rizzo G, Romanini C, et al: Fetal blood velocity waveforms as predictors of growth retardation. Obstet Gynecol 1987;70:7.
71. Gudmundsson S, Marsal K: Umbilical and uteroplacental blood flow velocity waveforms in pregnancies with fetal growth retardation. Eur J Obstet Gynecol Reprod Biol 1988;27:187.
72. Brar HS, Medearis AL, DeVore GR, et al: Fetal umbilical velocimetry using continuous wave and pulsed wave Doppler ultrasound in high risk pregnancies: Comparison of systolic and diastolic ratios. Obstet Gynecol 1988;72:607.
73. Yoon BH, Syn HC, Kim SW: The efficacy of Doppler umbilical artery velocimetry in identifying fetal acidosis: A comparison with fetal biophysical profile. J Ultrasound Med 1992;11:1–6.
74. Locci M, Nazzaro G, DePlacido G, et al: Correlation of Doppler and placental immunohistochemical features in normal and intrauterine growth-retarded fetuses. Ultrasound Obstet Gynecol 1993;3:240–245.
75. Bruinse HW, Sijmons EA, Reuwer PJHM: Clinical value of screening for fetal growth retardation by Doppler ultrasound. J Ultrasound Med 1989;8: 207–209.
76. Stuart IP, Lindow SW, and van der Elst CW: Fetal acidosis and Doppler velocimetry of the umbilical arteries in labor. Ultrasound Obstet Gynecol 1993; 3:256–259.
77. Brace RA: Amniotic fluid dynamics. In: Creasy RK, Resnik R, eds: Maternal-Fetal Medicine: Principles and Practice, 2nd ed. WB Saunders, Philadelphia, 1989, pp 129–133.
78. Planiol T, Pourcelot L, Pottier JM, et al: Etude de la circulatin carotidienne par les methodes ultrasoniques et al thermographie. Rev Neurol (Paris) 1972;126:127–141.
79. Manning FA: Dynamic ultrasound-based fetal assessment: The fetal biophysical profile score. In: Fleischer AC, Romero R, Manning FA, et al, eds: Ultrasound in Obstetrics and Gynecology, 4th ed. Appleton & Lange, 1991, pp 417–428.
80. Johnson JAM: Fetal biophysical profile scoring. In:

Rumack CM, Wilson SR, Carboneau JW: Diagnostic Ultrasound, vol 2. Mosby/Year Book, St Louis, 1991, pp 379–744.
81. Kay HH, Carroll BB, Dahmus D, et al: Sonographic measurements with umbilical and uterine artery Doppler analysis in suspected intrauterine growth retardation. J Reprod Med 1991;36:65–68.
82. Divon MY, Guidette DA, Braverman JJ, et al: Intrauterine growth retardation—a prospective study of the diagnostic value of real-time sonography combined with umbilical artery flow velocimetry. Obstet Gynecol 1988;72:611–614.
83. Wenstrom KD, Weiner CP, Williamson RA: Diverse maternal and fetal pathology associated with absent diastolic flow in the umbilical artery of high-risk fetuses. Obstet Gynecol 1991;77:374–378.
84. Rochelson BL, Schulman H, Fleischer A, et al: The clinical significance of Doppler umbilical artery velocimetry in the small for gestational age fetus. Am J Obstet Gynecol 1987;156:1223–1226.
85. Arduini D, Rizzo G: Fetal renal artery velocity waveforms and amniotic fluid volume in growth-retarded and post-term fetuses. Obstet Gynecol 1991;77:370–373.
86. Wladimiroff JW, Huisman TWA, Stewart PA: Intracerebral, aortic and umbilical artery flow velocity waveforms in the late-first-trimester fetus. Am J Obstet Gynecol 1992;166:46–49.
87. Guzman ER, Schulman H, Karmel B, et al: Umbilical artery Doppler velocimetry in pregnancies of less than 21 weeks' duration. J Ultrasound Med 1990; 9:655–659.
88. Gerson AG, Wallace DM, Stiller RJ, et al: Doppler evaluation of umbilical venous and arterial blood flow in the second and third trimesters of normal pregnancy. Obstet Gynecol 1987;70:622–626.
89. Stuart B, Drumm J, FitzGerald DE, et al: Fetal blood velocity waveforms in normal pregnancy. Br J Obstet Gynaecol 1980;87:780–785.
90. Schulman H, Fleischer A, Stern W, et al: Umbilical velocity wave ratios in human pregnancy. Am J Obstet Gynecol 1984;148:985–990.
91. Cleveland WS: The Elements of Graphing Data. Wadsworth Advanced Books and Software, Monterey, CA, 1985, pp 167–178.
92. DeVore GR, Medearis AL, Platt LD: The effect of altitude on the umbilical artery Doppler resistance. J Ultrasound Med 1992;11:317–320.
93. Kay HH, Carroll BA, Bowie JD, et al: Nonuniformity of fetal umbilical systolic/diastolic ratios as determined with duplex Doppler sonography. J Ultrasound Med 1989;8:417–420.
94. Trudinger BJ, Warwick BG, Cook CM: Uteroplacental blood flow velocity-time waveforms in normal and complicated pregnancy. Br J Obstet Gynaecol 1985;92:39–45.
95. Degani S, Paltieli Y, Gonen R, et al: Fetal internal carotid artery pulsed Doppler flow velocity waveforms and maternal plasma glucose levels. Obstet Gynecol 1991;77:379–381.
96. Tulzer G, Gudmundsson S, Wood DC, et al: Doppler in non-immune hydrops fetalis. Ultrasound Obstet Gynecol 1994;4:249–283.
97. Indik JH, Chen V, Reed KL: Association of umbilical venous and inferior vena cava blood flow velocities. Obstet Gynecol 1991;77:551–557.
98. Reed KL: Opinion: The role of venous Doppler in fetuses with non-immune hydrops. Ultrasound Obstet Gynecol 1994;4:268–269.
99. Bromley B, Harlow BL, Laboda LA, et al: Small sac size in the first trimester: A predictor of poor fetal outcome. Radiology 1991;178:375–377.
100. Drose JA, Dennis MA, Thickman D: Infection in utero: Sonographic findings in 19 cases. Radiology 1991;178:369–374.
101. Williamson MR, Williamson SL: Gamuts in Ultrasound. WB Saunders, Philadelphia, 1992, pp 165–168.
102. Yeh HC, Rabinowitz JG: Amniotic sac development: Ultrasound features of early pregnancy—the double bleb sign. Radiology 1988;166:97.
103. Benirschke K: Normal development. In: Creasy RK, Resnik R, eds: Maternal-Fetal Medicine: Principles and Practice, 2nd ed. WB Saunders, Philadelphia, 1989, p 117.
104. Filly RA: Ultrasound evaluation during the first trimester. In: Callen PW, ed: Ultrasound in Obstetrics and Gynecology, 3rd ed. WB Saunders, Philadelphia, 1993, p. 71.
105. Nyberg DA, Mack LA, Laing FC, et al: Distinguishing normal from abnormal gestation sac growth in early pregnancy. J Ultrasound Med 1987;6:23–27.
106. Nazari A, Check JH, Epstein RH, et al: Relationship of small-for-dates sac size to crown-rump length and spontaneous abortion in patients with a known date of ovulation. Obstet Gynecol 1991; 78:369–373.
107. Schats R, Jansen CAM, Wladimiroff JW: Embryonic heart activity: Appearance and development in early human pregnancy. Br J Obstet Gynaecol 1990;97:989–994.
108. Brace RA: Amniotic fluid dynamics. In: Creasy RK, Resnik R, eds: Maternal-Fetal Medicine: Principles and Practice, 2nd ed. WB Saunders, Philadelphia, 1989, p 129.
109. Brace RA: Amniotic fluid dynamics. In: Creasy RK, Resnik R, eds: Maternal-Fetal Medicine: Principles and Practice, 2nd ed. WB Saunders, Philadelphia, 1989, pp 128–135.
110. Benson CB, Warneke LA: Sonographic appearance of milestones of pregnancy. In: Berman MC, ed: Diagnostic Medical Sonography, Vol 1: Obstetrics and Gynecology. JB Lippincott, Philadelphia, 1991, pp 210–211.
111. Phelan JP, Ahn MO, Smith CV, et al: Amniotic fluid index measurements during pregnancy. J Reprod Med 1987;32:601–604.
112. Gohari P, Berkowitz RI, Hobbins JC: Prediction of intrauterine retardation by determination of total intrauterine volume. Am J Obstet Gynecol 1977; 127:255–260.
113. Kurtz AB, Goldberg BB: Obstetrical Measurements in Ultrasound. Year Book Medical Publishers, Chicago, 1988, pp 181–192.
114. Geirsson RT, Ogston SA, Patel NB, et al: Growth of total intrauterine, intra-amniotic and placental volume in normal singleton pregnancy measured by ultrasound. Br J Obstet Gynaecol 1985;92:46–53.
115. Goldstein RB, Filly RA: Sonographic estimation of amniotic fluid volume: Subjective assessment versus pocket measurement. J Ultrasound Med 1988;7: 363–369.
116. Manning FA, Hill LM, Platt LD: Qualitative amniotic fluid volume determination by ultrasound: Antepartum detection of intrauterine growth retardation. Am J Obstet Gynecol 1981;139:254–258.
117. Magann EF, Nolan TE, Hess LW, et al: Measurement of amniotic fluid volume: Accuracy of ultrasonography techniques. Am J Obstet Gynecol 1992;167: 1533–1537.

118. Ross MG: Amniotic fluid volume determination (letter). Am J Obstet Gynecol 1993;169:435–436.
119. Magan EF: Reply: Amniotic fluid volume determination (letter). Am J Obstet Gynecol 1993;169:435–437.
120. Rutherford SE, Smith CV, Phelan JP, et al: Four-quadrant assessment of amniotic fluid volume. J Reprod Med 1987;32:587–589.
121. Sepulveda W, Flack NJ, Fisk NM: Direct volume measurement at midtrimester amnioinfusion in relation to ultrasonographic indexes of amniotic fluid volume. Am J Obstet Gynecol 1994;170:1160–1163.
122. Jeanty P, Laucirica R, Luna SK: Extra-amniotic pregnancy: A trip to the extraembryonic coelom. J Ultrasound Med 1990;9:733–736.
123. Hennigan HW, DuBose TJ: Sonography of the normal female urethra. AJR 1985;145:839–841.
124. de Gonzales EL, Cosgrove DO, Joseph AE, et al: The appearances on ultrasound of the female urethral sphincter. Br J Radiol 1988;61:687–690.
125. Anthony CP, Thibodeau GA: Textbook of Anatomy and Physiology. CV Mosby, St Louis, 1979, p 557.
126. Garza RR, DuBose TJ, Hill L, et al: Evaluating ureteral jets with color Doppler in adults. J Diagn Med Sonogr 1991;7:198–200.

CHAPTER 17

BIOPHYSICAL PROFILE

Terry J. DuBose

A woman's perception of fetal movement or "quickening" has historically been considered a milestone of pregnancy.[1] Quickening usually occurs between the 16th and 20th weeks after the start of the last menstrual period (16 to 20 LMP weeks). Fetal movements increase in both frequency and intensity from quickening to a peak of activity between the 29th and 38th LMP weeks. Reduced activity, delayed quickening, and movement localized in one area of a woman's abdomen raise questions about fetal defects of the nervous system or extremities.[2] Persistence of complete absence of fetal motion in the latter half of pregnancy is, of course, an ominous sign.

For these reasons, observations of fetal activity have always been of interest to sonographers. Among the earliest and most extensive sonographic research of fetal movement was that conducted by Manning, Platt, and associates.[3-11] Their work was based on the same logic as the evaluation of multiple vital signs in an adult or assessment of a neonate by Apgar score. In the 1970s, it was recognized that accelerations of the fetal heart rate (FHR) with fetal movement (nonstress test [NST]) and the absence of FHR variation with uterine contraction stress test or in labor were important indicators of fetal well-being or of distress and asphyxia[6] (see Chapter 12 for additional discussion of FHR variability).

Manning and colleagues used five variables in their design of the biophysical profile (BPP) score. These five biophysical variables were fetal breathing movements (FBMs), fetal movements, fetal tone (FT), qualitative amniotic fluid volume, and the NST. Each variable was scored as a meristic or discrete variable arbitrarily having only one of two scores, 0 or 2. Therefore, if a variable is observed to be normal or reactive, it receives a score of 2. If the variable is not observed, it receives a score of 0 and is considered nonreactive. This method gives a normal fetus a score of a perfect 10; a score of 6 was considered equivocal, and 4 or less was abnormal. This initial BPP design was later modified slightly to a form similar to that in Table 17–1. The variables that are generally associated with acute asphyxia are the loss of FBM, FT, fetal movements, and heart rate variability (NST). Chronic asphyxia is indicated by oligohydramnios because the body has a natural priority, in hypoxic conditions, to shunt more blood to the fetal brain (also to the heart, adrenals, and placenta), thus reducing blood flow to the rest of the body.[12, 13] This reduced blood flow to the body results in impaired kidney function, which in turn reduces the urine contribution to the amniotic fluid.

It has been suggested that having a woman take sugar in some form before the BPP might

TABLE 17–1. **BIOPHYSICAL PROFILE***

BIOPHYSICAL VARIABLES	NORMAL SCORE = 2	ABNORMAL SCORE = 0	SCORES
Fetal breathing movements (FBMs)	At least one episode of FBM lasting at least 30 sec in 30 min	No fetal breathing motions or FBMs 30 < sec in 30 min	
Fetal movements (FMs): gross body movements	Three or more discrete FMs within 30 min	Fewer than three FMs in 30 min	
Fetal tone (FT): opening and closing hand, limb extension and flexion	One or more FT movements in 30 min	Absent or reduced FT movements	
Fetal heart rate: nonstress test (NST)	Two or more accelerations and decelerations > 15 B/M in 30 min	Fewer than two accelerations and decelerations in 30 min	
Amniotic fluid index (AFI): Sum of four quadrants =	AFI > 5.0 cm ________	AFI < 5.0 cm Sum of scores =	________

*Use this table to score the BPP.
Adapted from Manning FA, Morrison I, Lange IR, et al: Fetal assessment based on fetal biophysical profile scoring: Experience in 12,620 referred high-risk pregnancies. Am J Obstet Gynecol 1985;151:342–350.

shorten the examination time and give her fetus a better chance of getting a good score.[14–16] This is because fetal activities have been found to increase during glucose tolerance tests. I have noticed that fetal activity seems to increase approximately 1 to 2 hours after a woman has eaten. Although I have not tested this observation, it does make sense that if a fetus is more active after maternal glucose intake, then BPP observations of fetal activity would be shortened after a meal containing any sugar. Despite the apparent logic of this, one of the prime researchers of the BPP states that "Feeding a patient prior to an ultrasound examination will not increase the chance of observing fetal movements."[17] Perhaps more research into maternal diet, fetal activity, and the BPP is warranted. The converse of this diet-induced stimulation, maternal use of depressant drugs, reduces fetal biophysical activity.[12]

Another question is when should the BPP be performed (Table 17–2). Some physicians have requested the BPP as early as 25 LMP weeks.[16] With modern medicine, a fetus may be viable at 25 weeks. It must be recognized, however, that a fetus before 33 weeks is more likely to have an equivocal or nonreactive score because of abnormal fetal breathing, and such a score might lead to premature delivery of an otherwise normal fetus. For this reason, the BPP should be interpreted as a function of fetal age.[18]

Mandatory reading for any who make decisions about high-risk pregnancy management and the BPP is a report by Vintzileos and associates.[19] These investigators point out that the biophysical activities that develop earliest in gestation are the last to disappear with asphyxia.[19] They emphasize the importance of this order of priority for the interpretation of the BPP. For instance, before 30 LMP weeks, a fetus has very short sleep cycles and rarely produces a false-positive BPP. Later in gestation, however, sleep cycles become longer (40 to 60 minutes) and may well produce false positives in observation times as short as 30 minutes. This concept was confirmed by Devoe and associates using a large population and stepwise logistic regression.[20] This last study found that the best predictive model contained all the BPP variables except fetal movement. FT was 100% predictive for neurological abnormalities. As the number of abnormal BPP variables (0 to 5) increased, higher percentages of all abnormal outcomes

TABLE 17–2. **BIOPHYSICAL PROFILE INTERPRETATION AND MANAGEMENT***

SUM OF SCORES	INTERPRETATION	RECOMMENDED MANAGEMENT
10	Normal fetus, low risk for chronic asphyxia	Repeat as indicated weekly, or twice weekly, in diabetic or postterm pregnancies
8	Normal fetus, low risk for chronic asphyxia	Same as above; oligohydramnios is indication for delivery
6	Suspected chronic asphyxia	Repeat BPP in 24 hr. Oligohydramnios or BPP ≤ 6 is indication for delivery
4	Suspected chronic asphyxia	If < 36 wk and L/S ratio < 2.0, repeat BPP in 24 hr. Oligohydramnios or repeated BPP ≤ 6 is indication for delivery
0–2	Strong suspicion of chronic asphyxia	Extend testing time to 120 min. Indication for delivery = persistent BPP ≤ 4

*This is the suggested management protocol for various BPP scores according to Manning.
From Manning FA, Morrison I, Lange IR, et al: Fetal assessment based on fetal biophysical profile scoring: Experience in 12,620 referred high-risk pregnancies. Am J Obstet Gynecol 1985;151:343–350.

were predicted and a positive correlation was found with intrapartum and fetal death, low 5-minute Apgar scores, and acidosis. Devoe and colleagues also found a strong correlation between abnormalities and intrauterine growth retardation, because all cases with poor outcomes but without other abnormalities had birth weights less than the 10th percentile for age.[20] This point becomes important in the abbreviated BPP (discussed later).

Note that the two previous paragraphs contain an apparent contradiction. The first states that the BPP may be equivocal or nonreactive before 33 LMP weeks, whereas the second states that the BPP rarely produces false-positive scores before 30 LMP weeks. These statements are made by knowledgeable researchers, and I have not found references that can resolve this contradiction. Nevertheless, all researchers emphasize that the BPP score must be interpreted in view of the age of the fetus, sleep cycles and biorhythms, and the effects of disease, drugs, or other agents.

Other researchers have pointed out that different populations may have differences in the BPP variables that may lead to errors of interpretation.[21]

Because much of the BPP is relatively subjective, such as what constitutes true fetal movement versus true FT, some researchers have suggested modifications to the classical BPP described by Manning and colleagues. Basically, the modifications use more variables such as the placental grade and the resistive index of the umbilical artery, or the modifications establish a rank of importance for the variables. One important modification is an abbreviated, 5-minute profile. These modifications as well as other factors are addressed later, after the discussion of the classical BPP.

Biophysical Profile

NONSTRESS TEST

The NST is a measure of the beat-to-beat FHR in time. The FHR should vary in response to fetal body movements and pressure, either pressure of uterine contractions or other external pressure. A tocodynamometer, which estimates the force of uterine contractions, is used to monitor active labor. Pressure from the transducer during sonographic studies has been shown to induce intermittent fetal bradycardia.[22] Here a word of warning is in order. As Mimi Berman, Ph.D., RDMS, cautions (personal communication, 1991), "We do not need any 'Rambo' types pushing transducers." Although FHR variation is normal, excessive transducer pressure is not a necessary part of the test.

For a reactive NST result, a fetus should exhibit two or more FHR accelerations and decelerations of at least 15 beats/minute (B/M) during a period of 20 to 40 minutes of observation. These accelerations usually follow gross fetal body movements. The decelerations occur during fetal quiet times.

Heart Rate Monitoring

Strip Chart

A method of recording the FHR during the examination is needed to observe beat-to-beat accelerations and decelerations. The traditional way this is done is with a strip chart recorder that enables the observer to correlate uterine contractions (tocodynamometer) or fetal movements with changes in the FHR. This records both the FHR and uterine contraction forces as a change in amplitudes across time.[15] By marking on the strip chart when fetal activities are observed, one can later determine if normal FHR accelerations occurred after the movements. Because the FHR amplitude or beat-to-beat rate and time are recorded on the strip chart, it is simple to determine whether or not a fetus is reactive.

M-Mode

Although a tocodynamometer and fetal monitor may be common in labor and delivery suites, they may not be available in all sonographic suites. This equipment is most useful when a woman is in active labor. Because I have spent most of my time in radiographic laboratories, where such equipment was not available, my colleagues (EKP, DKD, and LP) and I developed the following method for performing BPPs.

At the start of the examination, a base line FHR is taken using M-mode. As a fetus is measured and observed for the BPP variables, the FHR is determined as soon as a fetal body movement is observed, as well as at other times. In this way, we are able to document variations in the FHR. Because there is no way to determine if the base line FHR was in acceleration or deceleration, it is compared with the later heart rates. For the result to be considered reactive requires that at least two changes in the FHR of at least 15 B/M occur during the 30-minute examination (some researchers allow 40-minute observations for reactivity, others only 20 minutes).[10,11,23] The changes can be increases or decreases, as long as they are at least 15 B/M.

The drawback of this M-mode technique is that the FHR may accelerate and decelerate between M-mode observations and may appear nonreactive. To compensate for this problem, M-mode FHR observations must be made fairly frequently, and the fetus continuously observed for movements. However, with experience, we have obtained good results.

BREATHING MOVEMENTS

FBM appears sonographically as a rhythmical movement of the chest, diaphragm, and abdomen. It appears just as one would expect, as if the fetus were breathing. This breathing motion normally has a mean breath-to-breath interval of approximately 1 second but may range from a rapid half second to a slower 2 seconds between "breaths."[24] FBM should occur for at least 30 seconds during a 30-minute observation time for a reactive score of 2 on the BPP.[18] Some researchers called for three episodes of FBM lasting at least 60 seconds within a 30-minute observation period for reactivity.[25] The 30-second episodes seem to be the prevailing criterion.

Some sonographers have sought a method of documenting FBM on hard-copy.[26] M-mode was suggested; however, FBM may be very subtle and difficult to show in all cases using M-mode. Another method that would produce dynamic results would be to use Doppler to visualize the rhythmic ebb and flow of the amniotic fluid in the fetal nasopharynx (see Fig. 13–33). Some reservations are still expressed about using Doppler in obstetrical sonography, and because the FBM episodes may last less than 1 minute, the time factor for adjusting the equipment for optimal Doppler may pose a problem. Fetal position often precludes Doppler documentation.

Because observations of FBM primarily fall within the purview of real-time sonography, it is suggested that visual confirmation of FBM is most efficient and accurate. Although some may question a nonphysician sonographer's visually documenting sonographic information without hard-copy, such is the nature of this modality. Sonographers and sonologists should have an honest, trusting relationship with open communications and the best interests of good health care at the center of their practice (see Chapter 6). In this way, if a sonographer sees FBM with real-time and states this to the physician, that should be all the documentation that is necessary. Although documentation of the examination on hard-copy is good practice and a necessary part of the standard of care, with real-time it may not always be practical or possible. Otherwise, videotaping every examination and maintaining voluminous files of the tapes for review is the only alternative, and an expensive alternative at that.

BODY MOVEMENTS

Gross fetal body movements are usually defined as three or more discrete extensions and flexions of the body or extremities within 30 minutes of observation. Simultaneous and continuous movements of the body and limbs are counted as a single movement.[10, 18, 25] Movement is considered to be more than just yawning- or breathing-type motions.[27]

FETAL TONE

FT was initially defined as full extension and flexion of the upper and lower extremities with return to the original position. The definition has been modified to include discrete hand movements.[12, 27] A reactive score requires at least one episode of extremity movement during the observation period. None of the references gives a time limit for the FT observations. Because most of the other BPP observations are expected within a 30-minute time limit, it is assumed that observation for that period of time is sufficient (see Chapter 15 for more discussion of normal limb and hand motion).

AMNIOTIC FLUID

BPP amniotic fluid volume was defined as "fluid evident throughout the uterine cavity; largest pocket of fluid greater than 1 cm in vertical diameter."[6] The estimate of volume was subsequently modified several times. I suggest use of the amniotic fluid index, which is the measurement of the vertical axis of the largest pocket of amniotic fluid in each of four quadrants of the maternal abdomen. The sum of these four measurements should be greater than 5 cm.[11, 29, 30]

Biophysical Profile Variations

MORE COMPLEX BIOPHYSICAL PROFILE

Vintzileos and colleagues add the placenta grades to the BPP because they have found that grade III (mature, inhomogeneous) placentas are associated with abnormal heart rate patterns and placenta abruption during labor.[19] They state, "The value of including placental grading is to alert the physician during the intrapartum period of the presence of a grade III placenta."

Another study that added to the BPP included two other variables, umbilical artery Doppler recording and abdominal circumference (AC) as an indicator of fetal growth.[31] This interesting study found that the order of deterioration was as follows: First the umbilical artery Doppler recording indicated increased resistance to perfusion or, worse, absent or reversed end-diastolic flow; second was reduced AC for age; last was an abnormal BPP score. The study noted that either an abnormal umbilical artery Doppler signal or a small AC alone was usually associated with a favorable prognosis; however, the worst outcomes were in the fetuses with an abnormality of all three.

ABBREVIATED BIOPHYSICAL PROFILE

Sim and colleagues have suggested that an abbreviated BPP could be performed in less than 5 minutes and is useful for screening studies.[32] They found that an AC below the 10th percentile for age and subjectively judged reduced aminotic fluid volumes identified 90% of small-for-gestational-age infants and five of six perinatal deaths in the study population (n = 662).

BIOPHYSICAL PROFILE RULE OF THUMB

I have found that if normal fetal activity is observed (breathing motions and extremity movements) during a normal obstetrical sonographic examination lasting 15 to 30 minutes, subsequent BPP scores are invariably normal. However, it must be noted that this rule of thumb has not been subjected to a controlled study but is based on 18 years' experience.

If oligohydramnios is noted or if the AC is less than −1 SD below the mean for size or approaches −2 SD, it may be wise to check the umbilical artery for increased resistance (reduced or reversed end-diastolic flow) using Doppler sonography. This is particularly true if the pregnancy is in the early to mid-second trimester because in cases of intrauterine growth rate the relative reduction in AC size is often progressive. If the AC is approaching −2 SD by midpregnancy, it may be below −2 SD by the third trimester (see Chapters 13 and 16 for discussion of the umbilical cord and Doppler and for a general discussion).

REFERENCES

1. Cunningham FG, MacDonald PC, Grant NF: Human pregnancy: Overview, organization, and diagnosis. In Williams Obstetrics, 18th ed. Appleton & Lange, Norwalk, CT, 1989, p 13.
2. Jones OW: Basic genetics and patterns of inheritance. In: Creasy RK, Resnik R, eds: Maternal-Fetal Medicine: Principles and Practice, 2nd ed. WB Saunders, Philadelphia, 1989, p 63.
3. Manning FH, Platt LD, LeMay M: Effect of amniocentesis on fetal breathing movements. British Med J 1972;2:1582–1583.
4. Manning FA, Platt LD: Maternal hypoxemia and fetal breathing movements. Clin Obstet Gynecol 1977; 53:758–760.
5. Manning FM, Platt LD: Fetal breathing movements: Antepartum monitoring of fetal condition. Clin Obstet Gynecol 1979;6:335–349.
6. Manning FA, Platt LD, Sipos L: Antepartum fetal evaluation: Development of fetal biophysical profile. Am J Obstet Gynecol 1980;136:787–795.
7. Manning FA, Baskett TF, Morrison I, et al: Fetal biophysical profile scoring: A prospective study in 1184 high-risk patients. Am J Obstet Gynecol 1981;140: 289–294.
8. Manning FA, Morrison MB, Harman CR, et al: Fetal assessment based on fetal biophysical profile scoring: Experience in 19221 referred high-risk pregnancies. Am J Obstet Gynecol 1987;157:880–884.
9. Manning FA, Platt LD, Sipos L, et al: Fetal breathing movements and the nonstress test in high-risk pregnancies. Am J Obstet Gynecol 1979;135:511–515.
10. Manning FA, Morrison I, Lange IR, et al: Fetal assessment based on fetal biophysical profile scoring: Experience in 12,620 referred high-risk pregnancies: 1. Perinatal mortality by frequency and etiology. Am J Obstet Gynecol 1985;151:343–350.
11. Walla CA, Platt LD: Observing fetal maturation through fetal movement and fetal breathing. In: Berman MC, ed: Diagnostic Medical Sonography: A Guide to Clinical Practice, Vol 1. JB Lippincott, Philadelphia, 1991, pp 445–457.
12. Manning FA: Dynamic ultrasound-based fetal assessment: The fetal biophysical profile score. In: Fleischer AC, Romero R, Manning FA, et al, eds: Ultrasound in Obstetrics and Gynecology, 4th ed. Appleton & Lange, Norwalk, CT, 1991, pp 417–428.
13. Johnson JAM: Fetal biophysical profile scoring. In: Rumack CM, Wilson SR, Carboneau JW, eds: Diagnostic Ultrasound, vol 2. Mosby/Year Book, St. Louis, 1991, pp 379–744.
14. Devoe LD, Searle N, Castillo RA, et al: Fetal biophysical testing: The effects of prolonged maternal fasting and the oral glucose tolerance test. J Reprod Med 1987;32:563–568.
15. Parer JT: Fetal heart rate. In: Creasy RK, Resnik R, eds: Maternal-Fetal Medicine: Principles and Practice, 2nd ed. WB Saunders, Philadelphia, 1989, p 339.
16. Craig M: Everything you need to know about biophysical profiles. J Diagn Med Sonogr 1989;5: 261–268.
17. Walla CA, Platt LD: Observing fetal maturation through fetal movement and fetal breathing. In: Berman MC, ed: Diagnostic Medical Sonography, vol 1: Obstetrics and Gynecology. JB Lippincott, Philadelphia, 1991, p 448.
18. Walla CA, Platt LD: Observing fetal maturation through fetal movement and fetal breathing. In: Berman MC, ed: Diagnostic Medical Sonography, vol 1: Obstetrics and Gynecology. JB Lippincott, Philadelphia, 1991, p 453.
19. Vintzileos AM, Campbell WA, Nichimson DJ, et al: The use and misuse of the fetal biophysical profile. Am J Obstet Gynecol 1987;156:527–533.
20. Devoe LD, Youssef AA, Gardner P, et al: Refining the biophysical profile with a risk-related evaluation of test performance. Am J Obstet Gynecol 1992;167: 346–352.
21. Johnson MJ, Paine LL, Mulder HH, et al: Population differences of fetal biophysical and behavioral characteristics. Am J Obstet Gynecol 1992;166:138–142.
22. Mendoza GJ, Almeida O, Steinfeld L: Intermittent fetal bradycardia induced by midpregnancy fetal ultrasonographic study. Am J Obstet Gynecol 1989;160: 1038–1040.

23. Manning FA, Morrison I, Lang IR, et al: Antepartum determination of fetal health: Composite biophysical profile scoring. Clin Perinatol 1982;9:285–295.
24. Patrick J, Gagnon R: Fetal breathing and body movement. In: Creasy RK, Resnik R, eds: Maternal-Fetal Medicine: Principles and Practice, 2nd ed. WB Saunders, Philadelphia, 1989, p 281.
25. Platt LD, Walla CA, Paul RH, et al: A prospective trial of the fetal biophysical profile versus the nonstress test in the management of high-risk pregnancies. Am J Obstet Gynecol 1985;153:624–633.
26. Kepple D: Personal telephone communications, Vanderbilt University, 1990.
27. Petrikovsky BM, Kaplan G: Assessment of fetal behavior. The Female Patient 1992;17:32–34.
28. Kurtz AB: The high risk obstetrical examination: Growth retardation and the biophysical profile, the leading edge in diagnostic ultrasound (lecture). Atlantic City, NJ, May 7–9, 1987.
29. Phelan JP, Ahn MO, Smith CV, et al: Amniotic fluid index measurements during pregnancy. J Reprod Med 1987; 32:601–604.
30. DalCompo S, Sabbagha RE: Intrauterine growth retardation. In: Berman MC, ed: Diagnostic Medical Sonography: A Guide to Clinical Practice, Vol 1. JB Lippincott, Philadelphia, 1991, pp 468–470.
31. James DK, Parker MJ, Smoleniec JS: Comprehensive fetal assessment with three ultrasonographic characteristics. Am J Obstet Gynecol 1992;166:1486–1495.
32. Sim D, Beattie RB, Dornan JC: Evaluation of biophysical fetal assessment in high-risk pregnancy to assess ultrasound parameters suitable for screening in the low-risk population. Ultrasound Obstet Gynecol 1993;3:11–17.

SECTION III

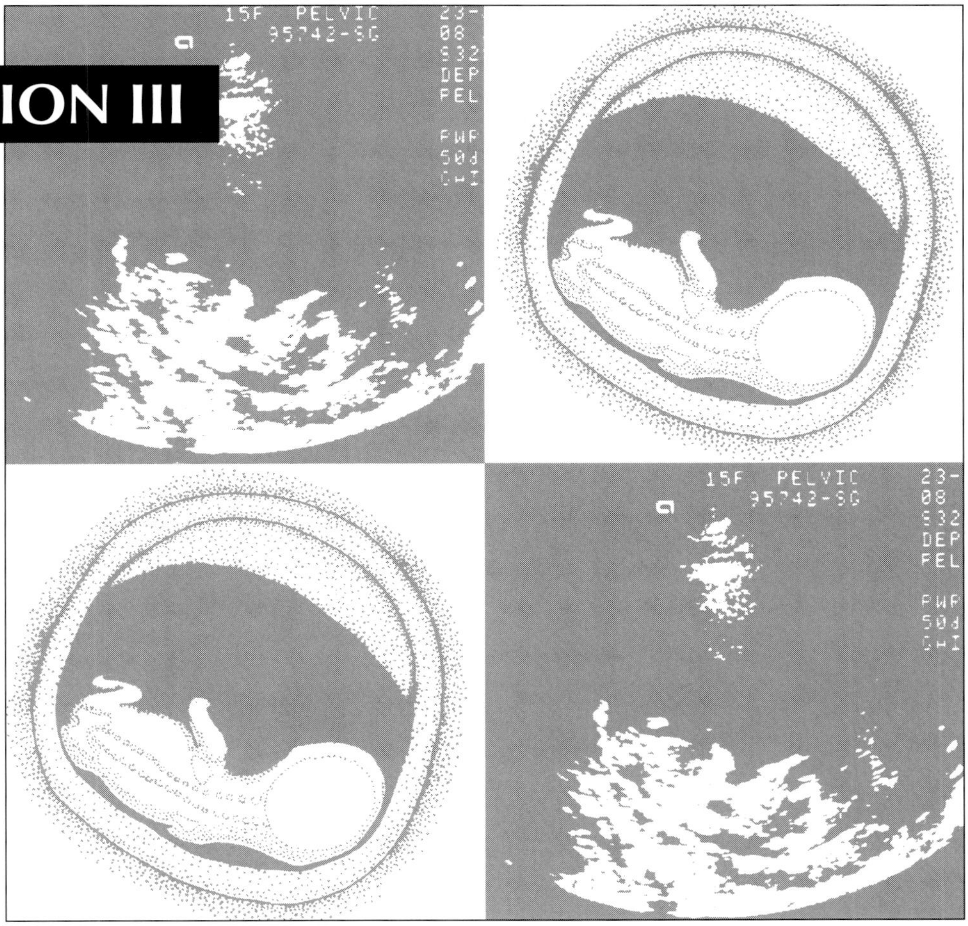

Fetal Sonography Throughout Pregnancy

CHAPTER 18

FIRST TRIMESTER

Terry J. DuBose

Because embryogensis occurs in the first trimester, any developmental problems during this period often result in spontaneous abortion. This trimester is also a period of rapid change as the fertilized egg develops into an embryo and the embryo becomes a fetus by the 10th last menstrual period (LMP) week. Figure 18–1 is a chart that correlates sonographic images and graphics to show the periods in which congenital anomalies occur.

To demonstrate the first trimester sonographically, this chapter uses representative examinations of normal pregnancies by week, starting with the fourth week after the LMP. These examinations were performed by registered diagnostic medical sonographers or students under supervision, and each examination was reviewed for diagnosis by a qualified sonologist. Each case includes representative sonographic images, some printed life-size.

Each week includes a computer screen of the various parameter size/ages and age range analysis (ARA). It is hoped that readers will in this way get some feel for the variability of fetal parameters at each stage of pregnancy. The sonographer who performed the examination and made the measurements is identified by initials in this computer screen. Figure 18–2*A* is a legend of the measurements used, and Figure 18–2*B* is a legend for the computer report screen that is used to estimate the fetal age. (For detailed discussion of each parameter, see the appropriate chapter, and see Chapter 7 for an explanation of the fetal parameter size/age and ARA method used here.)

Real-time sonography has become an integral part of modern obstetrical evaluations. Fetal motion is recognized as having relatively normal patterns. Activity is a reassuring sign of the well-being of the gestation. The biophysical profile requires observations of fetal motion as a part of its scoring system. A normal pregnancy lasts approximately 280 days from the start of the LMP. Historically, pregnancy has been thought of as divided into three equal parts. Each of the three divisions is 3 calendar months, or approximately 13 weeks.[1] This discussion follows this convention.

The advent of transvaginal or endovaginal transducers has opened a window on the earliest phases of human development that was not available just 10 years ago. This book uses transvaginal and endovaginal interchangeably to identify sonograms produced with this type of transducer. Until now, most understanding of embryonic development was based on animal models. It is now common knowledge that the embryo is much more active than most people believed. The fact that

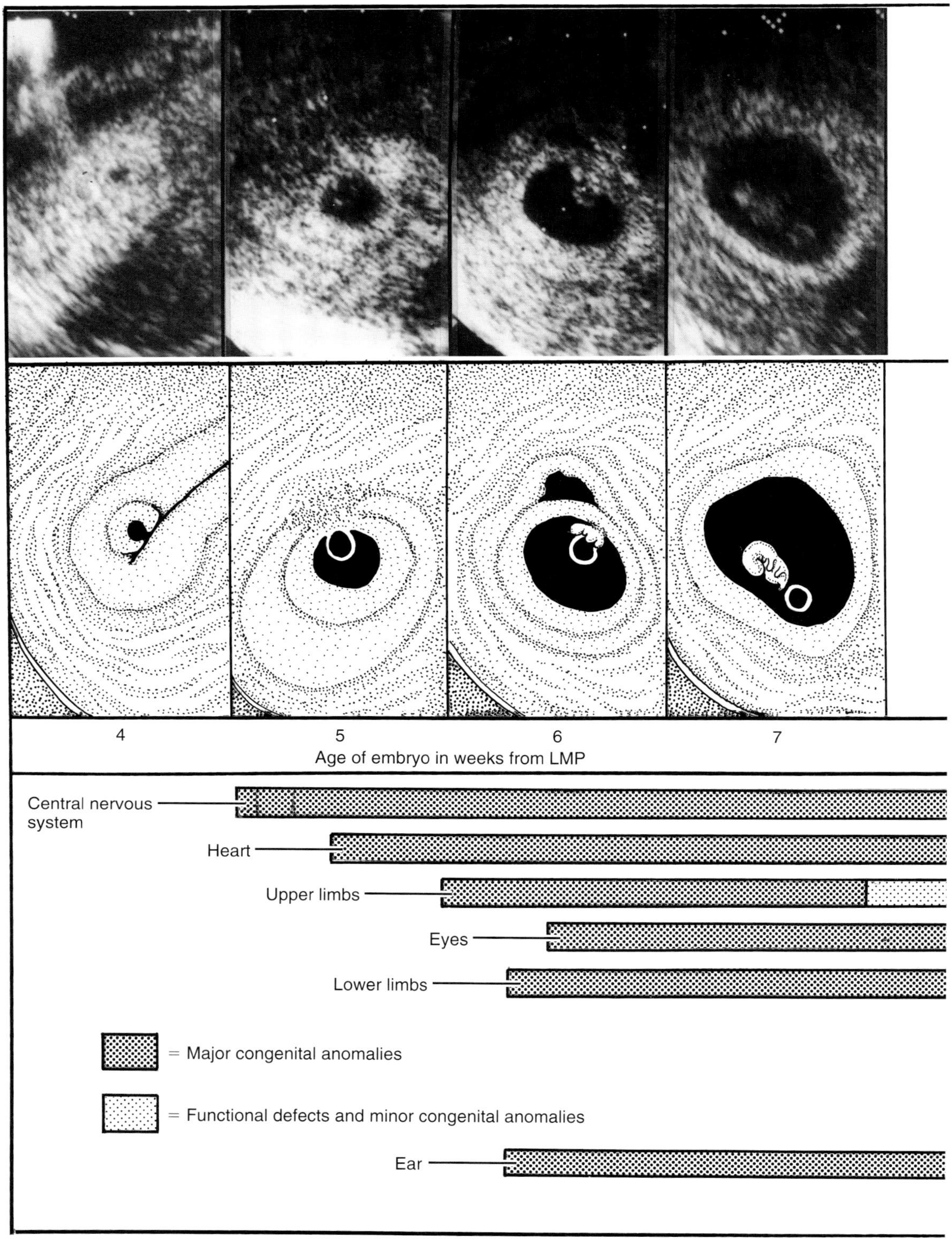

FIGURE 18–1.
This schematic illustrates the critical periods of development and compares the stages with the sonographic appearance. The critical period for the central nervous system continues until the 16th week. Note that the critical period for the heart rate ends near the end of the eighth LMP week, about the same time that the embryonic heart rate reaches its peak rate. The sonographic images and the schematic drawings are life-size, 1:1 scale. Also note that in week 8 the sonograph and embryo schematic are vertically reversed. (Adapted from Moore KL, Persaud TVN: The Developing Human: Clinically Oriented Embryology, 5th ed. WB Saunders, Philadelphia, 1993, p 156.)

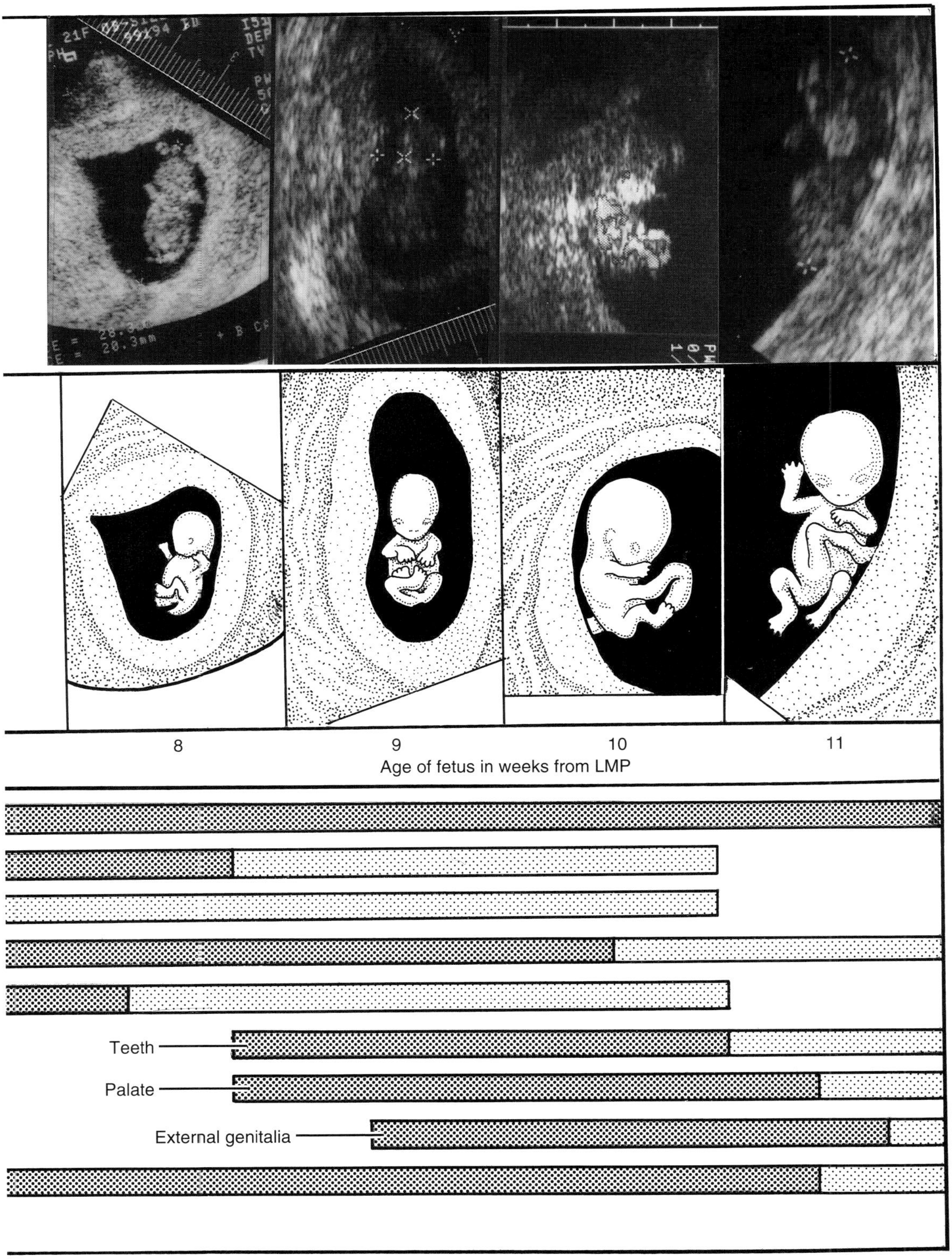
8
9
10
11
Age of fetus in weeks from LMP
Teeth
Palate
External genitalia

```
================================[ BASIC BABY  (c)]================================
        LEGEND OF MEASUREMENTS:

Acronym = Explanation
LMP     = Age from Last Menstrual Period in weeks.
GSD     = Gestational Sac (Chorionic cavity) Diameter(s) (mm).
CRL     = Crown-Rump Length (mm).
FOD     = Frontal-Occipital, mid-edge to mid-edge,(mm)(Long Skull Diameter).
BPD     = BiParietal Diameter (leading-edge to leading-edge)(mm).
VCD     = Vertical Cranial Diameter (mid-HBL to mid-vertex)(mm).
TAD     = Transverse Abdominal Diameter (at umbilical vein)(mm).
AAD     = Anterior-posterior Abdominal Diameter (at umbilical vein)(mm).
FemL    = Femur length (mm).
HumL    = Humerus length (mm).
HBL     = Hippocampal Base Line(bisquamae dia.tangential to bases of gyri)(mm)
Cerbl   = Cerebellar Diameter (tranverse width)(mm).
BiOcD   = BinOcular Diameter (outer to outer of both eyes)(mm).
Ang.Sd  = triAngle Side length (mid-vertex to squamae-HBL intersection)(mm).
FHR     = Fetal (or embryonic) Heart Rate (beats/min.).
HEARTc  = Number of Heart Chambers.
AvDEVIAT= Average of deviations from mean.


================================[   BBII   (tm)   ]================================
```

A

```
================================[ BASIC BABY  (c)]================================
                                LEGEND OF REPORT/GRAPH
Acronym    = HistoG = Explanation (HistoG are symbols in time-series histogram)
LMP          =    M = Age from Last Menstrual Period  (MP) in weeks.
ALL AGE      =    A = Average of all (n) fetal ages in MP weeks.
BRAIN AGE    =    b = Average of (n) fetal brain ages in MP weeks.
BODY AGE            = Average of (n) AC, HUM and/or FEM ages in MP weeks.
EDC                 = Est.Date of Confine.(40 Wk.LMP/38 Wk.Gest),(A/b=age used)
GSD          =    G = Gestational Sac (Chorionic cavity) Diameter(s) (mm).
CRL          =    R = Crown-Rump Length (mm).
BPD          =    B = BiParietal Diameter (mm).
TriCD        =    > = Triangle Circumference Diameter (mm)(approx.= BPD).
THC          =    T = Transverse Head Circumference (mm).
CHC          =    C = Coronal Head Circumference (mm)(approx.86% of true CHC).
CV           =    V = Cranial Volume (cc)(approx.90% of true volume.)
BiOcD        =    O = BinOcular Distance (outer to outer) (mm).
HumL         =    H = Humerus Length (mm).
FemL         =    F = Femur length (mm).
AC           =    a = Abdominal Circumference (mm).
          | |   | | = AGE RANGE ANALYSIS (approx.+-2SD RANGE of ALL & BRAIN ages)
EHR          =    E = Embryonic Heart Rate & appropiate age in weeks +-1.2.
 NOTE: BB does NOT COMPUTE beyond 41 weeks. 41+WKS means n measurements exceed
  BB look up tables & an abitrary 41 wks is used in AVE.WKS, use your judgment.
================================[   BBII   (tm)   ]================================
```

B

FIGURE 18–2.
A, A computer printout of the legend of the measurements used to evaluate the representative cases. These measurements may be used to directly estimate the fetal age, as with the biparietal diameter, or they may be used in other calculations such as circumferences or volumes, from which the age may be estimated. The measurements are taken as appropriate to the time in gestation (i.e., the crown-rump length is used early in pregnancy but not later, and head measurements are used later in pregnancy but not earlier). *B,* This legend shows the various parameters used to estimate the fetal ages. A computerized report with a time-series symbol histogram is presented for each representative case here. The characters used in the time-series symbolic histogram are the letters under *HistoG.* Each letter in the time-series histogram takes up 0.5 week of space; therefore, any characters that are less than 0.25 week apart are stacked in a bar-type graph or histogram. Each histogram is over the estimated fetal age in LMP weeks, and the dispersion increases with time in gestation as the fetuses become more individuated.

the human heart rate passes through a rapid acceleration phase that ends at precisely the time the interventricular foramen closes was not known just 5 years ago. The significance of the shape of the embryonic heart rate curve in time is still not understood. The embryonic phase of human development is a very interesting period for sonographic study.

Early research of the human embryo used a classification of *horizons* to track development.[2] These horizons were numbered consecutively and documented significant changes in the embryo. For this reason, the horizons are not necessarily correlated with calendar ages such as LMP weeks. More recent research has led to the adjustments of Streeter's original horizon dating system,[3] and the horizons are not generally used in the sonographic study of embryology. The following sonographic images and discussion of the week-by-week development of the embryo include Streeter's horizons in approximation with the weeks. These are approximate because of the recent adjustment in the original horizons and the fact that the horizons do not match the week-to-week developments. The horizon classifications are included in the hope that they will assist embryologists who may use this textbook. An excellent companion book to this section for the study of the developing human is Marjorie England's *A Colour Atlas of Life Before Birth: Normal Fetal Development*.[3] England's textbook uses color photographs of specimens to demonstrate fetal development just as this section uses sonography. It was from that text that the conversions of the horizons for the following section were developed.

LMP Weeks 1, 2, and 3

LAST MENSTRUAL PERIOD

The menstrual cycle and pregnancy are generally timed from the start of the LMP. Perhaps this should really be considered the end of the cycle previous to the current cycle, because menstrual flow is caused by sloughing of the endometrium that proliferated during that previous cycle. The problem with dating a pregnancy from the LMP is that not all women have menstrual cycles of the same length, and the time of fertilization and implantation after the LMP varies somewhat. For these reasons, the LMP has more variability in predicting the dates of a pregnancy than do the actual sonographic measurements. However, the equivalent LMP age as determined from ovulation, basal temperature, sonographic measurements, or other methods is still used when discussing the dates of a pregnancy.

Historically, pregnancy was mysterious and the date of the LMP was usually the only way to estimate the time of pregnancy. Indeed, even today, with all our understanding, a great deal of mystery and some unanswered questions about human fertility remain.[4] Sonography has made great contributions to this body of knowledge, providing still another reason why the last quarter of the 20th century is such an exciting time to be a sonographer.

LMP WEEK 2

The end of week 2, about 13 to 14 days after the LMP, is the normal date of ovulation, and fertilization generally occurs within 1 to 3 days. Sonographically, the endometrium should be proliferative and appear thickened. It is ready to receive the fertilized ovum.

The ovum develops in an ovarian cyst or dominant follicle, which ruptures when it reaches approximately 20 to 24 mm in diameter, releasing the egg.[5] Fertilization normally takes place in the distal end of the fallopian tube, and mitotic division begins during the tube travel before implantation. For this reason, scarring of the fallopian tube by previous pelvic inflammatory disease or other processes increases the likelihood of an ectopic implantation.

LMP WEEK 3

During horizons I to IV, gestational days 0 to 7, fertilization, fallopian tube travel, and implantation take place. The first week of the pregnancy, or week 3 after the last menstrual period (third LMP week), is the period of fertilization and implantation. There is little to visualize sonographically except a normal-appearing uterus with a proliferative endometrium. Unless a woman is in a fertility program, she usually has no reason yet to suspect that she is even pregnant.

LMP Week 4

MATERNAL

During horizons V to IX, gestational days 7 to 20, the blastocyst implants in endometrium and chorionic villi branching occurs. This is the end of the presomite period and the start of somite development (somite pairs develop into vertebrae).

Four weeks after the LMP is approximately 2 weeks after conception. Because this is the week in which the next menses is expected to start, it often is approximately the time when a woman begins to suspect that she may be pregnant.

It is not uncommon for a woman to have some spotting or light bleeding around the middle of the fourth LMP week, most often about 17 days after conception. This is medically thought of as threatened abortion. One of four or five women has early gestational bleeding in the first half of their pregnancy, and of these, about half abort. Some have considered light spotting in this week to be normal. Studies of rhesus monkeys found at least microscopic bleeding at this time.[6]

OBSERVATIONS

The most characteristic sonographic observation in the fourth LMP week is the early gestational sac or ring (Fig. 18–3*A*). Although the sonographic literature almost always refers to this early evidence of pregnancy as the *gestational sac*, it is more appropriately called the *chorionic cavity*.

Proliferation of the endometrium and often a double-ring sign are observed (Figs. 18–3*A* and 18–4*A*). This double ring is due to the layering effect of the decidua capsularis, or outer wall of the gestational sac, lying adjacent to the decidua parietalis, or opposite endometrium.

In the presence of pelvic pain or spotting, the double-ring sign is one of the best signs for ruling out an ectopic pregnancy. With an ectopic pregnancy, a small amount of blood in the uterine cavity may mimic an early gestational sac, but this pseudosac should not exhibit the double ring.

Figure 18–3*B* is magnified sonographically to a 4:1 scale. This scale can be observed on the centimeter ruler, at the edge of the sonographic field of view. Next to the 2-cm and 6-cm graduations are two white dots, which are the sonographic scale markers. The distance between these two dots is 1 cm; therefore, this image is enlarged to four times lifesize. This image shows early trophoblastic vascular flow away from the transducer, not that the direction is important at this time (see technical note below). This early flow can be helpful in recognizing an early intrauterine pregnancy versus a pseudosac, which might be associated with an ectopic pregnancy.

Figure 18–4 shows transabdominal sonograms of a normal 4.6-LMP-week pregnancy. Figure 18–4*A* demonstrates the long axis of the uterus, showing the gestational sac diameter (GSD) and characteristic double-ring layering effect of the decidua capsularis and decidua parietalis. Maternal bowel and its resulting bright reflections and distal shadowing can be observed just cephalad to the uterine fundus. Figure 18–4*B* is from the same examination and demonstrates the transverse sonographic plane of the pelvis. The GSD, myometrium, endometrium, and bilateral adnexa can be observed.

MOVEMENT

In the fourth menstrual week, no embryonic motion can usually be observed. The fourth week is from the 14th to the 21st day after conception.

According to embryologists, the human heart does not begin beating until 21 to 22 days after conception (35 to 36 LMP days, early fifth LMP week).[8] In one case, the embryonic heart rate (EHR) was measured at 75 B/M at 4.7 LMP weeks by GSD (10 mm), and a normal term delivery resulted. Some may debate that an embryonic heart can be observed sonographically this early in a pregnancy, and this question is valid. There are two problems with making this observation at this time. First is the issue of determining the dates; the LMP is not useful when the date must be resolved to less than plus-or-minus 3 or 4 days. The crown-rump length (CRL) is also not helpful at this time, although Schats states that "cardiac activity should be detected as soon as the embryonic pole has appeared."[9]

The other issue of EHR at this time is that the rate starts out below 90 B/M. This is approximately the same range as the maternal heart rate. For this reason, it may be very difficult to determine whether one is actually observing the embryonic heartbeat or the "body shock" or "tissue thump" from the maternal pelvic vasculature. It must not be forgotten that the maternal reproductive vessels are dilating to accommodate the needs of the pregnancy at this time (see Chapter 12 for more on the EHR). The embryonic heartbeat might be observed transvaginally at the end of the fourth LMP week; however, the heart rate is more likely to be discernible after this week.

SIZE/AGE

During the fourth LMP week, the mean GSD should be less than 10 mm. The greatest GSD should increase from about 10 mm at the start of the fourth week to approximately 15 mm at the end of this week. The embryonic pole or disk is usually not observed in the fourth week. At the very end of the fourth LMP week (days 20 to 21 after conception), the embryonic pole or disk is approximately 1.5 to 3.0 mm in length, at the lower limits of resolution of most sonographic equipment.[10]

For images of the fourth week, two examples were chosen, one early in the fourth week and one around the middle of the fourth week (see Figs. 18–3*A* to 18–4*B*). Both women were subsequently re-examined and found to have a sonographically normal pregnancy at 7.5 and 14.8 LMP weeks, respectively.

The first example is shown in Figure 18–3*A* and *B*. The transvaginal or endovaginal image in Figure 18–3*A* was printed to a 1:1 scale, as can be observed on the centimeter ruler that was attached to the easel during the photographic process. The GSD measured 5 mm in greatest diameter; no embryonic heartbeat was observed. In this endovaginal image (see Fig. 18–3*A*) the early gestational sac can be seen as a cystic, hypoechoic structure near the center of the endometrium and in a good uterine location. The sonographic line or stripe of the uterine cavum can be observed.

The mother had reported that her LMP had been 7.1 weeks prior; however, this 5-mm GSD computed to 4.0 LMP weeks (Fig. 18–3*C*). For this reason, the pregnancy was followed up 20 days later, at which time a sonographically normal embryonic pole was observed with appropriate heart rate and interval growth. The GSD was also appropriate. It was therefore concluded that the woman's originally reported LMP date was erroneous.

LMP Week 5

OBSERVATIONS

During horizons IX to XII, gestational days 21 to 27, the head and tail folds develop, the neural groove closes, and limb buds are present. The two heart tubes fuse, and the heart begins beating.

In the fifth LMP week (21 to 28 days after conception), the secondary yolk sac should become visible as a smooth, rounded, cystic structure. The primary or primitive yolk is not visible sonographically and by the fifth LMP week has become only a remnant embedded in the extraembryonic somatic mesoderm (inner lining of the chorion).[11] The secondary yolk sac, which is generally simply called the yolk sac, usually is adjacent to one edge of the chorionic cavity, as shown in Figure 18–5*A* and *B*. Figure 18–5*A* is life-size, with a 1:1 scale, whereas Figure 18–5*B* is enlarged to a 5:1 scale. A yolk sac that is not smooth and round or that is too large or is solid and hyperechoic is not a favorable sign for the pregnancy.[11] The yolk sac shown in Figure 18–5*A* and *C* is normal.

The decidua and endometrium continue to develop and proliferate in the fifth week. The gestational sac or, more correctly, the chorionic cavity should be clearly visible transvaginally and often transabdominally in the fifth week. In Figure 18–5*A*, the developing lacunae can be seen as hypoechoic areas in the endometrium. The lacunae are spaces that form in the syncytiotrophoblast and become the initial connection with the maternal side of the circulation.[11] These lacunae are the first indication of the location of the developing placenta.

It is common to note the strongest echoes from the two sides of the yolk sac; these are specular or perpendicular to the sonographic beam. The edges of the yolk sac that are more parallel to the beam do not reflect as strongly and therefore are less echogenic.

MOVEMENT

During the fifth menstrual week, the embryonic heartbeat may often be observed using transvaginal transducers. A beating embryonic heart located in the uterus is a

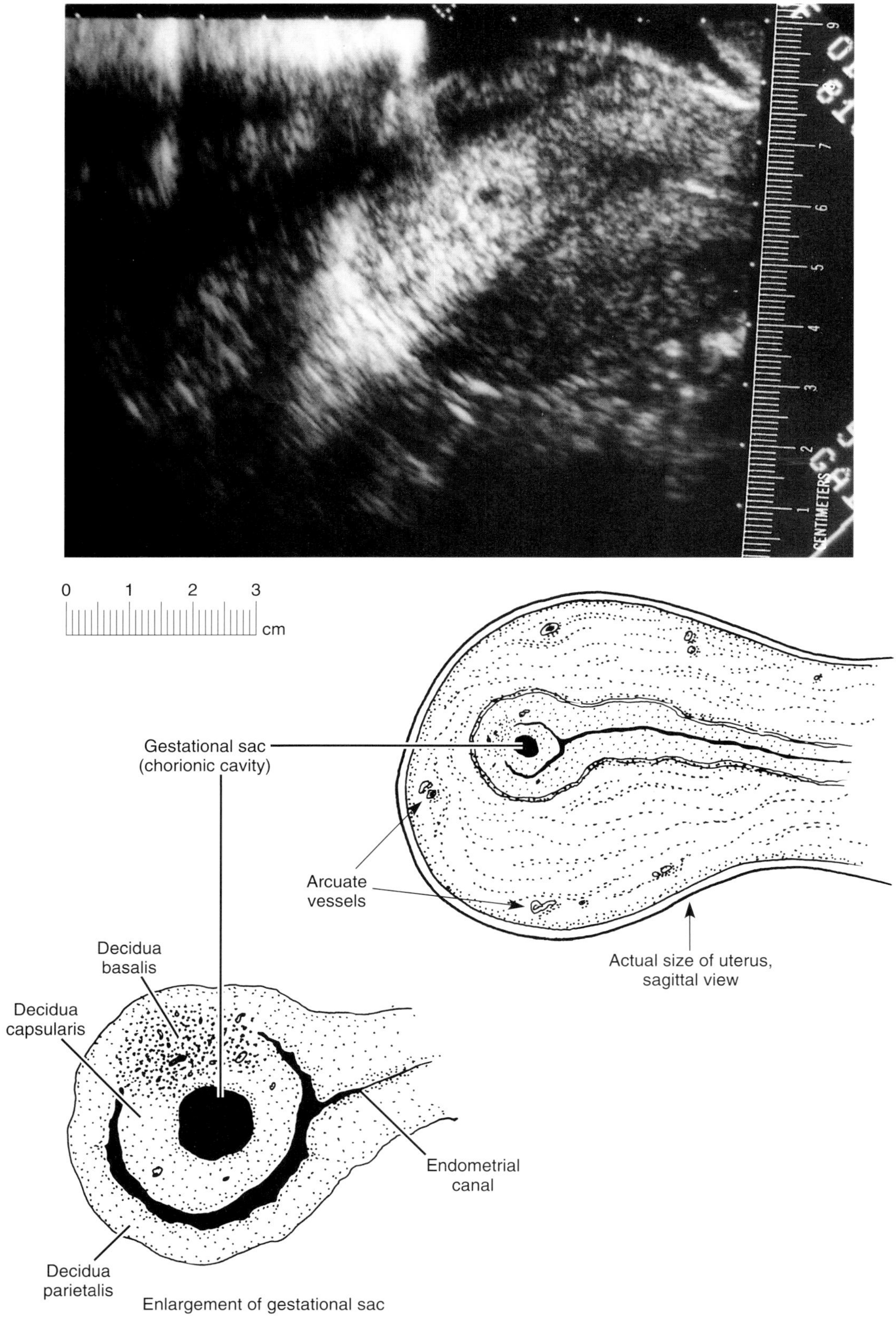

A

FIGURE 18–3.

A, Transvaginal sonogram of a 4.0-LMP-week chorionic cavity or gestational sac with a corresponding drawing. The gestational sac diameter (GSD) measures 5 mm. The sonogram is printed life-size (1:1 ratio).

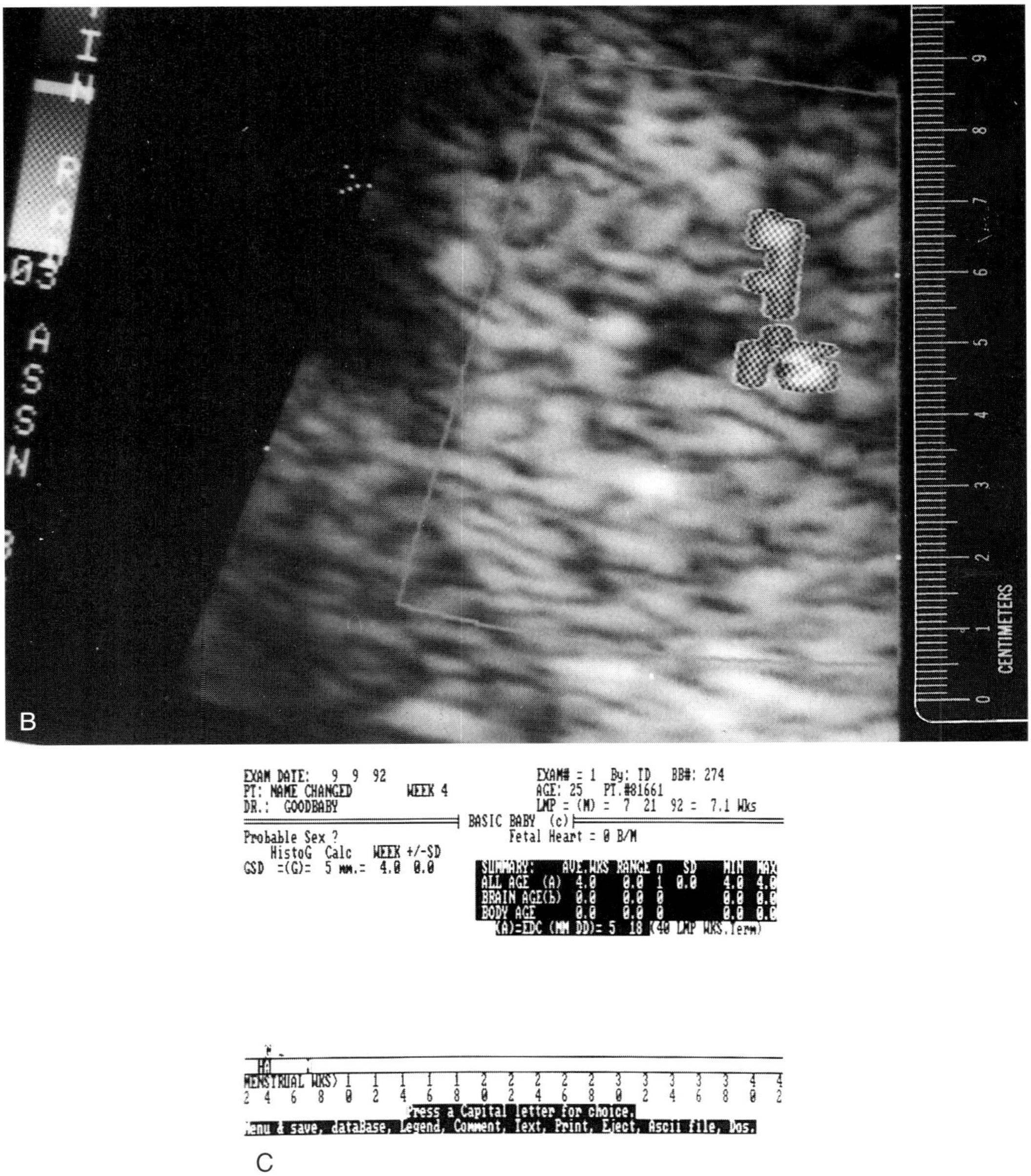

FIGURE 18–3 *Continued*
B, A 4:1 enlargement of the same case shown in *A*. This case was referred to rule out an ectopic pregnancy. Color Doppler was used to confirm trophoblastic flow at the implantation site. A slow-flow velocity tag was used to highlight the black-and-white color Doppler information, which is printed with a checkered pattern. *C,* Computer printout of size/age parameters. In this case, only the GSD was measured, and it evaluated to a 4.0-LMP-week pregnancy. The embryonic heart has not yet started to beat.

TECHNICAL NOTE: The black-and-white color Doppler demonstrated in Figure 18–3*B* is easily observable as a checkered area outlined by white. This checkered flow was a phenomenon that occurred when these sonographic laboratories installed a new imaging system that digitizes the images on magnetic media (5.25 rigid disks) for later transfer to film in the darkroom. The sales person was rather upset on first seeing the checkered Doppler flow, for it is visible in both black-and-white and color prints, and exclaimed, "I'll get the engineers to fix that!" However, with consideration, it was decided that in a black-and-white print of a color Doppler image, a smooth Doppler signal might be difficult to distinguish from the sonographic image background. It was therefore decided to keep the checkered Doppler.

This checkering of the Doppler does not help to determine the direction of flow in a black-and-white image as is possible with color. However, because color is much more expensive and black-and-white film processing is more common, the *slow-flow tag* outline method was de-

Technical Note continued on following page

TECHNICAL NOTE *Continued*

veloped.[7] This method uses a velocity tag, provided by many Doppler machine manufacturers, to highlight the very slowest flow in contrasting white. Because of the laminar nature of blood flow, the slowest velocities tend to be at the edges of the vessel wall; therefore, this method results in a contrasting outline of the flow. Direction can be determined in the black-and-white image because, in this case (see Fig. 18–1*B*), only the slow flow away from the transducer was tagged. Flow toward the transducer would not be outlined, and this particular image shows none. The slow-flow outlining works whether the black-and-white color Doppler signal is checkered or smooth.

These two handy techniques point out that the manufacturers have not exhausted the possibilities of sonographic displays. It can be imagined that multiple velocity tags might be provided with various types of dithering or vertical, horizontal, and diagonal contrasting lines for depicting the flow tags in black and white. Perhaps a color flow display could be developed to use tiny triangles or arrowheads pointing in the general direction of flow. This would make black-and-white color Doppler more economical and useful in areas where color processing might not be as available. It would also make publication costs much lower by eliminating the need for color separations.

favorable sign and gives confirmation of an intrauterine pregnancy. A more comforting finding is close correlation of the EHR age and the ages calculated from other parameters (see the size/age section later).

Inability to see a beating heart is not always an unfavorable sign, however; the embryonic heart may not become visible until the sixth week. In a study of 47 in vitro fertilization pregnancies, Shats found an interval of 5 days in which the embryonic heartbeat was initially observed.[13, 14] In this study, transvaginal sonography was used daily to search for heartbeats, starting from the 25th day after follicle aspiration. First observations of the embryonic heartbeats were as early as the 25th day, and the beating heart was first observed most often on the 27th day. If we assume that in an in vitro fertilization procedure, aspiration of the follicle is the equivalent of ovulation in a normal pregnancy, then the embryonic heart would be expected to be observed as early as 5.5 LMP weeks and most often at the end of the fifth week.

In Shats' study, during the fifth to eighth LMP weeks, the heart rate of embryos that continued to a normal-appearing fetus at the end of the first trimester was between 70 and 110 B/M, with a mean of approximately 100 B/M. This is similar to the findings in our large population study. In the fifth LMP week, it is not uncommon to detect heart rates less than 85 B/M.[13, 15–18]

When the EHR is observed, not much variation in the rate over a relatively short time of 60 minutes or less should be seen. Schats and colleagues found that interobserver variation in EHR measurements had a mean difference of 2.9 B/M (SD 1.7, range = 0 to 4, median=2, n = 47) during time intervals of 15 to 60 minutes between observations.[13] This is of a similar magnitude to my group's findings in 36 normal embryos, between 5 and 11.6 LMP weeks, in which the mean difference in the EHR was 1.3 B/M (1 SD = 3.3 B/M, range = 0 to 14 B/M, median = 0 difference B/M) with a mean interval between observations of 9.6 minutes (range = 15 seconds to 29.8 minutes, median = 6 minutes).

It was interesting that one embryo at 5.6 LMP weeks by CRL measurement of 3 mm (not included in the previous statistics) had a variation of 26 B/M in five observations in less than 8 minutes. This embryo's EHR was first

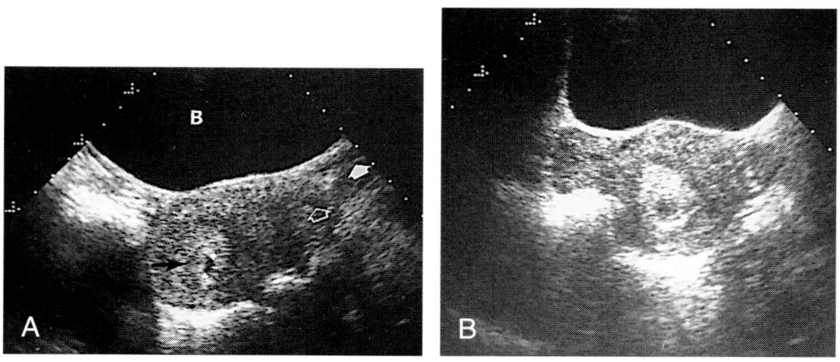

FIGURE 18–4.
A, A different 4-LMP-week pregnancy from the case shown in Figure 18–3. It is presented here to show the fourth LMP week by transabdominal sonography. In this sagittal plane, the full maternal urinary bladder (B) is anechoic and anterior to the uterus. The gestational sac diameter (GSD) is measured at 9.6 mm, which evaluated to 4.6 LMP weeks. The double-ring sign of the decidua parietalis and decidua capsularis is shown (black arrow). The external os of the cervix (open white arrow) and the vaginal tract (solid white arrow) are also seen. *B*, A transverse transabdominal sonograph of the same case as in *A*. The GSD within the echogenic endometrium is near the center of the uterus; the bilateral adnexa extend to the sides.

observed to be 88 B/M; subsequent observations were 95, 113, 87, and 97 B/M. The pregnancy ended in spontaneous abortion less than 2 weeks later. Although one case is not proof (this case with the small variations in the EHR shown by the two different studies previously mentioned), it appears prudent to watch closely any embryos with irregular heart rates.

SIZE/AGE

It is in the fifth LMP week that the first true embryonic measurements may be taken using transvaginal transducers. Figure 18–5*B* shows the measurement of this embryonic disk or pole to be 2.5 mm. This measurement calculated to the equivalent of 5.5 LMP weeks. It was possible to determine that this group of echoes was the embryo because the embryonic heartbeat could be observed and measured to be 92 B/M (see Fig. 18–5*C*).

During the fifth week, the embryonic length should grow from slightly less than 2 mm to about 3 to 4 mm at the end of the week. In the sonographic literature, the length of the embryonic pole is generally referred to as the CRL. This terminology grew out of early embryology long before sonographic equipment had been developed.[19] The accuracy of various tables for predicting the age of the pregnancy from CRL measurements has been discussed at length. There seem to be slight variations in all published tables, and only in the 1990s did CRL measurement tables become available before the seventh LMP week.[20, 21]

A new method for predicting the age of the embryo uses the EHR.[17] Many will find this surprising. The EHR accelerates linearly until the start of the 9th LMP week, which is near the end of the embryonic period (see Chapter 12 for details of the EHR and age). Let it suffice here that the EHR should accelerate from approximately 94 B/M to about 116 B/M at the end of the fifth week (± 20 B/M). The regression for predicting the embryonic age is as follows:

$$\text{LMP age in days} = (\text{EHR} \times 0.3) + 6$$

This age is accurate to within ± 8 days. Although the EHR does accelerate at a rate of 3.3 B/M per day until the start of the ninth week, it does not vary much during the period of a few minutes of an examination.[9] As stated before, the EHR is discussed in great detail in Chapter 12.

The greatest GSD increase is from approximately 16 to 23 mm during the fifth LMP week.[22] The average of three perpendicular measurements of the GSD increases from approximately 10 mm to about 16 mm.[23, 24] However, the shape of the chorionic cavity can be affected by the degree of filling of the maternal bladder and resulting pressure on the uterus, as well as by uterine fibroids and variable shapes of the uterus. This variability in the shape of the gestational sac makes the GSD a less desirable measurement for dating pregnancies (see Chapter 7).

LMP Week 6

OBSERVATIONS

During horizons XIII to XVI, gestational days 27 to 34, the head is flexed toward the chest, the heart bulges from the body, the four branchial arches are present, the cerebral hemispheres are enlarging, the hands have definite carpal and digital regions, and the leg buds have differentiated into thigh, leg, and foot.

In the sixth menstrual week (28 to 34 conceptual days), the embryo should be identifiable immediately adjacent to the spherical yolk sac by transvaginal scanning. Fig. 18–6*A* is an example of an embryo measuring 4 mm in length, which calculated to an equivalent 6.0 LMP weeks of age. This sonogram is printed in a 3:1 scale—that is, it is three times actual size. By the transabdominal/transvesical approach, through the maternal abdominal wall and full urinary bladder, these structures may not be discernible until the seventh week in obese patients or with poor resolution.

The yolk sac should be smoothly spherical and clearly cystic. A sac that is irregular, small, large, or internally echogenic is a sign that the pregnancy may not be progressing normally.

MOVEMENT

The embryonic heartbeat is the most reliable sign that the embryo has been identified. The heartbeat is the only motion observed in the 6th week (Fig. 18–6*B*).

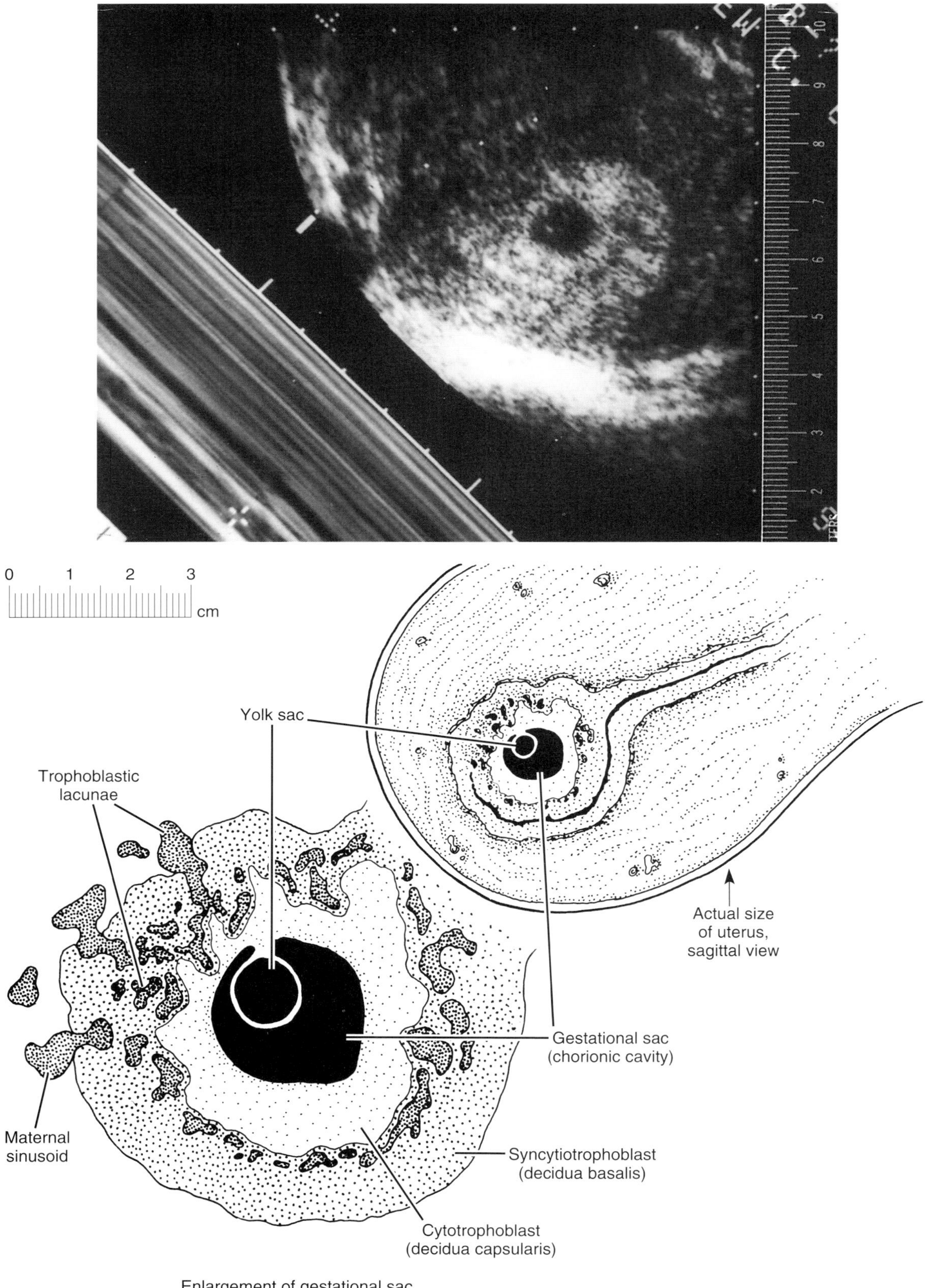

FIGURE 18–5. *See legend on opposite page*

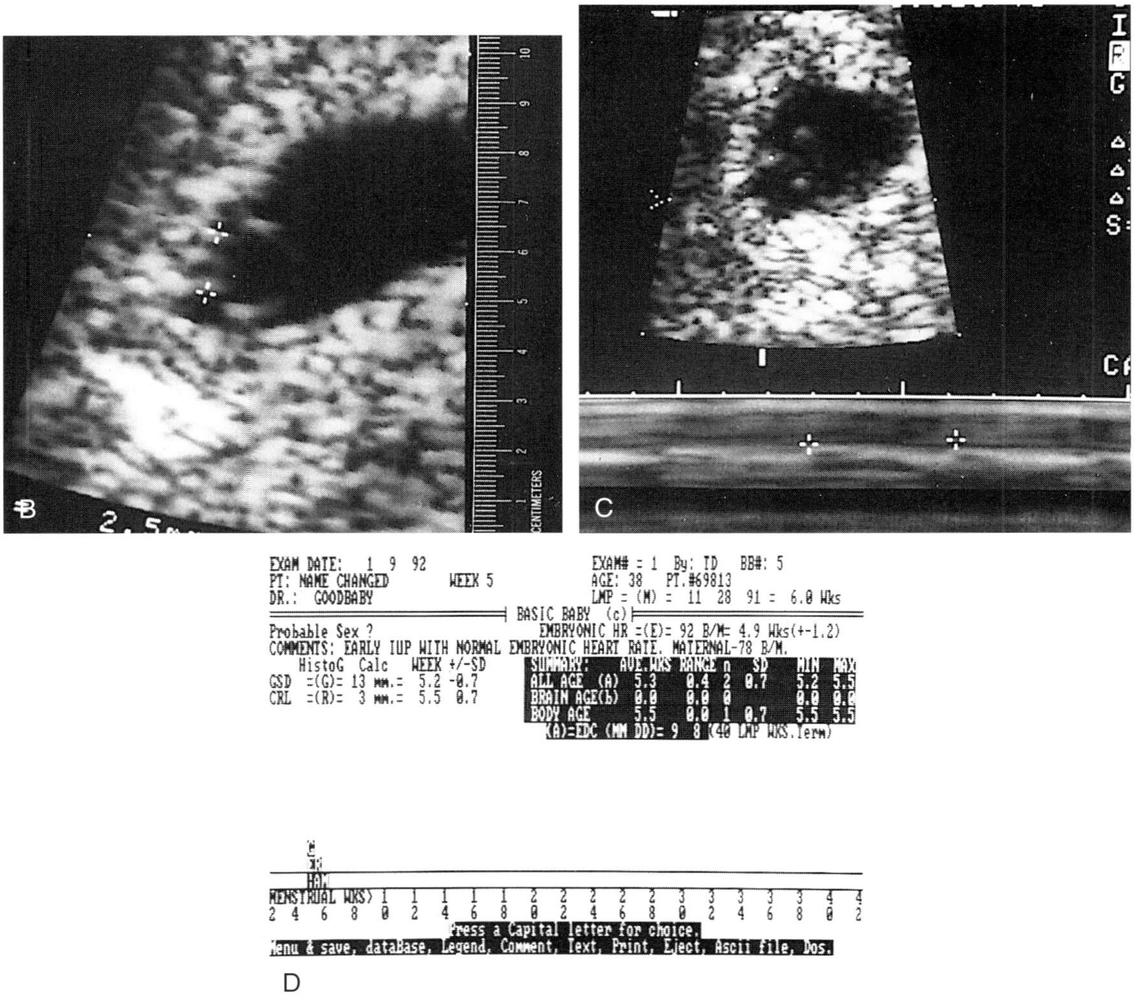

FIGURE 18–5.
A, The sonogram shows a life-size (1:1 ratio) chorionic sac that contains a yolk sac and live embryo. The embryonic heart rate (EHR) is measured by M-mode (see *C*). On the sonogram, the yolk sac edges, which are perpendicular to the sound beam, show clearly as specular echoes. The drawings show the anatomy. *B*, An enlargement (5:1) showing the yolk sac and embryonic measurement. The EHR could be observed and measured, allowing identification of the embryonic pole or disk. The length of the embryo, or crown-rump length (CRL), measures 2.5 mm. *C*, The EHR is being measured by M-mode at 92 B/M. Because this rate is slow enough to be confused with the maternal rate, the woman's heart rate was measured by transvaginal M-mode from vessels in the adnexa at 78 B/M (not shown). *D*, Computer printout showing the average age of two fetal parameters (gestational sac diameter and CRL) to be 5.3 LMP weeks. The EHR evaluated to 4.9 LMP weeks. The range of ages, including the EHR age, is only 0.6 weeks, well within the 2 SD of 1.1 week by age range analysis (ARA) (see Chapter 7).

The EHR normally is in the range of 93 to 166 B/M (± 2 SD), with the mean EHR increasing from approximately 118 at 6.0 LMP weeks to 141 B/M at the end of the week. Embryos with EHRs less than 93 B/M should be followed up in a week or two to confirm continued viability. Several researchers have found that if the EHR drops below the EHR acceleration curve, the pregnancy is likely to end in first-trimester embryonic demise.[13, 15, 17, 18, 25]

At this early age, the EHR may be slow

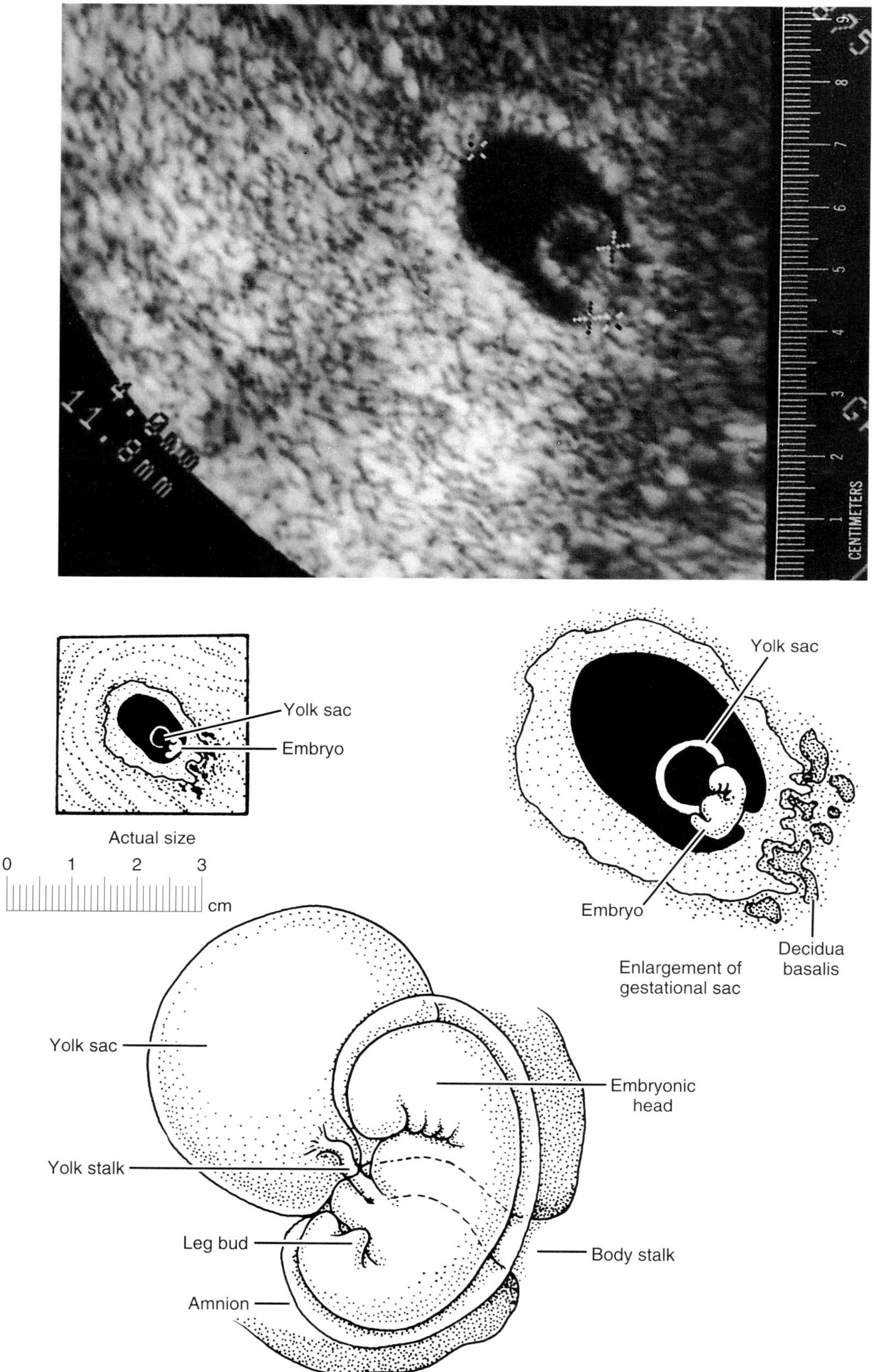

A

FIGURE 18–6.
A, The sonogram is a 3:1 enlargement of the chorionic cavity (gestational sac), yolk sac, and embryo. The drawings show the corresponding anatomy.

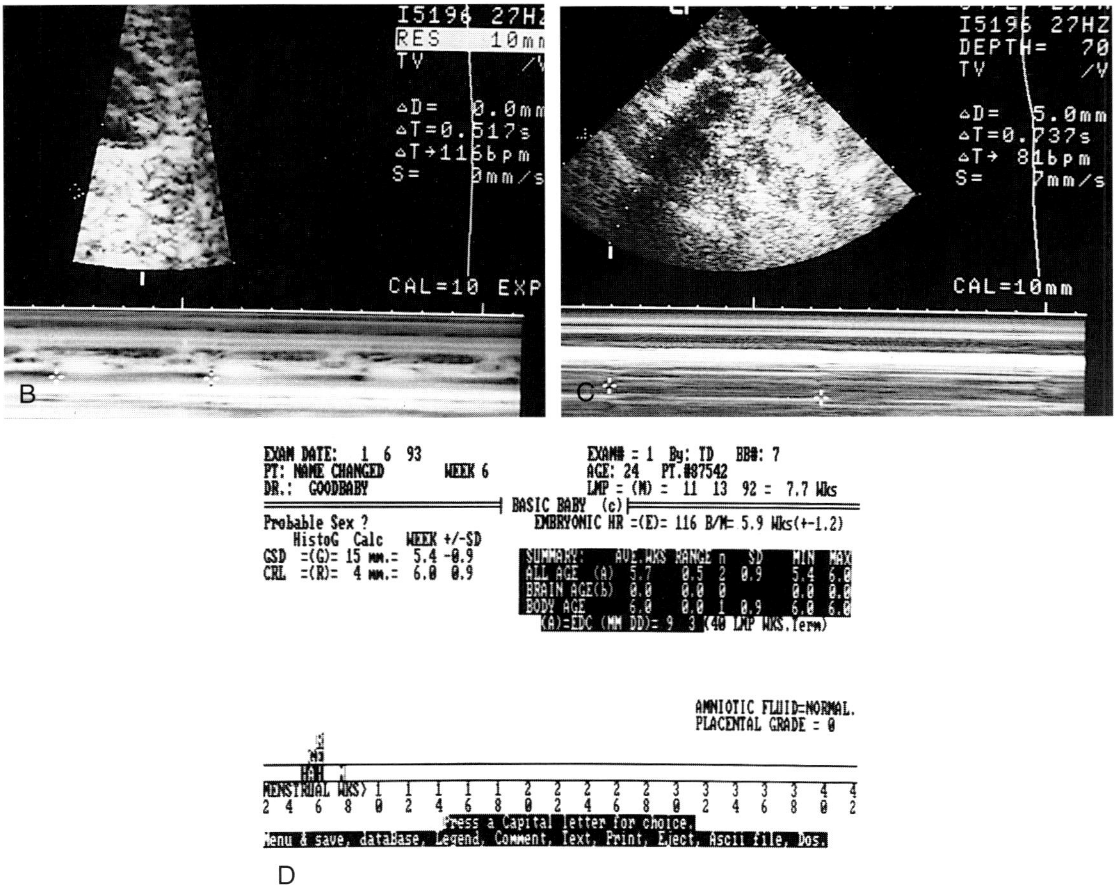

FIGURE 18–6 *Continued*
B, An enlargement of the embryo with the transvaginal (TV) M-mode tracing below. The embryonic heart rate (EHR) was measured at 116 B/M. One complete heartbeat is measured by M-mode between the small, dark dots just above the + cursors. These dots were used for the measurement because they form sharp demarcation of the beats. *C*, To confirm that the woman's heart rate was different from her embryo's, this TV M-mode tracing was produced from the right adnexa. The TV M-mode vector is seen as a line of dots in the sonogram while one complete beat is measured between the + cursors on the M-mode tracing. The maternal heartbeats were registered as faint tissue thump from the adnexal vessels and measured 81 B/M. *D*, In this computer analysis of the parameters' size/ages, the mean of two parameters (gestational sac diameter and crown-rump length) was 5.7 LMP weeks with a range of 0.5 weeks. The EHR age was 5.9 LMP weeks. These ages are well within the ±2 SD for age range (ARA) of ±10% of the age (see Chapter 7).

enough to be confused with the maternal, heart rate (see Fig. 18–6*B*). This is especially true if the woman smokes tobacco or is excited, both of which may accelerate her heart rate. If there is concern that the maternal, rather than the embryonic heart rate is being recorded, it is easy to determine the woman's heart rate by angling the transvaginal field of view and M-mode vector toward her adnexa and recording the maternal pulse from the many arteries located there. Figure 18–6*C* demonstrates this technique and found the maternal rate to be 81 B/M, clearly different from her embryo's, which was 116 B/M (see Fig. 18–6*B*).

SIZE/AGE

In the sixth LMP week, the embryonic length (CRL) grows from approximately 4 to about 9 mm, and the greatest chorionic cavity diameter (GSD) increases from about 18 to 26 mm.[20] The mean of three perpendicular GSDs normally increases from 17 to 23 mm during the sixth week.[23, 24]

The GSD, CRL, and EHR are the only reliable sonographic indicators of the dates of the pregnancy during the sixth LMP week. The woman's reported last normal menstrual period (LNMP) is, of course, another indicator of age, but it is not as reliable as sonographic measurements. The CRL is the most accurate measurement during the sixth week (± 3 to 4 days)[21] and the EHR is the next most accurate (± 8 days).[17] The chorionic cavity measurement (± 7 to 14 days),[23, 26, 27] depending on the researcher, is slightly more reliable than the LNMP (± 21 days or more)[28] for estimating the age of the embryo.

Close correlation between the ages calculated from the CRL, EHR, and GSD with the LNMP is comforting that the pregnancy is starting out well. If the CRL, EHR, and GSD ages correlate well but the LNMP does not, then one must consider that the LNMP may be unreliable.

In Figures 18–6*A* to *D*, a normal embryo is shown. The CRL measured 4 mm or 6.0 weeks and the EHR was 116 B/M, which evaluated to an approximate age of 5.9 weeks (see Fig. 18–6*D*). This is a difference of less than 1 day (0.1 week = 16.8 hours) in estimated ages. The mean sac size was approximately 9 mm, and the greatest GSD was approximately 12 mm, both of which calculated to approximately 5.4 weeks, indicating that the GSD is slightly small compared with the CRL and EHR. The difference in the means of the sac size and the CRL was 5 mm. Despite the relatively small GSD, this embryo was delivered by cesarean section at 38 weeks LMP age (by this sonographic examination) as a normal 8-pound boy, Apgar Scores 8 and 9.

Discrepancies between the estimated ages from the CRL and EHR greater than 8 days should be double-checked for accurate measurement and age calculations. If the discrepancies still exist, after re-estimating the ages, the pregnancy should be followed up in a few weeks to confirm continued viability. This is especially true if the calculated EHR age is less than the CRL age, which indicates that the EHR is not accelerating normally. I do not worry as much about discrepant GSD ages because of the large variability in chorionic sac shapes due to pressure from a full maternal bladder, uterine fibroids, and the variable shape of the uterus.

Of course, large GSD age differences from the CRL and EHR ages are of concern. Several studies have found that small GSDs are associated with abnormal karyotypes (genetic problems) and spontaneous abortion.[29–32] Opsahl and Pettit[32] found that differences between the mean GSD and CRL greater than 8 mm did not reflect an increase in the rate of spontaneous abortion in the normal control group, but these size differences were associated with an increase in rates in the couples with a history of recurrent spontaneous abortion.

LMP Week 7

OBSERVATIONS

During horizons XVII to XX, gestational days 34 to 41, the head remains flexed against the chest and the heart bulge. The midgut herniates into the umbilical cord. The paramesonephric ducts (müllerian) are present, as are the secondary bronchial branches of the lungs.

During the early seventh LMP week, the embryo can be observed transabdominally as demonstrated in Figure 18–7*A* to *C*. Figure 18–7*A* is life-size.

This pregnancy might appear to have two gestational sacs. However, the lower sac is thought to be an organizing blood clot rather than a twin gestation. This conclusion was reached because of the absence of a recognizable yolk sac, embryo, or cardiac activity. It also appears to be outside and below the echogenic ring of the chorion.

A normal gestational sac is ovoid or ellipsoidal and is surrounded by the echogenic chorion (see Fig. 18–7*A* and *B*). The implantation site may be predicted by observing the location of the thicker portion of the chorionic ring.[33]

In the late seventh LMP week, many more sonographic observations are possible than earlier in gestation. The embryonic head is clearly discernible from the body, and the arm and leg buds and the amnion may be seen. The heart rate can be easily observed.

Figure 18–8*A* to *E* shows a normal pregnancy at an average of 7.6 LMP weeks, calculated from the mean of three fetal parameters. In these images, the amnion is seen completely enclosing the embryo. This is best demonstrated in Figure 18–8*D* and *E*. The amniotic fluid contained within the amniotic membrane is clear, whereas the chorionic cavity outside the amnion appears speckled because it is not a true fluid but a gel. This slightly echogenic gel, called the *magma reticulare*, is described as "a gel that liquefies upon touching."[34]

The yolk sac is spherical and outside the amniotic cavity, suspended in the gel of the magma reticulare (see Fig. 18–8*D*). The EHR is normally rapid, 169 B/M (see Fig. 18–8*E*).

The rhombencephalon can be seen as a cystic structure in the superior and posterior portions of the head in Figure 18–8*B* and *C* (coronal plane) and *D* (sagittal plane). The rhombencephalon is a fluid-filled space that becomes the hindbrain and fourth ventricle.[35]

MOVEMENT

In the seventh LMP week, embryonic somatic motion as well as cardiac motion can be observed. These movements have been described as "just discernible movements" and "vermicular movement" or wormlike movements, as in peristalsis,[36] a slow shifting of the embryo lasting from a half second to 2 seconds at a time.[37]

The EHR is still rapidly accelerating at a rate of 3.3 B/M per day. It increases from a mean of 143 B/M early in the week to a mean of 165 B/M at the end of the seventh week (2 SD range = 118 to 168, to 149 to 190). The EHR should not vary much in the short term, as stated in the description of LMP week 5.

Late in the seventh week, the embryo becomes more active. The movements could be described as more of a jerky extension, followed by relaxation toward the normal embryonic curve with the developing face against the heart prominence (chest).

SIZE/AGE

During the seventh week, the embryonic length grows from approximately 10 mm to about 15 mm. The mean GSD increases from 24 to 30 mm, and the greatest GSD measurement is from 27 to 36 mm.[20, 23, 24]

Figure 18–7*A* to *C* shows a pregnancy that might be considered somewhat abnormal because of the organizing blood clot; however, the embryo appears normal by biometric standards. The greatest GSD was 27 mm, the CRL was 7.3 mm, and the EHR was 141 B/M, which evaluated to 7.0, 7.3, and 6.9 LMP weeks, respectively (see Fig. 18–7*D*). This is a mean age of 7.2 weeks, with a range of 0.3 week or approximately 2 days. At this time of the pregnancy, a range of 0.3 week is less than 0.5 SD (2 SD range = 20% of age) (see Chapter 7 for more on ARA).

Figure 18–8*A* is a life-size sonogram of a late seventh-week embryo. Note the increased size over the previous case (see Fig. 18–7*A* to *C*) in just under 1 week. The range of ages was 7.3 to 8.0 weeks. The CRL and EHR ages were closest at 7.9 and 8.0 weeks, respectively (Fig. 18–8*F*).

In the coronal view of the embryo (see Fig. 18–8*C*), the biparietal diameter (BPD) is measured at 5.6 mm, which evaluated to 7.3 LMP weeks. Although the BPD can be measured at this early age, its relatively small size means that any variation in measurements due to image resolution or placement of the cursors results in relatively large percent errors. For this reason, the BPD is best used later in pregnancy. In this case, the age from the BPD was 0.4 weeks less than the next smallest age (GSD) of 7.7 weeks. For comparison, it is noted that the range for the other three ages was only 0.3 week (EHR, 8.0 weeks − GSD, 7.7 weeks = 0.3 week range). Although the low BPD age more than doubled the range of ages in this case, a range of 0.7 weeks is still less than 1 SD and quite normal.

LMP Week 8

OBSERVATIONS

During horizons XXI to XXIII, gestational days 42 to 48, fingers and toes are formed, the superficial scalp plexus is spreading toward the vertex of the head, and embryonic motion is obvious.

In the eighth menstrual week (42 days or 6

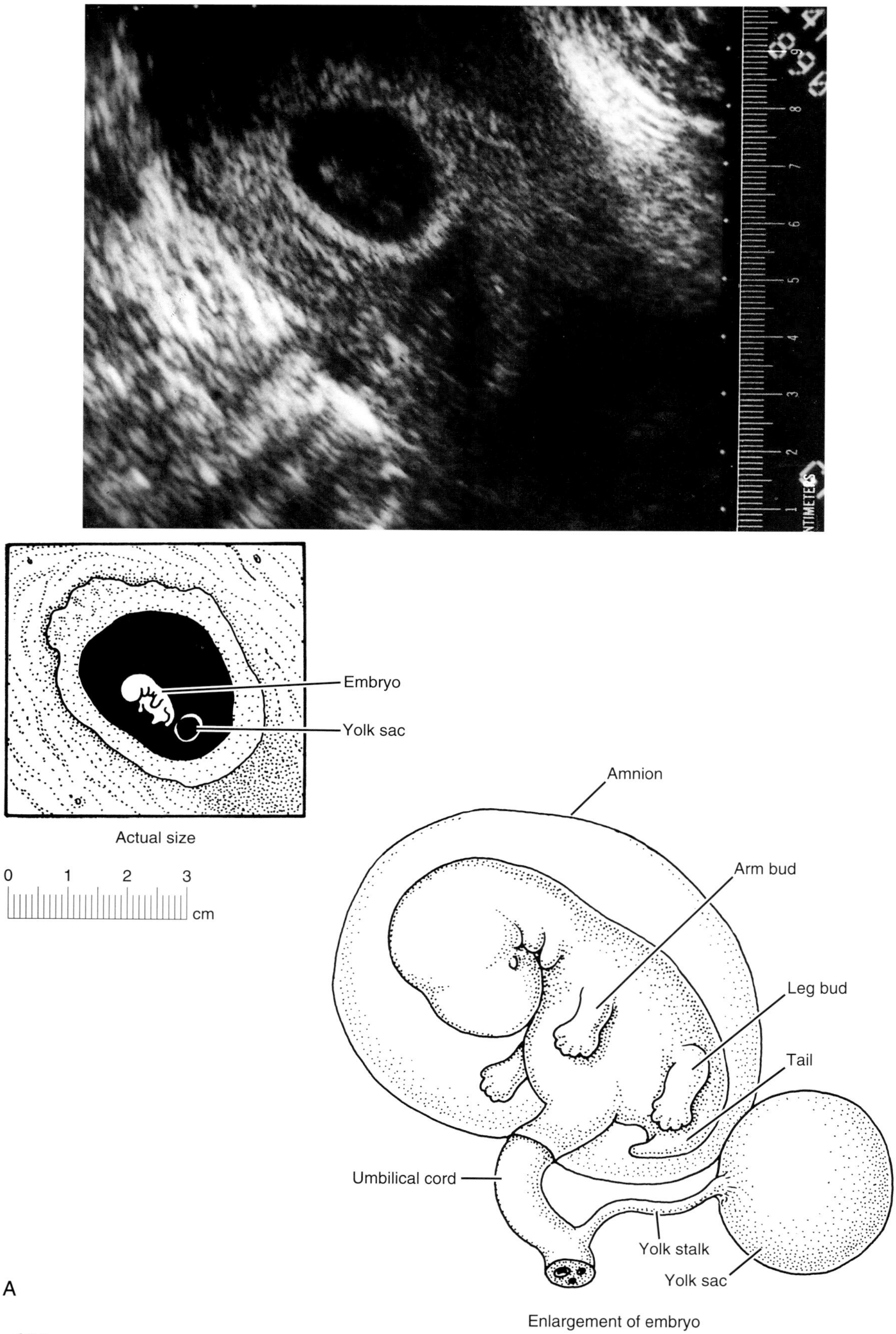

FIGURE 18–7 *See legend on opposite page*

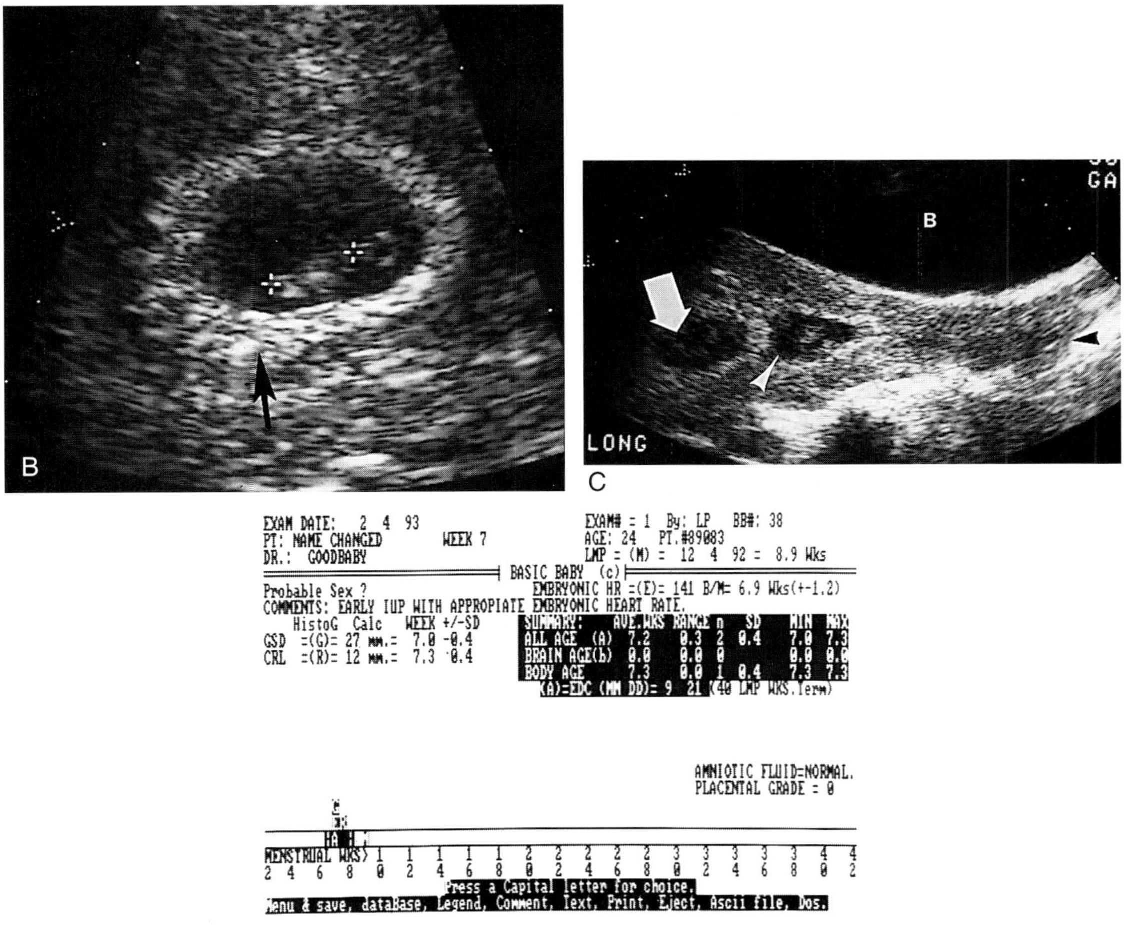

FIGURE 18–7.
A, A 1:1 life-size sonogram of a normal early 7-LMP-week pregnancy. The embryo and yolk sac can be seen in this transabdominal sonogram. *B,* The crown-rump length is being measured (+ cursors) at 10.2 mm. Note that the yolk sac is excluded from the measurement. The implantation site and thus the placental location can be predicted by the thicker part of the chorionic ring (arrow). *C,* Two hypoechoic areas are seen in the uterus. The large white arrow points to the chorionic cavity, which contained the live embryo (see A). The white arrowhead points to a second cavity, which was thought to be an organizing blood clot secondary to subchorionic bleeding. It is also possible that this could be a demised twin. The black arrowhead points to the external os of the cervix. The maternal bladder (B) is anterior to the uterus and vagina. *D,* This computer age range analysis has an average age of two fetal parameters (MFP) of 7.2 LMP weeks and a range of 0.4 weeks. The embryonic heart rate of 141 B/M evaluated to 6.9 LMP weeks.

weeks after conception), the embryo is clearly recognizable. The head, trunk, arms, and legs can be seen. The digits of the hands and feet are formed but are not yet complete. Figure 18–9*A* is a life-size sonogram of an early 8-LMP-week embryo.

It is easy to distinguish the head from the body in Figure 18–9*A* to *C*. The head is relatively large, as large as the body at this stage. In Figure 18–9*B*, a small appendage can be seen between the legs. This is not a penis but is the tail, which does not completely disappear until the end of the embryonic period in 2 more weeks.[38]

The amnion is easily seen with transvaginal sonography. The amniotic fluid should be anechoic, or clear of echoes. The extraembryonic coelom or chorionic cavity, which is the

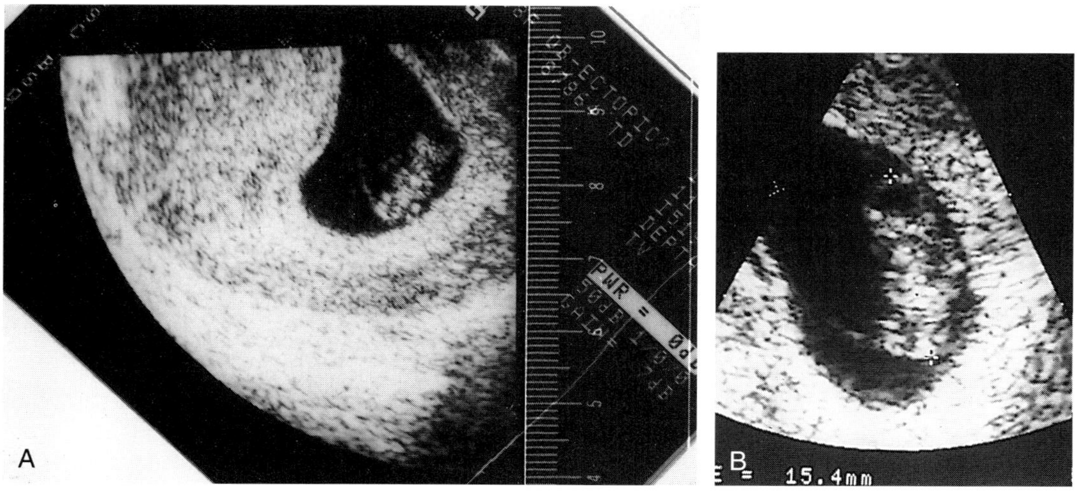

FIGURE 18–8.
A, A 1:1 life-size transvaginal sonogram of a normal late 7-LMP-week pregnancy. The embryo can be seen in coronal section. *B*, An enlargement of the embryo for the crown-rump length (CRL) measurement (15.4 mm). The rhombencephalon can be seen as an anechoic fluid cavity in the embryonic head.

space outside the amniotic membrane, normally contains diffuse echoes of the magma reticulare (discussed earlier) and becomes thinner and more spread out as the amniotic cavity begins to fill the chorionic cavity.

The rhombencephalon is still obvious in the posterior of the head (see Fig. 18–9*C*). This fluid space becomes the fourth ventricle as the hindbrain enlarges to fill it. This is one of the most sonographically distinctive features of the embryonic head during the eighth LMP week. This fluid cavity is, of course, normal and should not be mistaken for early hydrocephaly, meningocele, or other anomalies.

The spine can also be visualized sonographically during this week (Fig. 18–9*D*). The 8-LMP-week spine should appear as two parallel lines of echogenic dots.

The gut herniation into the umbilical cord is obvious as well during the 8th LMP week. In Figure 18–9*E*, this herniation can be seen as relatively lower-level echoes anterior to the more echogenic and circular abdomen. A short piece of the twisting cord is seen between the embryo and yolk sac (+ cursors). The yolk sac is outside the amniotic membrane.

As shown in Figure 18–9*E*, the umbilical cord is prominent during the eighth LMP week, although it is still too small to determine the number of umbilical cord vessels. The location of the placenta may also be suggested at this time (see Fig. 18–9*D*). However, it is too early to declare a placenta previa, even if a low-lying placenta is observed. This is because placental "migration," or trophotropism, often causes a low-lying placenta early in pregnancy to appear to move away from the internal os later in pregnancy[39] (see Chapter 17 for more on the cord and placenta).

MOVEMENT

The embryo becomes noticeably active during the LMP week 8 and can be observed to wiggle. These motions can be impressive.

The heart is also obvious now. The heartbeat is still accelerating and should be rapid, with a normal rate of 168 B/M early in the week to approximately 185 B/M at the end of the LMP week 8 (±15 B/M).[17] During this week, the EHR should not be less than 150 B/M in 95% of the population. A lower heart rate or one that is very irregular is not a favorable sign for the continuing pregnancy. It is at the end of the eighth and start of the ninth LMP week that the EHR abruptly stops accelerating.

SIZE/AGE

The CRL is still the most accurate estimator of dates for pregnancy during the eighth LMP week. Other measurements can be obtained, but because of their small size, their efficacy is questionable.

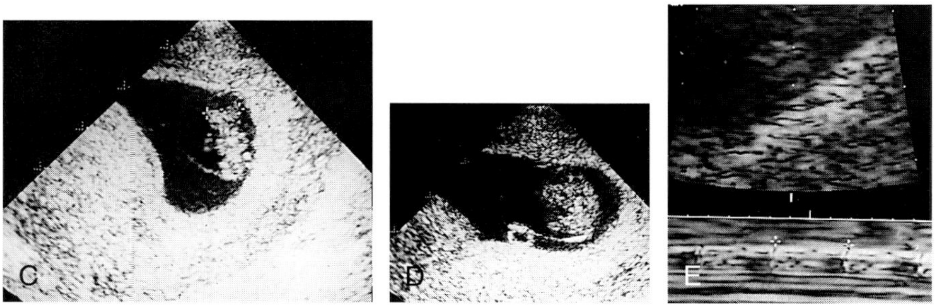

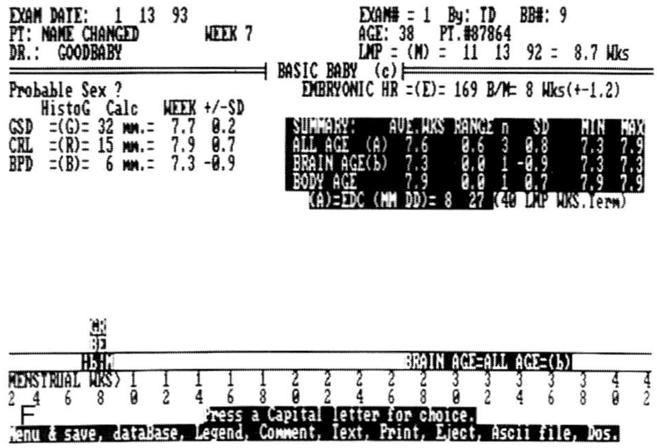

FIGURE 18–8 *Continued*
C, The embryo is clearly seen in coronal section. The + cursors are measuring the transverse head diameter or biparietal diameter (BPD= 5.6 mm). At this stage, the BPD is so small that any variance in cursor placement results in relatively large percent errors in age estimates. The CRL is the most accurate measurement for age at this time, followed by the embryonic heart rate (EHR) age. A portion of the amniotic membrane can be seen extending from the bottom of the embryo. The amniotic fluid around the embryo (inside the amnion) is clear and free of echoes, whereas the remainder of the chorionic cavity outside the amnion is filled with the gel of the magma reticulare, which is normally slightly echogenic. *D*, The amniotic membrane is clearly seen surrounding the embryo. The yolk sac is suspended in the gel of the magma reticulare outside the amnion. In this sagittal plane through the embryo, the rhombencephalon is seen as a hypoechoic area in the superior and posterior aspect of the head. *E*, The EHR is measured at 166 B/M and is normal for the late seventh and early eighth LMP weeks. EHR can be more accurately measured by using a fast M-mode sweep to elongate the beats and by placing the cursors at a sharp echo, as shown here. In this image, the + cursors measure one beat by being placed at the top of very narrow dark lines, which repeat in each beat of the M-mode. *F*, The age range analysis (ARA) has a mean age of 7.6 LMP weeks for three parameters and a range of 0.6 week. However, because the BPD is small and not normally measured at this time and because the CRL is the most accurate estimator of age, this embryonic age was placed at 7.9 LMP weeks based on the 15-mm CRL measurement. This was confirmed by the mean EHR of 169 B/M which evaluated to 8.0 LMP weeks. Even with the BPD and gestational sac diameter measurements, the range of ages was still within ±2 SD for range.

At this early age, most parameters may be measured when using transvaginal transducers. However, the femoral length (FemL) and humeral length (HumL) are simply bright spots (echoes) in the proximal portion of the extremity. In 7600 consecutive obstetrical sonographic examinations, three femurs and humeri were measured during the eighth menstrual week. The femurs measured between 2.4 and 3.9 mm, and the humeri measured between 2.1 and 3 mm. Because these parameters are so small, any slight variation in cursor placement results in very large percent errors; therefore, the clinical utility of measuring very small parameters is questionable.

In our example of a fetus in the eighth LMP week, five parameter age estimates were made (Fig. 18–9G). The greatest GSD underestimated the age at 7.8 weeks. The CRL and transverse head circumference were only 0.2 week apart or approximately 1.4 days different, at 8.3 and 8.5 weeks, respectively. The BPD was measured and found to be relatively

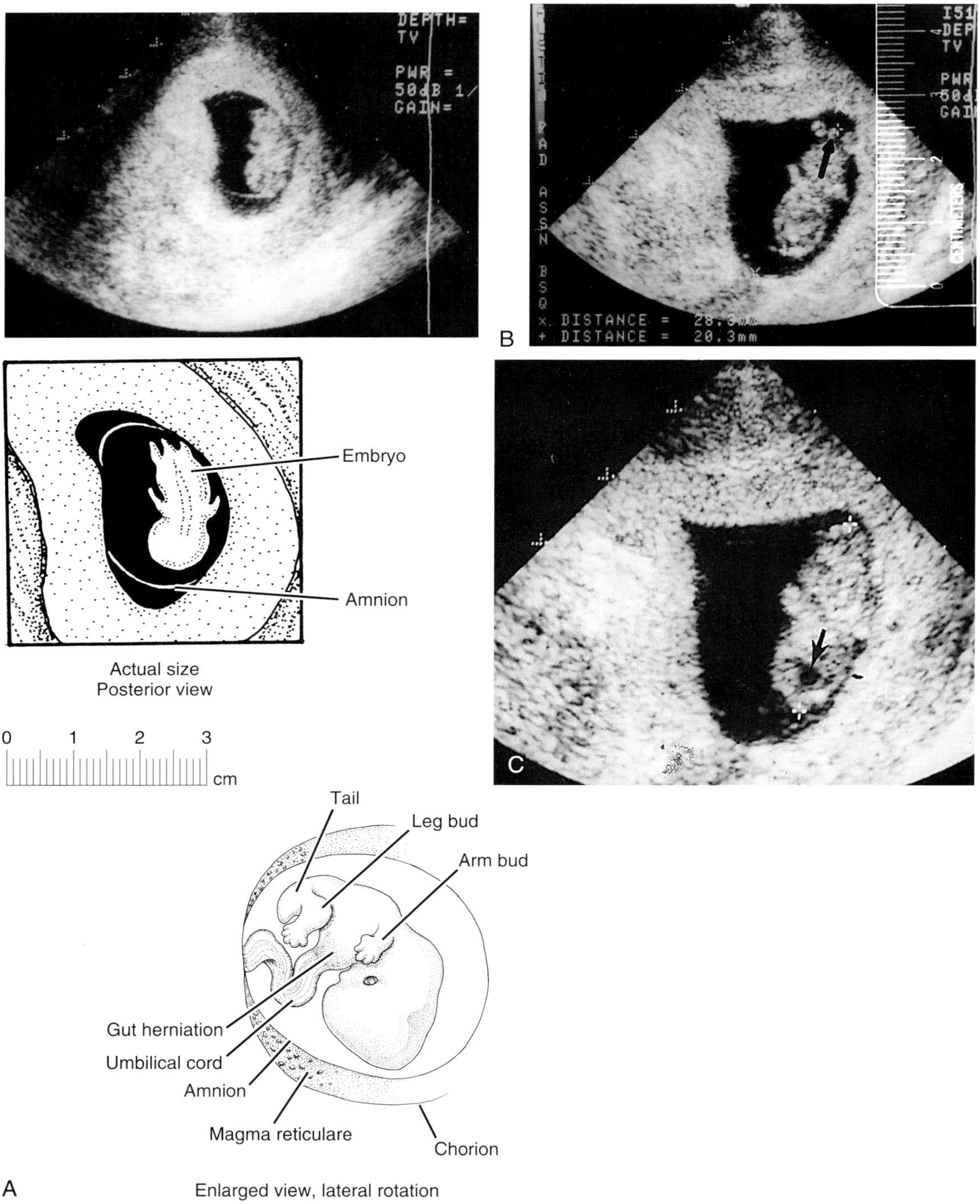

FIGURE 18–9.
A, Transvaginal sonogram of a normal 8.3-LMP week pregnancy. The embryo, amnion, chorion, and magma reticulare can be seen. *B*, The embryo is shown life-size in a coronal plane through the anterior head and body. The head is down, and the arrow points to the embryonic tail between the leg buds. The arms can also be distinguished. The arrow is on the embryonic abdomen. The + cursors measure the crown-rump length (CRL) at 18.3 mm. Note the relative sizes of the embryonic head and trunk. *C*, This coronal image is more posterior in the embryo and shows the rhombencephalon (arrow). The CRL measures 21.0 mm, just 0.7 mm more than in the previous image. The arms can be seen to extend to either side of the thorax.

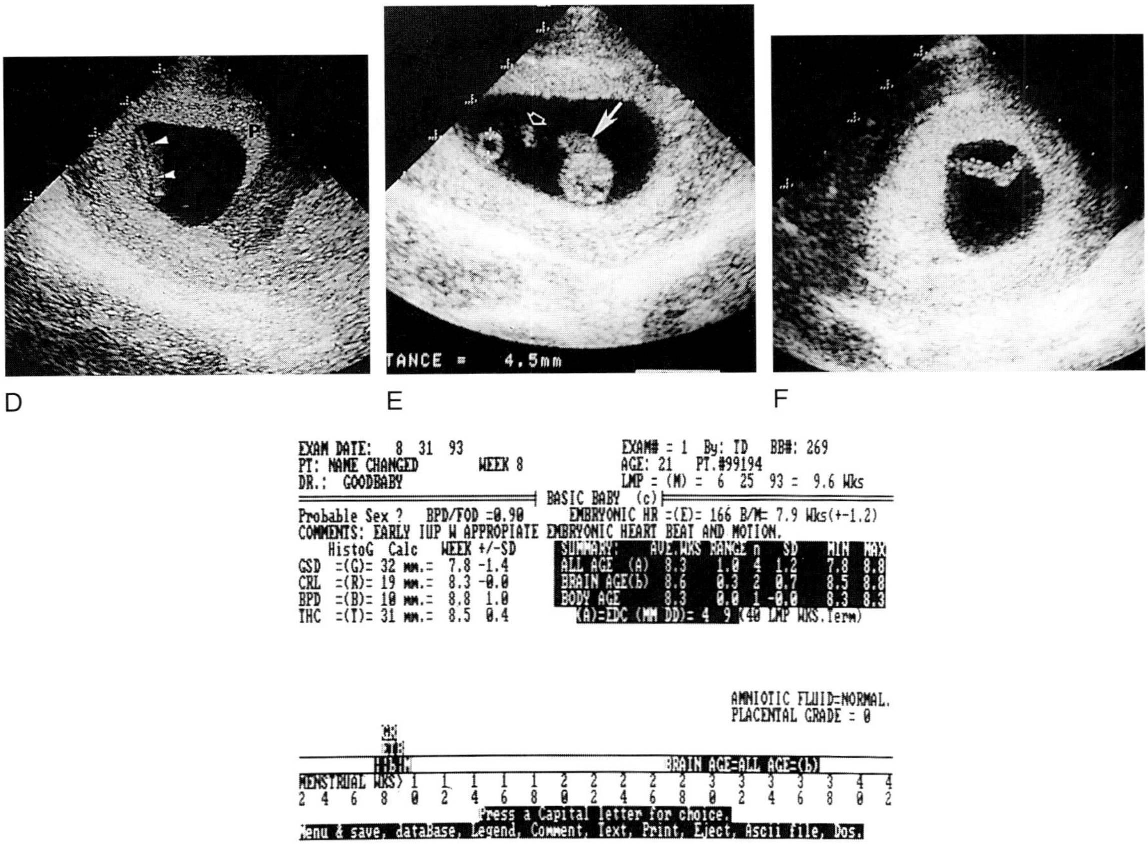

FIGURE 18–9 *Continued*
D, This coronal plane is through the posterior embryo and shows the double lines of echoes of the developing spine (arrowheads). The placenta (P) is seen as an echogenic layer around the chorionic cavity. *E*, A transvaginal sonogram of the transverse embryonic abdomen at the insertion of the umbilical cord. The midgut herniation into the cord (white arrow) is seen anterior to the abdomen. If abdominal measurements are taken at this time, they should exclude this gut herniation. A portion of the umbilical cord can be seen as a collection of echoes (open arrow). The yolk sac is measured at 4.5 mm and is normal. *F*, The umbilical cord is clearly seen. Although it is difficult to determine the number of vessels in this cord, the use of high-resolution endovaginal color Doppler may help in this endeavor if indicated. *G*, In this computer age range analysis, the mean age of four parameters is 8.3 LMP weeks, with a range of 1.0 week The embryonic heart rate of 166 B/M evaluated to 7.9 LMP weeks, still within ±2 SD for range (see Chapter 7).

large (10 mm) at 8.8 weeks of age. These four parameter ages averaged to a mean age of 8.3 weeks, which was exactly the same age as that from the CRL estimate. The EHR was 166 B/M, which evaluated to an LMP age of 7.9 weeks {LMP age = (EHR × 0.3)+6}, ± 8 days. Because the EHR age was only 0.4 weeks (3 days) less than the average and CRL age, the heart rate was considered normal. The range of ages was 1 week (8.8 to 7.8), or less than 2 SD, and therefore normal (see Chapter 7 for more on ARA).

If abdominal circumference (AC) measurements are desired, they should not include the umbilical herniation. In this case, the abdominal diameters measured 10.3 × 9.9 mm (not shown).

Because the embryonic parameters appeared normal and because all age estimates were within about 1 week of the LMP age, this pregnancy was considered normal (at this writing, term is still 7 months away). If clinical signs, such as maternal bleeding, required further investigation, a follow-up sonographic examination could confirm fetal viability.

LMP Week 9

OBSERVATIONS

In the ninth LMP week (seventh week after ovulation and conception), the embryo is more obvious, even transabdominally (Fig. 18–10). At this time, it is easy to distinguish sagittal and coronal sections through the long axis of the embryo (see Fig. 18–10*A* and *B*).

Figure 18–10*A* is a sagittal view and Figure 18–10*B* is the same embryo in the coronal view. The embryo is 9.3 LMP weeks by the average of seven embryonic parameters and the greatest GSD.

In Figure 18–10*B*, the interhemispheric fissure or midline of the brain is clearly visible. In this image, it can also be observed that the placenta is forming anteriorly. This figure is life-size. The interhemispheric fissure is less clearly seen in the transverse image in Figure 18–10*D* owing to the slightly oblique angle between the sonic beam and the fissure. The rhombencephalon can still be seen in the posterior cranium in Figure 18–10*A*.

The yolk sac can be faintly seen near the embryonic head in Figure 18–10*C* and *D*. The yolk sac and amniotic membrane are more difficult to image transabdominally than transvaginally. Parts of the amniotic membrane can be seen emerging from behind the embryo's head and abdomen in Figure 18–10*D* and *E*.

The umbilical cord is shown in Figure 18–10*C* as it emerges from the umbilical herniation in the abdominal wall just below. The umbilical cord and umbilical gut herniation are more clearly seen in the transverse view of the abdomen in Figure 18–10*E*. It is still difficult to determine the number of umbilical vessels at this early age, especially transabdominally. Color Doppler in the transvaginal approach might occasionally be able to demonstrate the number of umbilical vessels in the ninth LMP week.

MOVEMENT

The embryo becomes more active in the ninth week. The heartbeat is still the most obvious motion, but subtle, isolated arm or leg motions may occasionally be detected.[36] In general, vigorous motion is considered a favorable sign.

The EHR reaches its peak of approximately 170 B/M early in the ninth week.[25] In the first half of this week, EHRs between 150 and 190 B/M are considered normal (±2 SD). The EHR appears to peak on day 63 after the LMP, which is the first day of the ninth week, at a mean of approximately 177 B/M with a normal range (±2 SD) of 160 to 192 B/M. This is the fastest rate an embryo normally exhibits. After this peak, the heart rate abruptly stops its acceleration and slowly declines until term.[17]

It should be noted here that the EHR should never be less than 150 B/M at any time during the ninth LMP week, when using the CRL to determine the age. That is, when the CRL is between 25 and 31 mm, the heart rate should never be less than 150 B/M in 95% of the population. With normal heart rates as high as 190 B/M, a sonographer should never attempt to count the beats visually while watching the sonographic image with one eye and a clock with the other eye. This method produces large errors and may give the observer a headache. M-mode is the only accurate way to measure EHRs that are this rapid.

The EHR is easily measured in Figure 18–10*F* at 179 B/M. This is a normal heart rate at LMP week 9.

SIZE/AGE

Many measurements can be made of the various embryonic parameters during the ninth LMP week. Although the CRL remains the most accurate for age at this stage, the AC and several head measurements are also available.

Multiple GSDs (or chorionic cavity measurements) averaged 52 mm, or approximately 9.6 LMP weeks. This measurement, along with the AC and EHR age, were the most inaccurate but only slightly.

The CRL is most accurate because it is the largest embryonic measurement and therefore produces the smallest percent errors. The CRL increases from about 23 or 25 mm at the start of the ninth week to about 31 or 32 mm at the end of the week, depending on the report.

In the example offered here, the mean CRL measurement was 27 mm or approximately 9.2 weeks. Two of the CRL measurements used to arrive at this mean are shown in Figure 18–10*A* and *C*.

Figure 18–10*B* and *D* shows four cranial

measurements being taken. The vertical cranial diameter and hippocampal base line are measured in the coronal view of the embryo in Figure 18–10*B*. The BPD and the fronto-occipital diameter in the transverse view of the head are shown in Figure 18–10*D*. These, along with the sides of the equilateral triangle from Figure 18–10*B*, produced five different cranial age estimations shown in the computer printout of Figure 18–10*G*. These five cranial age estimations were averaged to produce a brain age of 9.1 LMP weeks with a range of 0.2 weeks.

In Figure 18–10*E* the AC is measured using the cursor ellipse-drawing function. The umbilical gut herniation is excluded at the top of the ellipse. The AC mean measurement was 36 mm or approximately 9.7 weeks.

In Figure 18–10*G*, the ARA put all eight parameters at less than ± 1.0 SD from the average age of 9.3 LMP weeks, well within a normal range. The EHR age at 8.5 LMP weeks is at −1.7 SD below the mean age, still within the normal ±2 SD. At less than 6 days below the average age, the EHR age is well within the ± 1.2 weeks (8 days), which represents the 5th and 95th percentiles.

The embryo in this case is at or slightly beyond the normal peak of the acceleration phase of the EHR; therefore, the EHR age estimate is low but the EHR is normal. This is because the EHR regression should not be used after the EHR peaks by the start of the ninth LMP week.[17] At this point and thereafter, the heart rate tends to decline until term. This slowing of the heart rate is more rapid from the ninth week until about the LMP week 15, and then it is more gradual and variable to term (see Chapter 12 for detailed discussion of the embryonic and fetal heart rates).

LMP Week 10

OBSERVATIONS

LMP week 10 (eighth week after conception) is the end of the embryonic stage of life. By the end of the 10th LMP week, a fetus has a distinct human appearance.[8] After this week, the developing human is called a fetus. Figure 18–11 shows an embryo in the very late 9th or early 10th LMP week.

Figure 18–11*A* and *B* shows an embryo reclining in a supine position in the dependent portion of the amniotic/chorionic cavities in the early 10th week. The amnion is not well demonstrated in these transabdominal images. Only a portion of the amniotic membrane is shown as a bright line of echoes in Figure 18–11*E*, just posterior to the embryonic body. The size of the uterus and gestational sac is normal; therefore, the quantity of amniotic fluid is considered normal also. The umbilical gut herniation is well demonstrated in this first image.

Figure 18–11*A* shows measurement of the CRL in the sagittal plane of the embryo. The yolk sac can be observed at the top of the head. The umbilical cord is shown near the front of the embryonic forehead as a series of parallel lines. Three umbilical vessels can be counted as spaces between four of these lines.

A transverse view of the fetal head is shown in Figure 18–11*C*, which is a transverse plane through the uterus. The developing placenta is shown as a hyperechogenic area on the maternal left uterine wall. The echoes extending anterior to the head in this image are the umbilical cord, which is more clearly seen in Figure 18–11*B*.

Figure 18–11*D* is a coronal view of the head. The echogenic area at the base of the head is the developing facial structures.

MOVEMENT

In LMP week 10, some sonographers have reported observing the onset of breathing motions and independent limb movements.[40] The embryo is noticeably active, with occasional body flexions and extensions; however, the heartbeat is still the most obvious movement.

The EHR in Figure 18–11*E* was measured at 172 B/M. This is slightly less than the LMP week 9 example. This EHR decelerates fairly rapidly for the next 5 weeks and then levels in a slow decline with more beat-to-beat variability toward term.

SIZE/AGE

By the 10th LMP week, most normally accepted parameters can be measured. However, the smaller parameters are still questionable owing to the large percent errors that

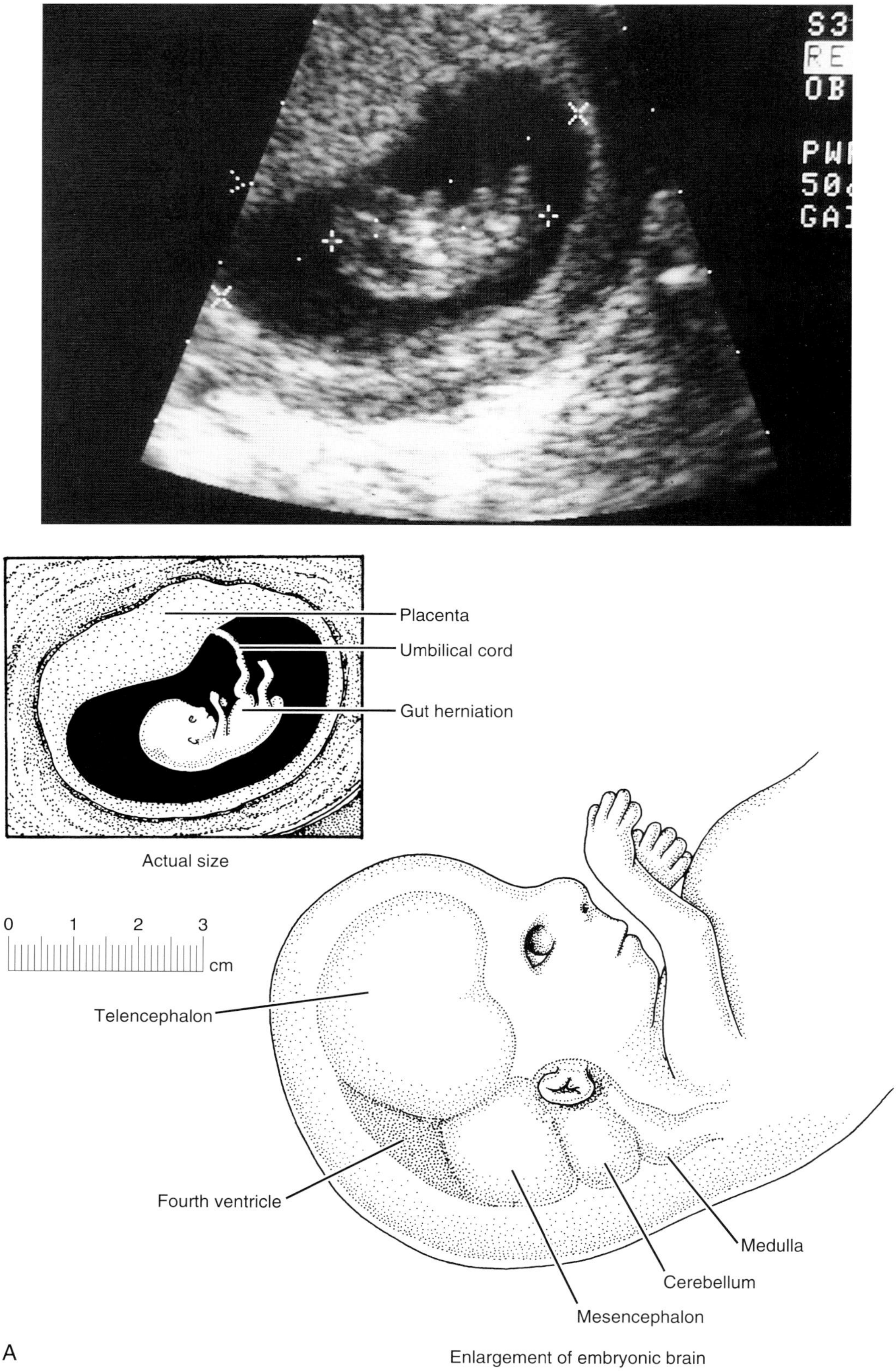

FIGURE 18–10

A, Sonogram showing a sagittal plane through the embryo at 9.3 LMP weeks. The drawings show corresponding anatomy. *B,* A 1:1 scale image of the coronal plane through the embryo. The midcoronal head can be observed to be circular in this plane, and the interhemispheric fissure of the brain can be seen (arrow) between the X cursors. In this im-

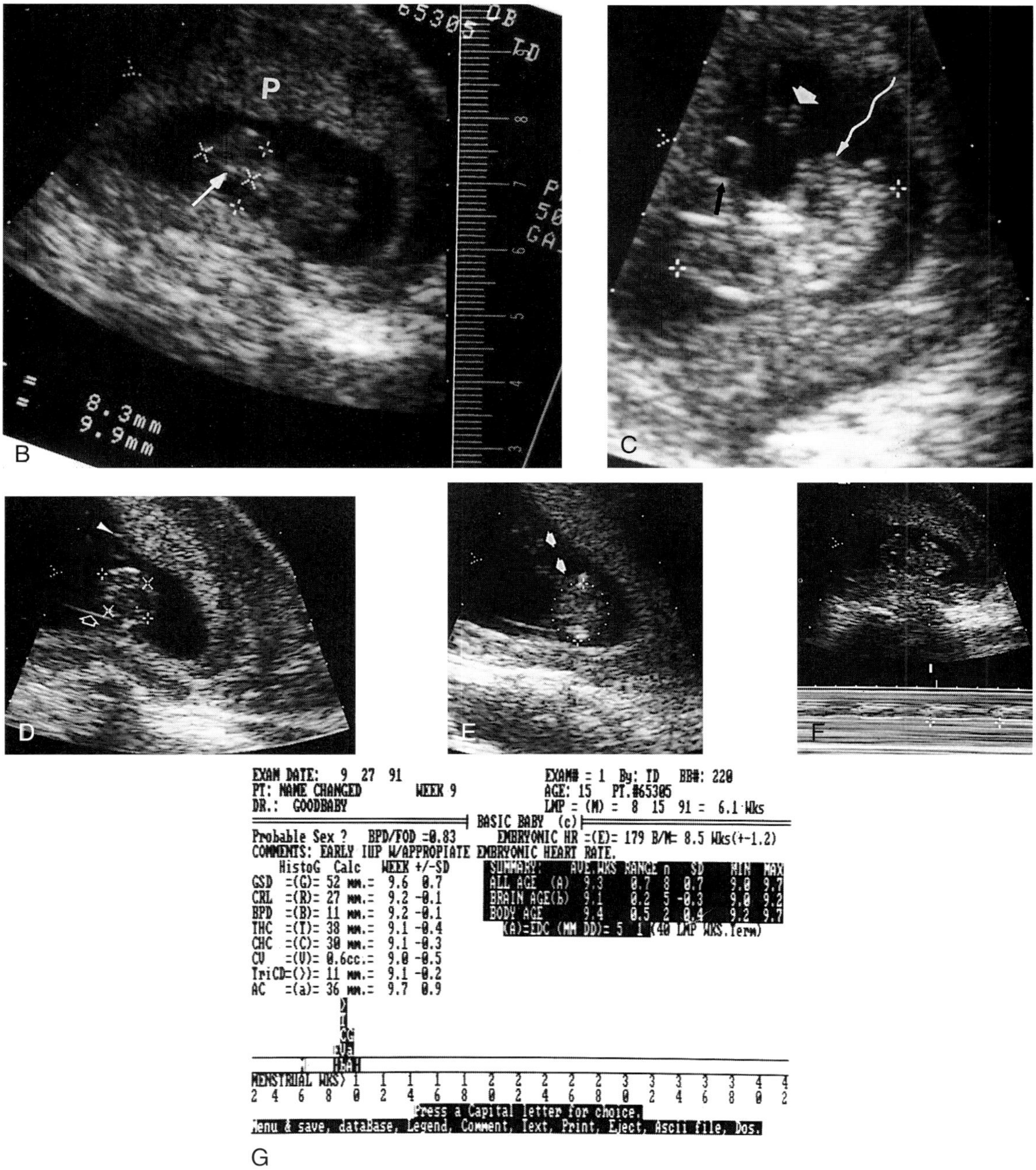

FIGURE 18–10 *Continued*
age, the coronal triangle of the head is measured; the + cursors measure the hippocampal base line (HBL), which is the base of the coronal triangle, and the X cursors measure the vertical cranial diameter from the mid-HBL to the vertex of the calvarium. The placenta (P) is seen anteriorly. *C*, A sagittal plane through the 9.3-week embryo. The crown-rump length is measured between the + cursors at 28.4 mm. The yolk sac (black arrow on the embryonic head) was excluded from the measurement. The gut herniation into the umbilical cord (wavy white arrow) and free loops of cord (solid white arrow) are seen. *D*, This image is perpendicular to B and shows the transverse head circumference (THC). The THC is normally called simply the head circumference. However, because this text discusses the head in three dimensions, it is necessary to distinguish the THC from the coronal head circumference. The X cursors measure the biparietal diameter at 10.3 mm, and the + cursors measure the fronto-occipital diameter at 13.6 mm. This produces a normal transverse cephalic index of 0.83. The interhemispheric fissure is seen as a line extending between the + cursors. The amniotic membrane (open arrow) can still be seen, as can the yolk sac (arrowhead). *E*, This image shows the measurement of the transverse abdomen. An ellipse-drawing function was used because all edges of the abdomen were not clearly seen. The gut herniation into the umbilical cord was excluded. Free loops of the umbilical cord are seen (arrows). *F*, This M-mode of the embryonic heart rate (EHR) measured 179 B/M. This very rapid heart rate is normal in the ninth menstrual week. This is at the time when the heart rate peaks and begins a slow decline to term. In this week, the EHR should normally be greater than 150 B/M. *G*, In the 9th LMP week, a large number of parameters become available. In this case, eight parameters produce an average age of 9.3 LMP weeks with a range of 0.7 week. This is well within ±1 SD for range at this time.

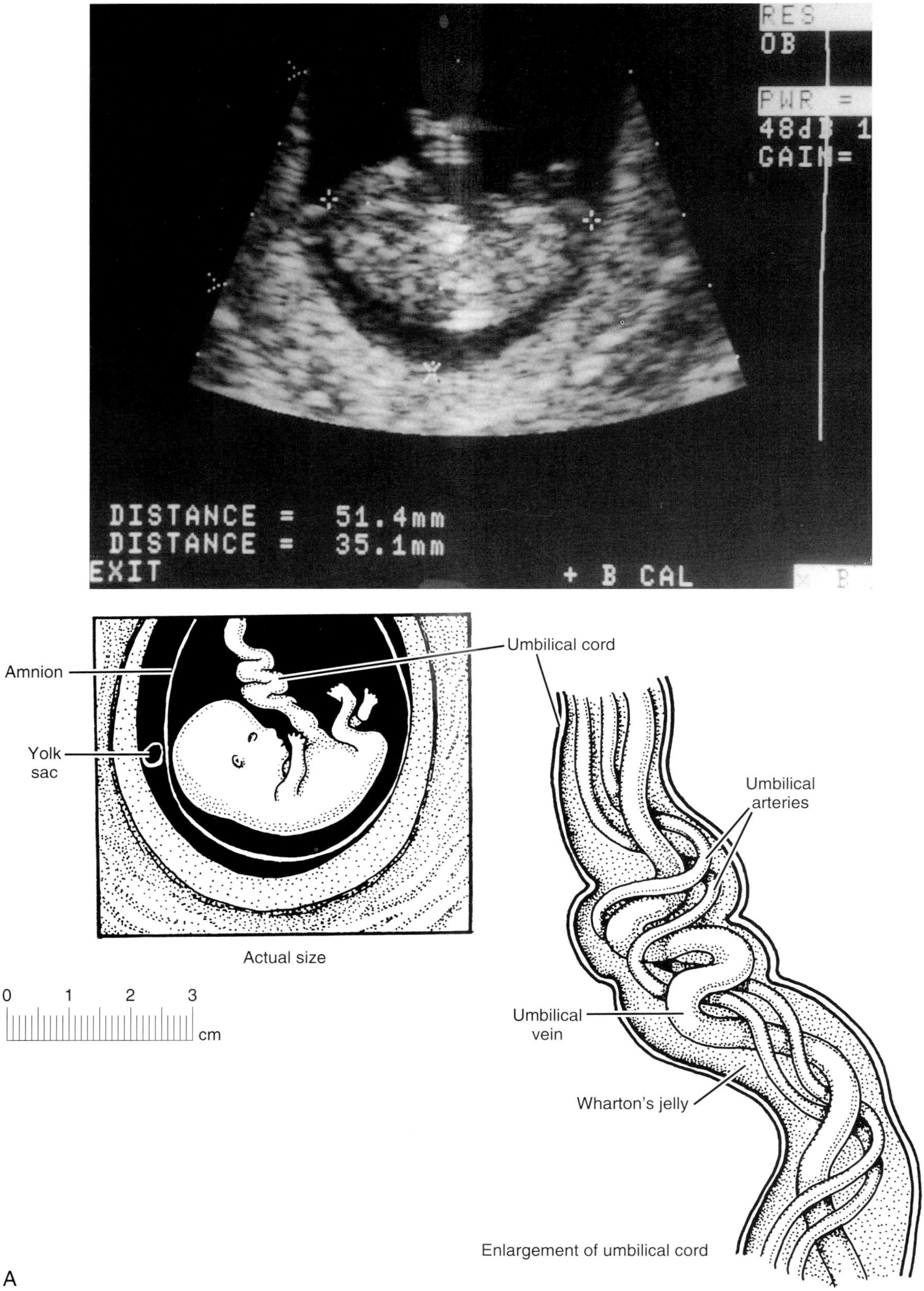

A

FIGURE 18–11.
A, Sagittal plane through a 10.0-LMP-week embryo. This is the last week of the embryonic period. The crown-rump length is being measured between the + cursors at 35.1 mm, excluding the yolk sac. The life-size drawing shows corresponding anatomy. The umbilical cord anatomy is also illustrated.

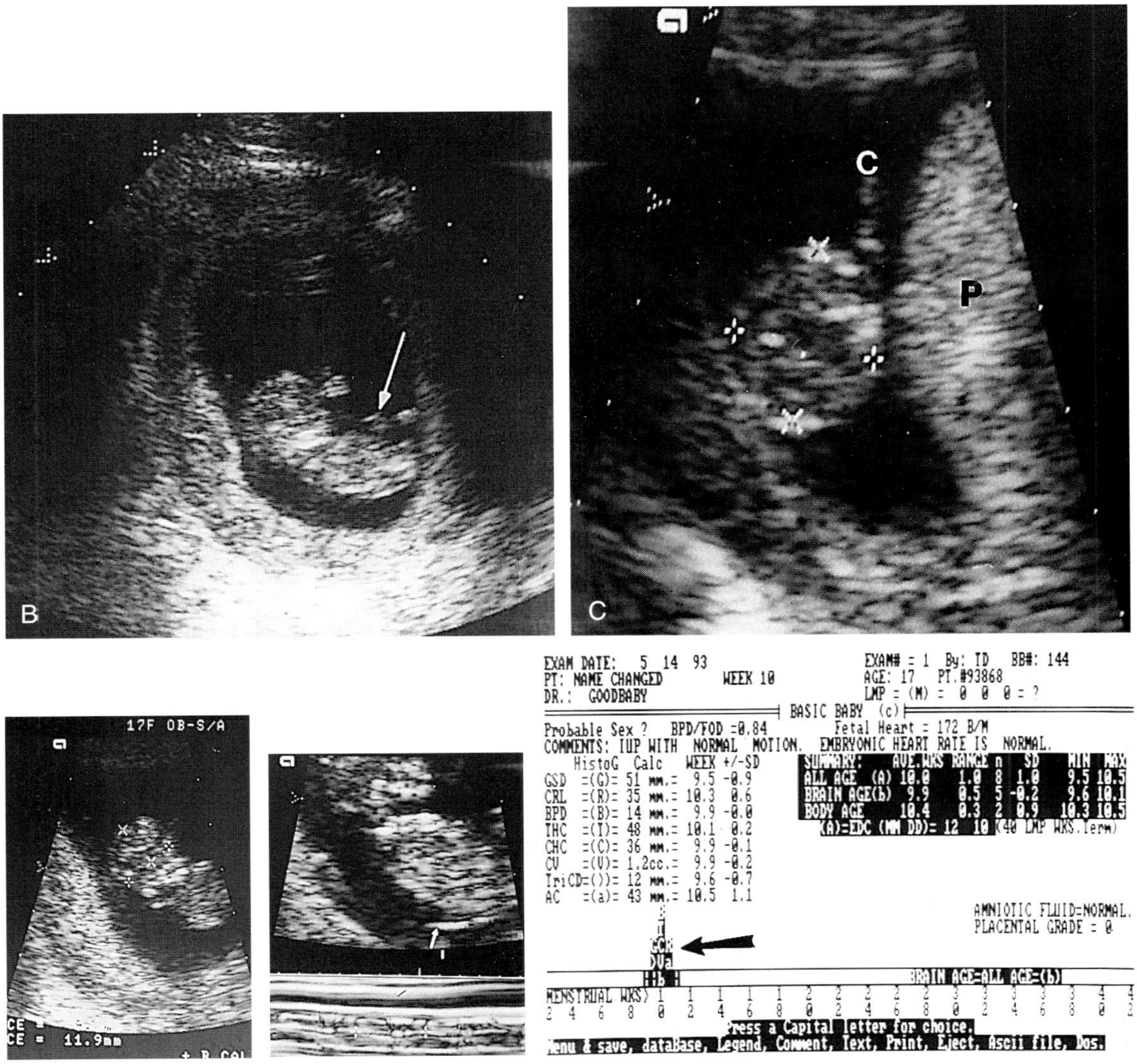

D E F

FIGURE 18–11 *Continued*
B, Sagittal plane through the uterus demonstrating the chorionic cavity and embryo. This is also a sagittal plane in the embryo and shows the gut herniation into the umbilical cord (arrow). *C,* The familiar transverse head circumference (THC) with the fronto-occipital diameter (FOD) measured at 14.5 mm and the biparietal diameter at 13.8 mm. A portion of the umbilical cord (C) can be seen in front of the skull, as can the placenta (P). *D,* A midcoronal image of the head. The + cursors measure the hippocampal base line and the X cursors measure the vertical cranial diameter at 11.9 and 9.3 mm, respectively. These measurements, along with the biparietal diameter and FOD, are used by the computer program to calculate cranial volume and other cranial parameters. *E,* The embryonic heart rate is measured at 172 B/M. This heart rate is past the peak and starting its normal decline toward term. A small portion of the amniotic membrane (arrow) is shown. *F,* In this case, eight parameters produced an average age of 10.0 LMP weeks with a range of 1.0 week. The parameters all are within ± 1 SD of the mean, with the exception of the abdominal circumference (AC), which is at +1.1 SD. The time-series symbol histogram (arrow) forms a normal bell curve that is narrow and peaked (leptokurtic), with the mean at 10.0 menstrual weeks.

they produce. In the population mentioned earlier (10,000+ consecutive obstetrical examinations), both the FemL and HumL were measured during the 10th week in 11 cases. All FemL measurements were between 3 and 4.6 mm, and all the HumL measurements were between 3 and 4 mm.

The CRL is still the largest and most accurate embryonic parameter available during this week. Figure 18–11*A* shows the CRL measurement at 35.1 mm. The GSD in this figure measured 51.4 mm; however, the GSD is affected by uterine morphology and maternal bladder pressure and therefore is less reliable for estimating age this late in the first trimester.

Figure 18–11*C* and 18–11*D* shows the transverse and coronal head measurements, respectively. The abdominal measurements are not shown in this case.

The average age was 10.0 LMP weeks in this case (see Fig. 18–11*F*). This is a normal embryo, and in the next week it will be a fetus.

LMP Week 11

OBSERVATIONS

In LMP week 11, the ninth week of gestation, the fetus is large enough to measure most parameters that are in common use for size/age estimations. Figure 18–12*A* shows an oblique coronal view of a fetus in the late 11th LMP week.

In this week, the uterus is still small enough to be viewed in its entirety with long linear array transducers. Figure 18–12*B* is a long-axis image of the uterus and was generated using a 12-cm linear array transducer with a correspondingly large field of view. In this image, the maternal bladder, vagina, and uterine fundus are visualized. The uterine cervix is also included but is not clearly appreciated owing to through-transmission or posterior enhancement of the sound beam passing through the maternal bladder, as well as shadowing from the anterior uterovesical wall. The posterior uterine wall is cut off at the cephalic edge of the field of view.

Figure 18–12*B* shows the chorionic cavity (gestational sac), and a transverse section of the fetal head with the occiput posterior. Figure 18–12*C* is transverse through the uterus but is a long-axis sagittal view of the supine fetus, which has its head to the maternal right. Again the occiput is posterior. The placental location can be appreciated in both images. In Figure 18–12*B*, the placenta is in the posterior fundal portion of the uterus, and in Figure 18–12*C*, the placenta is seen on the maternal right side of the uterus. Therefore, it can be deduced that this placental location is posterior, fundal, and extending to the maternal right side of the uterus.

The yolk sac can still be seen in Figure 18–12*D* and *E*, adjacent to the fetal head. Figure 18–12*E* was generated to demonstrate that this truly was the yolk sac and not a meningocele, because Figure 18–12*D*, which was useful for the CRL measurement, did not clearly separate the yolk sac from the head. In Figure 18–12*D*, portions of the spine, arm, and leg can be appreciated.

Figure 18–12*F* is another image of the transverse head circumference with BPD (+ cursors) and fronto-occipital diameter (X cursors) measurements. The head in this image is strongly echogenic because the sound beam is enhanced by passing through the amniotic fluid. This image is from a sector transducer from the same point of view as Figure 18–12*B*; however, during a hiatus of approximately 9 minutes, the fetal head rotated with the occiput more toward the maternal head, providing a transverse view of the head with the midline almost perpendicular to the beam.

In Figure 18–12*G*, the fetal abdominal diameters are being measured. The spine can be seen posteriorly. The small horizontal echoes just anterior to the abdomen are from the umbilical cord.

Figure 18–12*H* and *I* shows measurement of the extremities. Although it is recognized that these measurements are actually of the bone diaphysis and exclude the extreme ends of the bones, they are commonly referred to as the FemL and HumL in the literature. This is an accepted misnomer. In Figure 18–12*I*, small echoes from the umbilical cord are seen anterior to the abdomen, and some small echoes in front of the fetal face are from the hand.

In Figure 18–12*J*, the fetal mandible and maxilla can be seen. The early development of the parietal and occipital plates can also be observed.

MOVEMENT

A fetus is often active during the 11th week, and its movements are clearly evident. In a normal fetus, they include jumping, arm and leg movements, and the beating of the heart, of course. Jaw movements have been documented during the 11th menstrual week.[40]

Rotation of the head is documented in the change of position between Figure 18–12*F* and *B* (*F* was actually recorded 9 minutes before *B*).

The heart rate continues to decelerate slowly during the 11th LMP week, from a mean of 162 B/M to approximately 158 B/M at the end of the week. The mean heart rate in LMP week 11 should be 160 B/M, with a range for 95% of the population between 176 and 145 B/M.

The heart rate is measured by M-mode in Figure 18–12*K* at 157 B/M. This is well within the normal range at this age.

SIZE/AGE

In the 11th LMP week, the fetus is complete in its parts. The remainder of the pregnancy is spent in increasing the size or mass of the organs. Growth of the organs does not continue at the same rates. The head, which is still relatively large in the 11th week, grows more slowly than the body. This differential growth brings a fetus to more normal proportions at birth, with the body being larger than the head.

The upper portions of the embryo tend to develop somewhat in advance of the lower body parts.[41] In a large population, the average HumL normally but not always exceeds that of the femur until about the 16th menstrual week. This difference in size is demonstrated in Figure 18–12*H* and *I*. In the former image, the HumL measures 6.9 mm, whereas in the latter the FemL measures only 6.6 mm (see Chapter 15 for more discussion on this topic).

Figure 18–12*L* is an example of a computer printout for an 11-LMP-week fetus. All six parameters are within ± 2 SD of the mean age of 11.9 LMP weeks. In this case, six parameter age estimates were made, with the range of ages being between 11.1 and 12.5. This fetus was considered normal at this time; however, at this writing, delivery has not yet occurred.

The CRL is still a useful measurement for estimating fetal age during this week. This is true for only about 2 more weeks, however, because after 14 weeks, a fetus exceeds many transducers' fields of view and fetal torso flexion and extension introduce more variability in the linear measurement of the CRL.

LMP Week 12

OBSERVATIONS

Week 12 after the LMP (week 10 after conception) is the end of the first trimester. All organs are present, and the major changes in the fetus are increases in mass. During this early fetal period, the head is still relatively larger than the body, but the body begins a rapid growth spurt in comparison with the head (Fig. 18–13*A*). The amnion is infrequently observed during the 12th or subsequent weeks. The placental location can be established at this time, but a low-lying placenta may still migrate away from the internal os (see Chapter 16 for more on the placenta).

In Figure 18–13*B*, the lower uterine segment is shown with a posterior, low-lying placenta. Although this placenta appears to approach the internal os, it does not appear to cross the os and therefore should be of little concern unless vaginal bleeding or spotting occurs. The placenta is also seen in Figure 18–13*C*, but because the internal os is not demonstrated, little more than the posterior position could be concluded from this image alone.

In Figure 18–13*C* to *G*, a normal amount of amniotic fluid is appreciated. No satisfactory methods have yet been developed for quantitating the amount of amniotic fluid, especially during the first half of the pregnancy. A sonographer must still rely primarily on experience for making this subjective judgment.

Figure 18–13*C* shows a coronal section of the cranium and spine. The proximal portion of the central canal of the spinal cord can be observed extending into the cervical portion of the neck.

MOVEMENT

A fetus is strongly active at this time. Independent arm and leg movements as well as rotation of the head are observed.[40] A fetus can change position now. The hands may be observed to touch the face and head, an activity that occupies much of a fetus's time until after birth.

Text continued on page 424

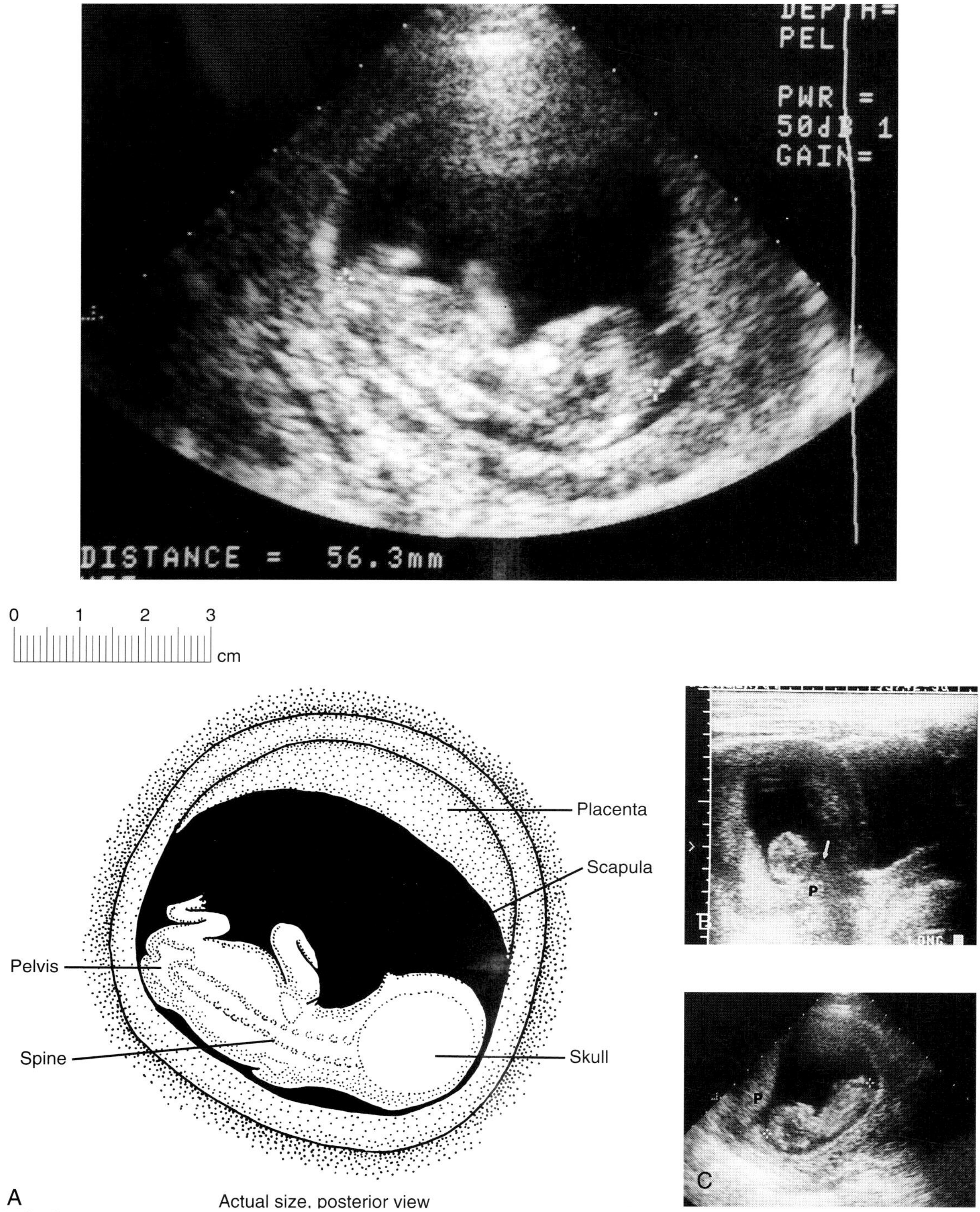

FIGURE 18–12.
A, An obliquely coronal plane of an 11.9-LMP-week fetus. This is the first week of fetal life. In this image, the crown-rump length (CRL) measures 56.3 mm. The drawing shows corresponding anatomy. *B*, A transabdominal sagittal plane through the uterus with a linear array transducer. The vagina and cervix can be observed. The placenta (P) is posterior to the fetal head and comes near the internal os of the cervix (arrow) but does not appear to cross the os. *C*, This image is perpendicular to that in *B*. The fetus is supine, and the CRL measures 58.9 between the + cursors. The placenta (P) is seen on the maternal right. Therefore, using this image and *B*, the placental location can be said to be posterior and to the right side of the uterus.

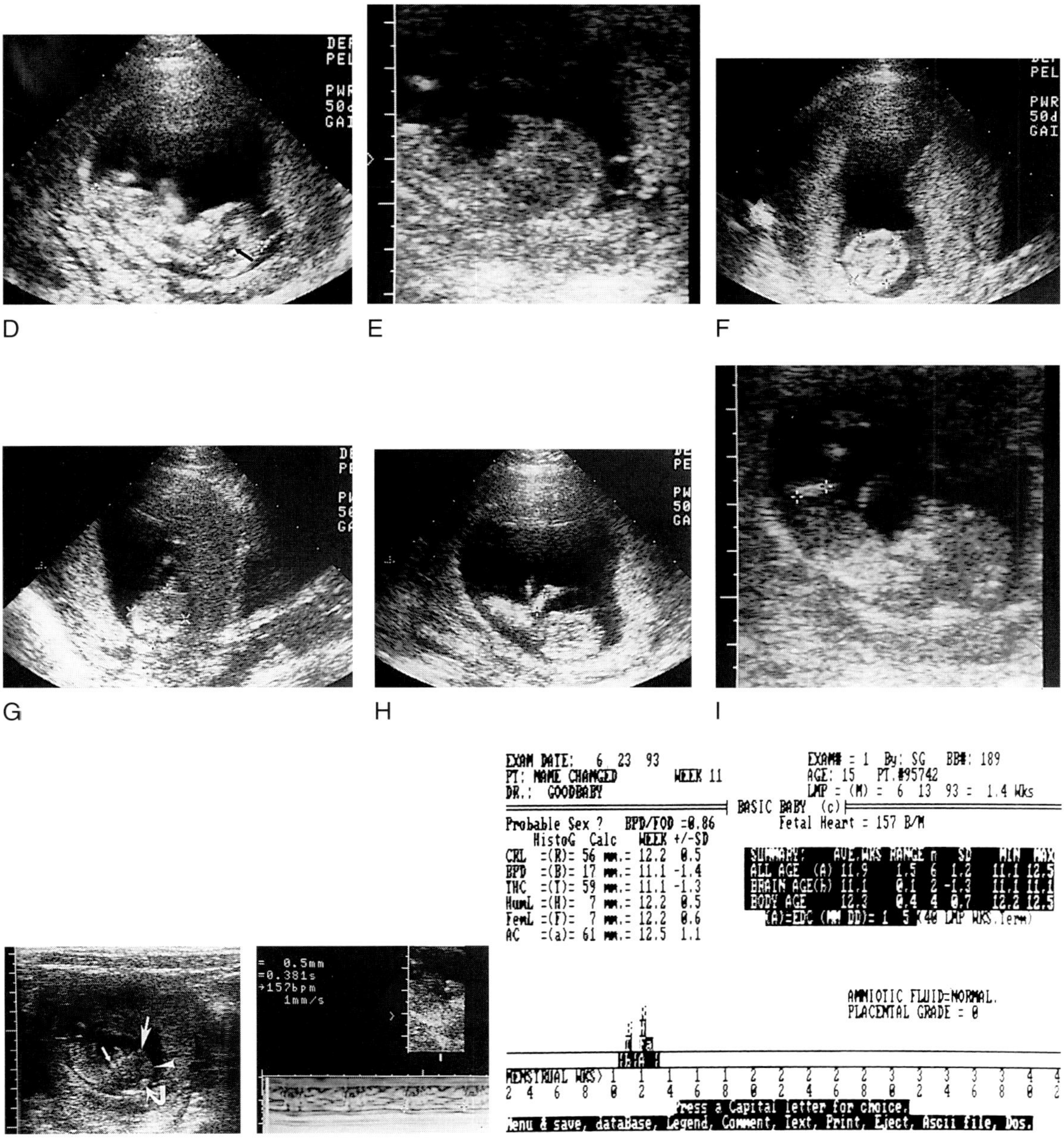

D E F G H I J K L

FIGURE 18–12 *Continued*
D, In this obliquely coronal plane, the CRL was measured (+ cursors) at 56.3 mm. The yolk sac is excluded at the top of the head. The rhombencephalon (arrow) is seen to be smaller than it was in earlier weeks, relative to the size of the cranium. *E*, This image was made to show the yolk sac as clearly separate from the fetal head. This was not as clear in *D*. *F*, This transverse head circumference shows the chorid plexus as echogenic tissue filling the cerebral ventricles. The biparietal diameter and fronto-occipital diameter measured 18.0 and 19.5 mm, respectively. *G*, The anteroposterior abdominal diameter (AAD) is measured between the + cursors at 18.1 mm and excludes the umbilical cord, and the transverse abdominal diameter (X cursors) measures 18.8. These diameters are used in the formula for the circumference of an ellipse {circumference = $(d_1 + d_2) \times 1.57$} to calculate the abdominal circumference (AC = 61.1 mm). *H*, The echogenic humeral diaphysis is measured between the – cursors as 6.9 mm. *I*, The femoral diaphysis is measured between the + cursors to be 6.6 mm. *J*, A sagittal plane through the head of an 11.9-LMP-week fetus. The mandible (small arrow) and maxilla are seen. The hand was seen to move on real-time just in front of the maxilla. The frontal (largest arrow), parietal (arrowhead), and occipital (curved arrow) plates of the skull are seen to be forming. *K*, The fetal heart rate (FHR) was measured to be 157 B/M. This is normal at this time. The FHR cannot be used to estimate fetal age in the way that the EHR can be used before the ninth LMP week. *L*, In this case, six fetal parameters were used to estimate the average fetal age at 11.9 LMP weeks, with a range of ages of 1.5 weeks. This range is within the ± 2 SD for range at this age.

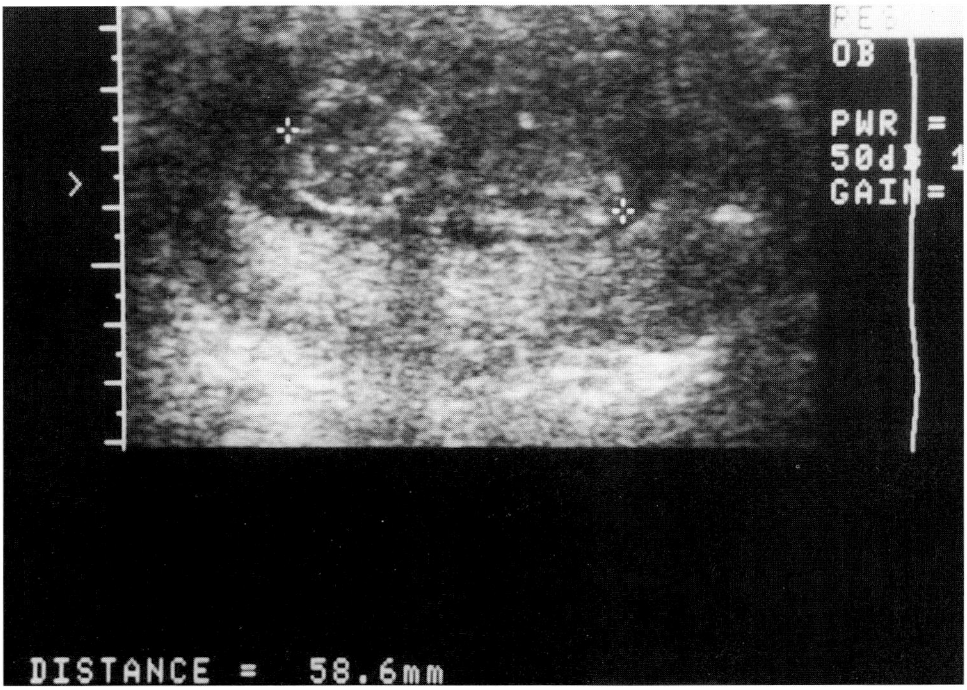

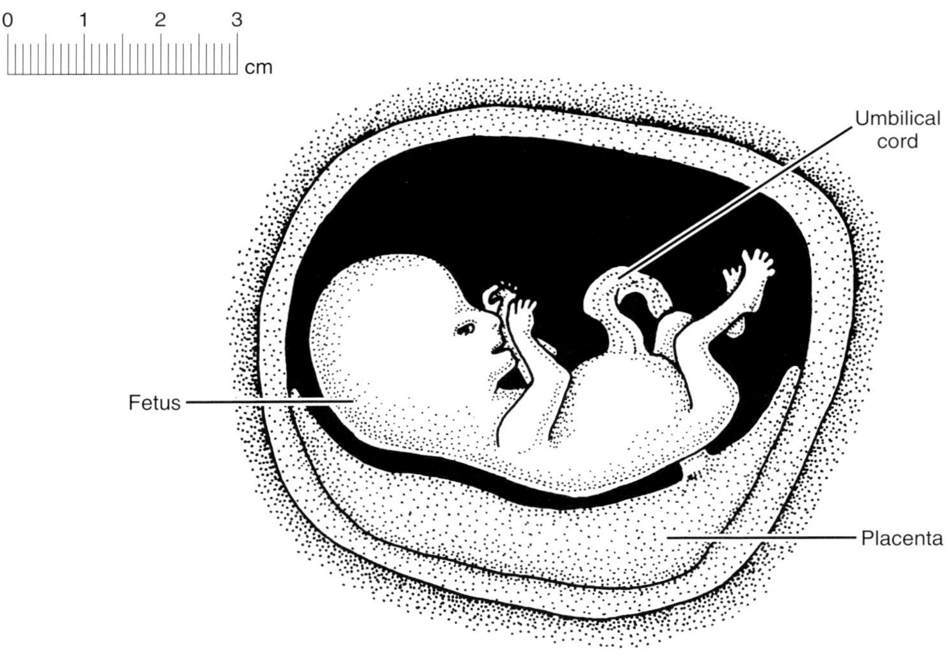

A Actual size, lateral view

FIGURE 18–13.
A, This sonogram shows a sagittal section through a 12.4-LMP-week fetus. This is toward the end of the first trimester, and the fetus should normally be quite active. The drawing shows the lateral view to scale.

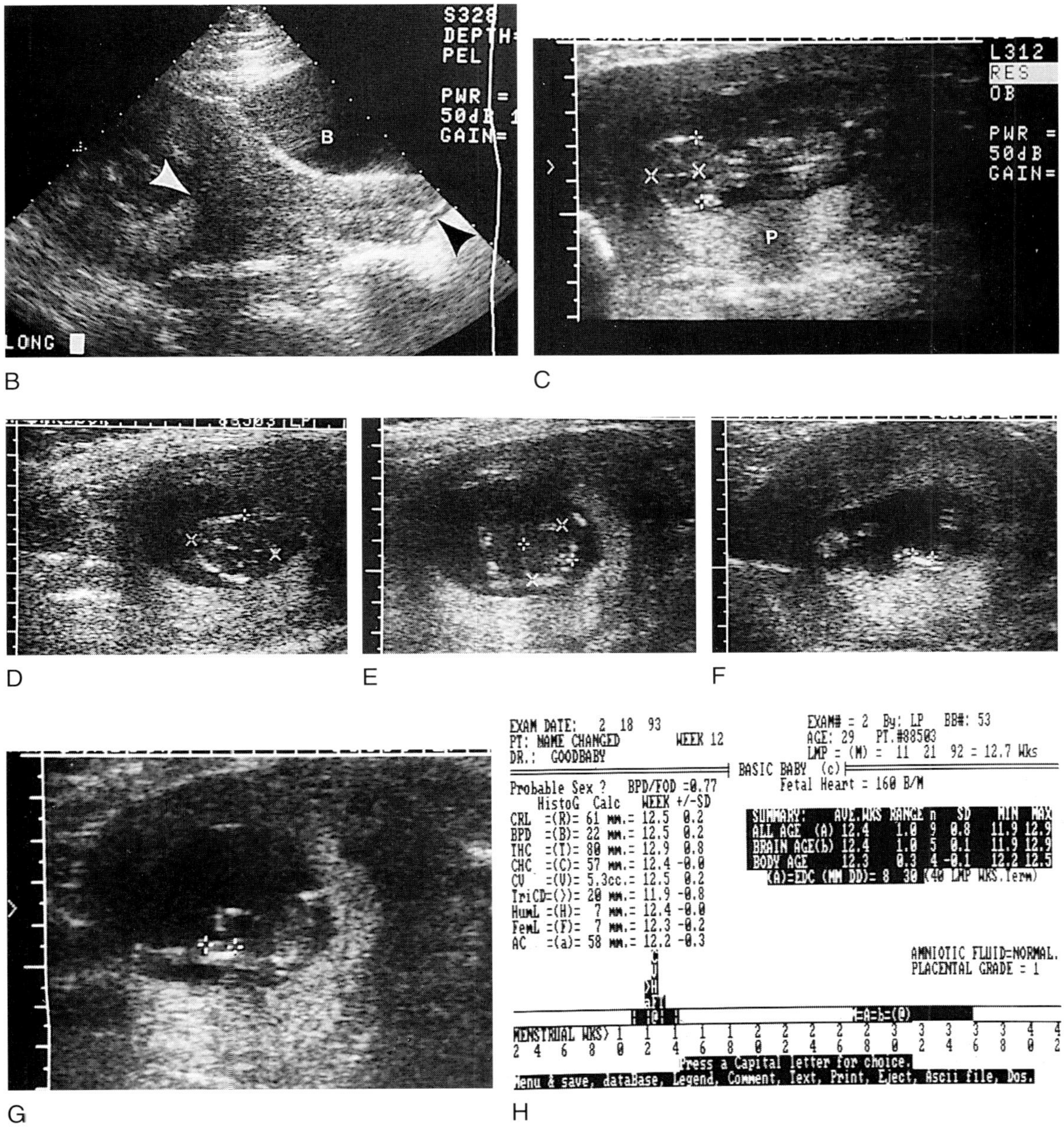

FIGURE 18–13 *Continued*

B. The endocervical canal is clearly shown in this transabdominal sonogram. The external cervical os (black arrowhead) and the internal os (white arrowhead) are easily seen posterior to the maternal urinary bladder (B). The fetal head is partially obscured by the white arrowhead. *C*, The coronal fetal head and portions of the spine are shown. The hippocampal base line and vertical cranial diameter are being measured. The thalamus can be seen at the center of the cranium with the interhemispheric fissure passing through it (between the X cursors). The placenta (P) is posterior and evenly distributed from side to side. *D*, This image is perpendicular to *C*. The biparietal diameter (+ cursors) is measured to be 21.2 mm, and the fronto-occipital diameter (X cursors) is 29.3 mm. The interhemispheric fissure is an intermittent echogenic line between the X cursors. *E*, The transverse abdominal diameters (TADs) are being measured. The anteroposterior abdominal diameter is 16.8 mm, and the TAD is 18.3 mm. Portions of the extremities are seen near the abdomen. *F*, The humeral diaphysis is measured to be 7.1 mm. The + cursors were placed adjacent and just above the ends of the diaphysis to avoid obscuring the ends of the bone. *G*, The femoral diaphysis is measured to be 7.0 mm. The + cursors are placed above and even with the ends of the bone to avoid obscuring the ends. *H*, In this computer analysis of the fetal parameter size/ages, it can be observed that all parameters are less than ±1.0 SD of the average age of 12.4 LMP weeks. This age was estimated from the average ages of nine fetal parameters. The average of all nine parameters (ALL AGE = A), five cranial parameters (BRAIN AGE = b), four somatic parameters (BODY AGE), and the mother's reported LMP age (M) all are less than 0.5 week different.

The fetal heart rate is slowing and declines from the high 160s to the low 160s during the 12th LMP week. This slow decline is not as linear as the accelerating embryonic period and exhibits more variability. The fetal heart rate can easily be determined using M-mode because of the larger size of the fetus.

SIZE/AGE

A fetus at LMP week 12 is large enough to allow several of the more common parameter measurements, as well as the coronal cranial measurements that permit cranial volume estimations. Figure 18–13*A* shows the CRL, which is still a very accurate estimator of age. Figure 18–13*C* and *D* shows the coronal and transverse cranial measurements, respectively. Figure 18–13*E* demonstrates the abdominal diameters' measurements, which are used to calculate the AC. Figure 18–13*F* illustrates measurement of the HumL, and Figure 18–13*G* shows FemL measurement.

Figure 18–13*H* is the computerized calculation of the parameter ages and averages and ARA for this case. For nine fetal parameters, the average age is estimated to be 12.4 weeks, with a range of 1.0 week, in which all parameters are less than ± 1.0 SD of the mean. This fetus has normal proportions.

The heart rate can be measured by M-mode; however, it cannot be used to estimate fetal age after the start of the ninth LMP week.

REFERENCES

1. Cunningham FG, MacDonald PC, Gant NF: Williams Obstetrics. Appleton & Lange, Norwalk, CT, 1989, p 258.
2. Streeter GL: Carnegie Institution of Washington Publications, Washington, D.C., 1940 and 1942; 30: 211–245 and 32:133–203.
3. England MA: A Colour Atlas of Life Before Birth: Normal Fetal Development. Wolfe Medical Publications, London, England, 1990, pp 12–18.
4. Creasey RK, Resnik R: Maternal-Fetal Medicine: Principles and Practice. WB Saunders, Philadelphia, 1989, pp 114–115.
5. Steurer K, Sanders RC: Role of sonography in infertility management and in contraception. In: Berman MC, ed: Diagnostic Medical Sonography: A Guide to Clinical Practice, vol I. JB Lippincott, Philadelphia, 1991, pp 176–181.
6. Cunningham FG, MacDonald PC, Gant NF: Williams Obstetrics. Appleton & Lange, Norwalk, CT, 1989, p 496.
7. DuBose TJ, Porter LM, Hill LW, et al: Black-and-white color Doppler sonography. AJR 1990;155:199.
8. Moore KL, Persaud TVN: The Developing Human. WB Saunders, Philadelphia, 1993, p 310.
9. Shats R: Transvaginal Sonography in Early Human Pregnancy. Universiteit Rotterdam, Roelof Shats, Rotterdam, 1991, p 69.
10. Moore KL, Persaud TVN: The Developing Human. WB Saunders, Philadelphia, 1993, p 78.
11. Moore KL, Persaud TVN: The Developing Human. WB Saunders, Philadelphia, 1993, pp 41–43.
12. Nyberg DA, Laing FC: Threatened abortion and abnormal first-trimester intrauterine pregnancy. In: Nyberg DA, Hill LM, Bohm-Velez M, et al, eds: Transvaginal Ultrasound. Mosby/Year Book, St Louis, 1992, pp 91–99.
13. Schats R, Jansen CAM, Waldimiroff JW: Embryonic heart activity: Appearance and development in early human pregnancy. Br J Obstet Gynaecol 1990;97: 989–994.
14. Shats R: Transvaginal Sonography in Early Human Pregnancy. Universiteit Rotterdam, Roelof Shats, Rotterdam, 1991, p 107.
15. Laboda LA, Estroff JA, Benacerraf BF: First trimester bradycardia: A sign of impending fetal loss. J Ultrasound Med 1989;8:561–563.
16. DuBose TJ, Porter L, Dickey D, et al: Sonographic correlation of fetal heart rate and gender. J Diagn Med Sonogr 1989;5:49–53.
17. DuBose TJ, Cunyus JA, Johnson LF: Embryonic heart rate and age. J Diagn Med Sonogr 1990;6:151–157.
18. Howe RS, Isaacson KJ, Albert JL, et al: Embryonic heart rate in human pregnancy. J. Ultrasound Med 1991;10:367–371.
19. Goldstein SR: Embryonic ultrasonographic measurements: Crown-rump length revisited. Am J Obstet Gynecol 1991;165:497–501.
20. DuBose TJ: Assessment of fetal age and size: Techniques and criteria. In: Berman MC, ed: Diagnostic Medical Sonography: A Guide to Clinical Practice, vol I. JB Lippincott, Philadelphia, 1991, pp 279–283.
21. Hadlock FP, Shah YP, Kannon DJ, et al: Fetal crown-rump length: Reevaluation of relation to menstrual age (5–18 weeks) with high-resolution real-time US. Radiology 1992;182:501–505.
22. DuBose TJ: Assessment of fetal age and size: Techniques and criteria. In Berman MC, ed: Diagnostic Medical Sonography: A Guide to Clinical Practice, vol I. JB Lippincott, Philadelphia, 1991, p 280.
23. Hellman LM, Kobayashi M, Fillisti L, et al: Growth and development of the human fetus prior to the 20th week of gestation. Am J Obstet Gynecol 1969; 103:784–800.
24. Goldberg BB, Kurtz AB: Atlas of ultrasound measurements. Year Book Medical Publishers, Chicago, 1990, p 252.
25. van Heeswijk M, Nijhuis JG, Hollanders HMG: Fetal heart rate in early pregnancy. Early Hum Dev 1990;22:151–156.
26. Sabbagha RE: Diagnostic Ultrasound Applied to Obstetrics and Gynecology. JB Lippincott, Philadelphia, 1987, p 95.
27. DuBose TJ: Assessment of fetal age and size: Techniques and criteria. In: Berman MC, ed: Diagnostic Medical Sonography: A Guide to Clinical Practice, vol I. JB Lippincott, Philadelphia, 1991, p 278.
28. Sabbagha RE: Diagnostic Ultrasound Applied to Obstetrics and Gynecology. JB Lippincott, Philadelphia, 1987, p 91.
29. Bromley B, Harlow BL, Laboda LA, et al: Small sac size in the first trimester: A predictor of poor fetal outcome. Radiology 1991;178:375.

30. Nazari A, Check JH, Epstein RH, et al: Relationship of small-for-dates sac size to crown-rump length and spontaneous abortion in patients with a known date of ovulation. Obstet Gynecol 1991;78:369.
31. Dickey RP, Olar TT, Taylor SN, et al: Relationship of small gestational sac–crown-rump length differences to abortion and abortus karyotypes. Obstet Gynecol 1992;79:554–557.
32. Opsahl MS, Pettit DC: First trimester sonographic characteristics of ptients with recurrent spontaneous abortion. J Ultrasound Med 1993;12:507–510.
33. Benson CB, Warneke LA: Sonographic appearance of milestones of pregnancy. In Berman MC, ed: Diagnostic Medical Sonography: A Guide to Clinical Practice, vol I. JB Lippincott, Philadelphia, 1991, pp 207–208.
34. Benirschke K: Normal development. In: Creasy RK, Resnik R: Maternal-Fetal Medicine: Principles and Practice, 2nd ed. WB Saunders, Philadelphia, 1989, p 117.
35. Goldstein SR, Woletz PS: Fertilization and embryology. In Berman MC, ed: Diagnostic Medical Sonography: A Guide to Clinical Practice, vol I. JB Lippincott, Philadelphia, 1991, pp 202–203.
36. Walla CA, Platt LD: Observing fetal maturation through fetal movement and fetal breathing. In Berman MC, ed: Diagnostic Medical Sonography: A Guide to Clinical Practice, vol I. JB Lippincott, Philadelphia, 1991, pp 446–447.
37. deVires JIP, Visser GHA, Prechtl HFR: The emergence of fetal behavior: I. Qualitative aspects. Early Hum Dev 1982;7:301–322.
38. Moore KL, Persaud TVN: The Developing Human. WB Saunders, Philadelphia, 1993, pp 84–91.
39. Finberg HJ: The placenta and umbilical cord: Recent observations. Official Proceedings, Society of Diagnostic Medical Sonographers (SDMS), 10th Annual Conference, Anaheim, CA. SDMS, 12770 Coit Rd, Suite 508, Dallas, TX 75251; pp 241–247.
40. deVries JIP, Visser GH, Prechtl HFR: Fetal motility in the first half of pregnancy. Clin Dev Med 1984;94:46.
41. Moore KL, Persaud TVN: The Developing Human. WB Saunders, Philadelphia, 1993, pp 84.

CHAPTER 19

SECOND AND THIRD TRIMESTERS

Terry J. DuBose

The 13th week after the last menstrual period (LMP) is generally considered the first week of the second trimester. This is an arbitrary division of pregnancy into three equal parts of approximately 3 calendar months.[1]

The second trimester lasts from approximately the end of the 13th week until the 26th week. Historically, fetuses delivered during the second trimester had little chance of surviving; however, modern medicine can often keep babies born during the late second trimester alive.

The third trimester is from the 26th to the 40th LMP week. This last phase of pregnancy varies because not everyone delivers at exactly 40 weeks. Normal human birth occurs approximately 280 days after the LMP. The time of term pregnancy is between 38 and 42 weeks after the LMP.[2] Almost all cases of pregnancy-caused hypertension become clinically apparent during the third trimester.[3]

In this chapter, normal pregnancy is sonographically followed through the second and third trimesters to term. These studies are not from the same pregnancy, except for the two studies at term, but include representative normal gestations. In this phase, observations are not made in consecutive weeks but at intermittent weeks. This is because after the embryonic phase (or first trimester), little actual change occurs in a fetus, only increases in size and mass. The descriptions for each week become rather redundant as we watch the measurements of the same organs grow. I have tried to point out interesting observations along the way to abate the tedium of "watching the pot boil." One of the prime lessons of this section is the observation of the increase of individuation with time in gestation. This individuation is best observed in the age range analysis (ARA) of the various parameters and is discussed at the end of each week. It is in the last half of pregnancy that fetuses that will be fat or long at birth gain in size more rapidly than fetuses destined to be thin or short. Ages estimated from the sizes of these variously growing parameters exhibit a distribution or range of ages about the average age of each fetus.

The two examinations chosen to illustrate normal term pregnancy are from the same pregnancy. One sonographic examination was performed at 38.4 LMP weeks, and the last was at 39.6 weeks by sonographic estimation. The mother did not know the date of her LNMP. Biophysical profiles (BPPs) were performed during the examinations and both times scored a perfect 10. It is hoped that these two studies of the same term fetus only 5 days apart give readers a good idea of what to expect sonographically at term.

LMP Week 15

OBSERVATIONS

By the 15th LMP week, the placenta can definitely be located. Figure 19–1*A* and *B* comprises sector scans of the lower uterine and upper uterine segments. In *A*, the top of the fetal skull can be seen near the internal os of the cervix, with amniotic fluid in between. The cervical canal, external os, vagina, and maternal bladder can also be seen. This is sufficient evidence that placenta previa does not exist. Figure 19–1*B* is a sagittal section near the fundus (top) of the uterus. The placenta is located anteriorly. This is a grade I placenta, which means that it has a homogeneous texture.

The 15th week is a particularly advantageous time for parents to observe the sonograms because the fetus is large enough to be recognizable and yet small enough that most of it fits into the field of view. Whether or not one believes both parents or others should be allowed in an examination room or should even receive a videotape of the fetus from a diagnostic examination, society exerts strong procreative pressure for parents to have "baby pictures." Whether the pictures are created with visible light or with sound, the baby picture is an icon and is ritualistic (see Chapter 6 for discussion of these issues).

Most fetal organs can be observed in most pregnancies. It is usually only in obese women or in cases of oligohydramnios (reduced amniotic fluid) that the fetal organs may be difficult to define. Figure 19–1*C* demonstrates a parasagittal section through the fetal left side. The spine is most obvious, but sections through the ribs, shoulder, lung, bowel, and portions of the pelvis are also discernible. The placenta is clearly an anterior grade I in this image. Between the anterior trunk and placenta, two parallel echoes are seen. These are the walls of one of the umbilical vessels. It is not possible to determine from this single image if this is one of the arteries or the vein. An ovoid structure just anterior to the lower third of the spine is most likely a kidney; however, without real-time, it is difficult to ascertain this retrospectively with any certainty.

It is noted here that many structures that can be readily identified with real-time sonography are almost impossible to identify at a later time on static images. The advantage of real-time sonography in the study of a very active fetus cannot be overemphasized. For this reason, taking the time to label images may be an absolute necessity for later recall, especially in cases of abnormalities, because the very definition of *abnormality* may mean that the sonographer may have never observed this particular configuration of anatomy before.

The orbits and nose are shown in Figure 19–1*D*. In this image, it would be possible to measure the outer binocular distance (BiOD). The wing of the left sphenoid bone can be seen as a bright echo just posterior to the more posterior orbit. Again, the anterior placenta is observed to be grade I, and the amnion can be seen as a thin line, indicating that it is still incompletely fused with the chorion.

Figure 19–1*E* is a coronal view of the head, neck, and upper torso. In the head, the bilateral choroid plexus is seen to be relatively large. The interhemispheric fissure can be seen as the falx cerebri at the top and extending down into the cervical spine area as the central canal of the spinal cord. The thalamus and brainstem are seen as a central hypoechoic area that extends toward the base of the skull. The bright echo at the center of the thalamus is the third ventricle. The circles around the hippocampal complex can be seen bilaterally. The cervical spine is obvious in this image, and the proximal ear is faintly seen. The ribs are also obvious, as are the scapula and shoulder. A portion of the descending aorta is shown in the midthoracic area. The placenta can be seen anterior to the fetus.

Figure 19–1*F* is a sagittal section of the fetal head. One of the choroid plexuses is shown in its entirety. The frontal and occipital bones are distinct, and the area from the anterior fontanelle to the posterior fontanelle is less clear. The nasal, maxillary, and mandibular bones are also seen.

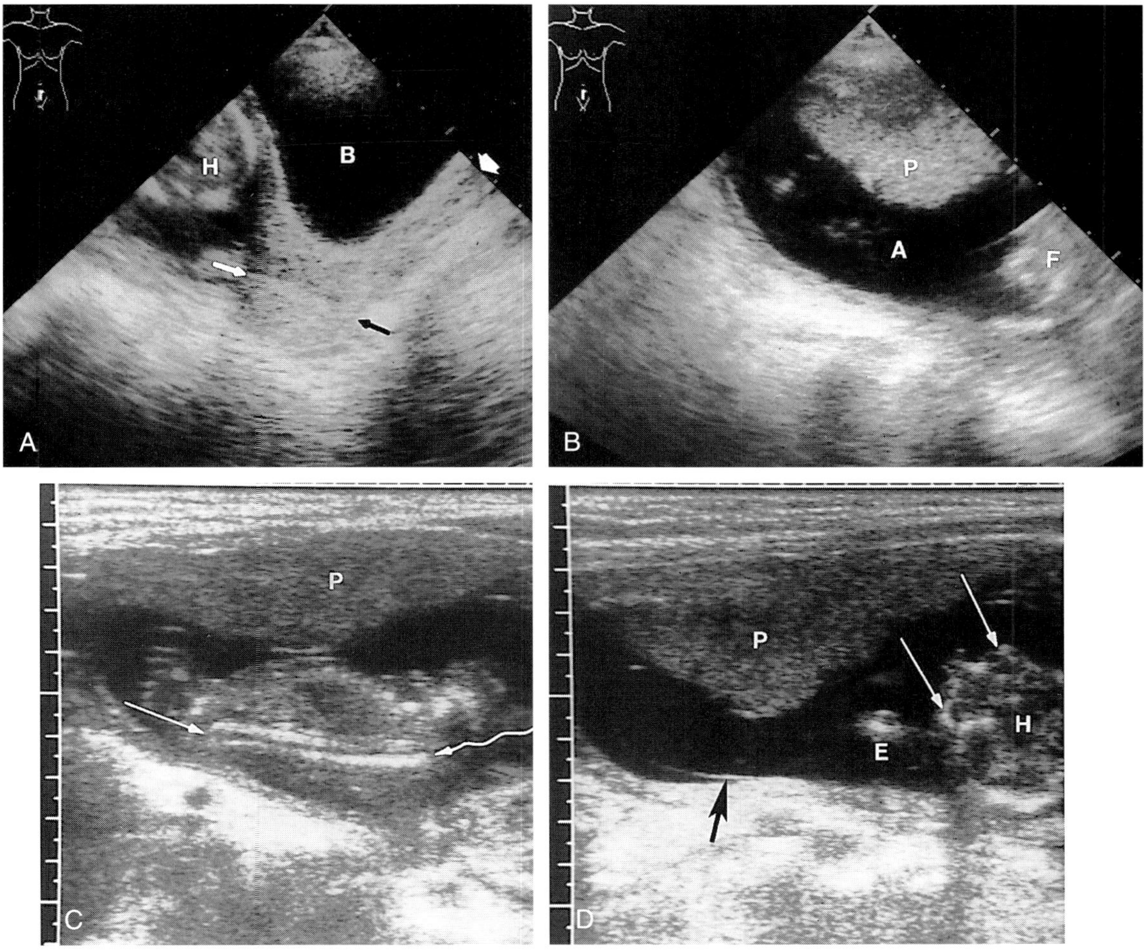

FIGURE 19–1. LMP WEEK 15.
A, The internal os (thin white arrow) is free of placenta, and the fetal head (H) is presenting. The cervical canal runs between the internal os and external os (black arrow) along the length of the cervix, which is posterior to the full maternal urinary bladder (B). The distal vagina (wide white arrow) can be seen.
B, A large pocket of amniotic fluid (A) is seen in the uterine fundus. The placenta (P) is anterior. Part of the fetus (F) is at the edge of the image.
C, A long portion of the fetal spine is shown from the upper thorax (wavy arrow) to the lower lumbar (straight arrow). This also provides an oblique, parasagittal view of the shoulder, ribs and lung and part of the abdomen. The placenta (P) is anterior.
D, A parasagittal plane in the uterus showing a transverse view of the fetal head (H) and face. The orbits (arrows) can be seen, with the bridge of the nose between. A cross section of one extremity (E) can be seen in the amniotic fluid. The placenta (P) is anterior. A very small portion of the amniotic membrane (black arrow) has not yet fused with the chorion.

One of the most common sonographic views of the fetal skull is shown in Figure 19–1G, the transverse head circumference (THC). This view is usually referred to as simply the *head circumference;* however, because this text discusses the head in three dimensions (3-D), the distinction is made between the THC and the coronal head circumference (CHC). In this image, the biparietal diameter (BPD) is measured between the + cursors. The BPD is measured from the leading edge to leading edge of the parietal bones. That is to say, the cursors are placed at the edge of the parietal bones that are nearest the transducer because these are the sharpest, specular echoes. The X cursors are measuring the longest skull diameter or the fronto-occipital diameter (FOD). The FOD measurement

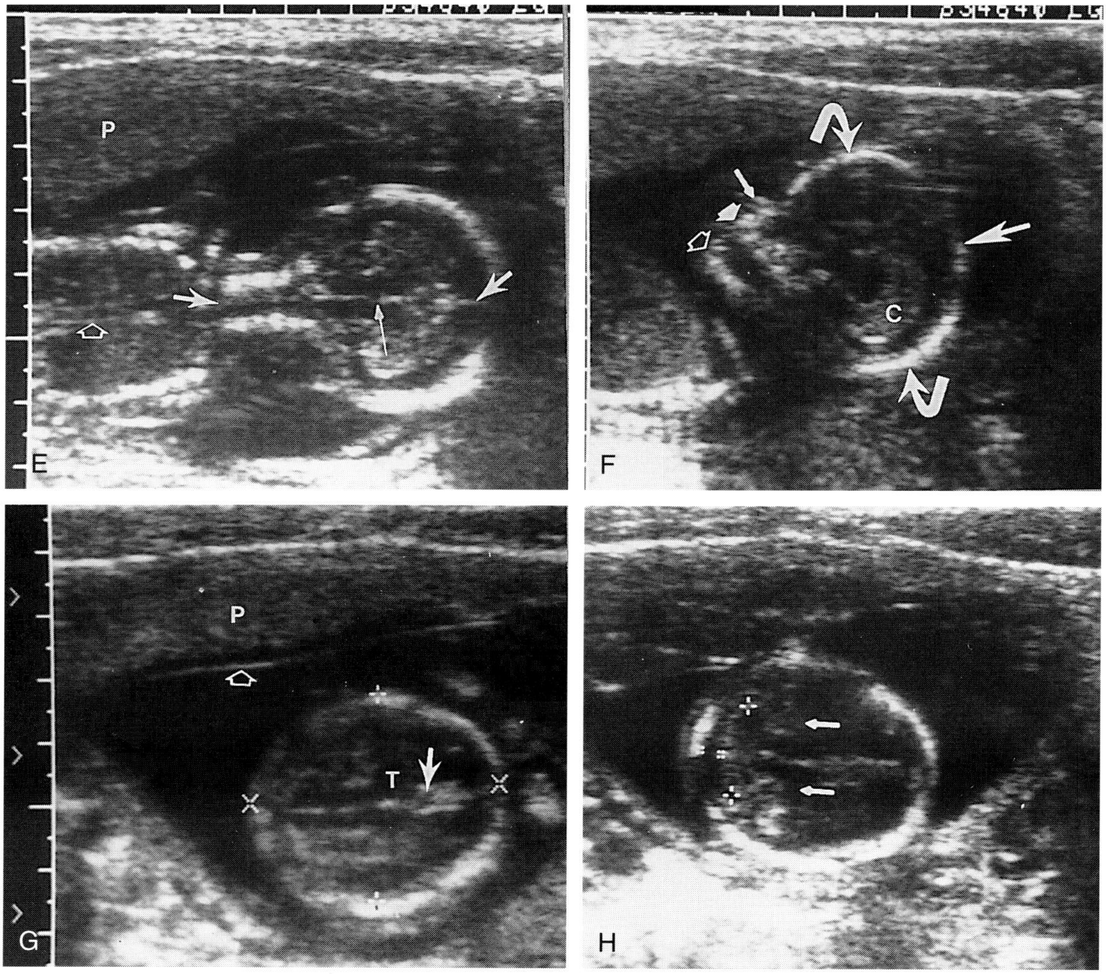

FIGURE 19–1. *(Continued)*
E, Coronal view of the fetal head and chest. The interhemispheric fissure extends from the top of the head and continues as the central canal of the cervical spinal cord between the large white arrows. The third ventricle is at the center of the thalamus (thin white arrow). The echogenic choroid plexus fills the bodies of the lateral ventricles lateral to and above the thalamus. The lateral ventricles extend beyond the sides of the coronal triangle until the 18th to 20th LMP weeks (see Chapter 8). A portion of the descending aorta (open arrow) is shown. The placenta (P) can be seen to taper off anterior to the head.
F, Parasagittal view of the fetal head. Structures identified are the mandible (open arrow), maxilla (closed arrow), and nose (small arrow). The choroid plexus (C) curves posteriorly. The frontal and occipital bones (curved arrows) are easily seen, but the anterior and posterior fontanelle areas (large straight arrow) are less distinct.
G, Transverse view of the fetal head showing the central thalamus (T) and the cavum septi pellucidi (white arrow), which is anterior to the thalamus. This is the common plane for measuring the biparietal diameter (+ cursors) and fronto-occipital diameter (X cursors). The amnion (open arrow) can be seen along the fetal surface of the anterior placenta (P).
H, This transverse plane is lower in the fetal head than *G* and is not appropriate for the transverse head circumference measurements. The + cursors measure the width of the cerebellum, and the small x cursors measure the anteroposterior diameter of the cisterna magna. The arrows point to the location of the bilateral hippocampal complexes. The top of one petrous ridge is the echogenic area just lateral to the distal hippocampal gyri.

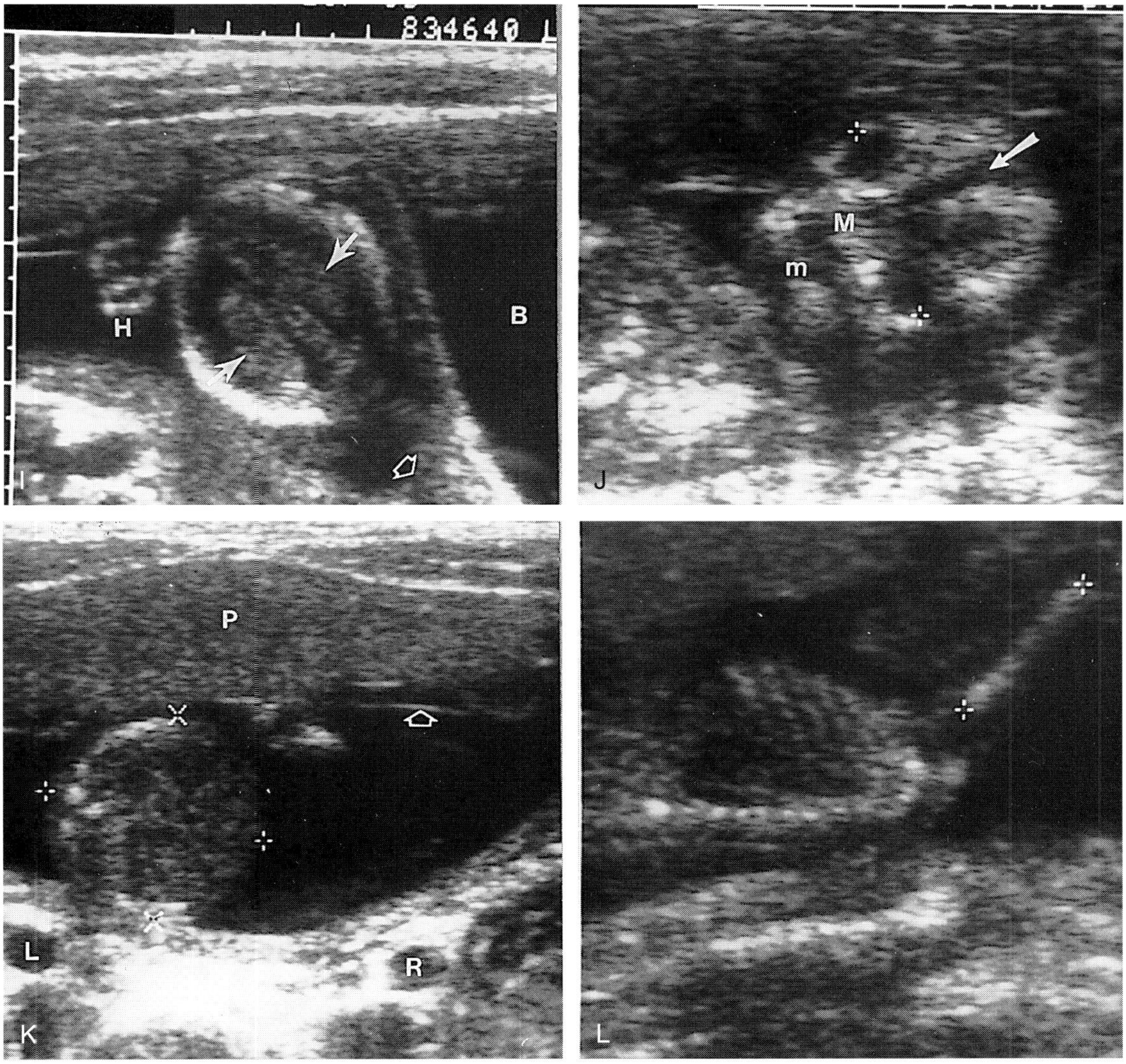

FIGURE 19–1. *(Continued)*

I, Sagittal plane through the lower uterine segment showing the internal os (open arrow) and full maternal bladder (B). This transverse view of the fetus is above the thalamus and too high in the head for measurement of the transverse head circumference. The chorid plexus (solid white arrows) can be seen in the bodies of the lateral ventricles. A portion of one fetal hand (H) is touching the area of the frontal bone with its thumb, as in a left-handed salute.

J, A coronal plane through the fetal face. The mandible (m) and maxilla (M) are seen. The + cursors measure the outer orbital distance, which is usually called the binocular distance (BiOD). The arrow points to the frontal or metopic suture, which widens into the anterior fontanelle; this is normal and should not be confused with a facial cleft.

K, Transverse section of both the uterus and the fetal abdomen. Note that the skin line of the abdomen is faint, and care must be taken not to underestimate the important abdominal measurements. Note that the anteroposterior abdominal diameter (AAD, + cursors) is measured to the skin line behind the spine and not to the more obvious ossification centers of the spine (three bright echoes). A portion of the amniotic membrane (open arrow) is still not fused with the fetal side of the placenta (P). Posterior to the uterus, the maternal iliac arteries (L, left; R, right) are seen on either side of the bright echogenic area of the anterior maternal spine.

L, Parasagittal view of the fetal thorax with the ribs faintly seen. The measurement of the humeral diaphysis is between the + cursors. The head of the humerus is the dark, hypoechoic area at the proximal end of the diaphysis.

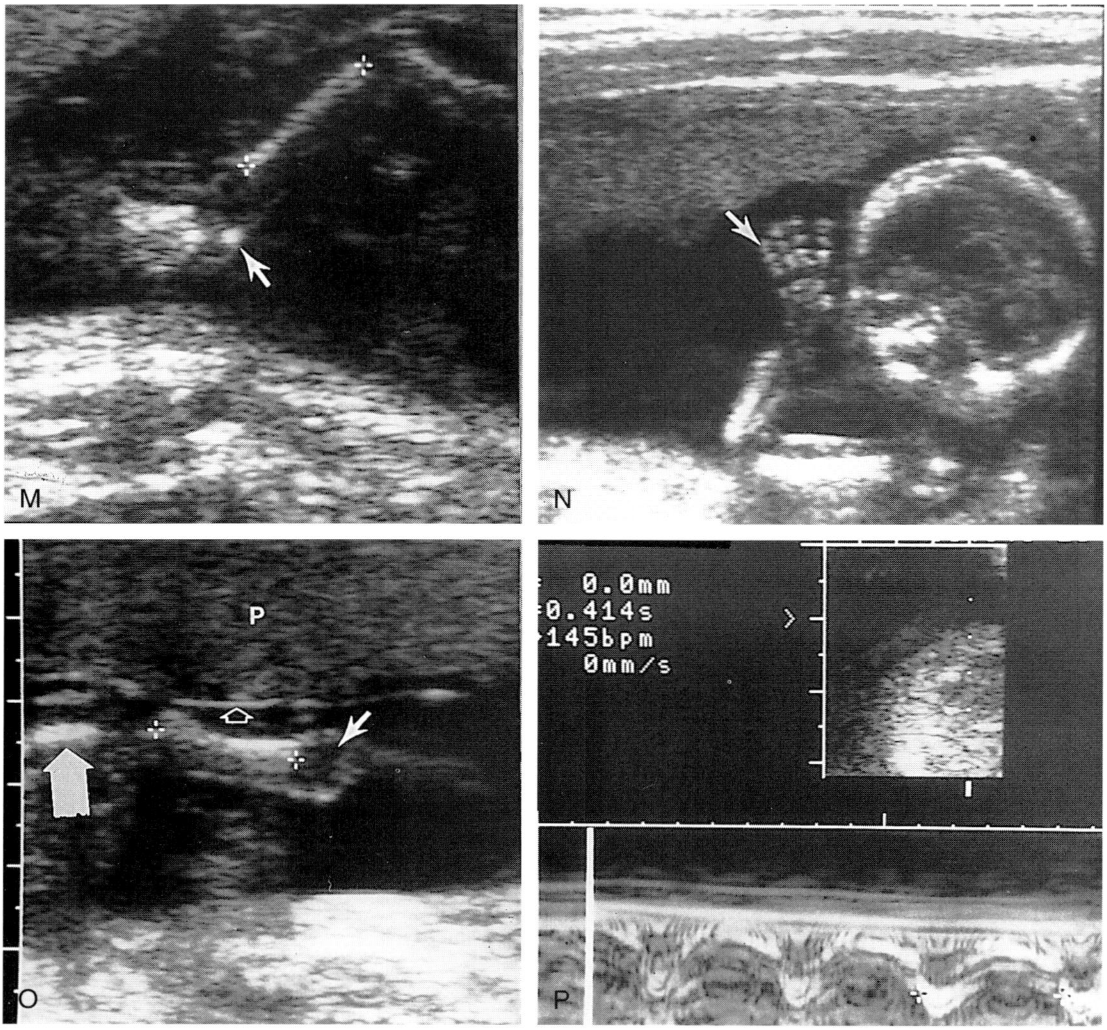

FIGURE 19–1. *(Continued)*
M, The humeral diaphysis measurement (+ cursors) is again seen. The fetal scapula is the trapezoidal and brightly echogenic area near the echo of the acromion of the scapula (arrow). The humeral head is hypoechoic and between these structures and the proximal end of the diaphysis.
N, The fetal hand is seen in front of the fetal face. Four of the fetal fingers can be seen. The arrow points to the fifth digit, or little finger. The thumb is out of this plane of view. A portion of the forearm, elbow, and humeral diaphysis is seen distally.
O, The femoral diaphysis length is measured between the + cursors. The hypoechoic cartilage of the distal femoral condyles (small white arrow) and one iliac bone (large white arrow) are seen at either end of the femur. The placenta (P) and amniotic membrane (open arrow) are anterior to the femur.
P, One complete heartbeat is measured between the + cursors. The image was enlarged to obtain the most accurate measurements possible

should be taken from the middle of the frontal bone to the middle of the occipital bone to minimize beam-width artifacts (see Chapters 5 and 8 for more explanation of this topic). The cavum septi pellucidi and the thalamus are the landmarks of anatomy for the correct THC view.

The placenta can be seen anteriorly in Figure 19–1*G*. The relatively bright line along the surface of the placenta is the incompletely fused amniotic membrane. This membrane usually fuses with the chorion by the 26th LMP week.[3] If this fusion does not take place, the fetus is at risk of becoming entangled in an amniotic band, resulting in severe birth defects.[4]

Slightly lower in the fetal skull than the previous section for the THC, the cerebellum

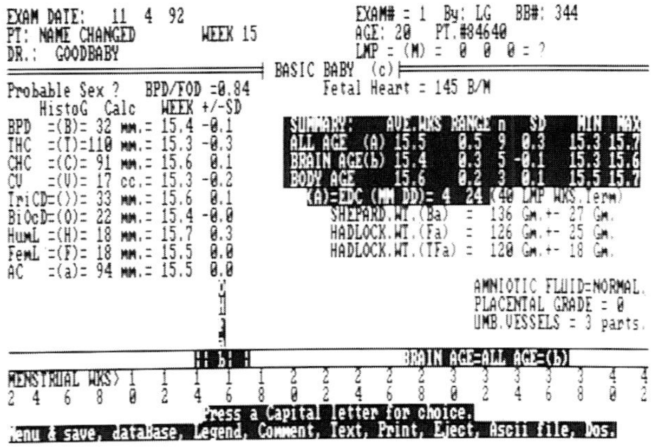

Q

FIGURE 19–1. *(Continued)*
Q, In this computer analysis of the multiple fetal parameters, sizes and ages, all ages are within 0.5 week of one another. Age range analysis puts all parameters within ± 0.3 SD of the mean age of 15.5 LMP weeks. Note that in the symbol histogram, all parameters stack vertically. This is a very well-proportioned fetus. The woman did not know the date of her LMP.

is shown in Figure 19–1*H*. The cisterna magna is measured between the posterior cerebellum and the occipital bone. The hypoechoic brainstem can be seen on either side of the midline near the center of the skull. The tops of the bilateral hippocampal complexes are seen just anterior to the lateral edges of the cerebellum.

Slightly higher than the proper section for the THC, the bodies of the lateral ventricles containing the choroid plexus are shown in Figure 19–1*I*. The falx cerebri can be seen as a faint line of echoes between the ventricles. A hand is located near the frontal bone. In this image, it can be seen that the fetal head is presenting near the internal os, just posterior to the full maternal bladder.

Turning the plane of view to the coronal plane and through the anterior skull, the facial bones can be seen in Figure 19–1*J*. The + cursors are measuring the BiOD. These cursors should be placed just inside the zygoma, which forms the outer orbits. The dark (hypoechoic) area in the middle of the frontal bone is the frontal or metopic suture, which leads down from the anterior fontanelle. The maxilla and mandible can also be seen.

The transverse abdominal diameters (TADs) are measured in Figure 19–1*K*. The + cursors measure the abdominal anteroposterior diameter (AAD) to be 32.8 mm, and the X cursors measure the TAD to be 30.2 mm. The abdominal diameters are among the most important and most often incorrectly measured of fetal parameters. These measurements are important because most formulas for estimating fetal weight rely on the abdominal circumference (AC). The abdominal diameters are frequently incorrectly measured because an inexperienced sonographer may measure to the brightest echoes, which are often the bony structures rather than the skin line. Measuring only to the spine or ribs excludes the subcutaneous "baby fat" and underestimates the true AC. In Figure 19–1*K*, note the three bright echoes of the fetal spine and the correct placement of the + cursor posterior to these, just at the edge of the faintly visualized skin. Also, note the X cursor at the distal side of the abdomen is at the interface of the uterine wall and the abdominal wall, not at the more obvious rib or peritoneal echo.

The importance of these types of errors cannot be overemphasized. Underestimating the abdominal girth can result in underestimation of the fetal weight, which could result in a misdiagnosis of intrauterine growth retardation (IUGR). A diagnosis of IUGR can be an indication for early delivery in some cases.

Two cystic-looking structures just posterior to the uterine wall in Figure 19–1*K* are cross sections of the left and right iliac arteries, which lie on either side of the anterior maternal spine. These are normal. Sonographers should be observant of the entire sonographic image and not just focus on some single small area of the sonogram.

In Figure 19–1*L* and *M*, two different views of the same humerus are shown. In *L*, the humeral diaphysis is being measured and the ribs are demonstrated. In *M*, with a slightly different angle, the length of the humerus is still correctly measured but the shoulder, especially the body of the scapula, is shown. The bright echo posterior to the hypoechoic humeral head is the acromion of the scapula. It is possible to determine that this structure is the acromion and not the more anterior coracoid process because in the previous image, the fetus is in the supine position. This places the echo posterior to the humeral head. Novice sonographers must learn to acquire a mental picture of the positions from various images in order to integrate and identify the anatomy.

By the 15th LMP week, the fetal hands become an interesting object of observation (Fig. 19–1*N*). Thumb sucking, ear pulling, eye poking, head rubbing, and other face and head palpations as well as umbilical cord grasping are fetal occupations that are often observed. In this figure, is this fetus giving us the "high five" or "blowing a raspberry"? The index finger (second phalanx) through the little finger (fifth phalanx) can be seen. On close observation, all three phalanges of the four fingers can be seen, as well as the navicular, greater multangular, lesser multangular, capitate, and hamate bones. Portions of the ulna and the humerus are seen below the hand and face.

Figure 19–1*O* shows the femur just below the amniotic membrane and anterior placenta. Note that the condyles of the distal femur are not calcified and appear hypoechoic or anechoic. The femoral diaphysis (shaft) becomes calcified at the end of the embryonic period; however, the condyles are solid cartilaginous tissue and do not become completely calcified until after birth.[5] Cartilaginous tissue is a homogeneous solid with few tissue planes to reflect echoes and therefore appears hypoechoic. The bright linear echo near the other (proximal) end of the femoral diaphysis is the ilium of the pelvis in cross section.

MOVEMENT

By the 15th LMP week, almost the entire repertoire of movements is present. Isolated movements of the arms, legs, body, and head and combined movements occur. The hands are most frequently touching the head and face. This remains true for the rest of pregnancy. It is uncertain when grasping the umbilical cord begins. It is definitely a frequent activity in the last half of pregnancy (see Chapter 16 for more on this topic). Breathing and swallowing motions can be observed in the 15th LMP week. Breathing-type movements become a more important indicator of fetal well-being in the BPP later in pregnancy. These expanding and retracting motions of the chest and abdomen appear to be the same as breathing.

In the 15th week, the mean fetal heart rate (FHR) is still declining and continues in a similar trend until about the 18th week, when the curve flattens more. The FHR this week is approximately 150 B/M (± 15 B/M) in a normal (95%) population (Fig. 19–1*P*). By term, the mean FHR is approximately 140 B/M (±27 B/M). Most discussion in the literature about variability of the heart rate relates to labor and fetal distress.[6] It appears that the beat-to-beat variability of the heart rate over short periods of time increases from early pregnancy until birth. This FHR variability has been associated with fetal movement by the nonstress test, with maternal eating, with the time of day, and with the phases of labor and fetal distress. Before week 15, the embryo/fetal heart rate correlates more closely with the time in gestation than it does with the more immediate stimulus/response–induced variabilities.[7,8]

SIZE/AGE

In the 15th LMP week, a fetus is large enough that its age can be estimated using any of the more commonly measured parts of the skeleton. In the current example of a 15-LMP-week fetus, nine parameters were measured and an average of multiple fetal parameters, (MFP) ages calculated. The average age was 15.5 weeks, with a range of 0.5 weeks (±0.3 SD) (Fig. 19–1*Q*). In the ARA histogram (see Fig. 19–1Q), all parameter symbols stack one above another because they are all less than ± 0.5 week from the average age. Not all of the parameters are shown in the symbolic histogram because the ± SD data column overwrites the symbols at the top; however, we know that they must be in a single column because otherwise the histogram would have more than one column of symbols. This means the fetus is normally proportioned.

The ARA histogram tends to exhibit a high

degree of kurtosis (peakedness) earlier in pregnancy. This is called a *leptokurtic* curve and has all parameters at or near the mean age, a narrow distribution. As pregnancy approaches term, the proportions of the fetal parameters become more variable owing to individuation, and histogram dispersion becomes greater, resulting in less kurtosis with fewer parameters at or near the mean age. This wider, flatter histogram is described as *platykurtic*.

The estimated fetal weight is about 127 g (see Fig. 19–1*Q*). This weight estimate is the average of the results from three regression formulas, Shepard's modification of Warsof's and two of Hadlock's.[9–11]

LMP Week 18

OBSERVATIONS

The 18th week after the LMP is the time that Filly has said is an opportune time to study a fetus. "At 18 weeks, one can characterize a large number of important features of a pregnancy that cannot be judged at all in early pregnancy."[12]

In the 18th LMP week, a fetus is large enough that most organs can be distinguished. Indeed, the overall crown-rump length (CRL) exceeds the field of view of most current sonographic transducers. In Figure 19–2*A*, it can be observed that if the fetus were not curved in the traditional fetal position, the CRL would exceed the field of view. The spine is curved in a breech fetal position in this figure. The lower spine is examined, and the fractional spine length (FSL) is measured in Figure 19–2*B* to include seven complete vertebral bodies and spaces.

The head can easily be measured and its anatomy studied during the 18th LMP week. In Figure 19–2*C*, the normal transverse view of a fetal head (THC) is shown. The interhemispheric fissure of the brain can be seen as an intermittent line of echoes in the long axis of the characteristic egg-shaped transverse section of the head. The cavum septi pellucidi can also be seen. This view of the fetus is probably the most commonly obtained, worldwide.

Figure 19–2*D* is parallel and slightly caudal in the fetus to the view shown in 19–2*C*. This view shows the sonographic base X of the fetal calvarium. The base X has been a guide to finding the plane for the correct THC since the early 1980s.[13–16] In this image, the fetal cerebellum and cisterna magna are being measured. The pons is just anterior to the cerebellum and appears as two hypoechoic ovals on either side of the midline. The base X is made up of four arms of echogenic tissues that extend anteriorly along the tops of the wings of the sphenoid bones and along the ridges of the petrous bones posteriorly. The petrous ridges are on either side of the cerebellum. The frontal lobes occupy the space between and above the wings of the sphenoids in the anterior skull. The echoes above the contralateral sphenoids and petrous ridges form more or less straight lines, which intersect at the center of the base of the fetal cranium.

In Figure 19–2*E* and *F*, the coronal view of the fetal head is obtained by turning the transducer 90 degrees from the planes described earlier. Figure 19–2*E* is absolute real-time with no frame averaging, producing a grainer image; *F* has a four-frame averaging. Frame averaging produces a smoother image in which the choroid plexus is more easily observed. Frame averaging also puts real-time into slow motion, which can cause an active fetus to become blurred. Sonographers should not use frame averaging for geometric measurements in very active fetuses. Changes in frame averaging give different perceptions of tissue textures depending on a patient's habitus. Observations of these differences provide a better understanding of the overall anatomy.

Note that in the midcoronal view, the fetal calvarium is a large arc in a nearly perfect circle. This view also reveals extensive cranial anatomy. The bilateral choroid plexus in the lateral ventricles and hippocampal gyri, the interhemispheric fissure, and the brainstem all may be observed in coronal views. These structures should be bilaterally symmetrical on either side of the midline. The nasopharynx is also shown in Figure 19–2*E* as a fluid-filled space. Figure 19–2*F* is slightly posterior to the previous image, revealing the proximal carotid artery passing though the carotid canal. The echogenic anterior occipital bone is just medial to the carotid canal and its artery. The distal carotid artery is less clearly shown

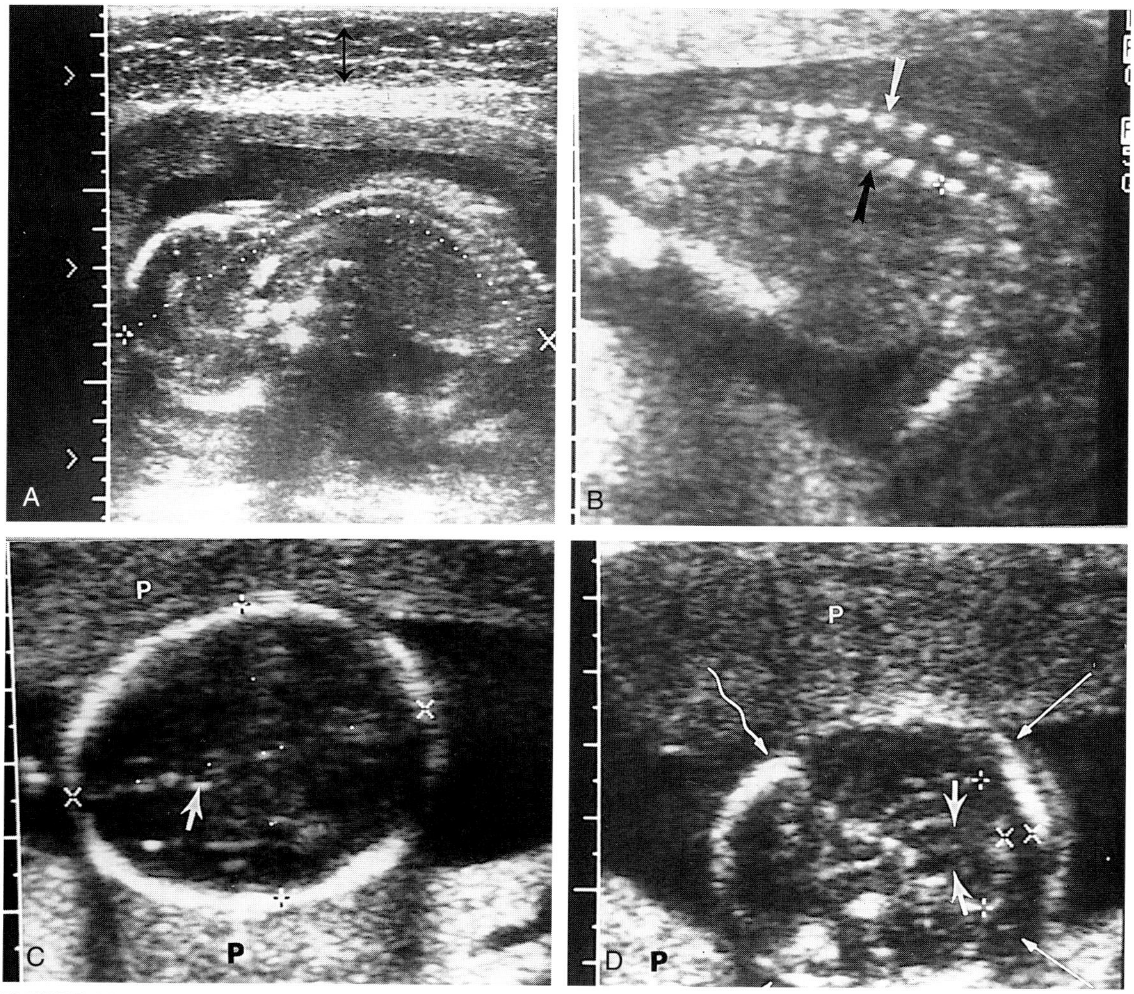

FIGURE 19–2. LMP WEEK 18.

A, This image illustrates why the crown-rump length (CRL) is not generally used to estimate age after the first trimester. This fetus is curled into a fetal position, and the CRL is being measured as a curve rather than as a straight line. Although this method can be used as late as the 18th LMP week (this is 17.8 LMP weeks), the variation becomes greater. This pregnant woman has a rather thick subcutaneous fat layer (double-headed arrow).

B, Long axis of the thoracolumbar spine (between arrows). The + cursors measure seven complete vertebral bodies and spaces to be 26 mm, which correlates to approximately 18.3 (± 1.8) LMP weeks (see Table 7–1).

C, The appropriate level for measuring the transverse head diameters. The biparietal diameter (+ cursors) and the fronto-occipital diameter (FOD) (X cursors) are shown. This plane, from which the FOD can be measured, always contains the cavum septi pellucidi (arrow) and thalamus. The fetus is breech, and the placenta (P) wraps around the uterine fundus and is seen both anteriorly and posteriorly to the head.

D, This plane is through the base of the fetal skull, showing the base X, and is below and parallel to the appropriate plane for the transverse head circumference (THC) measurement shown in *C*. The arms of this X are made up of the structures along the greater wings of the sphenoid bones (wavy arrows) anteriorly and the petrous ridges (straight arrows) posteriorly. The cerebellum (+) lies between the petrous pyramids. The two halves of the pons and brainstem (between arrows) are anterior to the cerebellum; the cisterna magna (X cursors) is posterior to the cerebellum.

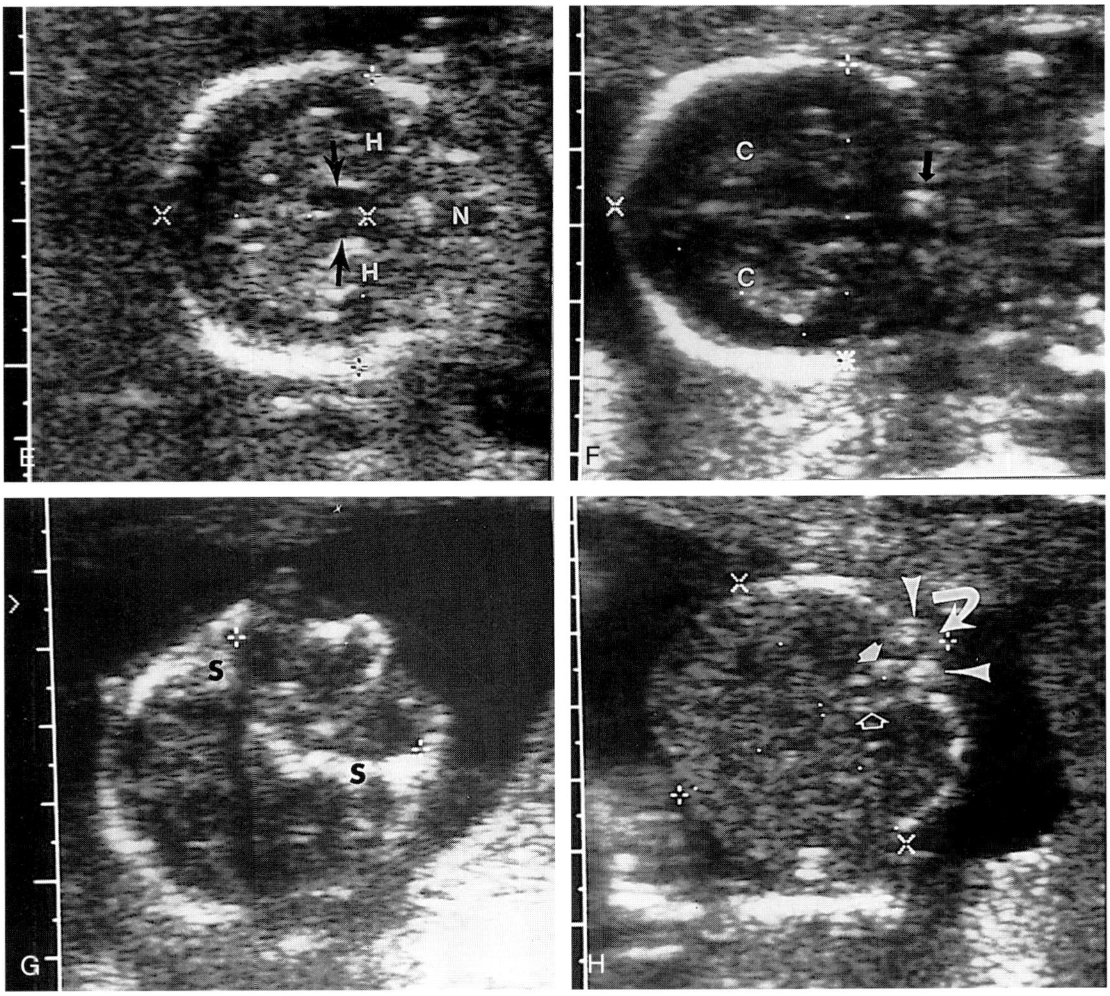

FIGURE 19–2. *(Continued)*
E, Coronal plane through the fetal skull. This is perpendicular to the transverse planes in *C* and *D*. Note the circular shape of the skull in this view. The + cursors measure the hippocampal base line (HBL) of the coronal triangle, and the X cursors measure the vertical cranial diameter along the interhemispheric fissure. The bilateral hippocampal complexes are just caudal to the two H's. The pons (between arrows) is also visualized in this plane, as is the nasopharynx (N).
F, another coronal view of the same fetal head. Again, note the circular shape of the skull. Here the HBL is again measured between the + cursors. The X cursors mark one side of the coronal triangle. Note that the side of the triangle is just tangential to the outer edge of the chorid plexus (C). Before 18 to 20 LMP weeks, the chorid plexus normally extends outside the sides of this triangle. After this time (20 weeks), the chorid plexus and lateral ventricles reside wholely within the apex of the coronal triangle. The carotid canal or jugular bulb (arrow) can be seen in the base of the skull.
G, Oblique, transverse plane showing the facial bones. The sphenoid bones (S) are posterior to the orbits. The outer binocular distance (BiOD) is measured between the + cursors. The bridge of the nose protrudes anteriorly, between the orbits.
H, Transverse plane through the fetal abdomen and perpendicular to the spine (curved arrow). Three ossification centers of a vertebral body can be seen, one anterior (solid white arrow) and two posterior (arrowheads). The open arrow points to a portion of the crux of the diaphragm, which is anterior to the spine and in intimate relationship with the aorta. The perpendicular diameters of the abdomen are measured between the + cursors and the X cursors. Note that these diameters are measured to the skin line rather than to the more obvious spine and rib echoes.

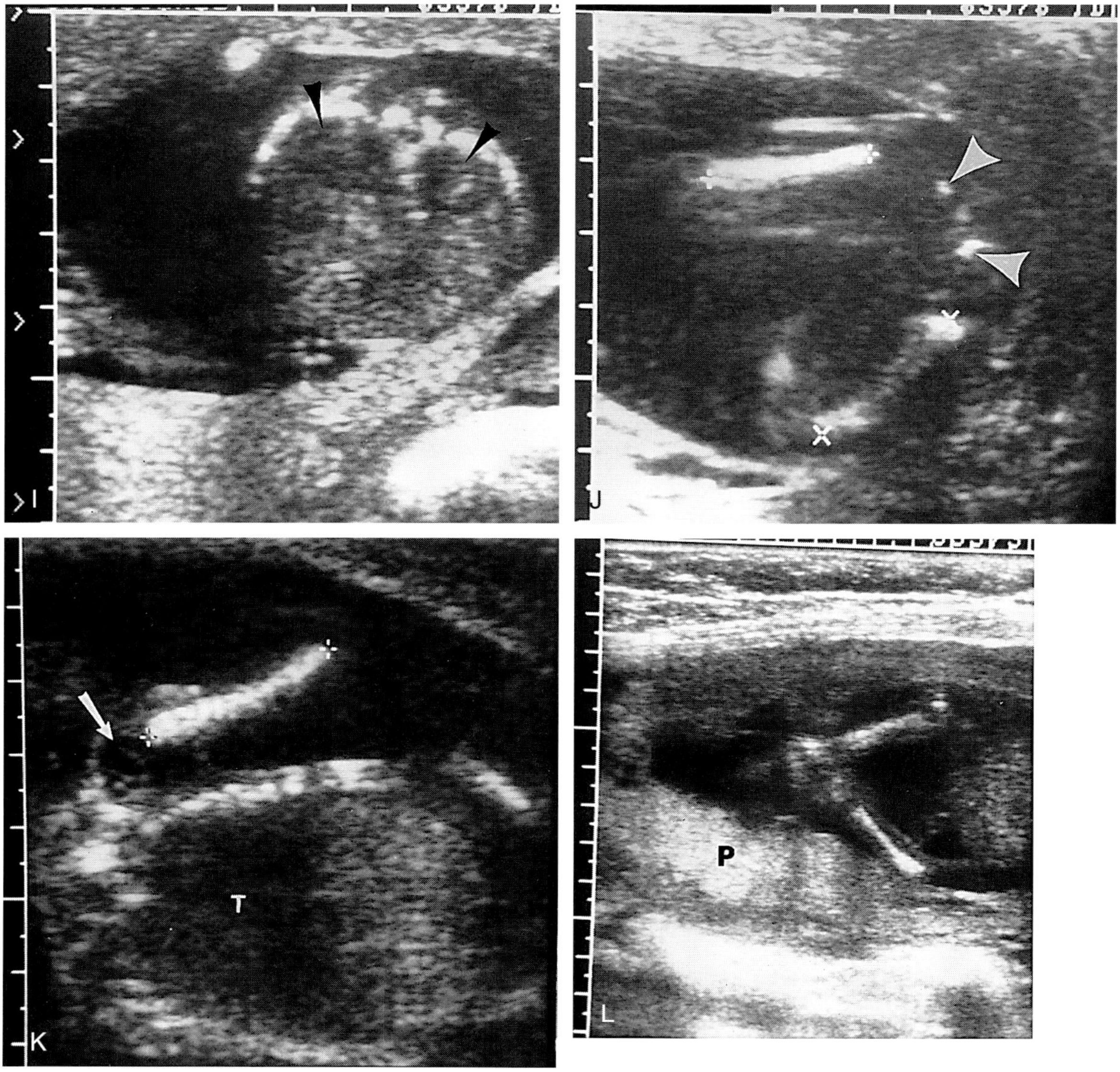

FIGURE 19–2. *(Continued)*
I, Transverse view of the abdomen slightly lower in the fetus than *H*. The bilateral kidneys (arrowheads) are located on either side of the spine. The three ossification centers are again seen, with the anterior center between the kidneys.
J, Lower in the fetal body, the pelvis and thighs are seen. Both femoral diaphyses are measured between the + and X cursors. Note that the more posterior femur (X) appears more curved than the anterior femur. This is because of the difference in shape of the femur's lateral and medial edges and is normal (see Chapter 15 for a discussion of the shape of these bones). The ossification centers of the ischium are seen as two bright echoes (arrowheads). The faint echo between the ischial echoes is most likely from the rectal tissues.
K, The humeral diaphysis is measured between the + cursors. The cartilaginous femoral head (arrow) is seen as a hypoechoic circle at the proximal end of the diaphysis. The trunk and ribs are posterior to the humerus. The thorax (T) is in the shadow of the diaphysis.
L, In this image, the fetal hands are seen clasped anterior to the abdomen. On real-time, the hands could be seen to move and manipulate the umbilical cord. The placenta (P) is posterior.

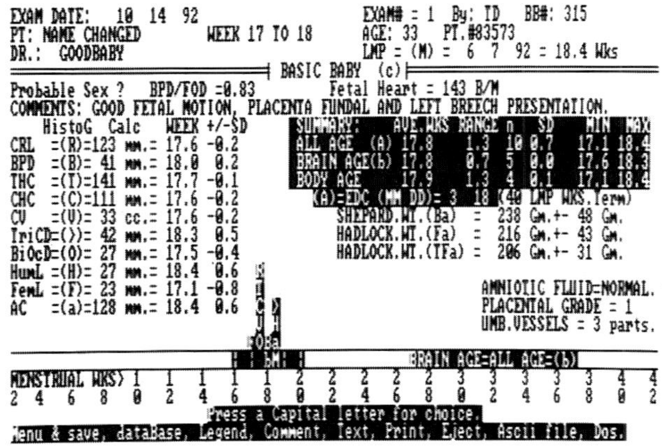

M

FIGURE 19–2. *(Continued)*
M, Computer age range analysis produced an average age of 17.8 LMP weeks from 10 fetal parameters, with a range of 1.3 weeks. This range is less than 10% of the age and places all parameters at less than ± 1 SD of the mean. The woman's reported LMP was 18.4 weeks earlier, which is only 0.6 week different from the mean age of 17.8 weeks. This is a normally proportioned fetus with a normal growth rate at this point in the pregnancy.

owing to shadowing from the more proximal tissues.

The base of the coronal triangle is the hippocampal base line (HBL) (see Chapter 8). The HBL is actually tangential to the circles around the hippocampal complex rather than the hippocampus itself. In Figure 19–2*E*, one side of the triangle is being measured. Note that the side of the triangle passes just tangential to the edge of the lateral ventricle and choroid plexus, which still occupies most of the bodies of the lateral ventricles. As the fetal head and ventricles grow, the size of the choroid plexuses does not grow as much and the relative size of the plexuses appears smaller. Earlier than the 18th week, the choroid plexuses and consequently the lateral ventricles extend beyond the sides of the coronal triangle. For the next 2 weeks, these structures should be approximately tangential to the sides of the coronal triangle. By the 20th LMP week, the lateral ventricles are well within the apex of the coronal triangle. After the 20th LMP week, the choroid plexuses should always be within the sides of the triangle. This indicates a preferential growth in the centrum semiovale and associated tissues of the cerebral hemispheres over the ventricles and midbrain structures. This has the potential of being a good guide line for evaluation of hydrocephalus, but more research is required to define the precise relationships throughout gestation. The HBL is a bisquamal diameter at or just caudal to the squamous suture, depending on the exact plane, and lies transversely in the base X.[16]

The fetal eyes and the bridge of the nose are seen in Figure 19–2*G*. The + cursors measure the outer orbital distance, often called the BiOD.[17, 18] The BiOD is often used to estimate fetal age if other cranial measurements are difficult to obtain owing to fetal position. The BiOD, however, is one of the most variable measurements. The bright echoes posterior to the orbits are the sphenoids.

A detailed study of any fetus should include both long and transverse sections through the spine (see Fig. 19–2*A*, *B*, *H*, and *I*). Figure 19–2*B* is a long axis of the thoracolumbar spine that is oblique to the sagittal plane from the left posterior to the right anterior in the fetus. Posteriorly in the fetus, one set of the two sets of posterior ossification centers is seen; more anteriorly are the ossification centers of the vertebral bodies. In Figure 19–2*B*, the plane of view is slightly oblique to the long axis and does not show the upper and lower ends of the spine.

Transversely, the spinal cord is located in the center of three ossification centers, two bilaterally and posteriorly, and the single vertebral body anteriorly (see Fig. 19–2*H* and *I*). The triangular arrangement of these ossification centers should be relatively uniform throughout the length of the spine, with very slight widening in the cervical spine and the lumbosacral region before the spine tapers to a point at the caudal end.

Figure 19–2*I* shows the kidneys bilaterally on either side of the vertebral body. These are normal-appearing kidneys in the 18th LMP week. A urinary tract obstruction below the kidneys causes some degree of hydronephrosis later in pregnancy, but at this time kidney function is not fully established. The relatively uniform speckled echogenicity of the anterior abdominal contents can be observed in Figures 19–2*A*, *B*, *H*, and *I*. This also is normal in the 18th week; later in pregnancy, fluid in the bowel becomes more obvious.

Both femurs are being measured in Figure 19–2*J*. The femur nearest the transducer appears straighter than the distal femur. This is an illusion because the anterior and lateral surfaces of the femurs are straighter than the medial and posterior surfaces of the femurs. Note that there is only 0.5 mm difference in the measurements, with the more curved-appearing bone measuring the longer. The knees are bent, and the lower legs are not visualized in this image.

The humerus is usually easy to locate by finding the skull, spine, and shoulder. In Figure 19–2*K*, the humerus nearest the transducer is measured.

In several of the images, it is possible to locate the placenta as being fundal (Fig. 19–2*L*) and circumferential from front to back (see Fig. 19–2*C* and *D*). The quantity of amniotic fluid can be observed to be normal. The amniotic membrane is normally completely fused to the chorion by the 18th LMP week.

MOVEMENT

Fetal motions become increasingly variable with age. Periods of active motion and quiet periods are observed. The fetus changes position, can turn over completely, and can move from a cephalic to a breech presentation during the time of a normal sonographic examination. When this occurs, the position is reported to be variable.

The hands become more obvious during LMP week 18. Figure 19–2*L* shows the fetus clasping its hands. By the 18th week, it is also possible to see the hands occasionally grasp the umbilical cord; however, head and face touching remains one of the most common activities for the hands.

A slight change in the rate of deceleration takes place at about the 15th LMP week. The rate has been declining since the start of the ninth LMP week. During the 18th week, the FHR is almost flat, with a mean heart rate of approximately 147 ± 16 B/M (95% population), which continues to decline to a rate of approximately 140 ± 27 B/M at term. After this time in gestation, the FHR exhibits more beat-to-beat variability depending on maternal diet, stimulus, and fetal activity.

SIZE/AGE

The fetus used in the example for the 18th week is actually a late 17- to 18-week fetus. The mother reported her LMP to have been 18.4 weeks prior, and the range of ages for 10 fetal parameters was between 17.1 and 18.4 LMP weeks, with a mean of 17.8 weeks (Fig. 19–2*M*). In the computer analysis of the ARA, it can be observed that the abdominal AC and HumL are relatively large, with sonographic size/ages of 18.4 weeks, whereas the FemL is relatively small at 17.1 weeks. By ARA, all parameters are within ± 1.0 SD of the mean age. This variation in parameter ages is considered normal.

When fetuses begin to flex and extend their bodies, the CRL is no longer a valid measurement in most cases. In Figure 19–2*A*, a CRL is being measured using a curvilinear measurement. This measurement was produced using the perimeter measuring function without closing the ends of the curve to form a circumference; thus, the measurement = 133.3 mm (see Fig. 19–2*A*) is actually the length of the curved line. This measurement is actually longer than the CRL measurement of record (123 mm), which was the average of several such measurements. Using this curvilinear function produces highly variable measurements depending on the placement of the curve. This method, as well as the CRL measurement, is not recommended after the 15th LMP week.

One study found that the relative size of the abdomen as early as 17 LMP weeks can be used to project birth weight.[19] This means that in the current example for the 18th week, the expected birth weight would be just above the average because the current AC is at + 0.6 SD relative to the mean of 10 fetal parameter ages using ARA (see Fig. 19–2*M*). Hadlock and associates found that fetal femurs tended to correlate with birth lengths, thus putting a slightly different twist on the earlier thesis of the AC and birth weight.[20]

The 18-week fetus in this example appears well proportioned using ARA. The AC is +0.6 SD, the FemL is −0.8 SD, and the HumL is +0.6 SD. The CRL and all five cranial parameters are within ± 0.2 SD of the mean. Thus, this fetus would be expected to deliver at term being slightly heavier and shorter than average based on the ARA of just the AC and FemL. However, because a correlation between humerus length and birth length has not been established, we cannot be sure if the slightly longer than average humerus mitigates the correlation between the relatively short femur and birth length. This kind of multivariate analysis deserves more research.

LMP Week 21

OBSERVATIONS

By midpregnancy, the entire fetus cannot be observed in a single sonographic real-time image. I like the approach of first observing the birth canal transabdominally through the maternal bladder. This allows one to rule out placenta previa, and once that is done, a patient may be allowed to empty her bladder and relax a bit. An extremely full bladder is not necessary after the first trimester, except in the occasional partial previa, and may make the sonographic experience quite unpleasant. Many humane sonographers justifiably argue that a full maternal bladder is no longer required for any obstetrical examination now that transvaginal transducers are available.

After placenta previa has been ruled out and the woman has relieved herself, the sonographic examination can continue by carrying out a general survey in which the fetal position, amniotic fluid, and placenta grade are assessed. Next a detailed study of the head, trunk, and extremities is conducted. By the time the head and abdomen observations are completed, the location of the extremities can be more easily anticipated. The positions of the extremities can vary markedly.

Examinations seem to progress faster and be more uniformly complete if one follows a routine as much as possible. If problems are encountered because of fetal position while obtaining some measurement or making certain observations, then one might of course go on to some other fetal observation and hope for a better position a little later.

In the example of a 21-week fetus, the examination was begun as shown in Figure 19–3*A*. The + cursors mark the internal and external ora. An image such as this can rule out an incompetent cervix and placenta previa.

In Figure 19–3*B*, a grade II placenta can be seen to be anterior. Loops of cord are evident as small linear echoes, which represent specular reflection from the anterior and posterior walls of the umbilical vessels. The fetal position was determined by real-time to be transverse, with the fetal head to the woman's right and fetal occiput toward her head (i.e., facing the mother's feet).

The standard THC is shown in Figure 19–3*C*. The thalamus, interhemispheric fissure, and cavum septi pellucidi define this plane. This is a normally shaped head with a normal transverse cephalic index (TCI = BPD/FOD = 0.79). The normal TCI is approximately 80% ± 10% in 95% of the population throughout pregnancy.[21]

The coronal view of the head in Figure 19–3*D* reveals that the cranium is nearly a perfect circle, which also confirms that the head is normally proportioned. The HBL (+ cursors) is passing just tangential to the bases of the circles that reside bilaterally around the hippocampal complexes. The HBL also passes just superior to the tops of the ridges of the petrous portions of the temporal bones. The transverse midportion of the bodies of the lateral ventricles can be faintly seen extending diagonally away from midline above the thalamus. The VCD (X cursors) is the distance from the vertex of the skull to the middle of the HBL in the brainstem, in this case 38.3 mm. By placing a straightedge from the vertex (X cursor) to the ends of the HBL (+ cursors), the bodies of the lateral ventricles can be observed to reside wholely within the apex of the coronal cranial equilateral triangle (CCET).

The CCET is a useful measurement. The height of the CCET is the VCD, a line in the interhemispheric fissure from the vertex of the skull to the midpoint of the HBL or base of this triangle. In normally shaped fetal

Text continued on page 446

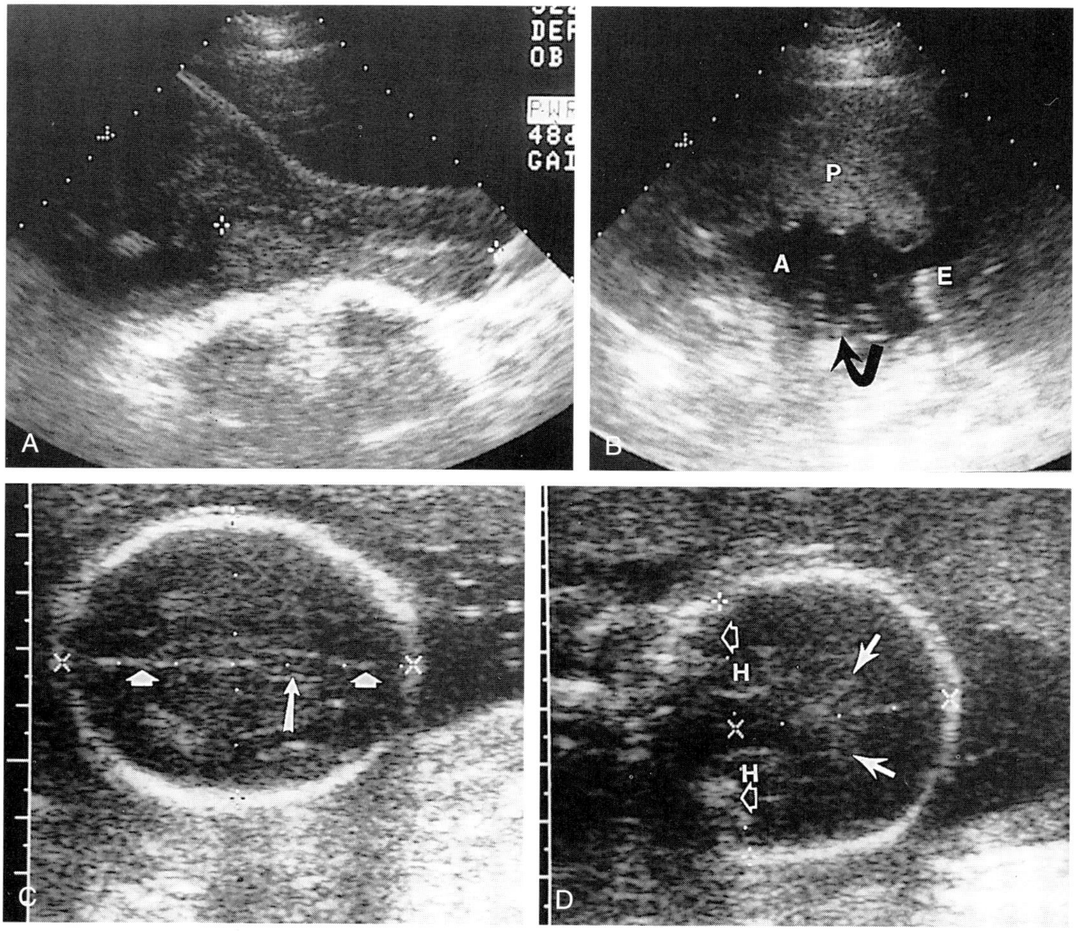

FIGURE 19–3. LMP WEEK 21.

A, Sagittal section through the lower uterine segment in the 21st LMP week of pregnancy. The endocervical canal can be seen between the + cursors. Note the shape of the external cervix and os at the edge of the image. The cervix measured 84.8 mm long and is normal.

B, In this image, near the uterine fundus, the only part of the fetus observed is an extremity (E). The placenta is a grade II. The slight suggestion of developing cotyledons can be seen as divisions of the placental tissue. The amniotic fluid (A) is adequate and appears clear except for a few free loops of umbilical cord (curved arrow).

C, The common view of the transverse head circumference (THC). The biparietal diameter (BPD) is measured (+ cursors = 49.4 mm) from the leading (outer) edge of the proximal parietal bone to the leading (interior) edge of the distal parietal bone. Note that the proximal + cursor is placed at the edge of the bone and not at the edge of the scalp, which is seen as a less echogenic layer around the skull. The fronto-occipital diameter (FOD) (X cursors) is measured from the middle of the frontal bone to the middle of the occipital bone to exclude beam-width artifacts and to preserve a more consistent transverse cephalic index (TCI) (see Chapter 8 for a discussion of this measurement method). The view for the THC always contains the cavum septi pellucidi (narrow arrow), and the interhemispheric fissure (wide arrows) is midline. The BPD is always perpendicular to the interhemispheric fissure and through the thalamus. In this case, the head is normally shaped with a THC of 0.79, which is only slightly on the dolichocephalic side of the mean TCI of 0.80.

D, This view of the fetal head again reveals a normally shaped skull, which is almost a perfect circle in the coronal view. The hippocampal baseline (HBL, + cursor) is the bisquamal measurement, which passes tangential to the inferior edges of the circles around the bilateral hippocampal complexes (H). The open arrows point to the top of the petrous pyramids. The faintly echogenic areas associated with the bodies of the lateral ventricles (solid arrows) are seen on either side of the midline. The vertical cranial diameter (VCD, X cursors) is measured from the midvertex to the middle of the HBL, at the center of the brainstem.

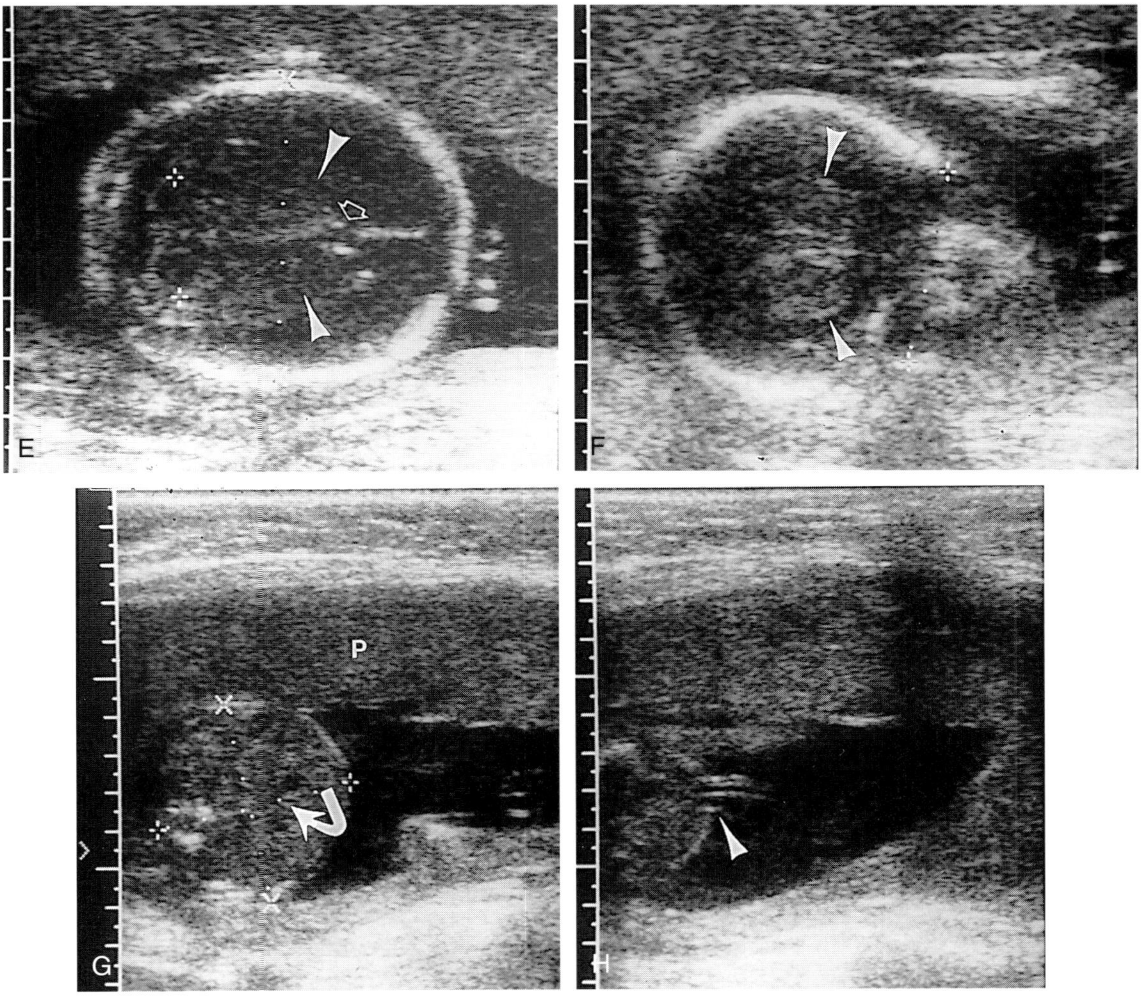

FIGURE 19–3. *(Continued)*
E, This transverse view of the head is oblique from low in the posterior to high in the frontal aspects of the skull. The cerebellum (+ cursors) is measured in the occipital fossa; the cavum septi pellucidi (open arrow), which is higher in the anterior head, is also seen. The arrowheads point to the area of the thalamus, and a BPD is measured (X cursors = 49.3 mm) only 0.1 mm different from the more traditional one in *C.* This is not an appropriate plane for measurement of the FOD.
F, This plane is from low in the anterior head (+ cursors = binocular outer distance [BiOD]), where the orbits and nasal bones are observed, to high in the posterior portion of the head. This view can be used for a valid BPD measurement because the thalamus (arrowheads) and interhemispheric fissure are midline. This view cannot be used for an FOD measurement.
G, A normal abdominal circumference is measured perpendicular to the spine and at the level where the umbilical vein curves into the liver (curved arrow). This faintly hypoechoic umbilical vein was more clearly appreciated with real-time. The placenta (P) is anterior, and the amniotic membrane is completely fused.
H, The umbilical cord insertion (arrowhead) into the anterior abdominal wall is clearly seen. This view is important to rule out abdominal wall defects such as gastroschisis or omphalocele.

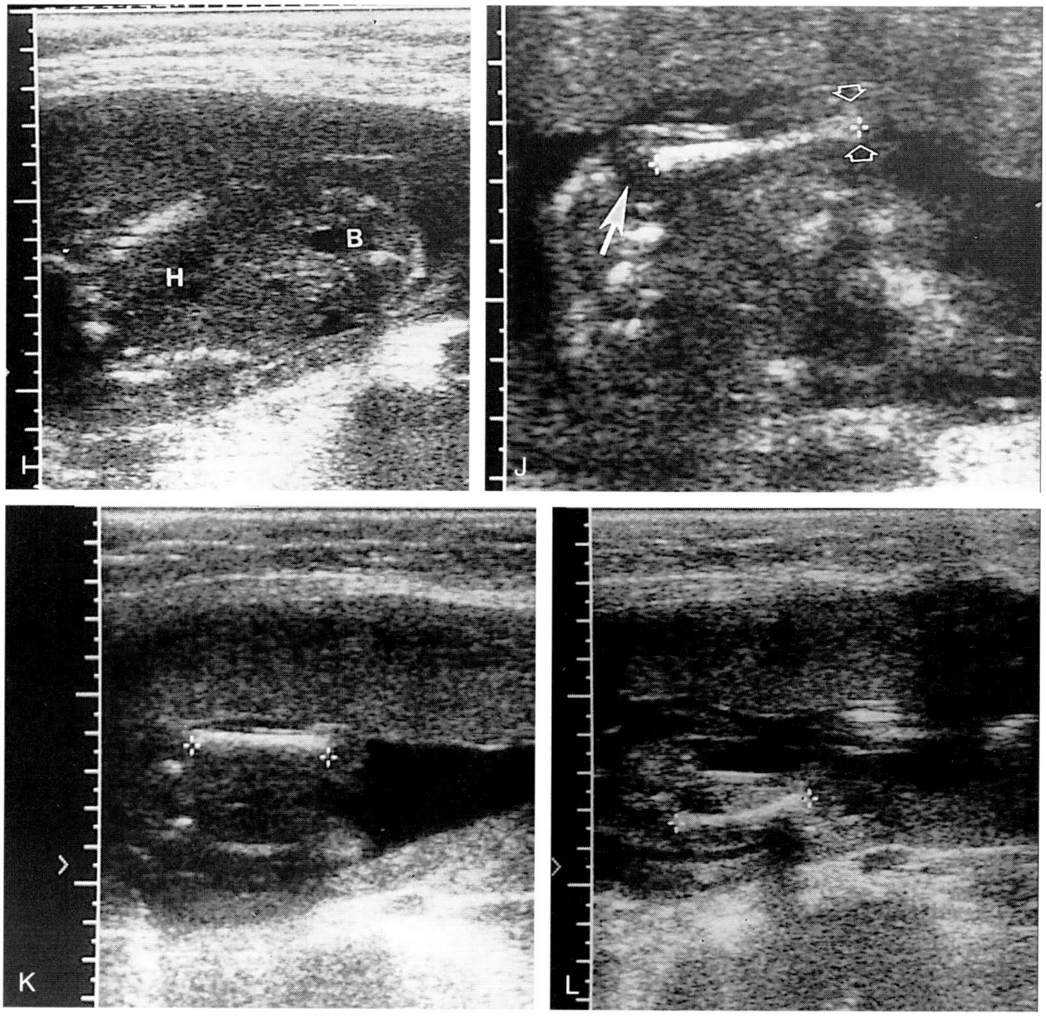

FIGURE 19–3. *(Continued)*
I, Coronal view of the fetal trunk showing the heart (H) in the thorax and the urinary bladder (B) in the pelvis. The stomach is not seen in this projection. This view can be helpful in assessing abdominal fluid cavities and the relationship of the organs.
J, The humeral diaphysis is measured (+ cursors). The hypoechoic, cartilaginous, proximal humeral head (solid arrow) and the widening of the distal lateral and medial humeral condyles (open arrows) can be observed.
K, The proximal femoral diaphysis is measured (+ cursors = 36.3 mm). Note the very straight appearance of the bone. The more distal femur is in the shadow of the measured femur.
L, By using cross-plane angling, the more distal femoral diaphysis is measured (+ cursors = 36.1 mm). Note the curved appearance of the medial surface of the diaphysis. Both femurs are normal; the difference in measurement is small (0.2 mm) and is probably due to the focal range (>) being set for the distal femur, resulting in some beam-width artifact addition to the proximal femur measurement. Compare this with *K*. The soft tissues of the thigh are shown in this image.

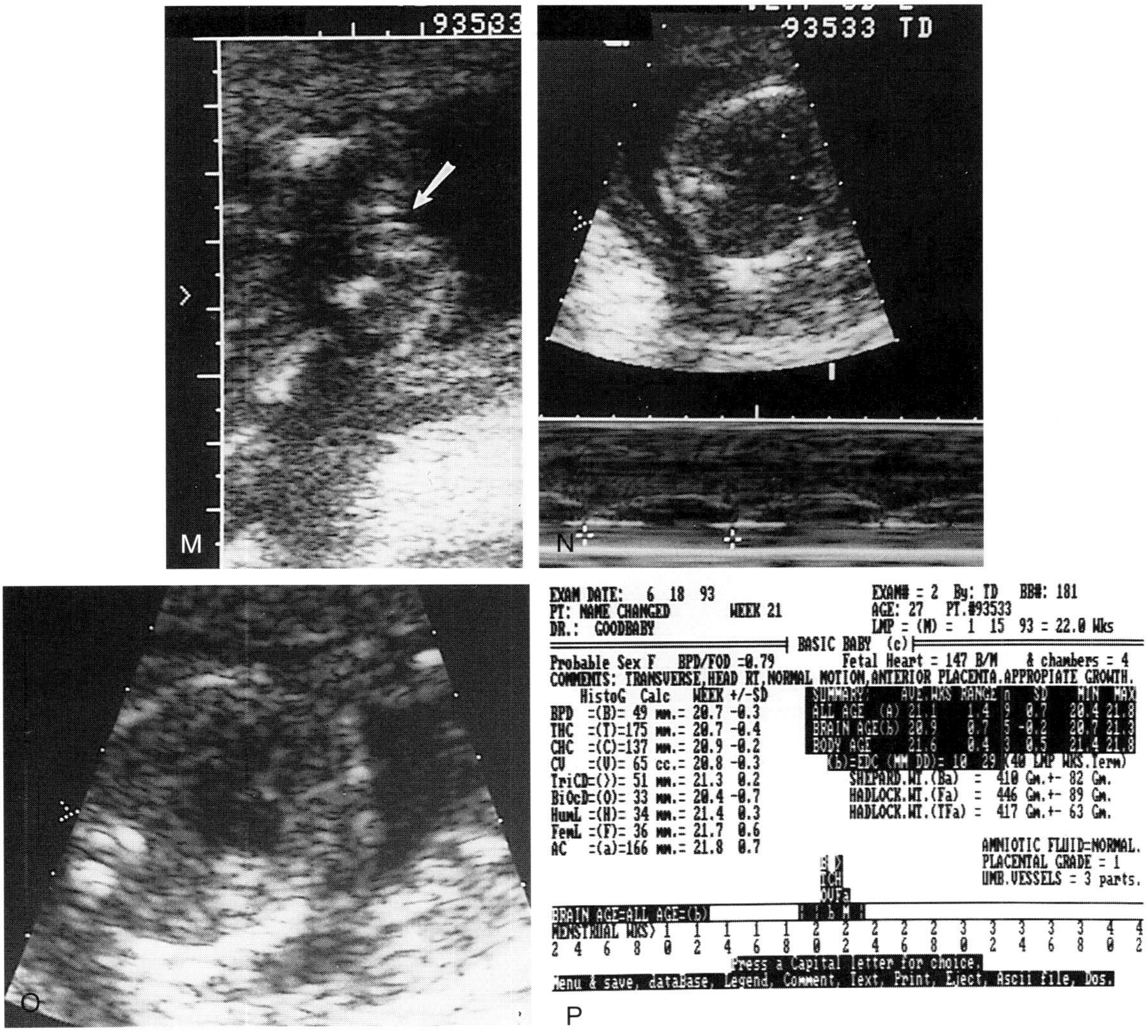

FIGURE 19–3. *(Continued)*

M, The female genitalia (arrow). The two parallel echogenic lines are specular echoes from the medial edges of the labia majora. The bright echoes on either side and posterior to the labia are from the pelvic bones.

N, The fetal heart rate (+ cursors, fetal heart rate [FHR] = 147 B/M) is measured and is normal. The M-mode vector (dots through heart) can be seen in the transverse section through the thorax.

O, An enlargement of the transverse section of the thorax reveals a normal four-chamber heart at 21 LMP weeks. In this image, the septa of the heart are indistinct; however, on real-time, the four chambers of the heart were obvious. Real-time motion often gives a much clearer impression of dynamic anatomy than do the still images.

P, Computer age range analysis produces an average age of 21.1 LMP weeks from nine fetal parameters with a range of 1.4 weeks. All parameters were within ± 1 SD of the mean, a normally proportioned fetus. Because the woman's reported LMP was 22.0 weeks prior, relatively normal growth is also assumed. However, if the LMP is a well-established date, the difference in the average age and the LMP age might possibly be due to mild intrauterine growth retardation (IUGR). If IUGR is clinically suspected, another examination at a later date helps determine if the growth rate is appropriate.

heads, the VCD, when averaged with the BPD and FOD, results in a 3-D BPD correction (3-D BPD) and is the basis of several equalities that I find interesting.[22]

$$\text{BPD} = \text{3-D BPD} = (\text{FOD} + \text{BPD} + \text{VCD})/3 = (\text{FOD} + \text{VCD})/2 = \text{TriCD}$$

The last equality, the TriCD, is the triangle circumference diameter. The coronal fetal skull forms the circle that circumscribes the CCET. The BPD is the diameter of this circle. (Chapter 8 discusses this solid 3-D geometry of the fetal calvarium in detail.)

In a fetal skull in which the linear array transducer face can be oriented parallel to the interhemispheric fissure, such as it is in Figure 19–3*C* and *D*, the transducer can be rotated around an axis that passes transversely through the fetal thalamus to arrive at either of the next two views (Fig. 19–3*E* and *F*). In Figure 19–3*E* the cerebellum (+ cursors, 19.7 mm) and BPD (X cursors, 49.3 mm) are measured. Notice that this BPD and the standard BPD measurement (+ cursors, 49.4 mm) in Figure 19–3*C* are only 0.1 mm different. If the reader uses mechanical dividers or marks on a piece of paper to compare the BPD, through the thalamus in Figure 19–3*F*, with the image scale on the side, a measurement of approximately 49 mm is again found.

These four images demonstrate that the only requirement for a valid BPD is that the measurement be perpendicular to the interhemispheric fissure and pass transversely through the thalamus (see Chapter 8 for more discussion of this and the various cranial measurements). The BiOD is being measured in Figure 19–3*F* between the + cursors. The nasal bones and septum can be seen midway between the orbits. The BiOD produces a relatively highly variable measurement, and I do not recommend it for use alone to date a pregnancy. It may be used in an average of dates established from other parameters.

The AC should be measured perpendicular to the spine at the level where the umbilical vein joins the left portal vein. In the proper plane for the AC, the umbilical vein appears to curve to the right into the fetal liver. This right-handed curve has been called the *hockey-stick sign* because of its shape. In Figure 19–3*G*, the anterior placenta is obvious.

Just caudal to the plane for the AC measurement, the insertion of the umbilical cord can be seen in Figure 19–3*H*. This type of view is helpful in ruling out omphalocele or gastroschisis, abdominal wall defects that generally occur just to the right of the umbilicus. With an omphalocele, the bowel and liver may protrude through the defect and be covered by a membrane. In gastroschisis, the bowel is free floating in front of the abdominal wall and is not covered by a membrane. Color Doppler imaging can be helpful in distinguishing a normal coil of umbilical cord in front of the abdomen from a mass of bowel of a gastroschisis.

The coronal view of the fetal abdomen (Fig. 19–3*I*) can help document the relative sizes and locations of the abdominal contents. In this image, the most obvious fetal fluid cavity is the urinary bladder. In the thorax, the heart can be located. Small movements of the real-time plane of view allow evaluation of the fetal renal kidneys and stomach to help rule out abnormal collections of fluid.

The humerus is viewed in Figure 19–3*J* in a coronal section. The epicondyles of the humerus can be seen as a widening of the bone at the distal end. The head of the humerus is cartilaginous and hypoechoic at the proximal end of the humerus.

Two different approaches to the fetal femur are demonstrated in Figure 19–3*K* and *L*. In *K*, the femur is viewed in a coronal section from the lateral side. Image *L* is again a coronal section but from the medial approach. Note that when viewed from the lateral side, the femur appears less curved than when viewed from the medial aspect. This is because the medial and posterior surfaces of the femur are more curved than the lateral and anterior surfaces. Because the surface of the bone reflects most of the sound, the shape of the side in the shadow generally cannot be appreciated. Also note that there is only 0.2 mm difference in the two measurements of the femurs. The first femoral length may measure longer because the area of greatest focus (> marker) is distal to the area of interest and the beam-width artifact may cause the ends of the diaphysis to be less distinctive.

The labia of the female genitalia are observed on either side of the vaginal opening in Figure 19–3*M*. The fetal labia can be affected by the maternal hormones and become prominent enough to be confused with a scrotum. Care should be taken to investigate whether the fetus has a penis to be more certain of the sex of the fetus. With experience, a sonographer should be able to determine the sex in most cases. In an unpublished study of 875 consecutive examinations in which 474 follow-ups were available to confirm sex (54.5% of the mothers returned self-addressed stamped postcards), three sonographers (TD, LP, and DKD) correctly identified males 96% and females 83% of the time, for a total of 90% correct predictions throughout the second and third trimesters. The predictions were incorrect 17% of the time for females and 4% for males. The earliest correct identification was in the 16th LMP week for a female and in the 12th week for a male. Of the total study group, the sonographers recorded a predicted sex in only 365 of the 875 cases (42%) and in only 47% of the follow-up cases. Reasons for not predicting fetal sex were a small fetus and insufficient resolution, inappropriate fetal position, and parents' request that the sex not be determined.

MOVEMENT

During the 21st LMP week, fetal motions include the entire repertoire of motions. Changes of position; extension and flexion of the extremities, neck, and trunk; breathing and swallowing motions; and grasping with the hands may be observed at any time until term. Also observable are periods of quiet when a fetus appears to be sleeping. According to the requirements for a normal score on the BPP, a fetus should exhibit three discrete movements during at least every period of 30 minutes.[23]

As a general rule of thumb, I expect to see normal motions during the course of an examination lasting at least 15 minutes. An active fetus is reassuring. A fetus in which the beating heart is the only noticeable motion should become the object of close scrutiny for longer periods. Although this rule of thumb has not been subjected to rigorous scientific method, it is the result of almost 20 years of sonographic observations.

A fetus most often touches the face and head, sucks its thumbs and fingers, pulls its ears, and appears to touch the eyes and nose as well as the scalp. A fetus can also be observed to clasp its hands and to grasp its feet and other parts of its body. Because the umbilical cord attaches to the anterior abdomen at the level of the elbows and between the hands, it is not surprising that grasping the cord is the activity second only to face and head touching. (see Chapter 17 for more on fetal hand activities).

By midpregnancy, the fetal heart rate is quite variable, depending on fetal activity and environmental influences. The mean rate is in the mid-140s but varies as much as ± 25 B/M or more (Fig. 19–3*N*). By this time, the four chambers of the heart should be easily observed (Fig. 19–3*O*).

The fetal heart has been observed to skip several beats completely. This brief, total cessation of heartbeats during a sonographic examination can be startling to the sonographer and especially to the patient if she is watching the monitor. By M-mode, I also have rarely observed the fetal heart rate to reach as high as 200 B/M and then return to a more normal rate in the 150s in a matter of minutes. The exact clinical significance of occasional cardiac arrhythmias is uncertain. They are most common between 25 and 35 LMP weeks and are benign if not persistent; however, they are of concern if they do persist.[24]

SIZE/AGE

In the current example of a 21-LMP-week fetus, the mean of nine fetal parameter ages was 21.1 weeks, with a range of 1.4 weeks. Using ARA, all parameters are less than ± 1.0 SD from the mean age, indicating a normally proportioned fetus. The fact that the mean age of 21.1 weeks is less than 1 week different from the reported LMP age (22.0 weeks) is also reassuring (Fig. 19–3*P*).

Because the ARA indicates that the range of ages for 95% of the population is normally (±2 SD) equal to ±10% of the mean age, the total range of ages could be as much as 4.2 weeks in the 21st week. Because the mean size/age of nine parameters is trailing the reported LMP by 0.9 week, one could suspect mild symmetrical IUGR. However, because the difference is less than the normal variation in the LMP as a predictor of age, this is of little concern without other collaborating clinical information. The fact that the AC has the largest size/age at +0.7 SD also weighs against IUGR.

In this case, an earlier, collaborating sonographic examination was performed at 15.0 LMP weeks. In that examination, difference between the MFP mean age for 10 parameters and the reported LMP was precisely the same as the difference in the current examination, 0.9 week. This very close correlation of the fetal size/ages and time interval between the two examinations confirms a normally proportioned fetus with a normal growth rate. It should be noted that in both studies, the ARA indicated all parameters in this fetus to be no more than ± 0.7 SD from the mean age.

The TCI (BPD/THC) in this case at 21 LMP weeks is 0.79. At 15 weeks, the TCI was 0.82. Fetal heads have a very slight tendency to become moderately dolichocephalic at midpregnancy. The reason for this tendency is not understood (see Chapter 8 for more discussion on this topic).

LMP Week 34

OBSERVATIONS

The third trimester begins in the 26th LMP week. Most of the third trimester is much the same as the late second trimester; however, in the late third trimester or at term, sonographic fetal observations become more difficult. A fetus triples its mass in the third trimester; weight gain is from around 1200 g to approximately 3600 g. As a fetus becomes more cramped, head molding begins. Fetal observations are more tedious because the arms, legs, face, body, placenta, and uterine wall all are often pressed together.

It has been reported that the length of the cervix should not be less than 40 mm in the second and early third trimesters.[25] Others have suggested that the cervix should be at least 3 cm in length.[26] The cervical length can range between 6 and 1.9 cm.[27] The degree of maternal bladder filling can affect the cervical measurement because the bladder may press the anterior uterine wall toward the posterior wall. This pressure may make it difficult to determine the exact location of the internal os. This same bladder pressure effect may also press the opposite uterine wall against a low-lying placenta, thus giving the appearance of a placenta previa. If a sonographer suspects that this is happening, allowing the mother to empty her bladder partially or completely may eliminate the appearance of placenta previa. The degree of bladder filling for adequate sonographic evaluation in the third trimester is debatable. A woman's bladder certainly needs to be no more distended than is demonstrated in Figure 19–4*A*. The fetal head is pressed against the internal os, thus ruling out placenta previa.

Figure 19–4*B* is a sagittal section of the uterine fundus. In this image, the placenta can be observed to be anterior and a grade II. Small echogenic calcifications are seen. This placenta is approximately 4 cm thick, which is normal. In the last half of pregnancy, the placenta should be between 1.5 and 5.0 cm thick.[28] A noticeably thin placenta may be due to hydraulic pressure in polyhydramnios. A noticeably thick placenta may be due to maternal diabetes, in which case the placenta has a smooth, homogeneous texture of a grade I, even at term. A focal uterine contraction, Braxton Hicks contraction, can have the appearance of placental tissue. Focal contractions should subside after a period of 15 to 30 minutes. Extending the observation time helps resolve questions about the contractions and placenta.

The hypoechoic band between the placenta and the anterior uterine fundus in Figure 19–4*B* is the retroplacental complex of uterine vessels and should not be confused with placental abruption or subchorionic bleeding. Amniotic fluid quantities are adequate in this case. The left fetal knee is the rounded object touching the posterior edge of the placenta.

A transverse view of the left side of the uterus shows the bulk of the placenta to be in an anterior left location in Figure 19–4*C*. The field of view cuts obliquely through the distal portion of one of the extremities. Without real-time sonography, it cannot be determined from this single image if this is the fetal shin or forearm. The two echogenic dots represent either the ulna and radius in the forearm or the tibia and fibula in the leg. A vessel of the umbilical cord can be observed in the space between the extremity and placenta as a small circle of echoes.

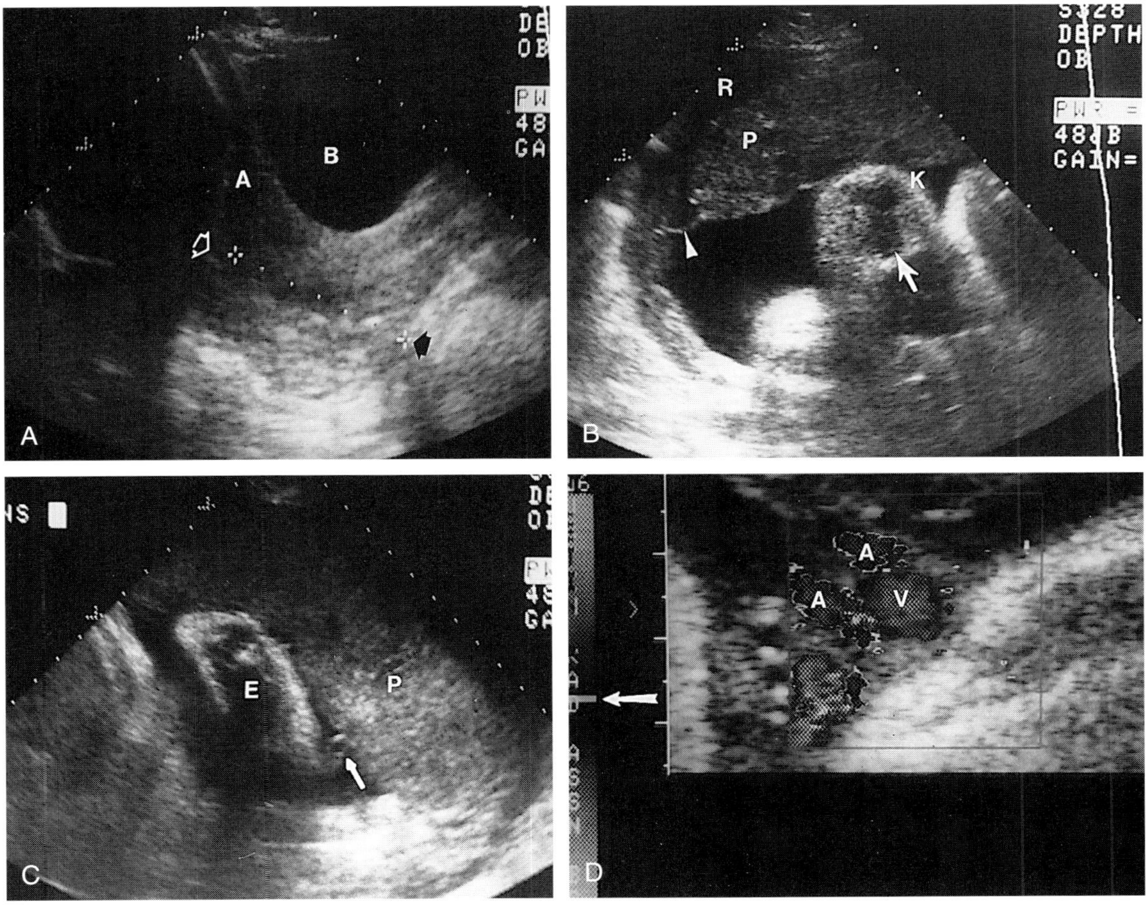

FIGURE 19–4. 34TH LMP WEEK.

A, A normal cervix in the 34th LMP week. The cervical length is measured (+ cursors = 60.6 mm). The external os (black arrow) is seen, as well as the approximate location of the internal os (open arrow). The full maternal bladder (B) is anterior to the cervix and vagina. The fetal skull is faintly seen, with an area of amniotic fluid (A) between it and the cervix, ruling out placenta previa.

B, Sagittal section through the uterine fundus. The placenta (P) is anterior, and a thin line of the chorionic plate (arrowhead, fused amnion and chorion) can be seen crossing the edge of the hypoechoic retroplacental complex (R) of vessels.The fetal knee (K) in cross section contains the hourglass-shaped, hypoechoic, cartilaginous condyles (arrow) of the distal femur.

C, Transverse section near the uterine fundus showing a portion of one extremity (E) and a small part of the umbilical cord (arrow) next to the placenta (P). The retroplacental complex is the hypoechoic area on the maternal surface of the placenta. This image shows the placental location to be anterior and left.

D, An enlargement of the umbilical cord showing the two arteries (A) and one vein (V). In this black-and-white color Doppler image, the flow toward the transducer (arteries) is outlined using the white slow-flow (arrow).

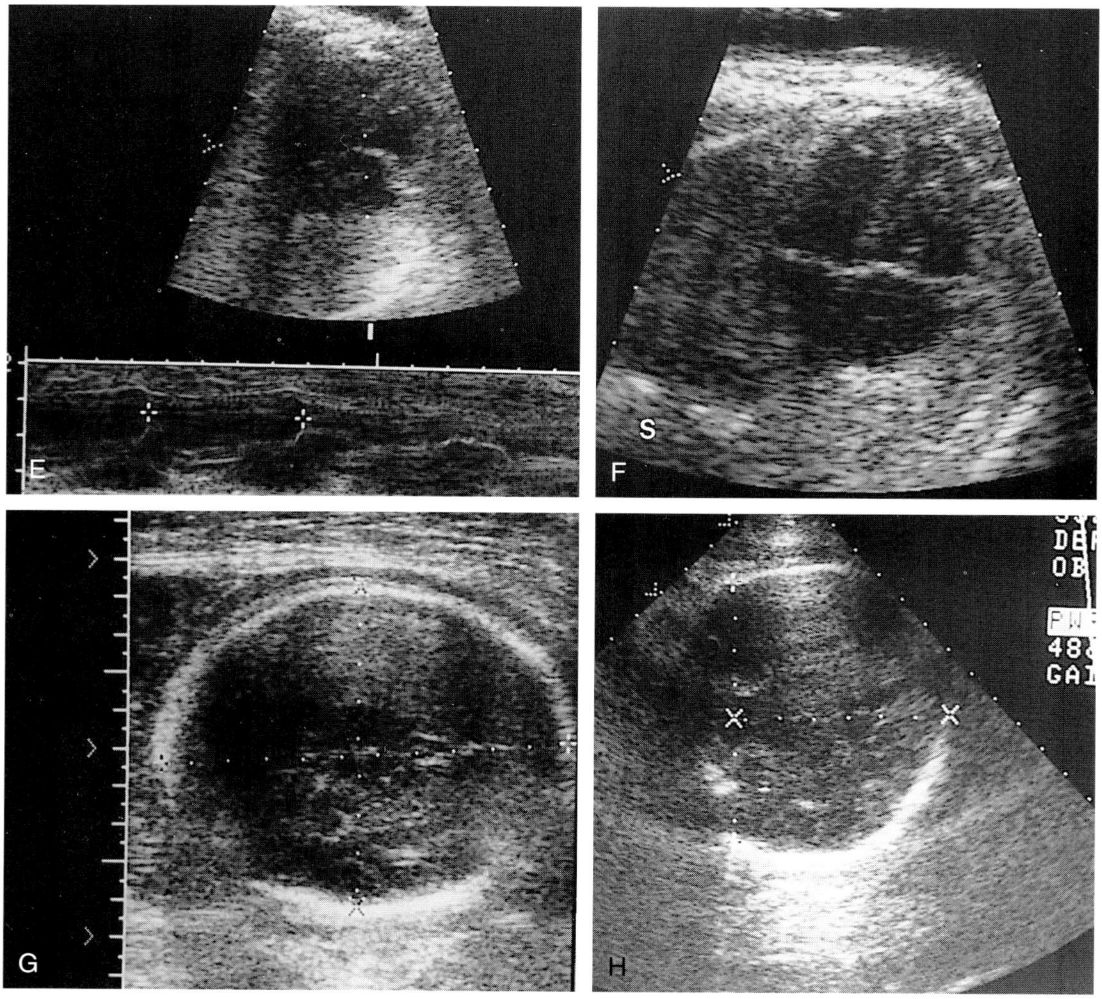

FIGURE 19–4. *(Continued)*
E, This fetal heart rate is normal at 137 B/M. By placing the M-mode vector at or near one of the valves (mitral valve in this case), a rapid or steep angle is achieved in the M-mode tracing, yielding more accurate beat-to-beat measurements.
F, Four-chamber view of the heart with the apex toward the top of the image and the atrium or top of the heart toward the bottom. The left atrium is nearest the spine (S), and the right atrium is slightly larger. The atrial septum is only faintly seen. The ventricles are clearly shown, as are the specular echoes from the atrioventricular septa and valves. The right ventricle is slightly larger and nearest the anterior chest wall at the top of the image. This heart is normal.
G, The two diameters of the transverse head circumference are measured. Note that the biparietal diameter (X cursors) does not include the scalp, and the fronto-occipital diameter (+ cursors) measures from the middle of the frontal and occipital bones. This is a normally shaped head.
H, Sector image of the coronal head circumference. The hippocampal base line (+ cursors) and the vertical cranial diameter (X cursors) are measured. This coronal view of the skull is almost a perfect circle, which is normal. Note that with the sector transducer, the edge of the skull that is parallel to the beam does not image well because of reflection and refraction of the sound.

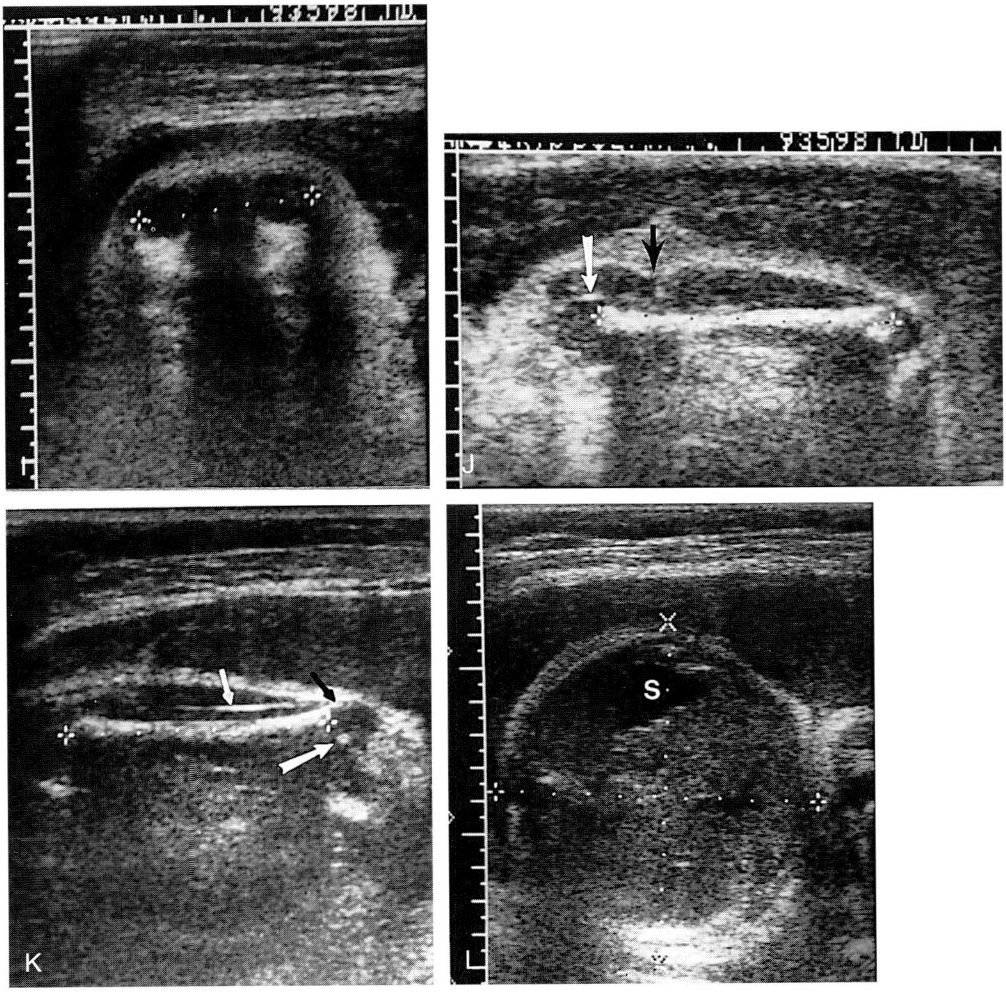

FIGURE 19–4. *(Continued)*
I, In this image, the fetus is facing toward the transducer, facilitating measurement of the outer orbital binocular distance (+ cursors). The fetal eyes appear cystlike, with smooth walls and posterior enhancement, sometimes called *through-transmission*. The nasal bones cast an acoustic shadow.
J, Posterolateral section through the long axis of the fetal arm. The humeral diaphysis is measured (+ cursors) to be 64.1 mm. The hypoechoic, cartilaginous humeral head is at the proximal end, and the proximal humeral point (PHP, white arrow) is seen as specular echoes from the surface nearest the transducer. The PHP should not be included in the measurement of the diaphysis. At the distal end of the humerus, the capitulum can be seen to project anteriorly (away from the transducer). This is the main clue that this view is from the posterior of the arm. The black arrow points to a notch between the deltoid muscle (beneath white arrow) and the triceps muscles distal to this notch.
K, Coronal view of the femur with measurement of the diaphysis (+ cursors = 69.5 mm). The widening of the cartilaginous condyles can be observed. The echogenic femoral epiphyseal ossification center (larger white arrow) is near the center of the femoral condyles. The femoral ossification centers usually appear around the 33rd LMP week and should always be present by the 36th week. The distal femoral point (DFP, black arrow) is seen as specular echoes from the surface of the condyle nearest the transducer and should not be included in the diaphyseal measurement. The bright linear echo (smaller white arrow) in the soft tissue lateral to the femur is thought to arise from the medial edge of the iliotibial band or tract, which extends from the lateral condyle of the tibia and widens superiorly, lateral to the femur, and finally attaches to the outer surface of the iliac bone of the pelvis.
L Normal transverse view of the abdomen. The anteroposterior abdominal diameter (+ cursors = 97.3 mm) and the transverse abdominal diameter (X cursors = 102.5 mm) are measured from the skin line. Note that a knee is pressed against the anterior abdominal wall, making precise location of the skin more difficult. The stomach is a fluid-filled, anechoic area (S).

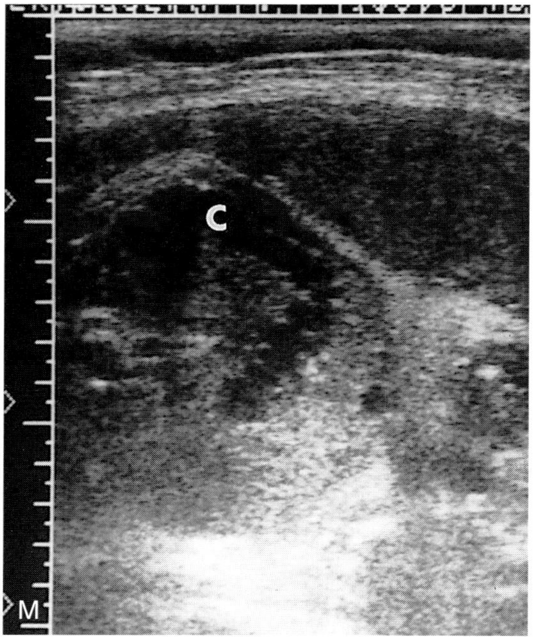

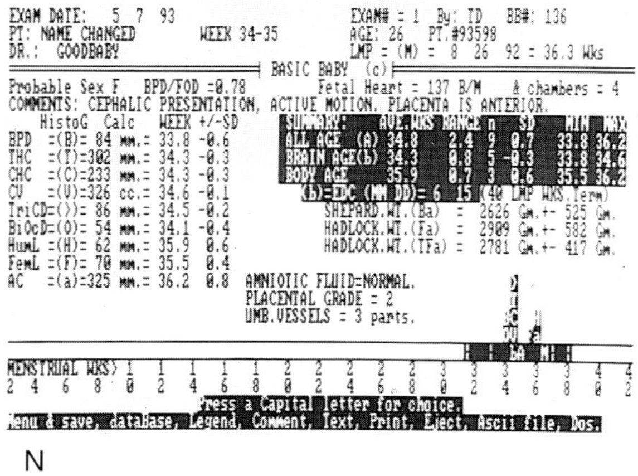

FIGURE 19–4. *(Continued)*
M, This transverse plane is lower in the fetal abdomen than *L.* The colon (C) can be seen curving around the gastric flexure. Notice the echoes inside the edges of the colon; these are from colonic haustra, bands or folds of the colon wall. This is a normal appearance in the third trimester.
N, Computer age range analysis calculated an average age of 34.8 LMP weeks from nine fetal parameters with range of 2.4 weeks. All parameters were within ± 1 SD of the mean. It is noted that the symbolic histogram is bimodal, with the distribution split between the cranial parameters and the abdominal circumference, femur and humerus. Interpretation of this situation can be troublesome. Does this indicate a fetus with a relatively large body or with a slight degree of microcephaly? More research in this area is clearly needed. This case was unavailable for follow-up.

The umbilical cord is examined by enlargement and color Doppler in Figure 19–4*D*. The use of color Doppler may aid in counting umbilical vessels in some cases. Two-vessel cords are more frequently associated with other fetal anomalies. In this image, a velocity tag in a contrasting shade is used to mark the slowest echoes moving toward the transducer. This slow-flow tag[29] is visible as a white band across the center of the color bar at the left of the image and as a contrasting white outline of the two umbilical arteries. In this image, flow in the vein is away from the transducer. The vein has no white outline and is larger than the two umbilical arteries. Color Doppler can also be valuable in differentiating between twists in the umbilical cord near the fetal abdomen and the free loops of bowel of a gastroschisis.

MOVEMENT

A fetus is vigorously active in the third trimester. Breathing, sucking, swallowing, and changes of position are common. An active fetus is expected and reassuring.

The heart rate can be quite variable, with a mean of approximately 140 B/M. Occasional variations of the heart rate are expected; even arrhythmias are considered benign if they are brief and do not persist.[24] In Figure 19–4*E*, the fetal heart rate is measured at a steady 137 B/M. Fetal heart rates can be more accurately measured if the M-mode vector passes through a valve. Rapidly moving valves give sharp changes in the M-mode tracing, making beat-to-beat cursor placement easier and more accurate.

The morphology of the heart should be

studied, and a four-chamber heart should be documented. The four chambers of the heart can be observed in Figure 19–4*F*. The fetal spine is at the lower part of the image. The left atrium of the heart is normally nearest the spine, and the right ventricle is beneath the anterior chest wall. The two sides of the heart should be approximately equal in size, with the right being very slightly larger as demonstrated in Figure 19–4*F*.[24,30]

SIZE/AGE

The fetal head is a good place to begin measuring parameters for estimation of fetal age and size. One of the most common fetal measurements is shown in Figure 19–4*G*, THC, which is more often referred to as simply the *head circumference*. In this case, the THC is being calculated from the measurements of two diameters. This circumference is characterized as being the widest point above the fetal ears in the transverse axis (BPD) and the longest skull diameter front to back (FOD) and containing the cavum septi pellucidi and thalamus. The measurements should not contain the scalp, which can be observed as a layer of echoes around the near side of the skull in this image. The protocol used here calls for the FOD to be measured to the middle of the skull echoes (see Chapter 8 for more on this topic).

This fetus has a normally shaped head with a TCI (BPD/THC) of 0.78. The normal THC is approximately 0.80 ± 0.10 in 95% of the cases. This THC of 0.78 is only slightly on the dolichocephalic side of the mean but well within the normal range of 0.70 to .090.

A coronal view of the fetal skull is shown in Figure 19–4*H*. This view is perpendicular to the plane of view in Figure 19–4*G*. The HBL is measured at 76.2 mm, and the VCD is 63.6 mm. The HBL passes just tangential to the inferior edges of the bilateral circles around the hippocampal complexes (H) and just superior to the petrous pyramids. Note the nearly perfect circle of the skull in this image, indicating a normally shaped calvarium. The coronal cephalic index (CCI = VCD/BPD) is also in the normal range at 0.83; mean CCI = 0.77, with the normal (95%) range being between 0.64 and 0.89. The interpretation of the indexes (TCI and CCI) is that the skull is being only lightly molded, with the BPD being slightly compressed (shortened). As a result, the TCI is slightly reduced and the VCD is compensatingly exaggerated; thus, the CCI is slightly greater than the mean. Although this fetal skull is well within normal limits for shape, this demonstrates the sensitivity of 3-D measurements to skull molding.

In the coronal view of the fetal skull, the thalamus is a faint hypoechoic heart shape at the center of the skull. It can also be noted in Figure 19–4*H* that the bodies of the lateral ventricles, located just above the thalamus, are not enlarged.

The fetal spine is not demonstrated here but was viewed in real-time. The spine should be examined in both the longitudinal and transverse views. Because the transverse view of the spine demonstrates only one vertebra at a time, it is more practical to examine the transverse spine in real-time rather than to photograph still frames.

In Figure 19–4*I*, the fetus is imaged facing straight toward the transducer. This position makes measurement of the BiOD particularly easy. The BiOD exhibits a relatively large degree of variation throughout pregnancy. The reason for this is unclear but is attributed to individual variations, hypertelorism (widely set eyes) and hypotelorism (narrowly set eyes), and slight changes in the plane of view, which may not always be in the largest diameter of one or the other of the orbits. Although intuition may tell one that the BiOD should be as accurate a measurement as any other because the eyes are bounded by bony structures, this is not the case. The BiOD is one of the most variable of measurements and therefore one of the least accurate for age estimation. (see Chapter 7).

Figure 19–4*J* and *K* demonstrates measurement of the humeral and femoral diaphysis, respectively. These long bones are good indicators of fetal size and age. Some variations are noted among individuals. Long birth lengths tend to correlate with longer extremity bones, and short birth lengths with shorter bones.[20] However, despite these individual variations, the long bones are relatively easy and accurate to measure sonographically if the sonographer understands the sonographic anatomy. Both the femur and humerus have cartilaginous tissue that does not calcify until after birth. This cartilaginous tissue has a sharply marginated surface that produces strong echoes on the surface nearest the transducer. Because the long bone measurements are only of the diaphysis, these surface echoes or points should not be included.

In Figure 19–4*J*, the humeral diaphysis is measured in an image from a posterolateral plane. The elbow is bent away from the transducer, and the forearm is out of the plane of view. At the proximal end of the bone, the spherical humeral head is seen with its bright surface echo or proximal humeral point (PHP). In this case, the PHP is easily distinguishable from the proximal diaphysis; however, on some occasions this distinction is not as easy to make. This plane of view of the distal end of the humerus is through the medial epicondyle, which has the characteristic club shape. The hypoechoic muscle and hyperechoic skin of the dorsal arm can also be seen.

Descriptions of the shapes of these bones becomes wordy, and readers should compare these and other sonographic images of fetal anatomy with standard anatomical textbooks for a more complete understanding.

The femoral diaphysis is measured in Figure 19–4*K* in a straight coronal plane of view. The femur appears only slightly curved in this projection. The hypoechoic condyles of the distal femur are easily observed with their bright surface echo, which has been called the *distal femoral point* (DFP).[31] This DFP should not be included in the femoral length (diaphysis) measurement. A bright echo can be observed near the center of the cartilaginous condyles. This is the ossification center of the distal femoral epiphysis. This ossification center can often be visualized after 32 weeks and should always be visualized by the 36th LMP week.[32] This echogenic center should not be included in the femur measurement.

Figure 19–4*L* and *M* shows transverse sections through the fetal abdomen. The former image is in the upper abdomen at the level of the umbilical vein and portal venous confluence in the liver. The stomach is the anechoic area in the left lateral abdomen nearest the transducer. The stomach is filled with the amniotic fluid that the fetus has swallowed. The AAD is measured from the skin line just behind the spine to the skin line at the anterior abdominal wall. The TAD is measured to the skin line at either side of the abdomen. Note that the measurements are to the skin and not to the echogenic ribs and peritoneal surfaces. In this single image, it is difficult to determine if the more distal X cursor is actually at the abdominal wall or beyond. With real-time sonography at the time of examination, this distinction was more easily made.

The AC is an important measurement for estimating fetal weight and is used in most published formulas for making this estimation. The AC can be calculated by using the two diameters (AAD and TAD) in the standard formula for the circumference of an ellipse or by using the ellipse-drawing functions provided by most modern sonographic machines. These ellipse-drawing functions can be very helpful for estimating the AC when the field of view is too narrow or when shadowing makes it impossible to visualize the entire circumference (see the later term case examples and Chapter 14 for more discussion on this topic).

In Figure 19–4*M*, the fetal aorta is seen in cross section just anterior to the spine. The fetal colon is seen as a curving hypoechoic structure with irregular edges. This appearance is normal late in pregnancy. The umbilical vein can be seen just inside the anterior abdominal wall near the umbilical cord attachment (not shown).

The fetal age and ARA are shown in Figure 19–4*N*. The average age of nine fetal parameters was 34.8 LMP weeks, with a range of ages between 33.8 and 36.2 weeks. All parameters were within ± 1 SD of the mean age. Although this is not a wide distribution of fetal ages and is decidedly normal, it is noted that the ARA histogram has a bimodal split between the head parameters and body parameters. This bimodal distribution may indicate either slight microcephaly or macrosomia. Because the average of the body ages (35.9 weeks) is closer to the woman's reported LNMP at 36.3 weeks, slight microcephaly might be suspected if the LNMP date is reliable. However, this pregnancy resulted in birth of a normal neonate at 38.3 weeks as determined by sonographic age. The birth weight was 3239 g (7.12 lb), which is slightly less than normal. The Apgar scores was 7 and

9. The use of the ARA requires further research to clarify its usefulness and sensitivity to the subtle differences in fetal proportions that are demonstrated in this case.

Term

The word *term* refers to the end of pregnancy. It is during this period that individual fetuses show their greatest parameter-to-parameter variability as well as population variability. A fetus may be fat or thin and short or long in any combination of these four generalized descriptions. The term of a normal pregnancy varies between 38 and 42 LMP weeks because not everyone delivers at exactly 40 weeks. A normal human birth occurs approximately 280 days after the LMP.[2]

The example of a term pregnancy offered here includes two examinations of the same fetus at 38 and 39 menstrual weeks. The example case was referred for BPPs twice in 5 days and scored a perfect 10 both times. The neonate was delivered 15 days after the first sonographic examination and 10 days after the second. The birth was at 40.0 LMP weeks based on the estimated age from the first examination and at 40.6 based on the second. The neonate weighed 4147 g (9 lb 2 oz), and the crown-heel length was 52 cm (19.5 in). Although redundant, it is hoped that these two studies so close together and so near to birth provide some understanding of normal variability in the fetal parameter sizes and the resulting age estimations. Readers are encouraged to compare the resulting birth weights and sizes with the two computer estimations for these examinations.

LMP WEEK 38

Observations

The general survey found the fetus in a cephalic presentation (head down), with the occiput to the woman's left. The placenta was posterior fundal and mature, as shown in Figure 19–5*A* and *B*. The amniotic fluid was adequate, and fetal motion was active, exhibiting breathing and extensions and flexions and heart rate changes as expected. The overall BPP score was 10.

In Figure 19–5*A*, one pocket of amniotic fluid is measured at 4.9 cm. Other pockets were found (not shown), yielding an amniotic fluid index (AFI) well over the required 5.0 cm but not considered excessive.[33]

The twisted umbilical cord is shown to have three vessels, two arteries and one vein (Fig. 19–5C). If convolutions of the cord such as this are near the fetal abdomen, it is possible to overlook the abnormal free loops of bowel of a gastroschisis. Color Doppler can help to distinguish a twisted cord from loops of bowel. Because high-resistance flow in the umbilical arteries has been associated with mature placentas and because a BPP was requested, it was believed that Doppler analysis of the cord was indicated. Figure 19–5*D* shows normal low-resistance flow in the umbilical artery (see Chapters 13 and 16).

Examination and measurement of the fetus began at the head. Figure 19–5*E* shows the THC with a TCI of 0.84. This TCI is well within normal limits, with a BPD that is only slightly wider and a THC slightly shorter than expected. The third ventricle is clearly seen as a hypoechoic line between two linear echoes at the center of the thalamus. It is not enlarged. The internal anatomy of the head in this image is normal.

The image in Figure 19–5*F* was obtained by rotating the transducer 90 degrees around the axis of the BPD in the previous image. The bilateral circles about the hippocampal complexes can be observed. The HBL is tangential to the bases of the hippocampal circles. The VCD extends along the midline from the vertex of the calvarium to the center of the HBL. The head is against the maternal bladder.

The internal anatomy of the fetal cranium is seen in Figure 19–5*G* to *I*. In *G*, the antrum of the lateral ventricle and choroid plexus is measured and found to be below the 10-mm threshold for ventricular enlargement. The cerebellum is measured in *H* and is observed more clearly in *I*. In *I*, the cisterna magna is measured. It is important that the cisterna magna be observed. If the spinal cord is tethered by a lower spinal defect, the cerebellum is pulled down into the posterior fossa and obliterates the cisterna. The bright echo just behind the most posterior + is the internal occipital protuberance and low portion of the falx cerebri.

Text continued on page 461

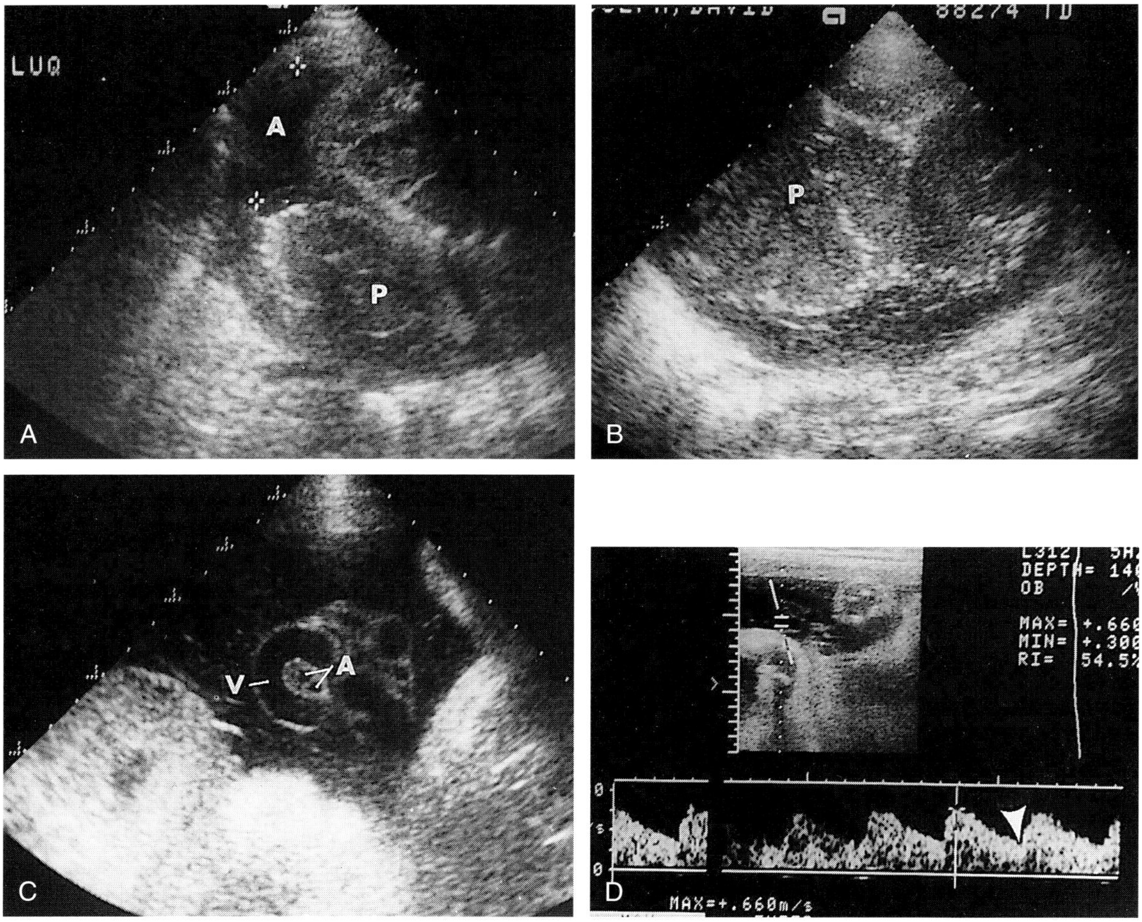

FIGURE 19–5. LMP WEEK 38.
A, Parasagittal plane through the left uterine fundus reveals a pocket of amniotic fluid that measures 4.9 cm in the vertical diameter. The placenta is posterior and observed to be maturing.
B, Sector scan through the placenta reveals a normal grade III placenta with well-defined cotyledons.
C, Another pocket of amniotic fluid containing free loops of umbilical cord. The umbilical vein (V) can be seen to curve around the two arteries (A). The echogenic material around the arteries is Wharton's jelly. Faint echoes from within the amniotic fluid arise from floating vernix and could be seen to swirl in the fluid with real-time.
D, Spectral Doppler study from one umbilical artery. The tracing across the bottom of the image shows the oscillating velocities of the blood flow, with the peak systolic velocity at 0.66 m/sec and the end-diastolic velocity (arrowhead) at 0.3 m/sec. All the flow is continuously toward the transducer (above the base line) at 0.0 m/sec. It has been found that the umbilical arterial end-diastolic flow should not stop (touch the base line) or reverse (cross the base line). Zero or reversed end-diastolic flow has been associated with reduced placental perfusion and does not bode well for the fetus.

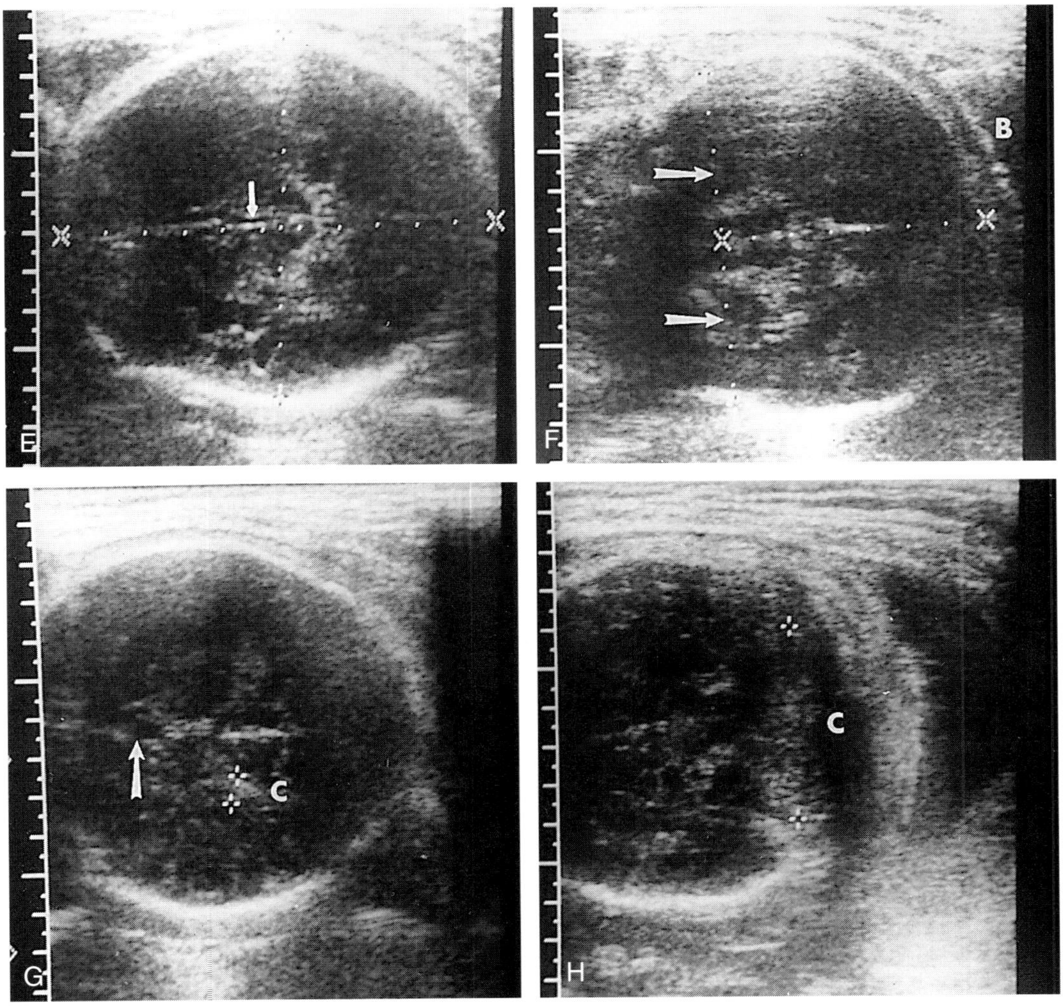

FIGURE 19–5. *(Continued)*
E, Normal transverse head circumference with a transverse cephalic index of 0.84, only slightly to the brachycephalic side of a normal 0.80. The third ventricle (arrow) is seen as a narrow slit at the center of the thalamus. This image could have been improved by lowering the gain in the near field to visualize more clearly the difference in the scalp and skull echoes.
F, Coronal view of the skull again shows a normal circular appearance. The hippocampal base line (HBL, + cursors) passes tangential to the inferior edges of the circles around the hippocampal complexes (arrows). The nearest hippocampal complex is not well visualized. The vertical cranial diameter is measured from the midvertex to the mid-HBL. The maternal bladder (B) can be seen at the edge of the image.
G, Oblique transverse view of the fetal cranium with measurements of the antrum of the lateral ventricle (+ cursors = 7.2 mm) and chorid plexus (C). This measurement should not be greater than 10 mm at any time in pregnancy. The arrow points to the cavum septi pellucidi.
H, Transverse plane through the posterior occipital fossa with transverse cerebellar diameter measurement (+ cursors = 49.8 mm). The cisterna magna (C) is not well visualized owing to acoustic shadowing from the skull.

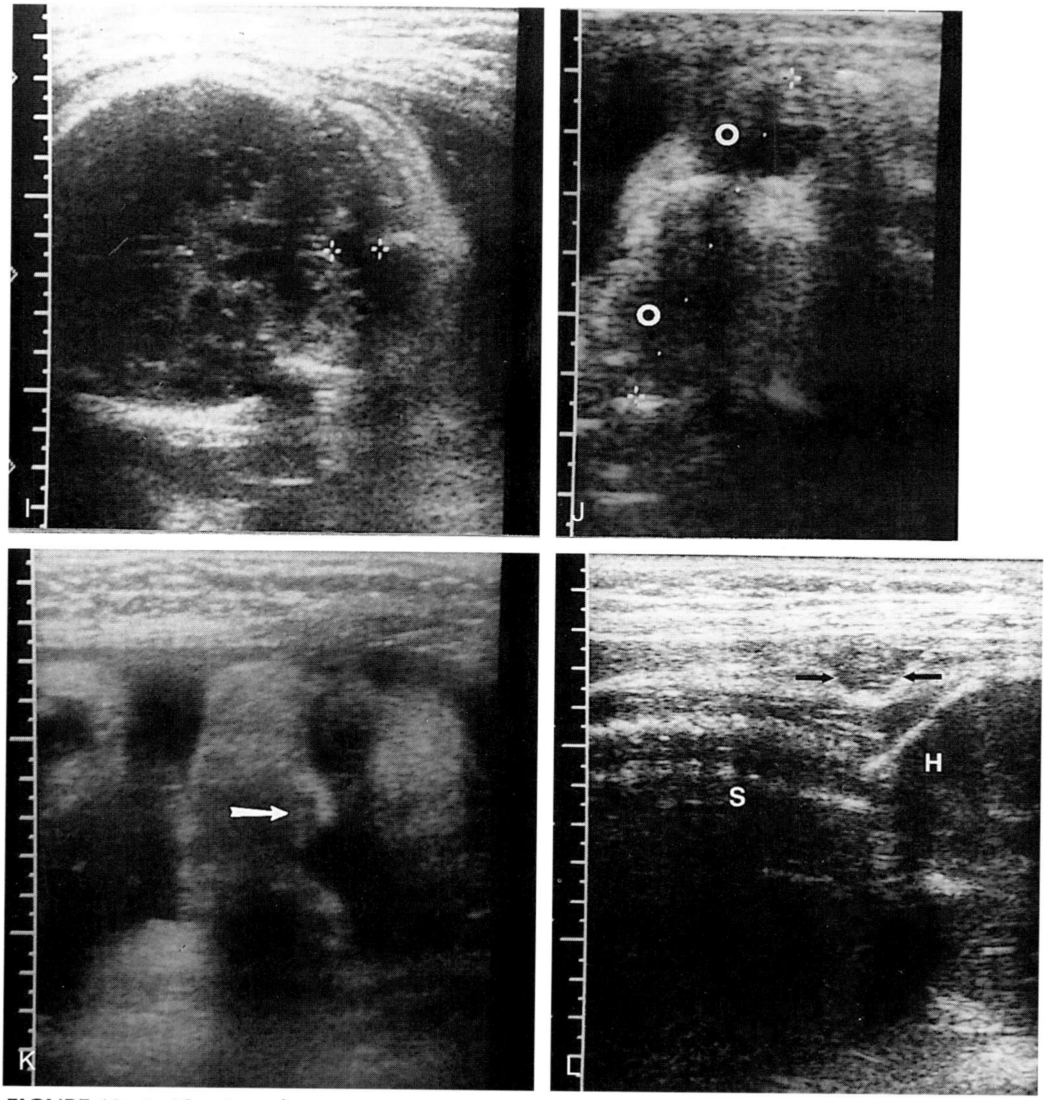

FIGURE 19–5. *(Continued)*
I, The cerebellum and cisterna magna (+ cursors) are better seen. In cases of spinal defects, the spinal cord may be tethered, resulting in a downward pressure on the brainstem and cerebellum that obliterates the cisterna magna.
J, The orbits (O) may be difficult to image as the cranial bones become more dense late in pregnancy. The more distal orbit in this figure is partially shadowed by the nasal bones. The + cursors measure the outer orbital binocular distance to be 58.0 mm, or 36.9 LMP weeks size/age.
K, Coronal plane through the face. The nose (arrow) can be seen, but the eyes are not shown well. The lips are under the arrow.
L, Posterior view of the head (H) and spine (S) shows a depression (arrows) in the skin behind the neck. This depression is caused by a nuchal cord, or a loop of umbilical cord that is across the shoulder or around the neck. Although many will worry about a cord around the neck, this is a fairly common occurrence and is not a particular cause for concern unless the cord is clearly looped twice around the neck. Color Doppler can help to assess the location of the cord. The nuchal skin does not appear thickened.

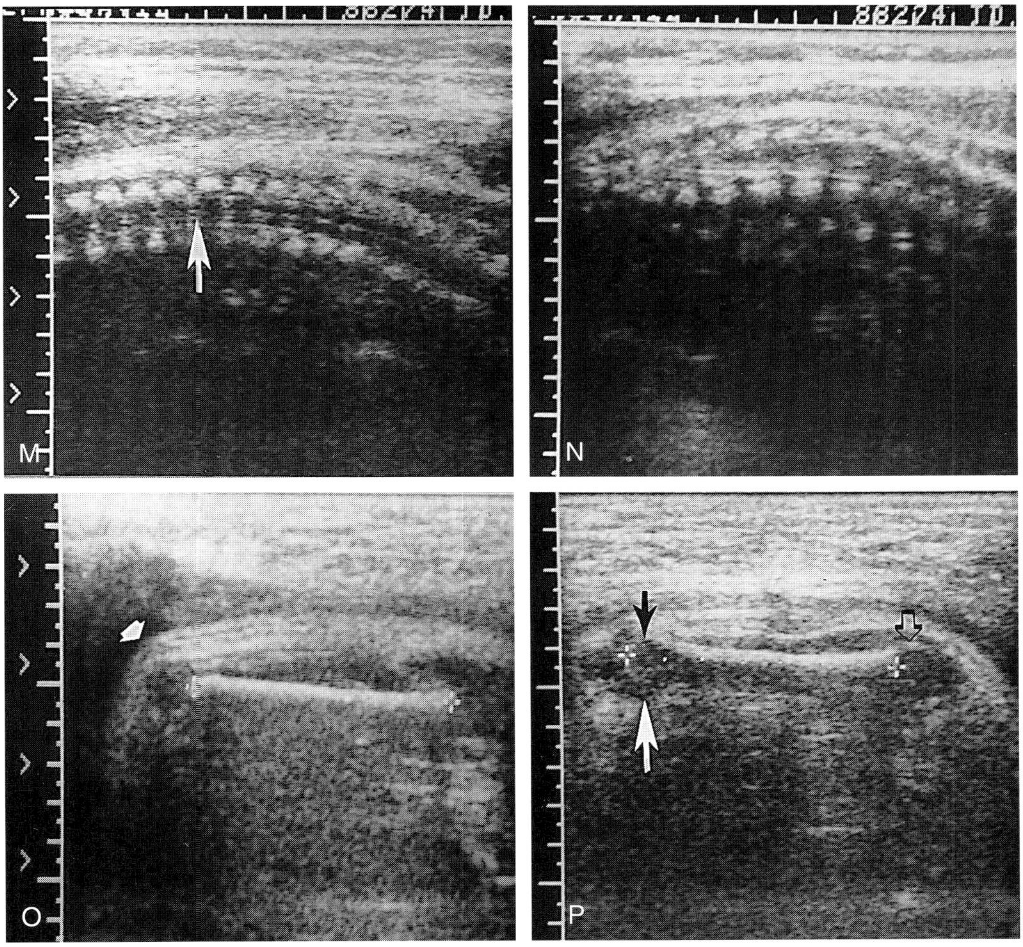

FIGURE 19–5. *(Continued)*
M, Thoracic spine. The cord (arrow) can be seen at the center. The spinal echoes should be regular in spacing in both the transverse and long axis.
N, The lumbar and sacral spine should smoothly taper to a point. The slightly wider portion of the lower lumbar spine and sacrum contains the cauda equina (horse's tail) of the cord.
O, Sagittal section of the arm with measurement of the humeral diaphysis (+ cursors = 66.5 mm). The image is from the posterior of the arm, and the elbow (arrow) is bent with the forearm away from the transducer. The deltoid muscle can be seen around the head of the humerus.
P, Coronal section of the same arm as in O. The diaphysis is measured (+ cursors = 69.5 mm). Note that the hypoechoic cartilaginous head of the humerus and its proximal humeral point (open arrow) are not included in the measurement. The distal end of the humerus can be difficult to locate because an image may contain one condyle or the other or the more protuberant trochlea. The lateral condyle (black arrow) and the medial condyle (white arrow) can be observed to widen at the distal end of the humerus.

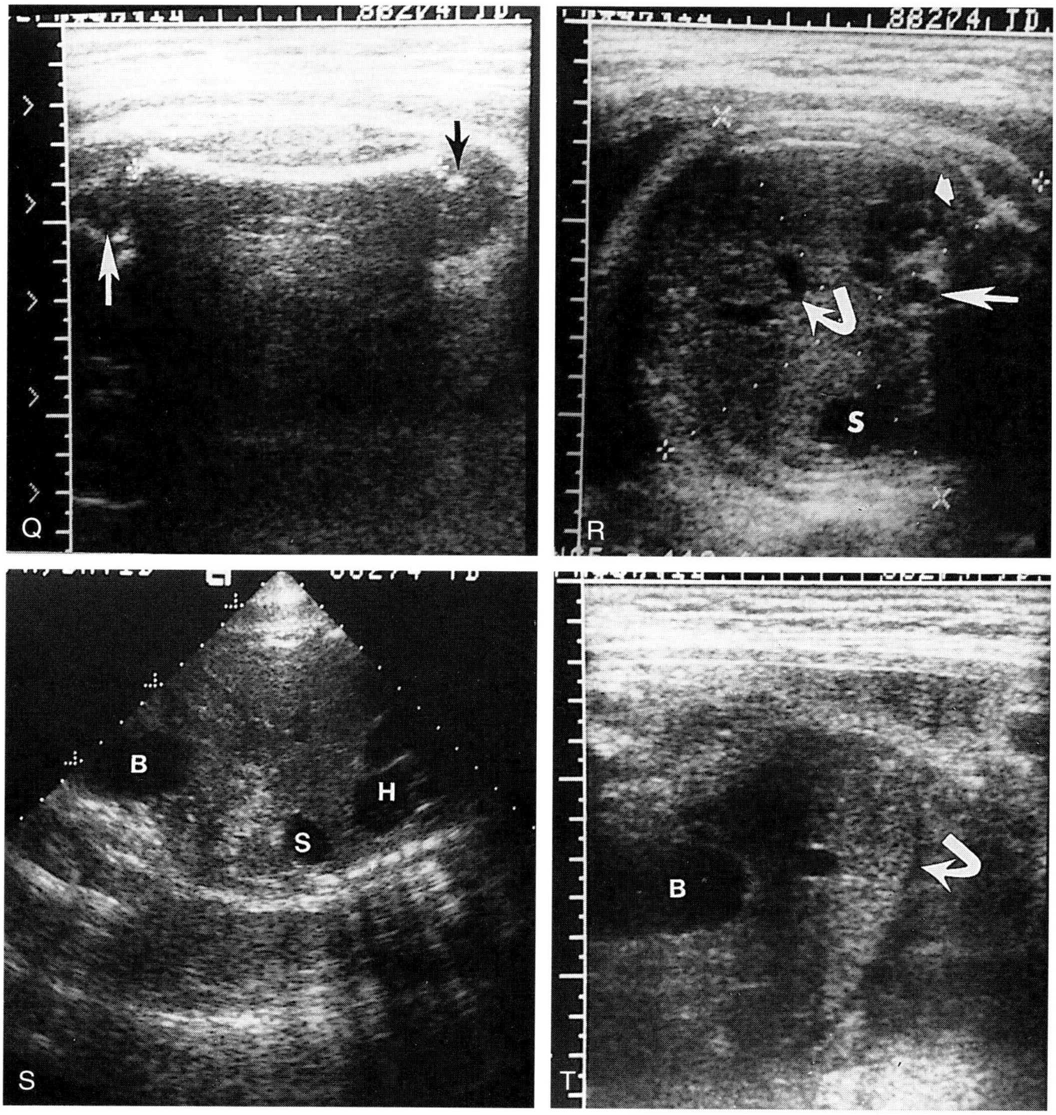

FIGURE 19–5. *(Continued)*
Q, The femoral epiphyseal ossification center (black arrow) is seen in this coronal section of the thigh. The femoral head (white arrow) can be seen at the proximal end of the bone. The measurement of the diaphysis (+ cursors = 78.5 mm) is actually from the top of the greater trochanter at the proximal end to the distal end, excluding the distal femoral point. The acoustic shadowing, posterior to the femoral diaphysis, may help to locate the ends.
R, The curve of the umbilical vein (curved arrow) into the liver is well demonstrated in this image of the abdominal circumference. The stomach (S) is in the distal part of the abdomen. The direction of the umbilical curve and the location of the stomach help sonographers to orient themselves so that other organs may be identified. The right kidney (wide white arrow) and aorta (long white arrow) are also seen. From these anatomical references, the reader should be able to locate the inferior vena cava as an anechoic oval just anterior and to the right of the aorta.
S, Coronal section through the fetal trunk, showing the three fluid cavities in appropriate relationship. The urinary bladder (B), stomach (S), and heart (H) are the primary fluid spaces in the abdomen and should always be identified. The bowel may also contain some fluid but is not as prominent as these three structures. Note the appearance of the liver and the echogenicity of the small bowel. If the stomach were to appear adjacent to the heart, a diaphragmatic hernia would be suspected.
T, This coronal section through the trunk is more anterior than *S.* The urinary bladder (B) is again visualized, and the hypoechoic line of the diaphragm (curved arrow) is shown.

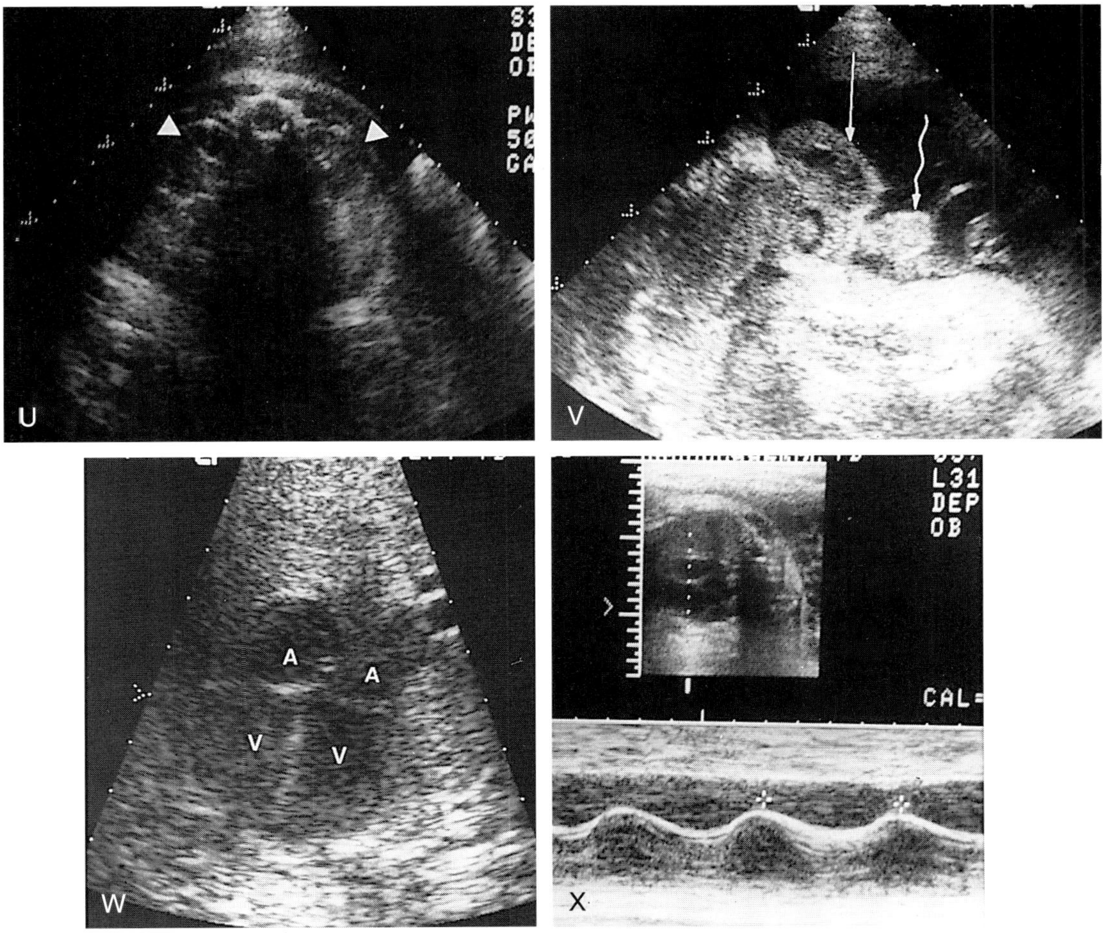

FIGURE 19–5. *(Continued)*
U, Both kidneys (arrowheads) are normal. The spine between the kidneys casts a strong acoustic shadow.
V, The male genitalia, including the scrotum (straight arrow) and penis (wavy arrow), are shown. Small hydroceles are seen as fluid around the testicles. They generally resolve by or at birth. The penis is against a normal three-vessel umbilical cord.
W, The four chambers of the heart are clear in this image. The left atrium (A) is nearest the spine and aorta at the edge of the image. The right ventricle (V) is nearest the anterior chest wall.
X, This heart rate was measured by M-mode at a normal 139 B/M. Note that the beats have very regular spacing.

Figure 19–5*J* illustrates BiOD measurement. Late in pregnancy, the facial bones are more dense and are thick enough to cause severe shadowing. Measurement of the BiOD is thus more difficult, probably adding to the variability of the measurements.

Turning the field of view 90 degrees from the BiOD measurement plane, the fetal face can be observed in a tangential view (Fig. 19–5*K*). This view allows observation of the nose and lips to detect clefts. Although a cleft lip could not be ruled out from this image alone, the image does document that the face was observed with real-time. It is often impossible to capture one picture that provides absolute proof of the presence or absence of small defects. In these cases, the observations must be made with real-time. If documentation is required, a videotape of the examination is indicated.

After the head was examined in this case, the spine was studied. Figure 19–5*L* shows the lower skull and the cervical and thoracic spine. A nuchal cord is observed. This is a common occurrence that has been reported in 25% of all normal deliveries.[34] Unless the cord

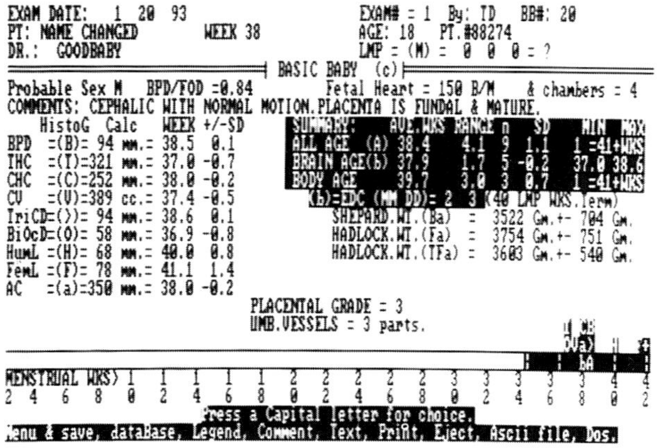

Y

FIGURE 19–5. *(Continued)*
Y, The computer age range analysis produced an average age of 38.4 LMP weeks from nine fetal parameters with a range of 4.1 weeks. This range is just over 10% of the age, placing the range at 1.1 SD. The femur was rather long and slightly exceeded the values in Table 7–1; therefore, an arbitrary 41.1 weeks was used for the femur, placing it at + 1.4 SD above the mean. The woman did not know the date of her LMP.

is looped twice around the neck, which would be evidenced by seeing two adjacent depressions of the neck, there seems little cause for concern.

In Figure 19–5*M*, the thoracic and upper lumbar spine is viewed. The vertebrae continue to be regular in spacing both along and across the spine. The central spinal canal can be observed as a thin intermittent line of echoes at the center of the cord. The intermittence of the echoes is due to shadowing from the surrounding bony structures of the spine.

The lower lumbar spine and sacrum are observed in Figure 19–5*N*. In the lumbar region is a very slight widening of the spinal cord and the vertebral echoes. This should be a smooth, gradual widening, and the spaces between the vertebral bodies should be constant. It is possible to measure seven complete thoracolumbar vertebral bodies and spaces for a close estimation of fetal age (see Chapter 7).

Figure 19–5*O* and *P* shows two different views of the humerus. A parasagittal plane from the posterior of the arm is shown in *O*. The elbow is bent away from the transducer. *P* is a coronal section through the same humerus. The proximal humeral point (PHP) is clearly seen around the hypoechoic, cartilaginous humeral head. This PHP is always on the side nearest the transducer and should not be included in the measurement of the humeral diaphysis. At the other end of the bone, at the elbow, the lateral epicondyle can be seen nearest the transducer. The medial epicondyle is more faintly seen owing to shadowing of the more proximal lateral condyle. The hypoechoic coronoid fossa between the two condyles often gives the appearance of a Y or split end of the bone.[35] Because the two distal condyles of the humerus are not symmetrical, measurement of the humerus from different planes may result in some variability. The measurements shown in these two images, 66.5 mm in the first versus 69.5 mm in the second, are actually measured to the end of the trochlea between the two condyles. These measurements were averaged for the measurement of record for age estimation (see the later section on size/age).

The diaphysis of the femur is measured in Figure 19–5*Q*. At the proximal (hip) end, the hypoechoic femoral head is clearly seen. At the distal (knee) end of the bone, we can see the ossification center. The measurement does not include the femoral head or the ossification center. This measurement is the *femoral length* (FemL), although this is a misnomer because it is really the length of the femoral diaphysis.

The abdomen is larger than the field of view, as demonstrated in Figure 19–5*R*. Because of this problem, the image was manipulated so that the true anteroposterior and transverse diameters were at a diagonal to the axis of the image. In this way, two perpendicular diameters could be measured at the visible skin line. Note that the cursors are placed at the skin line and not at the more obvious peritoneal or rib echoes. This measurement is taken perpendicular to the spine at the level of the confluence of the umbilical and the portal veins in the liver. The fluid-filled stomach is visible as an anechoic area. The aorta and upper pole of the right kidney can be seen in cross section.

A coronal view of the fetal trunk is demonstrated in Figure 19–5*S*. This view is very often overlooked because the transverse view is more commonly used to estimate the fetal weight. However, the coronal view is very useful in assessing the fetal trunk cavity and its three normal fluid spaces, the heart, stomach, and urinary bladder. This view allows a sonographer to judge the relative positions and sizes of these three fluid cavities. In general, they usually have the relationships shown here, although the stomach may be on the other side if the fetus is lying with its right side down. If any of the cavities are out of place, appear too large, or are not seen, further study is required. This is a subjective assessment that requires some experience.

A slight change of angle from the coronal view in Figure 19–5*S* produces the image shown in Figure 19–5*T*. In this view, the diaphragm is seen as a thin, hypoechoic line over the liver and under the heart. These two views rule out a diaphragmatic hernia, in which the stomach pulls up into the chest next to the heart.

A complete study of a fetus requires observations of the kidneys. The kidneys are among the organs most likely to have relatively large variations or anomalies. In Figure 19–5*U*, both kidneys are shown in cross section on either side of the spine. The more medial parts of the kidneys are in the shadow of the spine, but enough is seen to determine that there is a small amount of urine in the renal pelvis of each kidney. With real-time, changes of angles allow each kidney to be seen in full circumference. The amount of fluid demonstrated in 19–5*U* is not abnormal.

Figure 19–5*V* shows the scrotum and penis of the fetus. The penis is pressed against the umbilical cord. It is common to observe the cord adjacent to the genitalia, probably because the lower extremities act as a funnel to trap the cord between the legs.

The heart can be studied in Figure 19–5*W* and *X*. A four-chamber heart is shown in *W*, and the two sides appear to be normally symmetrical. The aorta and inferior vena cava are seen in cross section at the edge of the image. In normal placement of the heart, the left atrium is nearest to the aorta and spine.[24,30]

Figure 19–5*X* is an M-mode tracing of the heart rate at 139 B/M, a normal rate. Two measurements exceeding 155 B/M were recorded in association with fetal movements.

Movement

A fetus is more crowded in the uterus at term than earlier in pregnancy. As a result of this crowding, a fetus appears to become less active. A fetus is active but is less likely to make complete crown-rump reversals of positions as term approaches. This is an observation of experience and has not been tested in a controlled study. Most of the research on fetal movements has addressed either specific movements such as breathing, heart rate accelerations, or body movements during specific time periods or hourly means throughout the day.[36] Breathing motions and body and extremity motions all can be observed.

A term fetus responds to sounds, and all fetal activities are generally increased after acoustic stimulation. A fetus also responds to changes in maternal sugar intake, and fetal breathing motions peak between 15 and 60 minutes after a peak in maternal glucose concentrations.[37] This means that a fetus usually is more active for about an hour or two after meals.

At term, the FHR has an average rate of about 140 B/M but ranges from 100 to 170. Episodes of heart rates that are higher and lower are noted, but these are less common. The FHR varies in response to fetal movements, acoustic stimulus, maternal sugar ingestion, and normal variations throughout the day. These daily variations tend to parallel the woman's heart rates, with peak rates between 8:00 AM about 10:00 PM. After about 10:00 PM, there is a slow decrease to the lowest rates of the day in both the maternal and fetal heart rates between midnight and 6:00 AM.[38]

Although this text is primarily concerned with sonographic examination of a normal fetus, it should be mentioned that the variability of the FHR is important. Pressure on the fetal head or pressure from uterine contractions of labor normally causes decelerations of the FHR. The timing of the decelerations in relationship to the contractions is the basis for fetal monitoring during labor (see Chapter 12). It is important to recognize that the absence of FHR variability is considered sinister, whether it is within or outside of the normal range of rates.[39]

Size/Age

The 38-LMP-week fetus in our example is 38.4 LMP weeks of age by averaging nine parameter ages. The ARA for all parameters was 4.1 weeks or 10.7% of the age. All parameters are within ± 1.0 SD except for the femur, which was + 1.4 SD. This is still normal but long. The ARA for the AC size/age places it just − 0.2 SD below the average age, or very near the mean. The FemL was 78 mm, and the AC was 350 mm (Fig. 19–5*Y*), producing a FemL/AC ratio of 22.3, which is precisely the same as Hadlock's 38th week FemL/AC ratio of 22.3.[40] Both methods indicate an average AC just below or at the mean and would be predictive of an average birth weight. However, the birth weight exceeded 9 lb (4147 g) at 40 weeks, well above the 50th percentile and approaching the 90th percentile for weight, according to Hadlock and associates' sonographic weight standard.[41] In addition to the weight, the length at 52 cm was slightly greater than average.

The question arises, How could both the FemL/AC ratio and ARA make the fetus appear so nearly normal when the birth would occur in just 15 days and the resulting baby be so large? The problem is that the ratio compares one fetal parameter with another, and if both are relatively large, the ratios will be normal. One critical piece of information is missing—the actual age of the fetus. Without an accurate LNMP or a very early sonographic age, it is impossible to determine if this was a normal fetus or one that was large for dates. The one clue is that the weight estimates at 38.4 weeks' sonographic age based on the parameter sizes indicated an estimated weight of approximately 3626 g. This is the 50th percentile for weight 1.6 weeks later, at 40 weeks, according to Hadlock and associates.[41]

This case points out the need to establish early, accurate dates for a pregnancy. It is a complicated undertaking to determine at term whether a fetus is large, small, or normal in size without accurate dates (see Chapter 7).

LMP WEEK 39

Observations

The example here is the same fetus that was discussed previously but 5 days later. The average age of nine fetal parameters is now 39.6 LMP weeks. This would indicate about 1.2 weeks' increase in size/age in just 5 days or 0.7 week, suggesting accelerated growth. The BPP score was again a 10.

The placenta is a grade III, which was established in the previous week. In Figure 19–6*A*, the retroplacental complex of vessels can be observed as a hypoechoic band beneath the placenta.

The amniotic fluid is normal, as exhibited in Figure 19–6*A* and *B*. In *B*, the three vessels of the umbilical cord are easily observed. The two smaller vessels are the arteries, and the larger one is the vein.

Figure 19–6*C*, and *D* shows the same cranial measurements that were taken in the first examination. The head is still relatively normally shaped, with a TCI of 84%, and in the coronal view the head is still circular. This indicates that little molding is being caused by pressure on the head.

In Figure 19–6*E*, the BiOD is measured. The bridge of the fetal nose is seen between the orbits. By turning the plane of view 90 degrees from *E*, we arrive at a view tangential to the face (Fig. 19–6*F*). This view rules out a cleft lip. Eyes, nose, and lips are shown.

A normal term spine is imaged in Figure 19–6*G* to *I*. It can be seen in *G* that the umbilical cord is no longer across the back of the neck, as it was in the previous week. The spine appears regular in spacing and without abrupt angles. The uniformity of the spine was also confirmed in transverse sections by real-time.

The humerus of the upper extremity is measured in Figure 19–6*J*. This is a near coronal view, which can be determined because

Text continued on page 469

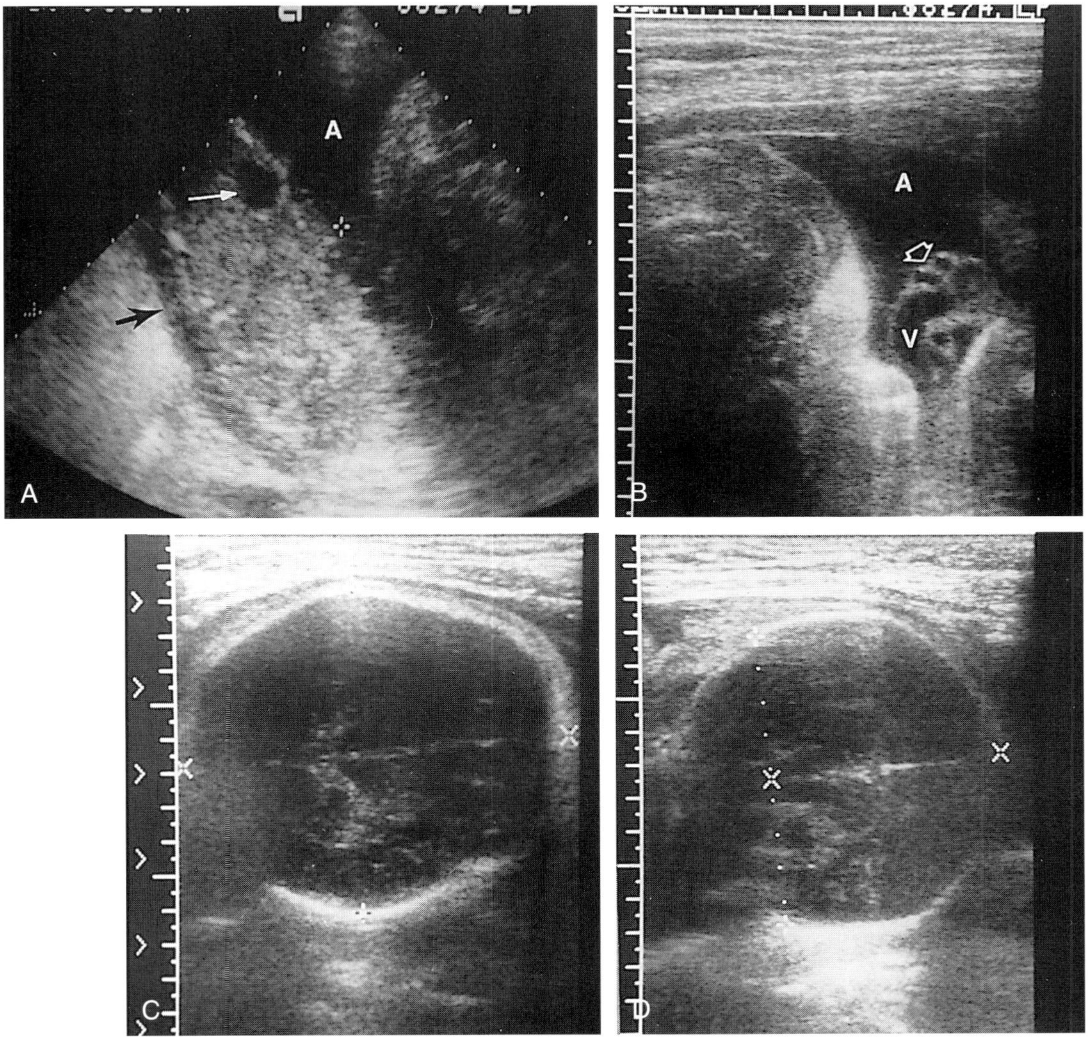

FIGURE 19–6. LMP WEEK 39.

A, The same pregnancy as in Figure 19–5, 5 days later, in the late 39th LMP week. Here the grade III placenta is seen to have a maternal lake (white arrow) and clearly defined cotyledons. The hypoechoic band of retroplacental complex of vessels (black arrow) is well visualized. The amniotic fluid was ample, with this single pocket measuring 6.7 cm in vertical diameter.

B, The umbilical cord has three vessels. The two umbilical arteries (open arrow) coil around the single vein (V). Again, the amniotic fluid (A) is normal.

C, A normally shaped term fetal head. The biparietal diameter (BPD) is measured from leading edge to leading edge of the parietal bones, excluding the scalp over the proximal side of the head. The fronto-occipital diameter (FOD) is measured from the middle of the frontal bone to the middle of the occipital bone. The narrow slit of the third ventricle can be seen at the center of the hypoechoic thalamus. The FOD is at the limits of the field of view for this transducer. Many transducers cannot visualize the entire fetal skull at term. In those cases, the next view can be helpful.

D, Normal coronal section of the fetal head. Note the circular shape of the skull. The thalamus and brainstem are well visualized. This image would yield a valid BFD measurement. The hippocampal baseline and vertical cranial diameter are measured.

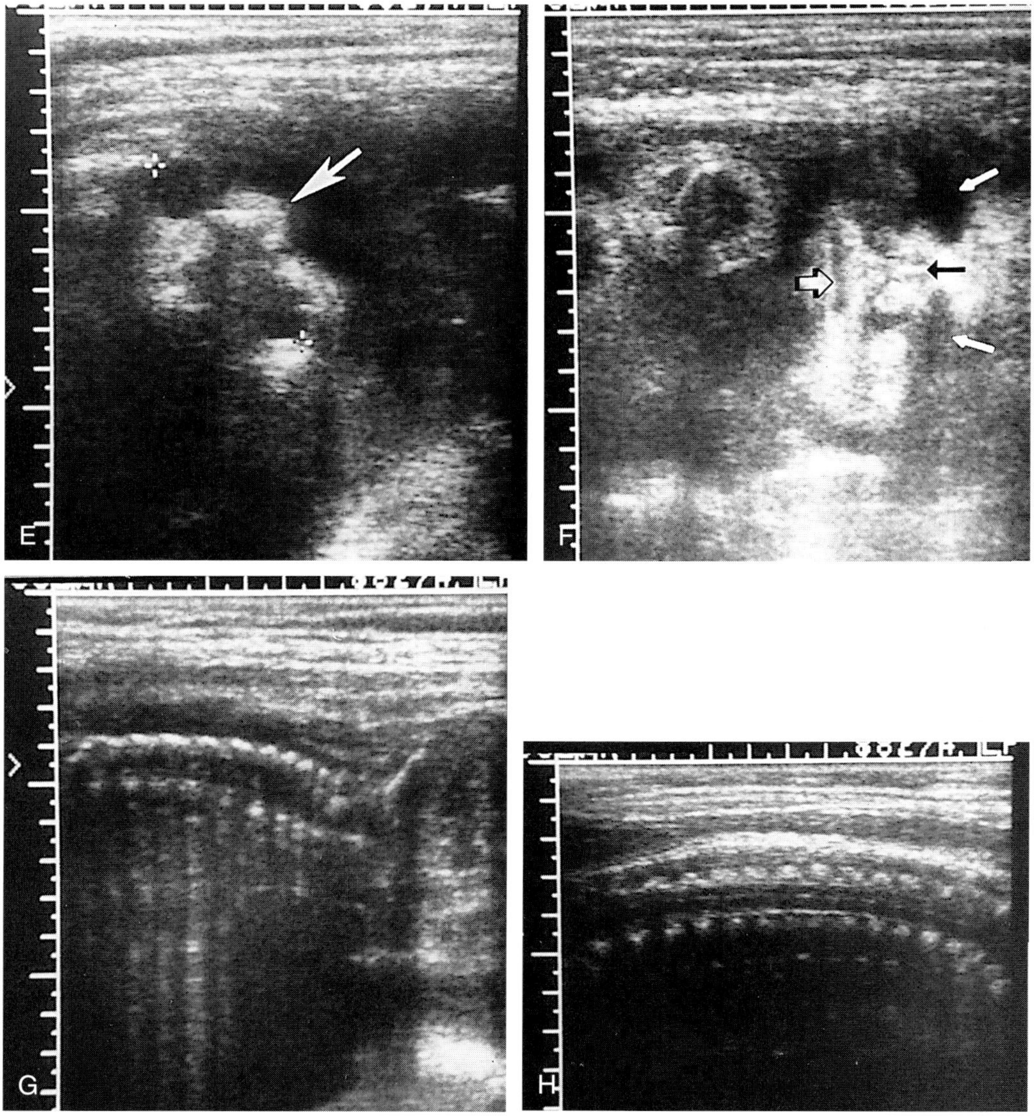

FIGURE 19–6. *(Continued)*
E, Oblique, transverse view of the fetal orbits. The + cursors measure the outer binocular distance to be 58.2 mm, or approximately 39 LMP weeks size/age. The bridge of the nose (arrow) is between.
F, This image is perpendicular to *E* and shows the fetal face. The eyes (white arrows) are not well visualized. The lips (open arrow) and nose are better visualized. The black arrow points to the nasal septum. This view is important for ruling out cleft lips.
G, The back of the skull and cervical spine. The nuchal skin is not thickened, and the spine appears normal.
H, The thoracic spine also appears normal. The vertebral bodies are evenly spaced in both the transverse and long axes. The faint central echoes of the median fissure of the spinal cord can be seen intermittently.

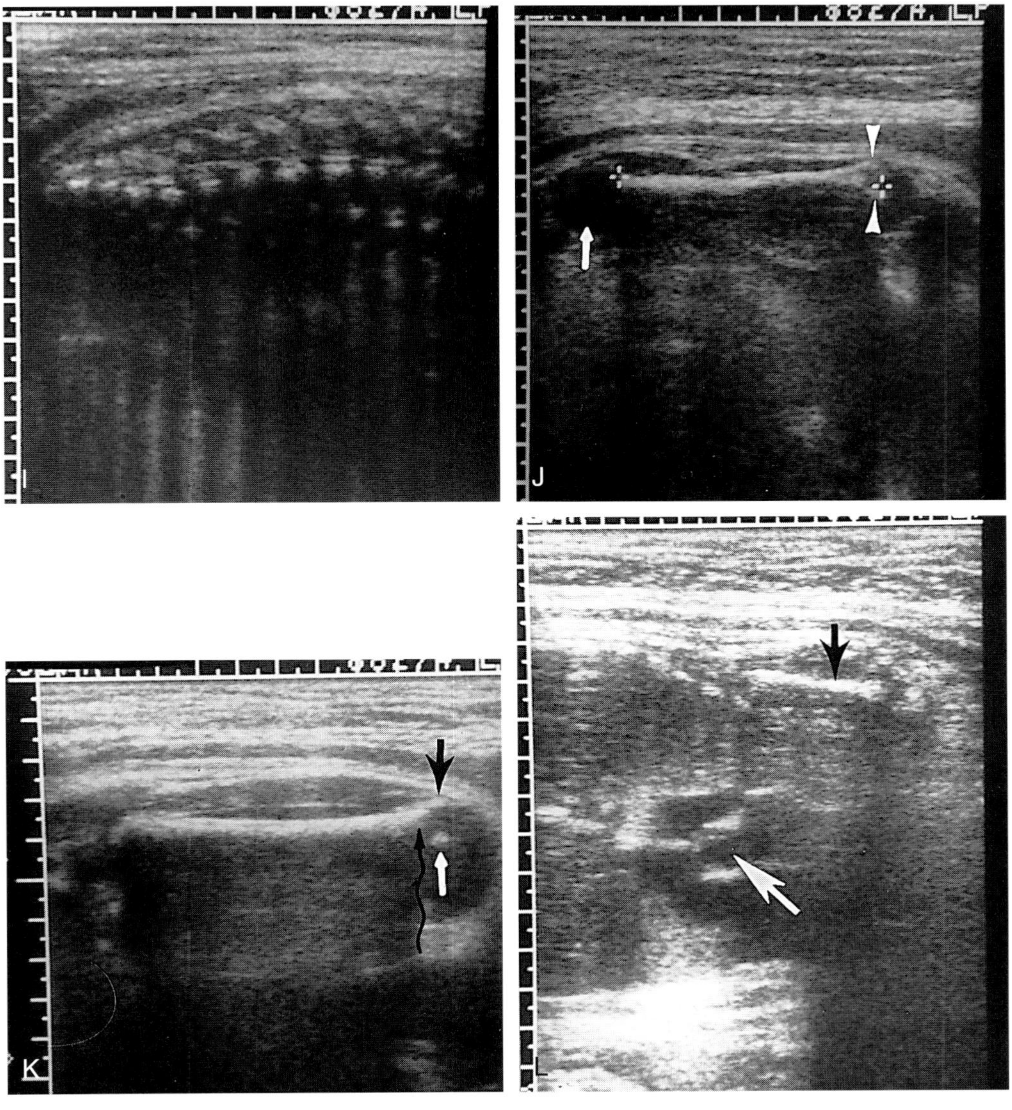

FIGURE 19–6. *(Continued)*
I The normal lumbosacral spine can be seen to taper to a point. The skin is smooth and uninterrupted along the fetal back. The vertebral bodies cast intermittent acoustic shadows posteriorly.
J, Coronal section through the fetal arm. The hypoechoic cartilaginous humeral head (arrow) is circular at the proximal end of the diaphysis, and the thicker deltoid muscle is lateral to the head. The distal end of the humerus appears split or Y shaped (arrowheads) because the coronoid fossa is imaged between the lateral condyle (top arrowhead) and the longer medial condyle (bottom arrowhead). The humeral diaphysis is measured to the end of the longer condyle.
K, The femoral diaphysis. The image clearly shows the distal femoral point (DFP, straight black arrow) and the epiphyseal ossification center (white arrow). The DFP and the ossification center should not be included in the diaphysis measurement. Note that the distal end of the diaphysis cast a distinct acoustic shadow, which helps to determine the location of the end of the calcified shaft (wavy black arrow).
L, Coronal section of the fetal thorax showing the scapula (black arrow) and cross sections of ribs below it. The heart in the short-axis view and its central, circular aortic root (white arrow) are also seen.

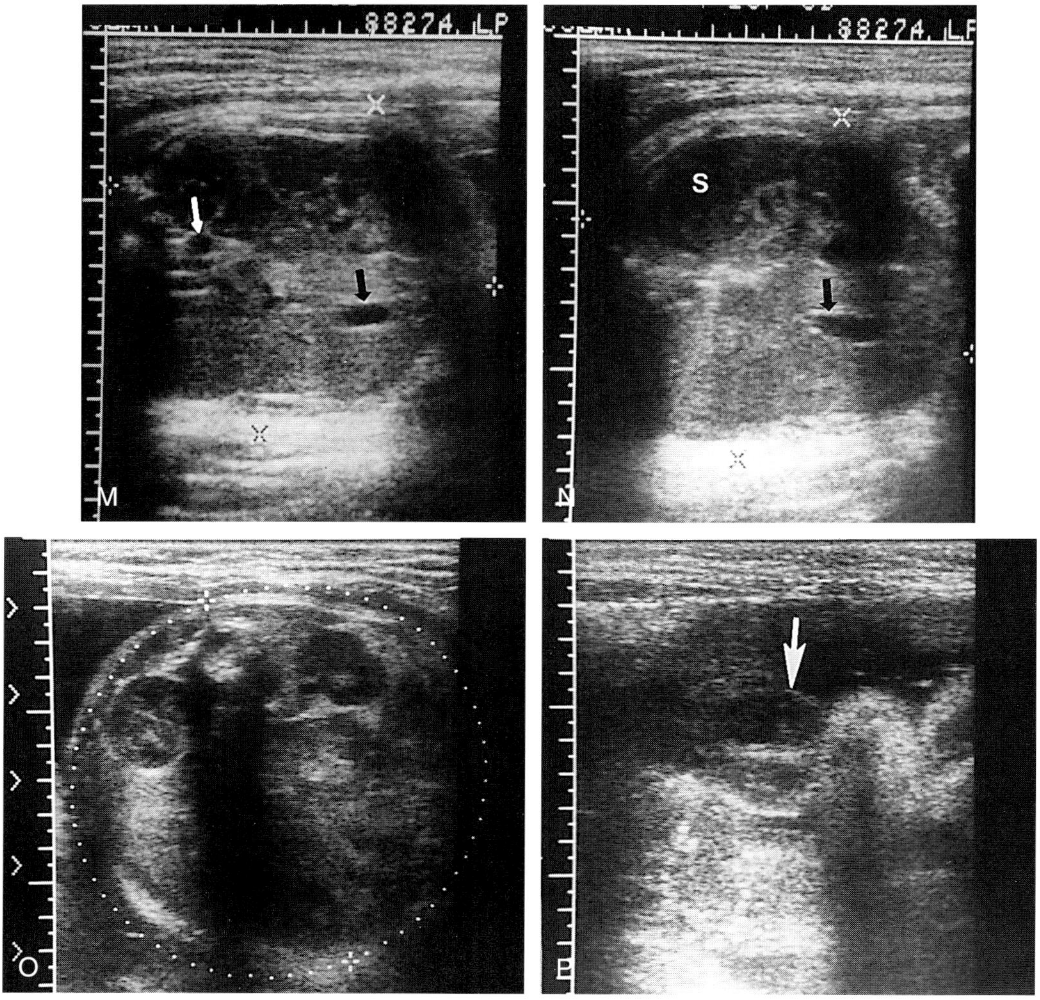

FIGURE 19–6. *(Continued)*
M, Transverse section of the fetal abdomen at the level of the liver and umbilical vein (black arrow). The aorta (white arrow) is anterior to the spine at the edge of the field of view. Measurement of the diameters is difficult in this case because the abdominal dimensions exceed the field of view. Here the abdominal circumference (AC) is 352 mm.
N, Another example of the difficulty of abdominal measurements at term. The greater and lesser curvatures of the stomach (S) are clearly seen, as is the umbilical vein (black arrow). However, almost none of the edges of the skin are clearly visualized, making accurate measurement almost impossible. Because these measurements are important for fetal weight estimates, all possible accuracy is needed. This AC measures 356 mm.
O, One solution to measuring a fetal abdomen (or head) that exceeds the field of view is to use an ellipse-drawing function, as demonstrated here. Many modern sonographic manufacturers provide this function. By using the smooth ellipse, the contour of the anatomy can be approximated very well. Because the kidneys are well visualized and the umbilical vein and liver are not visualized, this is not the best section for the AC measurement, 371 mm in this figure.
P, At term, the fetal genitalia may be difficult to visualize because the fetus is relatively large and crowded for space. The thighs are often pressed together, making visualization more difficult. Here the scrotum (arrow) is visualized but would be difficult to identify if real-time sonography had not been used to confirm the anatomy. Serendipitously, just 5 days earlier, in the first examination, the genitalia were much easier to visualize.

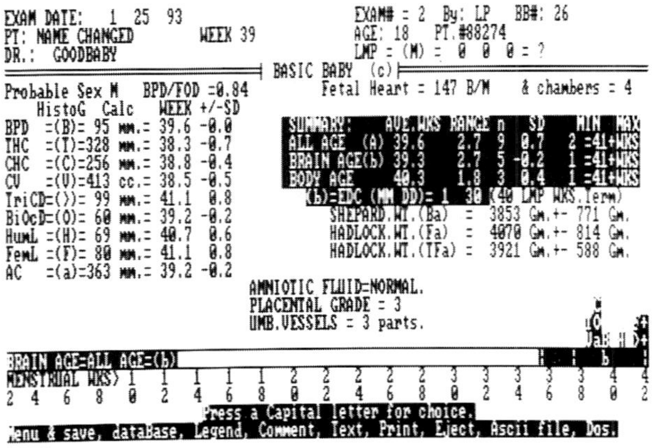

Q

FIGURE 19–6. *(Continued)*
Q, The computer age range analysis produced an average age of 39.6 LMP weeks from nine fetal parameters with a range of 2.7 weeks. This places all parameters within ± 1.0 SD of the mean. However, it must be noted that at this time, two parameters exceed the values in the computer look-up tables (see Table 7–1), and an arbitrary 41.1 weeks was used for the femur length [FemL (F)] and coronal triangle circumference diameter of the head [TriCD (>)].

the epicondyles with their intercondylar fossa are seen. The cartilaginous head of the humerus is again demonstrated as a hypoechoic sphere at the proximal end.

The DFP is obvious on the side of the cartilaginous condyles of the knee that is nearest the transducer. The ossification center near the center of the condyles is demonstrated again (see Fig. 19–6*K*).

Figure 19–6*L* is a coronal view of the thorax. The aortic root can be seen at the center of the heart. The scapula and cross sections of ribs are also shown.

Figure 19–6*M* to *O* demonstrates the difficulty of measuring the AC at term. In all three of these images, one portion of the abdomen is not well visualized because it is larger than the field of view. In *M*, the abdomen appears somewhat flattened side to side and elongated in the anteroposterior diameter. The umbilical vein and a cross section of the aorta are seen.

The larger portion of the stomach is imaged in 19–6*N*. The umbilical vein is also shown. Again it is difficult to determine the precise point to place the cursors owing to the small field of view relative to the large abdomen.

The use of the ellipse-drawing function in Figure 19–6*O* helps to estimate the skin line but still produces only an estimate. In addition, the kidneys on either side of the spine are well seen, but the umbilical vein is not. This may indicate that the image is too low in the fetal abdomen for the AC measurement. However, the measurements obtained were as large or larger than those in *M* and *N*. Because none of these AC measurements were clearly satisfactory owing to the relative size of the transducer and the fetal abdomen, it is preferable to make several measurements and average them for the measurement of record.

The fetus is again confirmed to be male in Figure 19–6*P*. In this image, only the scrotum is visualized. Real-time observations provided a complete view of the genitalia.

Movement

The fetal motion was normal. Breathing motions, flexions, extensions, and a normal heartbeat with variations were observed. In Figure 19–6*Q*, the heart rate is recorded by M-mode to be 147 B/M. This was one of the lower rates recorded during the examination.

Size/Age

This fetus can now be measured to be the size of a 39.6-LMP-week fetus. Although the AC appears relatively normal in size, both the humerus and femur appear relatively long (see Fig. 19–6*Q*). As discussed earlier, the birth weight exceeded 9 lb and the relative size/age increase during the 5 days between the two examinations was the equivalent of 1.2 weeks. For this reason, accelerated term growth was suggested.

The software used to estimate the parameter ages does not calculate beyond 41.1

LMP weeks; therefore, the femur size/age appears to remain at 41.1 weeks. The size/age analysis of a term fetus is problematic because one parameter or another often exceeds the measurements shown on a particular table. Perhaps someone will eventually develop a comprehensive table for sonographic measurement of postterm fetuses.

In cases in which it is difficult to obtain clearly accurate measurements, such as those of the abdomen in Figure 19–6*M* to *O*, it is advisable to take several measurements and average them for the measurement of record. If one of the measurements does not cluster with the majority of the measurements, the outlier can be excluded from the average. This process usually produces more consistent measurements.

REFERENCES

1. Cunningham FG, MacDonald PC, Gant NF: Williams Obstetrics. Appleton & Lange, Norwalk, CT, 1989, p 258.
2. Reskin R: Post-term pregnancy. In: Creasy RK, Resnik R, eds: Maternal-Fetal Medicine: Principles and Practice. WB Saunders, Philadelphia, 1989, pp 505–506.
3. Nyberg DA, Hill LM, Bohm-Velez M, et al: Transvaginal Ultrasound. Mosby/Year Book, St Louis, 1992, p 73.
4. Sabbagha RE: Diagnostic Ultrasound: Applied to Obstetrics and Gynecology, 2nd ed. JB Lippincott, Philadelphia, 1987, pp 246–250.
5. Moore KL, Persaud TVN: The Developing Human: Clinically Oriented Embryology, 5th ed. WB Saunders, Philadelphia, 1993, pp 354–359.
6. Parer JT: Fetal heart rate. In: Creasy RK, Resnik R, eds: Maternal-Fetal Medicine: Principles and Practice. WB Saunders, Philadelphia, 1989, pp 314–343.
7. Fine C, Cartier M, Doubilet P: Fetal heart rates: Values throughout gestation (abstract 1569). Official Proceedings WFUMB. J Ultrasound Med 1988; 7:S105.
8. DuBose TJ, Cunyus JA, Johnson L: Embryonic heart rate and age. J Diagn Med Sonogr 1990;6:151–157.
9. Warsof SL, Gohari P, Berkowitz RL, et al: The estimation of fetal weight by computer-assisted analysis. Am J Obstet Gynecol 1977;128:881.
10. Shepard MJ, Richards VA, Berkowitz RL, et al: An evaluation of two equations of predicting fetal weight by ultrasound. Am J Obstet Gynecol 1982; 142:47.
11. Hadlock FP, Harrist RB, Sharman RS, et al: Estimation of fetal weight with the use of head, body and femur measurements: A prospective study. Am J Obstet Gynecol 1985;151:333–337.
12. Filly R: Editorial. Radiology 1988;166:274–275.
13. Athey PA, Hadlock FP: Ultrasound in Obstetrics and Gynecology. CV Mosby, St Louis, 1981, pp 23–26.
14. Bowie JD: Real-time ultrasonography in the diagnosis of fetal anomalies. Clin Diagn Ultrasound 1982; 10:228.
15. Fisk CE, Filly RA: Ultrasound evaluation of the normal and abnormal fetal neural axis. In: Callen PW, ed: Ultrasonography in Obstetrics and Gynecology. Philadelphia, WB Saunders, 1983, p.100.
16. DuBose TJ: Assessment of fetal age and size: Techniques and criteria. In: Berman MC, ed: Diagnostic Medical Sonography: A Guide to Clinical Practice, Vol I, JB Lippincott, Philadelphia, 1991, pp 282–285.
17. Jeanty P, Cantraine F, Cousarert E, et al: The binocular distance: A new way to estimate fetal age. J Ultrasound Med 1984;3:241–243.
18. DuBose TJ: Assessment of fetal age and size: Techniques and criteria. In: Berman MC, ed: Diagnostic Medical Sonography: A Guide to Clinical Practice, vol I. JB Lippincott, Philadelphia, 1991, pp 295–296.
19. Santonja-Lucas JJ, Armero C, Martinez-Gonzalez L: Long-term prediction of birth weight. J Ultrasound Med 1993;12:431–436.
20. Hadlock FP, Deter RL, Roecker E, et al: Relation of fetal femur length to neonatal crown-heel length. J Ultrasound Med 1984;3:1–3.
21. DuBose TJ: Assessment of fetal age and size: Techniques and criteria. In: Berman MC, ed: Diagnostic Medical Sonography: A Guide to Clinical Practice, vol I. JB Lippincott, Philadelphia, 1991, p 288.
22. DuBose TJ: Coronal BPD revisited. J Ultrasound Med 1992;11:84.
23. Manning FA, Platt LD, Sipos L, et al: Fetal assessment based on fetal biophysical profile scoring: Experience in 19,221 referred high-risk pregnancies. Am J Obstet Gynecol 1987;157:880–884.
24. Cyr DR, Guntheroth WG, Mack LA: Fetal echocardiography. In: Berman MC, ed: Diagnostic Medical Sonography: A Guide to Clinical Practice, vol I. JB Lippincott, Philadelphia, 1991, pp 257–262.
25. Benson CB, Warneke LA: Sonographic appearance of milestones of pregnancy. In: Berman MC, ed: Diagnostic Medical Sonography: A Guide to Clinical Practice, vol I. JB Lippincott, Philadelphia, 1991, pp 215–216.
26. Hansmann M, Hackeloer B-J, Staudach A: Ultrasound Diagnosis in Obstetrics and Gynecology. Springer-Verlag, Berlin, 1985, p 345.
27. Parisi VM: Cervical incompetence. In: Creasy RK, Resnik R, eds: Maternal-Fetal Medicine: Principles and Practice. WB Saunders, Philadelphia, 1989, pp 450–451.
28. Chase LM, Cayea PD: The placenta and umbilical cord. In: Berman MC, ed: Diagnostic Medical Sonography: A Guide to Clinical Practice. JB Lippincott, Philadelphia, 1991, pp 313–314.
29. DuBose TJ, Porter L, Hill LW, et al: Black-and-white color Doppler sonography. AJR 1990;155:199.
30. DeVore G: Cardiac imaging. In: Sabbagha RE, ed: Diagnostic Ultrasound: Applied to Obstetrics and Gynecology, 2nd ed. JB Lippincott, Philadelphia, 1987, pp 326–328.
31. Goldstein RB, Filly RA, Simpson G: Pitfalls in femur length measurements. J Ultrasound Med 1987;6: 203–207.
32. Chinn DH, Bolding DB, Callen PW, et al: Ultrasonographic identification of the fetal lower extremity epiphyseal ossification centers. Radiology 1983; 815–818.
33. Walla CA, Platt LD: Observing fetal maturation through fetal movement and breathing. In: Berman MC, ed: Diagnostic Medical Sonography: A Guide to Clinical Practice, vol I. JB Lippincott, Philadelphia, 1991, pp 451–455.

34. Finberg HJ: The placenta and umbilical cord: Recent observations. Official Proceedings, Society of Diagnostic Medical Sonographers, 10th Annual Conference, Anaheim, CA, 1993, pp 241–247.
35. DuBose TJ: Assessment of fetal age and size: Techniques and criteria. In: Berman MC, ed: Diagnostic Medical Sonography, A Guide to Clinical Practice, vol I. JB Lippincott, Philadelphia, 1991, p 293.
36. Patrick J, Gagnon R: Fetal breathing and body movement. In: Creasy RK, Resnik R, eds: Maternal-Fetal Medicine: Principles and Practice. WB Saunders, Philadelphia, 1989, pp 268–287.
37. Patrick J, Gagnon R: Fetal breathing and body movement. In: Creasy RK, Resnik R, eds: Maternal-Fetal Medicine: Principles and Practice. WB Saunders, Philadelphia, 1989, p 274.
38. Patrick J, Gagnon R: Fetal Breathing and body movement. In: Creasy RK, Resnik R, eds: Maternal-Fetal Medicine: Principles and Practice. WB Saunders, Philadelphia, 1989, p 284.
39. Patrick J, Gagnon R: Fetal breathing and body movement. In: Creasy RK, Resnik R, eds: Maternal-Fetal Medicine: Principles and Practice. WB Saunders, Philadelphia, 1989, pp 330–331.
40. Callen PW: Ultrasound in Obstetrics and Gynecology, 3rd ed. WB Saunders, Philadelphia, 1993, p 734.
41. Hadlock FP, Harrist RB, Martinez-Poyer J: In utero analysis of fetal growth: A sonographic weight standard. Radiology 1991;181:129–133.

CHAPTER 20

CONCLUSIONS

When this book was first conceived, a chapter devoted to the use of computers was to have been included. Some discussion of computers is appropriate for a topic that is so measurement and calculation intensive as is fetal sonography. After some reflection and trying to intelligently decipher and give advice about the current computer hardware and software scene, I decided that a chapter would not provide enough discussion of the topic—if I could shed intelligent light on the topic at all in the current market. Therefore, this chapter offers a minimum of discussion of some computer basics, particularly software. Also briefly discussed is diagnostic medical sonography as a profession.

The foregoing topics require some crystal ball gazing as I give my opinions of what may be in store for sonography, including hardware, software, and some socioeconomics. The opinions that follow are mine and do not necessarily reflect the opinions of anyone else involved in producing this book.

Computers

CURRENT STATE OF COMPUTERS

Trying to decide where the personal computer (PC) industry is going is what discouraged me from trying to explain this subject in a full chapter. It cannot be done both completely and briefly. Because this book is about fetal sonography and not computers, we are left with only a brief PC discussion.

In the 1980s, this topic was much simpler. In the 1990s, several things make it much more difficult to discuss. The rapidly changing architecture of computer chips, the competition between operating systems, the availability of more software, and finally the InterNet have taken the PC to a level of complexity that may be beyond the grasp of an individual or simple discussions. If you want to know what is happening with PCs, you must pursue the current periodical literature and specific paperback books. The field is changing so rapidly that it simply cannot be followed by a single reference book. Some magazines describe not only specific PC brands and software but also specific uses of specific software. For instance, Visual Basic is a MicroSoft Corporation programming language for the Windows environment. Some magazines are devoted to Visual Basic, and there are numerous publications about the Windows graphical user interface (GUI). To become moderately computer literate takes energy, time, and money.

It is hoped that this chapter gives the novice a starting place and provides some useful information for the more experienced. I try not to be too basic; it seems everyone in medicine now has some familiarity with PCs.

COMPUTER HARDWARE

A PC is generally thought of as a box, a keyboard, a monitor, a printer, and some cables. Because of the many available varieties of each component, the subject is no longer simple.

The box contains circuit boards, chips, power supplies, cooling fans, and other electronic components. This is the central processing unit (CPU), and it is usually referred to by the type of CPU chip that acts as the "brains." In the 1980s, two main families of PC CPUs were in use. The Intel Corporation's family of chips operated the IBMs and those compatible with the IBM. The Motorola Corporation produced the chips used in the Apple brand of computers. There were a few others, but most were not in general use by the public. A number of other manufacturers produce "clones" of these chips that operate in the same way.

These chips are referred to by a name, which is often a number, in conjunction with a clock speed expressed in megahertz per second (MHz). In 1995, the most common speeds are somewhere between 50 and 100+ MHz, up from 8 to 16 MHz just 10 or 12 years ago. When considering a new computer, the general wisdom is that faster is better. Some of the other chips in the CPU box are random access memory (RAM) chips. These store the software, commands, and current working files for immediate use. Any document being typed is held in RAM until it is saved to disk. If the computer is turned off without saving them, the files in RAM are lost. A word to the wise is to save often to disk memory. Computers using a GUI should have a minimum of about eight megabytes of RAM, more if you can afford it.

The disk memory is usually in the CPU box also, although it may be external and connected by a cable. The two main types are the hard disk and the floppy disk. The hard disk usually stores large numbers of files and amounts of data. The hard disk usually cannot be removed or changed easily. The term *floppy disk* is a holdover from when diskettes were actually made of a thin, flexible, floppy plastic material 5.25 inches square. Today most diskettes are rigid plastic 3.5 inches square. Floppy diskettes can be removed from the disk drive. Diskettes are one of the best ways to save data and move it from one computer to another. Many different formats of permanent memory that are becoming available are faster and hold more data. These new technologies are starting to blur the differences between hard disks and floppy disks. In general, get the fastest, largest hard-disk memory you can afford.

In addition to the CPU, the PC must have input devices such as a keyboard, and nowadays a mouse or trackball is necessary. Keyboards come in many configurations with different feels. Try out different keyboards and get one that feels good to you. If your new computer comes with one you do not like, most reputable dealers will exchange it for a different one for free or at most for the difference in prices.

The mouse or trackball is a pointing device for point-and-click types of commands in GUI environments such as the Macintosh or Windows. Again, get one that feels good to you. Some prefer the mouse for its tactile, spatial response. I prefer a trackball with a large ball because I keep a fairly cluttered desk and a mouse needs too much clear space to run around in, and the large trackball gives me good spatial control. The pointing device comes with software known as *drivers* or *mouse drivers*. This is usually the most problematic part of installing the devices in an IBM-type PC. The IBM-compatible PCs have three "com ports" for communicating with peripheral devices such as mice and modems. If you attempt to communicate with two peripheral devices through the same com port, the PC locks up or functions erratically. Because ports may be software assignable or hardware switchable, it is fairly easy to have a conflict. Apple PCs are easier to install, but you have fewer choices and pay more for those few choices. It is hoped that by the time this is published, the IBM PC world will have a user-friendly "plug-and-play" standard in place to allow the addition of peripheral devices without the tedious hardware and software driver configurations.

A wide variety of monitors are available: large and small, expensive and inexpensive, high resolution and lower resolution, color and monochrome. In general, you should get the highest-resolution and largest monitor you can afford. People with visual problems may want to sacrifice resolution for larger sizes, but they are probably not sonographers.

Printers also are available in wide variety. The most common produce black print, but color printers are becoming more inexpensive. The main decision for most people is whether to get a dot matrix, ink jet, or laser printer. If economy is important, then a dot matrix is without question the cheapest, but don't get anything less than a 24-pin letter-quality dot matrix in this day and age. The ink jet or bubble jet printers squirt microdot drops of ink at the paper. The resolution is good, almost as good as from a laser, but the ink tends to smudge or run if it gets moist. Ink jet printers are medium priced. The laser printers are without a doubt the best for most people who want high-resolution, professional printing. Lasers are also the most expensive. A 300-dot-per-inch laser serves for most correspondence, but if you are going to do fancy graphics, then 600 dots or more may be required. There are many laser manufacturers, and most produce good products. The laser works much like a modern photocopy machine by fusing (melting) a plastic powder (toner) onto the paper. The main caution with laser printers is to select one that is not too difficult to maintain. The easiest to use requires inserting a single toner cartridge; the most difficult requires replacing a cartridge and a couple of other items. Some are delicate and start dropping out springs, clips, and pieces of plastic if you are not careful. When looking at laser printers, consider the long-term cost per copy; they can have a wide range of toner capacities and costs.

In most large hospitals or institutions, PCs are simple workstations linked to a central server computer by a network. These institutional networks are usually known as *local area networks* (LANs). Simple networks of two or three PCs are available. These are called peer-to-peer networks, but most large institutions have a client-server network. These client-server systems are complex and require an experienced person as the system operator who does the routine tasks such as backing up work so that it is not lost.

Those are the basic components for a standard PC system. As a sonographer, you may also want a modem for telecommunications on InterNet or a frame grabber to download sonographic images. There are many other peripheral devices, including compact disks (CDs), read-only memories (ROMs), sound cards, video acceleration cards, small computer system interface (SCSI, pronounced "scuzzy") connectors, and many others too numerous for this space. You can find peripheral devices for PCs to do almost anything you can imagine, from personal voice mail, to monitoring your home security system, to downloading satellite weather images. You are really limited only by your imagination. When you come up with a task, go to a good computer store and talk to a sales person about what you want to do, but do not buy anything at first. Listen and note the words and jargon; then go to a book store with a large periodical section and look for magazines that cover your topic. You can often find mail-order items at a fraction of the local retail price; of course, you may get only a fraction of the service and support. As with everything else, there are tradeoffs.

COMPUTER SOFTWARE

Software Basics

Computer hardware is useless without the software instructions to operate it. Software is usually called a *computer program*. This program contains all the instructions for making the PC usable as a word processor, number processor (spreadsheet), or any other task for which it may be used.

The software is what gives the PC tasks their look and feel. Several basic types of software are discussed here. Most software comes on several diskettes that have to be used to load the software into the computer.

The best advice for the use of PCs is to use your manuals for your PC and software. You cannot learn to use a computer by osmosis. The manuals for a different program or even a different version of the same program do not help very much. Different software uses different command sets. However, many contemporary software manufacturers include a fairly complete help menu of commands that is available as you use the program. You may have to read the manual to learn how to use the help file.

One of the major drawbacks of using pirated (copied) software is that you do not have the manuals. The other drawback is that pirated software is the easiest way to give your computer a virus. If you do not know what a computer virus is, read the last three chapters of Clifford Stoll's intriguing book about real-life computer espionage, *The Cuckoo's Egg*.[1] The last reason for not copying software is that it is illegal—it is theft. The computer manufacturers may prosecute. They can take your computer and software, make you pay stiff fines, and put you in jail. A legal precedent says that all documents processed by a piece of stolen software belong to the software manufacturer. This means that if a hospital or clinic buys one copy of a word processing program and then copies it for use in each department, it is in jeopardy of having to buy all of its own medical records back from the software company if it gets caught.

Operating Systems

The operating system (OS) software is the first piece of software loaded into the PC. In most cases, this process is automated to occur when the PC is first turned on and, except for the time it takes, is fairly invisible to the operator. The OS is the most basic set of instructions for the computer. Currently, the operating software is specific to the family of CPU in your computer. IBM-type PCs use the disk operating system (DOS) or operating system (OS/2). Apple computers use the system software. In general, the latest version of operating system available for your computer is the most desirable.

A complication will soon arise in making decisions about operating systems. MicroSoft Corporation is developing a new Windows-type system, and IBM has a new OS available. Others produce variations on these, and some people are devoted to variations of UNIX. A new chip, the Power PC chip, will eventually allow the user to select any operating system. When these PCs are fully developed, they will be Macintosh or IBM depending on the OS and the desires of the user.

Word Processing

Simple Word Processing

Word processing software or programs provide the most common use for a PC. These programs turn the PC into a very sophisticated typewriter. Contemporary word processors allow the user not only to type and move blocks of text around and do spelling checking but to select various fonts and type faces. They may contain a thesaurus, do grammar checking, and allow standardized templates or style sheets to be set up.

Word Processing in the Clinical Setting

Most modern word processors come with a macrolanguage. This is a computer software language that allows the user to preprogram certain repetitive tasks. These allow automatic entry of such things as inside addresses, greetings and salutations, or signature blocks. "Macros" can also be used to enter normal or standard paragraphs into medical reports, and these can be used over and over. Macros can be real time savers in medical typing stations. Once a person learns to use macrolanguages and implements the macrocommands for the system, other typists can be taught to use the commands without having to learn the complete system; they learn only those commands that they need.

Because macrolanguages are specific to the word processor, efficiencies are gained by everyone in the same hospital or institution using the same software. This way, people can move from job to job and department to department without having to relearn the word processor. I have found that people are very resistant to learning to use a new word processor once they have invested the time and energy into some other processor. These skills do have a steep learning curve, but once learned they are real time savers and make one more productive. I personally would never go back to a typewriter now.

Spreadsheets

Spreadsheet Basics

A spreadsheet is an electronic accountant's sheet of rows and columns for performing numerical operations. The rows are generally called *records*, and the columns are called *fields*. Where a record (row) and field (column) intersect is a cell, the place where a number exists. A cell can also contain a formula written in macrolanguage; the result of the formula is displayed in the cell. Modern spreadsheets also allow interpretation of the data in graphical ways such as bar graphs and pie charts. Many spreadsheets that have been released in the early 1990s can perform sophisticated statistical operations that in earlier times were available only on mainframe computers.

Spreadsheets are handy for keeping household records and checkbook information. They allow quick reference when paying bills to determine when a debt was last paid. The graphing capabilities can also enable one to visualize such things as water or electricity use when looking for trends and places to economize.

Spreadsheets also have macrolanguages similar to those discussed with word processing. These can be used to automate any repetitive tasks.

Sonographic Data

Spreadsheets are particularly useful for evaluating fetal parameter measurements. The original statistics, graphs, and tables used in this textbook were developed using five different software programs. As an example of how data can be used, the following gives the reader some idea about how the information in this book was manipulated.

The data were accumulated using a dedicated fetal analysis spreadsheet/database program (Basic Baby II).[2] The Basic Baby II program allowed for export of the fetal files in American Standard Code for Information Interchange, more commonly called ASCII text files. Once the data are in ASCII format, it is possible to read the files into any spreadsheet or database. We used dBASE IV.[3] In our case, new Basic Baby II files were started at the first of each year. Copies of last year's files were taken on diskette to a computer and concatenated (joined together) into a single database file. Statistical analysis was performed by using a spreadsheet to import the selected database information. The spreadsheets and word processing used for this textbook were primarily Framework IV (FWIV), which is an integrated software program of word processing, spreadsheets, databases, telecommunications, business graphics, and other useful tools.[4] The statistical analysis was done using a newer spreadsheet, MicroSoft Excel version 5.0.[5] The dating curves and formulas in Chapter 7 and other chapters were created using the curve-fitting software Tablecurve.[6]

Several software programs perform the foregoing operations, and these are not necessarily promoted here as the best available or as better than the others. They are simply the ones used to produce most of this book.

DATABASES

Uses

A database is an electronic sheet similar to the rows and columns of a spreadsheet. The main difference is that databases are designed to manipulate text data as in a phone book or in medical records. The database can perform some numerical operations such as counting items in a column or adding up the numbers of a column, but spreadsheets are much more powerful at numerical operations. Databases are better at sorting and manipulating large files of records including things such as patient information.

Like a spreadsheet, a database also is made up of records (rows) and fields (columns). At their intersection is the cell that contains specific information. For example, if the first column of fields is for a patient's last name and if John Doe's information is the 347th patient record, then the first field (cell) of his record (the 347th row of the database) contains his last name, Doe. The second field of the 347th record would probably contain John, his first name. A phone book is the most commonly used database, although it is usually on paper and less often electronic.

A database is useful not only for accumulating and storing data but also for "mail-merging" data with a word-processing document to send out individualized bills, letters, invitations, and so forth. In the report-generating system that I designed for a medical group, two databases were used. The first was a database of all referring physicians' addresses and phone numbers. This "DOCS-LIST" was used to mail-merge the report form so that the referring physicians' addresses were in the correct placement for the window envelope. The other database was the patient listing of identifying information, referring physician, dates, and examinations to be performed. The "PTSLIST" information was also mail merged into the report heading. If the report was normal, canned paragraphs could be called up with a two-key command. This system allowed for very fast transcription of normal reports. Abnormal reports were also expedited because the heading was automatically merged from the two databases. Even the dictating physician's signature block was automatically typed by a macrocommand. The DOCSLIST could also be used for fast look-up of physicians' telephone numbers, and the FWIV integrated software even dialed the number. It is also possible to transmit reports electronically by modem.

Sonographic Data

By having fetal measurement information in a database, prior examinations can be recalled quickly for growth series analysis. The database text-handling power makes it ideal for storing and recalling such information. It is also useful for archival information for statistical analysis by spreadsheet because most spreadsheets read the common database file types.

It was interesting at the end of the year to determine which referring physicians sent us most of our patients, to which laboratory, and for what reasons. This kind of information is useful for staffing and marketing.

SONOGRAPHIC COMPUTER USE

The field of sonography has been slow to integrate the PC with the sonographic machine. A few manufacturers have started providing options for connection, but they usually require that the PC and software be purchased from them at a price considerably higher than the same PC in the retail market. The software provided is preprogrammed, and the user has little ability to modify the program and no ability to integrate the user's own spreadsheet or software. This may mean that the user has to tie up the sonographic equipment in order to perform any statistical analysis of fetal data. I have long envisioned a sonographic machine that would allow me to connect any kind of PC and set up my choice of spreadsheet or database program to receive the fetal measurements automatically rather than have to read and transcribe the data into a PC. Transcription offers another opportunity to make errors.

We have found that having a PC with fetal growth analysis software in the sonographic scanning laboratory has distinct advantages. By entering the fetal measurements directly into the software, we are able to observe the proportionality and growth of a fetus as the examination is being performed. If a parameter measurement was entered incorrectly, the error is immediately detected and corrected without any commotion. If the data were entered correctly and the fetus appeared abnormal, however, the measurement could be quietly double checked. In this way, when the sonographer leaves the room, he or she knows that the measurements are correct and whether there are any questions about fetal growth or proportions.

The only drawback to this method is that an occasional patient insists on knowing the results. We found that explaining that this is only part of the examination and that the diagnosis must be given by a physician satisfied most. The advantage is that we do not have to go back into the scanning suite later, after calculation, to check whether a parameter was mismeasured or misentered or whether the parameter was really abnormal. Previously, before we used fetal analysis software in the laboratory and occasionally had to double check a measurement, a patient usually assumed that something was wrong with her pregnancy. It was rare that a patient would assume that we had made an error. It took more time to recheck the parameter, and we also had to calm and reassure the patient.

Another advantage is less obvious. The use of a computer to accumulate large amounts of data allows one to compare machine and operator performance. It was not until we accumulated several hundreds of fetal heart rates in a single file that we discovered that some sonographic machines are less accurate for calculating M-mode heart rates than others (see Fig. 12–2 for the results of that heart rate study). In 1989, the equipment manufacturer provided a software update that corrected the M-mode calculation error.

It is also possible to study interoperator performance. This is particularly important with students. Although subtle, errors such as placing the cursor at the surface of the fetal scalp rather than the skull in head measurements might be overlooked on an occasional basis. If a student is persistent in these errors, they show up when other students' or sonographers' results are examined in comparison. This is often easily observed with spreadsheet graphs comparing several operators.

Several specific obstetrical and fetal software programs are available. Some are collections of macrocommands that require you also to purchase and learn the parent program. Others are stand-alone compiled .EXE (execution) programs, which do not require anything but the OS to operate.

Diagnostic Medical Sonography as a Profession

SONOGRAPHY PAST AND PRESENT

This section does not rehash the history of fetal sonography (see Chapter 2). The intent here is to discuss the current events of the profession.

In the 1970s, sonographers decided to change the name of the society from the American Society of Ultrasound Technologists (ASUT) to the Society of Diagnostic Medical Sonographers (SDMS). This was done in large measure because they realized that sonographers do more than just take pictures. Sonographers look at hundreds of images (thousands when using real-time) during an examination and must decide if the images they are going to record tell the diagnostic story. Does the image show normal anatomy or does it document pathology? Any skillful sonographer can record images in a way that gives a false impression of the medical situation. Of course, a capable sonographer does not intentionally produce false impressions. The point is that the early sonographers realized that they were doing more than simply taking pictures. They realized that sonographers must have the knowledge and experience to interpret the image and must establish a diagnosis with the images that they record. This does not mean that a sonographer issues the diagnosis—that is up to the supervising physician—but the sonographer does make the diagnosis (see Chapter 6).

Currently, many people want to use this wonderfully powerful diagnostic tool, although many do not have adequate training to use it safely. This is not to imply that sonographic energy is dangerous, but a missed or wrong diagnosis harms a patient just as surely as an overdose of radiation. Many people—physicians, nurses, and others—are starting to use sonography. This is to be expected with such a useful tool. If they do not get proper training, however, they cannot understand the image. Knowledge of the physics of the interaction of sound energy with human tissues is necessary to decipher the information contained in the image. Just as Roy Filly decried promulgation of ever-increasing levels[7] of sonographic examinations because of lack of experience and claims that a level I examination is less diagnostic than a level II, III, IV, or V, a limited examination that misses a diagnosis still harms the patient.

The threat of health care reform has set off a frenzy of mergers, downsizing, and right-sizing of health care organizations. They are reducing staffs and using temporary help as needed when very busy or to cover vacations and holidays. This is done because the employer is not required to provide health insurance, retirement programs, or other benefits to part-time employees. It appears that we are going to become a nation of "temps," constantly looking for the next contract. The concept of the health care team seems to be a thing of the past. No one really knows the abilities of his or her coworkers in this situation.

CURRENT TURMOIL

The discussion of health care reform has included much consideration of multiskilled health care workers. It is presumed that having workers who can do more than one job saves money. However, at the same time there is talk of universal health care coverage. This means more work, not less, for the caring professions. It is my opinion that we will need more workers with better skills, not fewer workers who are jacks-of-all-trades and masters of none.

The SDMS endorses the concept of multicredentialing as the method to ensure competency and attain a high standard of quality health care. Voluntary certification currently is the only method available to assess the parameters on a standardized, international basis.

It appears that the drive for cross-trained allied health workers results from the belief that it is not cost-effective for rural areas and small health service organizations (HSOs) to maintain complete staffs for all specialties. On the surface, it is logical to have a few workers trained in all areas to fill this inadequacy. However, breaking down structured professions across the nation in order to assess the rural shortage is counterproductive in the urban areas (approximately 90% of the United States population is urban). Although this approach may fill a rural need, it certainly does not seem to increase efficiency in a hospital such as Massachusetts General in Boston or Parkland in Dallas or any other large metropolitan HSO.

Health care has become very complex; one person cannot be proficient at all tasks, and many do not desire to be so. The most highly skilled professionals usually have specific interests that drew them into their field. To expect people not to follow their interests and to become generalists of all professions is naive of human nature. It also goes against the logic of the division of labor and the efficiency it brings to complicated tasks. If the drive succeeds in making all health workers generalists, it is probable that in a short time the workers will spontaneously divide the work up among themselves again, each taking the tasks in which they are most interested, knowledgeable, and skilled.

The needs of rural and urban settings are different. It may be more logical and less disruptive to health care to reorganize the financing of health care and to use incentives to spur individuals who want to generalize to move to rural settings. This type of channeling has been used by the government in the past to encourage people into needed professions by providing draft deferments and scholarships to them.[8,9] There is no reason why incentives, whether financial or otherwise, cannot fill the more general needs of rural communities and small HSOs.

In addition, relaxation of the restrictions on the definition of the practice of medicine to allow very highly trained and skilled allied health care professionals to provide interpretations and perform procedures for which they are qualified but that are currently restricted to physicians will go a long way toward reducing the cost of health care. This will especially apply to remote rural areas that may not be able to offer the financial rewards expected by some contemporary medical doctors.

The Future

SONOGRAPHIC EQUIPMENT

What will the future hold? We know that 3-D sonography is a reality and will soon be available commercially. Will 3-D sonographic imaging improve diagnosis? We will not know until it is in use. It may make measurement of 3-D fetal parameters easier by allowing one to rotate a single image for the proper measurement of each axis.

Our understanding of hemodynamics will greatly increase through the use of Doppler. This is already starting to happen with the fetus, and Doppler has long been a good diagnostic tool for assessing arterial and venous diseases in adults. Blood flow is intimately related to life and health care.

We can also expect continued improvement of image resolution and better equipment, it is hoped at a reduced cost. PCs have doubled in capacity at about the same price every year for more than 10 years.

SONOGRAPHIC COMPUTERS

Although future science is unpredictable, I hope that in a few years a radically different sonographic machine will be available. The sonographic instrument I imagine would be peripheral to a standard PC, preferably a small but powerful laptop. The transducer(s) and associated electronics would acquire the sonic information and perhaps format it to a video signal. The PC, however, would display the image, be scaled for measurements, and allow labeling and image manipulation, and the measurements would be entered directly into a database or spreadsheet of the user's choice. The images could be saved to disk or transmitted by modem anywhere in the world. The PC would also be used to type in all the patient data for later recall through a network. As newer, faster, and better computers and software become available, sonographic peripherals could be moved by simply plugging into the new PC, much like a printer or monitor of today.

I believe that there is no logical reason why this type of integration cannot be achieved. Indeed, I think some sonographic machines are already doing this. Perhaps these sonographic PC peripherals will be less expensive than the machines we have today but with more utility. I do not want to ignore the fact that manufacturers have expended great resources for research and development of the wonderful machines we now have. It does seem, however, that acquisition of the data from these machines could be more user friendly and economical.

TELECOMMUNICATIONS

As the 20th century closes and we move into the 21st, health care workers will be among the first to see and use tools of the future. If the current debate about health care reform is any indication, people are going to give the priority to health that was reserved throughout the past 50 years for nuclear war and its deterrence. With any luck, we are entering a period in which health and life are given a central position in our society and in our budgets.

Anyone who has surfed through the worldwide web of InterNet can see the possibilities. We can now exchange images and information with anyone on Earth. What this ability will mean to health care and to society as a whole can only be guessed. We are just now seeing a glimmer of the possibilities.

The ability to store all medical records and images on digital media and to have instant access and recall will certainly change the way we work. It will also mean fewer lost records and images, as well as the ability to elicit expert opinion from anywhere.

All this sounds wonderful, but of course, problems will arise, many unforeseen. Anyone on InterNet who has received hundreds of misdirected messages from an errant "listserver" knows it is not a perfect system. Humans must direct the computers, and humans do make mistakes. Still, the future for the use of computer technology in health care looks bright.

DIAGNOSTIC MEDICAL SONOGRAPHY

Diagnostic sonography is a wonderful tool. It is very economical when compared with other new diagnostic tools. It is also very efficient, portable, and relatively easy to use on difficult patients. It is no wonder that its use has increased exponentially for more than 10 years. Diagnostic sonography is here to stay; it is a very valuable tool.

Currently, however, controversy is expressed about who should perform sonograms. It is such an attractive medium that it seems everyone wants in on the act. Obstetrical nurses want to perform limited sonographic examinations, family practitioners want to use it like a stethoscope, and some people even want to make fortunes with entertainment videos of the fetus.

I think that this trend will continue. The only thing that the American Registry of Diagnostic Medical Sonographers (ARDMS) and the SDMS can do is to maintain high educational and professional standards. People with limited training and limited examinations will make their mistakes and be revealed. Then we can encourage them to join the fold and take the appropriate ARDMS examinations to prove and improve their knowledge. It would seem that the HSOs, insurance companies, third-party payers, and especially patients would want experienced workers who can give them more diagnostic information for their dollar.

A major problem is the conflict between providing good health care and the drive to economize. In one way, saving money means using people who are less experienced to do the work, but that does not always result in the best health care. This basic conflict of economics must be dealt with before we can see a resolution of the health care reform issue. On the one hand we want good health care for everyone, and on the other we all want a good lifestyle. However, there are those who view life as a game in which the score is kept by counting dollars. In that kind of game there will never be enough. Those who die with the most toys are still dead. There are those who are creating unjustifiable inequities in the field of health care. I think it is important at this time for us to think about how to bring excellent health care to all people, not just to those who were more fortunate by birth. Attaining this goal will mean more business for all health care workers and better health care for society.

REFERENCES

1. Stoll C: The Cuckoo's Egg. Doubleday, New York, 1989, pp 317–339.
2. DuBose TJ: Basic Baby II: Obstetrical Software (BBII), copyright 1986–1994. Mind's Eye Imaging, 811 West 31st Street, Austin, TX 78705–2109.
3. dBASE IV, copyright 1990. Ashton-Tate Corporation, 6411 Guadalupe Mines Road, San Jose, CA 95120.
4. Framework IV integrated software, copyright 1991. Ashton-Tate Corporation, 6411 Guadalupe Mines Road, San Jose, CA 95120.
5. EXCEL, version 5.0, copyright 1993. MicroSoft Corporation, PO Box 3021, Bothell, WA 98041–3021.
6. Jandel Scientific: Tablecurve v3.10. Jandel Scientific, 2591 Kerner Boulevard, San Rafael, CA 94901.
7. Filly R: Editorial. Radiology 1988;166:274–275.
8. The Selective Service System: The Selective Service: Its Concepts, History, and Operation. US Government Printing Office, Washington, DC, 1967, 1967–0–267–285.
9. Waterhouse LG, Wizard MG: Turning The Guns Around: Notes on the GI Movement. Praeger Publishers, New York, 1971, pp 203–210.

INDEX

Page numbers in *italics* refer to illustrations; page numbers followed by t refer to tables.

ISBN 0-7216-5432-0

90038

9 780721 654324